DATE DUE

MAY 12 1999	
MAY 17 2000	

GAYLORD PRINTED IN U.S.A.

AF678313

CRC HANDBOOK SERIES IN CLINICAL LABORATORY SCIENCE

David Seligson, Sc.D., M.D.
Editor-in-Chief

SECTIONS AND SECTION EDITORS

SECTION A: NUCLEAR MEDICINE

Section Editor
Richard P. Spencer, M.D., Ph.D.
Chairman, Department of Nuclear Medicine
University of Connecticut School of Medicine

SECTION B: TOXICOLOGY

Section Editor
Irving Sunshine, Ph.D.
Chief Toxicologist
Cuyahoga County Coroner's Office (Ohio)
Case Western Reserve University

SECTION C: PATHOLOGY

Section Editor
Raymond Yesner, M.D.
Chief Pathologist
Yale University School of Medicine
Veterans Administration Hospital

SECTION D: BLOOD BANKING

Section Editors
Tibor J. Greenwalt, M.D.
Director, Blood Program
American National Red Cross

Edwin A. Steane, Ph.D.
Assistant Professor
University of Texas Health Science Center

SECTION E: CLINICAL MICROBIOLOGY

Section Editor
Alexander von Graevenitz, M.D.
Professor of Laboratory Medicine
Yale University School of Medicine

SECTION F: IMMUNOLOGY

Section Editors
Alexander Baumgarten, M.D.
Director, Immunology Laboratory
Yale University School of Medicine

Frank F. Richards, M.D.
Professor of Medicine
Yale University School of Medicine

SECTION G: CLINICAL CHEMISTRY

Section Editor
Mario Werner, M.D.
Professor of Laboratory Medicine
George Washington University Medical Center

SECTION H: VIROLOGY AND RICKETTSIOLOGY

Section Editors
Gueh-Djen Hsiung, Ph.D.
Professor of Laboratory Medicine
Yale University School of Medicine

Robert H. Green, M.D.
Professor of Medicine
University of Connecticut School of Medicine
Yale University School of Medicine

SECTION I: HEMATOLOGY

Section Editor
Robert M. Schmidt, M.D., M.P.H.
Medical Director
International Reference and Research Center for Blood Diseases
Lihue, Kauai, Hawaii

Each section contains one or more volumes.

CRC Handbook Series in Clinical Laboratory Science

David Seligson, Editor-In-Chief

Chairman and Professor
Department of Laboratory Medicine
School of Medicine
Yale University

Section I: Hematology
Volume II

Robert M. Schmidt, Section Editor

Medical Director
International Reference and Research
Center for Blood Diseases
Lihue, Kauai, Hawaii

Formerly: Director, Hematology Division
Center for Disease Control
Atlanta, Georgia

CRC PRESS, INC.
Boca Raton, Florida

Barry College Library
Miami, Florida

Library of Congress Cataloging in Publication Data (Revised)

Main entry under title:

CRC handbook series in clinical laboratory science.
Spine title: Handbook series in clinical laboratory science.
Includes bibliographies and index.
CONTENTS: Section A. Nuclear medicine. v.—Section E. Clinical microbiology. v.—Section I. Hematology.
1. Medical laboratories. 2. Diagnosis, Laboratory. L. Seligson, David. II. Chemical Rubber Company, Cleveland, III. Title: Handbook series in clinical laboratory science.

RB37.C18 616.07'56 76-27688
ISBN 0-8493-7000-0 (set)

This book represents information obtained from authentic and highly regarded sources. Reprinted material is quoted with permission, and sources are indicated. A wide variety of references are listed. Every reasonable effort has been made to give reliable data and information, but the author and the publisher cannot assume responsibility for the validity of all materials or for the consequences of their use.

All rights reserved. This book, or any part thereof, may not be reproduced in any form without written consent from the publisher.

Direct all inquiries to CRC Press, 2000 N.W. 24th Street, Boca Raton, Florida, 33431.

© 1980 by CRC Press, Inc.

International Standard Book Number
Complete Set 0-8493-7000-0
Hematology Section, Volume II 0-8493-7092-2

Library of Congress Card No. 76-27688
Printed in the United States

RB
45
.S4

122105

PUBLISHERS PREFACE

In 1913, when the First Edition of the *Handbook of Chemistry and Physics* appeared, scientific progress, particularly in chemistry and physics, had produced an extensive literature but its utility was seriously handicapped because it was fragmented and unorganized. The simple but invaluable contribution of the *Handbook of Chemistry and Physics* was to provide a systematic compilation of the most useful and reliable scientific data within the covers of a single volume. Referred to as the "bible", the Handbook soon became a universal and essential reference source for the scientific community. The latest edition published represents more than 65 years of continuous service to millions of professional scientists and students throughout the world.

In the years following World War II, scientific information expanded at an explosive rate due to the tremendous growth of research facilities and sophisticated analytical instrumentation. The single-volume Handbook concept, although providing a high level of convenience, was not adequate for the reference requirements of many of the newer scientific disciplines. Due to the sheer quantity of useful and reliable data being generated, it was no longer feasible or desirable to select only that information which could be contained in a single volume and arbitrarily to reject the remainder. **Comprehensiveness** had become as essential as **convenience.**

By the late 1960's it was apparent that the solution to the problem was the development of the multi-volume Handbook. This answer arose out of necessity during the editorial processing of the *Handbook of Environmental Control.* A hybrid discipline or, to be more precise, an interdisciplinary field such as Environmental Science could be logically structured into major subject areas. This permitted individual volumes to be developed for each major subject. The individual volumes, published either simultaneously or by some predetermined sequence, collectively became a multi-volume Handbook series.

The logic of this new approach was irrefutable and the concept was promptly accepted by both the scientist and science librarian. It became the format of a growing number of CRC Handbook Series in fields such as Materials Science, Laboratory Animal Science, and Marine Science.

Within a few years, however, it was clear that even the multi-volume Handbook concept was not sufficient. It was necessary to create an information structure more compatible with the dynamic character of scientific information, and flexible enough to accommodate continuous but unpredictable growth, regardless of quantity or direction. This became the objective of a "third generation" Handbook concept.

This latest concept utilizes each major subject within an information field as a "Section" rather than the equivalent of a single volume. Each Section, therefore, may include as many volumes as the quantity and quality of available information will justify. The structure achieves permanent flexibility because it can, in effect, expand "vertically" and "horizontally". Any section can continue to grow (vertically) in number of volumes, and new sections can be added (horizontally) as and when required by the information field itself. A key innovation which makes this massive and complex information base almost as convenient to use as a single-volume Handbook is the utilization of computer technology to produce up-dated, cumulative index volumes.

The *Handbook Series in Clinical Laboratory Science* has the distinction of being the prototype for the "sectionalized, multi-volume Handbook series". Currently underway are additional information programs based on the same organizational design. These include information fields such as Nutrition, Energy, and Agricultural Science which are of critical importance not only to scientific progress but to the advancement of the total quality of life.

We are confident that the "third generation" CRC Handbook comprises a worthy contribution to both information science and the scientific community. We are equally certain that it does not represent the ultimate reference source. We predict that the most dramatic progress in the management of scientific information remains to be achieved.

B. J. Starkoff
President
CRC Press, Inc.

PREFACE
CRC HANDBOOK SERIES IN CLINICAL LABORATORY SCIENCE

According to the *Webster 4 — Merriam Dictionary,* 3rd ed., a handbook is

1a. a book capable of being conveniently carried as a ready reference,
1b. a concise reference book covering a particular field of knowledge,
2a. a bookmaker's book of bets.

In order to accommodate the information in the field of clinical laboratory science we shall need more than 20 volumes. A series of volumes such as these, that will weigh in the order of 24 kg (53 pounds), will not fit the meaning of la: nor will 2a fit, although we are gambling that we can get the appropriate information together in a reasonable time. Definition 1b is more appropriate to our goal which is to accumulate, arrange, and present the qualitative and quantitative clinical laboratory data related to men and women (of all ages), so that anyone who needs to extract some information from the vast amount available will have it at his or her fingertips, provided he or she is within arm's length of these volumes.

To understand the biology of man, to know man, sick and well, requires knowledge of the body constituents and their interrelationships; the dynamic relationships of these constituents; and information about tools, chemicals and techniques used to get these data. Notation of the source of the data is important to scholars. It is our purpose to present this information in tabular and graphic form in a systematic way in order to help readers retrieve it.

If we are successful, we will make it possible for a user to find any information related to constituents of blood, body fluids, body tissues, and so on, whether they be organic or inorganic molecules, viruses, bacteria, or parasites. Users of these volumes should be able to find easily the composition of a buffer, the half-life of an isotope, or the life cycle of a parasite if that information has been used to study man or if the chemicals or particles are found in man.

We shall consider this *Handbook Series in Clinical Laboratory Science* successful if it meets most of our goals and if it provides the nidus for continuing growth. The editor of the series, the executive editor of each volume, the advisory boards, contributors, and publisher will make every effort to improve subsequent editions of this *Handbook*. The user will undoubtedly find errors of omission and commission or will have new information (all of which we hope will be called to our attention). All of us should strive to improve these volumes so that users and contributors the world over will find them useful in knowing more about man.

David Seligson
Editor-in-Chief

DAVID SELIGSON, EDITOR-IN-CHIEF
CRC HANDBOOK SERIES IN CLINICAL LABORATORY SCIENCE

Dr. David Seligson is Professor and Chairman of the Department of Laboratory Medicine (Clinical Pathology) and Professor of Pathology in the School of Medicine at Yale University. He is the Director of the Department of Clinical Laboratories of the Yale-New Haven Hospital. He has an Sc.D. in Biochemistry from Johns Hopkins University (1942) and an M.D. from the University of Utah (1946). He has been a President of the American Association of Clinical Chemists and the Academy of Clinical Laboratory Physicians and Scientists. He is a Fellow of the American Society of Clinical Pathologists, College of American Pathologists, American College of Physicians, and American Board of Clinical Chemistry.

He has been editor of *Standard Methods of the American Association of Clinical Chemists* (Volumes 2,3, and 4) and he is a member of other editorial boards.

Dr. Seligson has an honorary Masters degree from Yale University and has received the following awards:

John G. Reinhold Award, Philadelphia Section of the American Association of Clinical Chemists, 1966

Fellowship of Medici Publici, University of Utah College of Medicine and Medical Alumni Association, 1966

Donald D. Van Slyke Award, American Association of Clinical Chemists 1971 Ames Award, American Association of Clinical Chemists, National Meeting, Seattle, Washington, August 1971

Gerald T. Evans Award, Academy of Clinical Laboratory Physicians and Scientists, June 1974

Honorary Member Association of Clinical Biochemists, London, April 1976

PREFACE
SECTION I: HEMATOLOGY
VOLUME II

The Hematology section of the *CRC Handbook Series in Clinical Laboratory Science* provides a single ready reference for information on hematology which is now found in a wide variety of textbooks, laboratory manuals, monographs and journal articles written to reach specialized audiences. Organization of the section was performed with the assistance of an Editorial Advisory Board whose members represent the subspecialty areas of hematology. The eleven Board members are authorities from the major hematologic disciplines including internal medicine, pathology, pediatrics, laboratory medicine and basic research. Contributors to the Hematology Section are international experts selected by the Advisory Board members. It has been necessary to divide the material into four volumes to ensure in-depth coverage. Volume II includes blood cell morphology, quality control in hematology, data processing in hematology, principles of cell sizing and counting, red cell production, and the white blood cell. Board members who edited chapters in the second volume are Lemuel W. Diggs, John A. Koepke, Thomas F. Necheles, Frank E. Trobaugh, and Onno W. van Assendelft. The factual contents of each chapter have been chosen by the individual contributors.

Publication of the Hematology Section would not have been possible without the enthusiastic support of the Editorial Advisory Board and the Efforts of our contributors.

RMS

ROBERT M. SCHMIDT
SECTION EDITOR
SECTION I: HEMATOLOGY

Robert M. Schmidt, M.D., M.P.H., is Medical Director, International Reference and Research Center for Blood Diseases, Lihue, Kauai, Hawaii, where he is also President of the Board of Trustees of the International Health Resource Center of Hawaii and Medical Director, International Center for Health Education and the Kauai Preventive Medicine Program. Prior to accepting these positions in 1979, he was Director, Hematology Division, National Center for Disease Control, U.S. Public Health Service, Department of H.E.W., Atlanta, Georgia. He also holds faculty appointments in Medicine, Preventive Medicine and Community Health, and Pediatrics, at Emory University, Morehouse Medical School, and Tufts University.

Dr. Schmidt received an A.B. degree from Northwestern University, and M.D. degree from Columbia University College of Physicians and Surgeons, where he received several honors including the microbiology, pharmacoloy, urology, Upjohn Achievement and Borden Undergraduate Medical Research awards, and an M.P.H. degree in health services administration, international health and laboratory medicine from Harvard University. He also trained in internal medicine at the University of California at San Diego and is completing a Ph.D. degree in Law, Medicine and Public Policy at Emory University. He received the United States Public Health Service Commendation Medal while at CDC. He is a diplomate of the National Board of Medical Examiners and the American Board of Preventive Medicine, a Fellow of the American Society of Clinical Pathologists, a Fellow of the American College of Preventive Medicine, and a member of numerous scientific and medical societies including the American Association for the Advancement of Science, the American Sciety of Hematology, the American Society for Microbiology, the American College of Physicians, the American Public Health Association, the Academy of Clinical Laboratory Physicians and Scientists, and the American Medical Association. He is past chairman of the Area Committee on Hematology of the National Committee for Clinical Laboratory Standards and chairs the Clinical Chemistry and Hematology Committee of the American Public Health Association. He is also a member of the Secretariat and Managing Board of the International Committee for Standardization in Hematology (ICSH) and served as their representative to the International Committee on Thrombosis and Hemotasis, Secretary of the ICSH Expert Panel on Abnormal Hemoglobins and Thalassemia, Executive Secretary of the ICSH Expert Panel on Oral Anticoagulant Control, and Secretary of the ICSH Committee on Training; he is Secretary of the American Society of Hematology Committee on Clinical Hematology Laboratory Standards and a member of numerous other professional, national and international committees, advisory boards and panels. He serves as a consultant to the Biologics, Genetics and Health Laboratory Services units of the World Health Organization. He is a member of the editorial board of the *American Journal of Clinical Pathology* and serves as a referee for other professional journals. His medical interests span a wide area including laboratory medicine, especially hematology, preventive medicine, international health, and interdisciplinary public health aspects of these fields. He is the author of numerous publications including ten books and manuals.

While continuing these activities, Dr. Schmidt is currently developing the international health centers in Hawaii whose purpose is to promote world health through improved preventive health education, health professional continuing education, and medical laboratory reference services, in an atmosphere of basic and applied research.

ADVISORY BOARD MEMBERS
SECTION I: HEMATOLOGY
VOLUME I

Kenneth M. Brinkhous
Alumni Distinguished Professor of Pathology
University of North Carolina
School of Medicine
Chapel Hill, North Carolina

Lemuel W. Diggs
Goodman Professor of Medicine, Emeritus
University of Tennessee
Center for the Health Sciences
Memphis, Tennessee

Harvey R. Gralnick
Chief, Hematology Service
Clinical Center
National Institutes of Health
Bethesda, Maryland

John A. Koepke
Professor and Vice-Chairman
Department of Pathology
University of Iowa
College of Medicine
Iowa City, Iowa

John B. Miale
Professor of Pathology
University of Miami
School of Medicine
Miami, Florida

Thomas F. Necheles
Chief of Pediatric Hematology
Professor of Pediatrics
Tufts-New England Medical Center
Boston, Massachusetts

Walter A. Schroeder
Research Associate in Chemistry
Division of Chemistry and Chemical Engineering
California Institute of Technology
Pasadena, California

Douglas A. Triplett
Staff Pathologist
Ball Memorial Hospital
Associate Professor of Pathology
Indiana University School of Medicine
Muncie, Indiana

Frank E. Trobaugh, Jr.
Director, Section of Laboratory Hematology
Professor, Rush Medical School
Rush-Presbyterian-St. Luke's Medical Center
Chicago, Illinois

Onno W. van Assendelft
Chief, Hematology Branch
Hematology Division
Center for Disease Control
Atlanta, Georgia

Maxwell M. Wintrobe
Distinguished Professor of Medicine
University of Utah Medical Center
College of Medicine
Department of Internal Medicine
Salt Lake City, Utah

CONTRIBUTORS
SECTION I: HEMATOLOGY
VOLUME II

Maurice M. Albala
Division of Clinical Hematology
Rhode Island Hospital
Providence, Rhode Island

Andreas Athanasiou
Department of Pediatrics
Tufts-New England Medical Center
Boston, Massachusetts

James W. Bacus
Section of Laboratory Hematology
Rush-Presbyterian-St. Luke's Medical Center
Chicago, Illinois

William S. Beck
Harvard Medical School
Massachusetts General Hospital
Boston, Massachusetts

Ann Bell
Department of Medicine
University of Tennessee
Center for Health Sciences
Memphis, Tennessee

Richard D. Brunning
Departments of Laboratory Medicine and Pathology
University of Minnesota Hospitals
Minneapolis, Minnesota

Brian S. Bull
Department of Pathology and Laboratory Medicine
Loma Linda University
School of Medicine
Loma Linda, California

Lemuel W. Diggs
W. Department of Medicine
University of Tennessee
Center for Health Sciences
Memphis, Tennessee

James Crowley
Division of Clinical Hematology
Rhode Island Hospital
Providence, Rhode Island

Russell J. Eilers
BioScience Labs
Van Nuys, California

Ralph L. Engle, Jr.
Department of Public Health
The New York Hospital
Cornell Medical Center
New York, New York

Allen J. Erslev
Cardeza Foundation for Hematologic Research
Thomas Jefferson University
Philadelphia, Pennsylvania

Betty J. Flehinger
IBM Thomas Watson
Yorktown Heights, New York

David S. Gordon
Immunology Division
Center for Disease Control
Atlanta, Georgia

A. Richardson Jones
Regulatory Compliance
Coulter Electronics
Hialeah, Florida

Emin Kansu
Cardeza Foundation for Hematologic Research
Thomas Jefferson University
Philadelphia, Pennsylvania

F. Louis
Departments of Medical Research and Laboratories and Pathology
St. Margaret's Hospital for Women
Dorchester, Massachusetts

Paul N. Marshall
Medical Automation Research Center
Rush-Presbyterian-St. Luke's Medical Center
Chicago, Illinois

Elaine L. Mills
Department of Pediatrics
University of Minnesota Medical School
Minneapolis, Minnesota

G. W. Mitchell
Department of Medical Research and Laboratories and Pathology
St. Margaret's Hospital for Women
Dorchester, Massachusetts

Thomas F. Necheles
Pediatric Hematology
New England Medical Center Hospital
Boston, Massachusetts

Janet L. Parkin
Departments of Laboratory Medicine and Pathology
University of Minnesota Hospitals
Minneapolis, Minnesota

B. B. Paul
Department of Medical Research and Laboratories and Pathology
St. Margaret's Hospital for Women
Dorchester, Massachuestts

Waldemar Pruzanski
Immunology Diagnostic and Research Center
Department of Medicine
University of Toronto
Toronto, Ontario
Canada

Paul G. Quie
Departments of Pedicatrics and Microbiology
University of Minnesota
Minneapolis, Minnesota

Alex M. Saunders
Geometric Data
Wayne, Pennsylvania

Anthony Sbarra
Departments of Medical Research and Laboratories and Pathology
St. Margaret's Hospital for Women
Dorchester, Massachusetts

R. J. Selvaraj
Departments of Medical Research and Laboratories and Pathology
St. Margaret's Hospital for Women
Dorchester, Massachusetts

James D. Simon
Division of Clinical Hematology
Rhode Island Hospital
Providence, Rhode Island

Onno W. van Assendelft
Hematology Division
Center for Disease Control
Atlanta, Georgia

Lung T. Yam
Hematology Section
Veterans Administration Hospital
Louisville, Kentucky

TABLE OF CONTENTS
SECTION I: HEMATOLOGY
VOLUME II

* Additional information on the red cell will appear in Volume IV.

Morphology

BONE MARROW

L. W. Diggs and Ann Bell

Indications

Bone marrow examination is indicated for any disease in which there are abnormalities in the number and/or the morphology of blood cells in the peripheral blood that cannot be adequately explained on the basis of history, physical examination, and standard laboratory tests. Examination of the bone marrow is especially useful in the diagnosis of blood diseases in which the number of cells is decreased as in leukopenic, hypoplastic anemic, and thrombocytopenic states.

General indications include fever of undetermined origin, unexplained weight loss, tiredness and weakness, unexplained enlargement of lymph nodes, spleen, or liver, and unexplained pains in the back and other bones.

A list of some of the specific diseases in which the bone marrow examination may be of value in confirming or excluding a given diagnostic possibility is given in Table 1. From the standpoint of the patient the bone marrow puncture is of greatest value when a suspected dreaded and incurable disease can be excluded.

In private practice, where the patient is available for continued observation and follow-up studies of peripheral blood, it may be justified to delay bone marrow examination until the indication is sharply defined. When a patient is referred to a consultant in hematology, bone marrow examination is usually considered an essential constituent of the initial examination by the consultant in order to establish the diagnosis and prognosis, to furnish a base for future examinations, and to yield information of value in determining treatment and other diagnostic procedures to be performed.

Patients with an established diagnosis of leukemia, Hodgkin's disease, or other malignancy may need repeated marrow examinations in order to follow the course of their disease, and to evaluate the effectiveness of therapy and their toleration of cytotoxic drugs and other forms of therapy.

Bone marrow examinations are indicated in patients with thrombocytopenia, to exclude leukemia and aplastic anemia, and to determine the number and morphology of megakaryocytes. If there are numerous megakaryocytes that are not producing platelets, it is assumed that the decrease in platelets is due to antiplatelet antibody, that splenectomy, adrenocorticosteroids, and/or cytotoxic drugs are justified, and that platelet transfusions are likely to be ineffective. If there is a paucity of megakaryocytes (amegakaryocytic thrombocytopenia), platelet transfusions are needed and may be livesaving, but splenectomy and cell poisons are contraindicated.

There are numerous hereditary and acquired diseases other than primary diseases of the blood and blood-forming organs, which may reveal lesions in the marrow that are of academic interest, are confirmatory of or compatible with a given diagnosis, but in which bone marrow examinations are not needed, since the diagnosis can be established with confidence by the clinical manifestations and peripheral blood abnormalities. The practicing physician is obligated to give the patient the advantage of essential diagnositic procedures, but is also obligated to spare the patient the pain, the inconvenience, and the expense of procedures that are not necessary.

Marrow examination for the purpose of establishing diagnosis is seldom needed when there are numerous abnormal and immature cells in the peripheral blood.

Examination of bone marrow smears and tissue sections is of no value in the diagnosis of hemorrhagic diseases such as hemophilia and fibrinogenopenia. If marrow examination is ever indicated in a patient with a deficiency of a coagulation component

Table 1
DISEASES IN WHICH EXAMINATION OF BONE MARROW MAY BE INDICATED

Leukemia
Non-Hodgkin's lymphoma
Hodgkin's disease
Primary bone malignancy
Myeloma
Metastatic malignancy
Myleofibrosis
Hypersplenism
Refractory anemia
Aplastic anemia
Agranulocytosis
Essential neutropenia
Thrombocytopenic purpuras
Fungal diseases
Kala-azar
Granulomatous disease
Lipid histiocytoses
Amyloidosis
Hemochromatosis
Collagen diseases
Hyperproteinemia
Sarcoidosis
Cystinosis

because there is a superimposed nonhemorrhagic blood dyscrasia, the risk of postoperative bleeding is minimal if the puncture site is the sternum, if a small needle is used, if care is taken to control the depth of the puncture, and if pressure is applied to the wound until coagulation occurs.

Sites

Posterior Iliac Crest

The site of choice for bone marrow aspiration and for biopsy in children and adults is the posterior iliac crest (Figure 1). At this location the bone is near the surface, the cortical bone is relatively thin, and the marrow space is wide (Figure 2). There are no major blood vessels, nerves, or vital organs in the immediate vicinity; there are only muscles, tendons, and fat, so the risk of needle puncture is minimal. Patients prefer this site over the sternum because they cannot see the needle or the procedure. They are less apprehensive when the needle is pushed under pressure through the pelvic bone than through the breast bone. An advantage to the patient is that the scar is inconspicuous.

For the puncture of the posterior iliac crest, many operators prefer to have the patient lie on one side with the upper leg slightly flexed and the back near the edge of the bed or examining table. Others prefer to have the patient in a prone position with a small pillow under the pelvis in order to elevate the lower back. Movements of children during the procedure are restrained more easily when they are in the face-down position than when they are lying on their side.

The site of puncture of the posterior ilium can be located in some patients by inspection of the skin surface, because at the lateral points of the diamond-shaped sacral quadrangle (Rhomboid of Michaelis), there is a skin depression or dimple that overlies the posterior superior iliac spine. In this area the subcutaneous tissue is relatively thin, fibrous, and nonfatty, and the skin is more firmly fixed than in the surrounding more fatty and muscular areas. The superior spine can also be located by palpation. In most

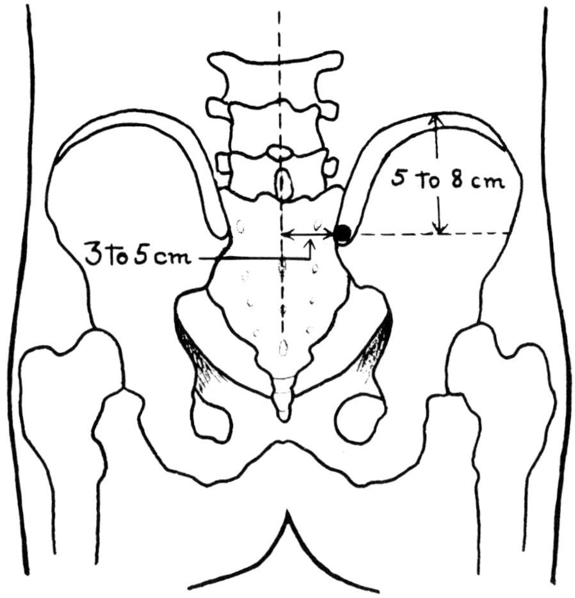

FIGURE 1. Location of point of needle puncture into marrow space; posterior superior iliac spine.

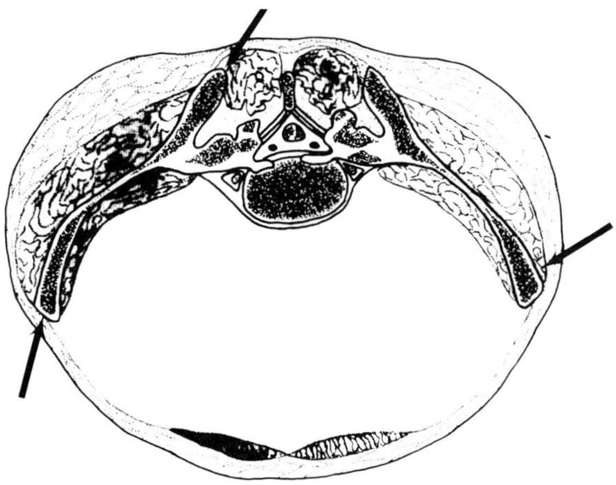

FIGURE 2. Drawing showing bony and anatomical structures in a cross section of the pelvis in the region of the posterior superior iliac spine. Arrows indicate direction of needle into marrow spaces of the ilium. (Modified from Carter, B. L., Morehead, J., Wolpert, S. M., Hammerschlag, S. B., Griffiths, H. J., and Kahn, P. C., *Cross-Sectional Anatomy: Computed Tomography and Ultrasound Correlation,* Appleton-Century-Crofts, New York, 1977, Section 38.)

adults the preferred site of needle entry into the skin is approximately 2 finger breadths (3 to 5 cm) from the midline of the spine on a horizontal line approximately three finger breadths (5 to 8 cm) below the highest point of the iliac crest (Figure 1). The needle is advanced slightly upward and laterally in the direction of the anterior crest (Figure 2). The cortical bone is reached usually several millimeters below the skin surface, but the distance varies considerably depending on the amount of fat. Long needles are needed for obese patients.

Anterior Iliac Crest

The anterior crest in the region of the superior iliac spine is recommended as the second choice for aspiration or biopsy if the first attempt to obtain marrow from the posterior crest is unsuccessful or if the patient is grossly obese. The patient lies on his back. The needle may be inserted directly into the crest in the line of the pelvic bone or at a right angle to the flat surface approximately 1 cm medial to the superior iliac promontory and 2 cm below the crest.

Spinous Process of Vertebra

The lower thoracic or upper lumbar spinous processes may be used for marrow aspirations in children as well as in adults. The patient may sit up with the back arched or may be in a prone position with a pillow under the pelvis. The point of entry of the needle should be at the midpoint of the spinous process and at a right angle to the surface of the skin. The spinous process is not suitable for biopsy because the marrow space is too narrow.

Sternum

The sternum has been widely used in the past and is still preferred by many for marrow aspiration because the bone is near the surface and the landmarks are readily visible. The anterior lamina of the body of the sternum of adults at the level of the second interspace is thin (1 to 3 mm) and easily penetrated. The amount of fat in the sternal marrow is less than that in marrow from the ilium, and the yield of hematopoietic cells and marrow particles is greater than that obtained from other bones. The sternum is the site of choice for obese and elderly patients, for patients with hemorrhagic diseases, for patients who have received whole body irradiation, and for surgical biopsies.

Before the skin surface is cleansed, the sternal area should be washed with soap and water and shaved if necessary. A pillow placed under the shoulders helps to elevate the chest and to tilt the head backward. Some prefer to use the manubrium as the site of choice, but the majority favor the body of the sternum in the second interspace 1.5 to 2 cm below the sternomanubrial prominence (angle of Louis) and slightly off center (Figure 3). The width of the cancellous bone in adults is usually in the 6 to 12 mm range. The advancing needle is slanted at a 45° angle (Figure 4) in order to minimize the chance of traversing the posterior cortical bone and puncturing underlying major blood vessels. Aspirations should not be attempted in the third or lower interspaces.

Needles for sternal puncture should be relatively small (16 to 19 gauge) and short. If longer needles are used they should be equipped with moveable guards in order to control the depth of puncture. Sternal aspirations are not recommended for children. Biopsy needles should not be used unless there is a focal lesion involving the sternum.

Tibia

The upper and anterior tibia, several centimeters below the greater tuberosity, is the preferred site for marrow puncture in infants less than 6 months of age. The tibia is not suitable for aspiration or core biopsy for children after the first few months of life, because the cortical bone is thick and hard, and the marrow contains a predominance of fat and relatively few blood cells.

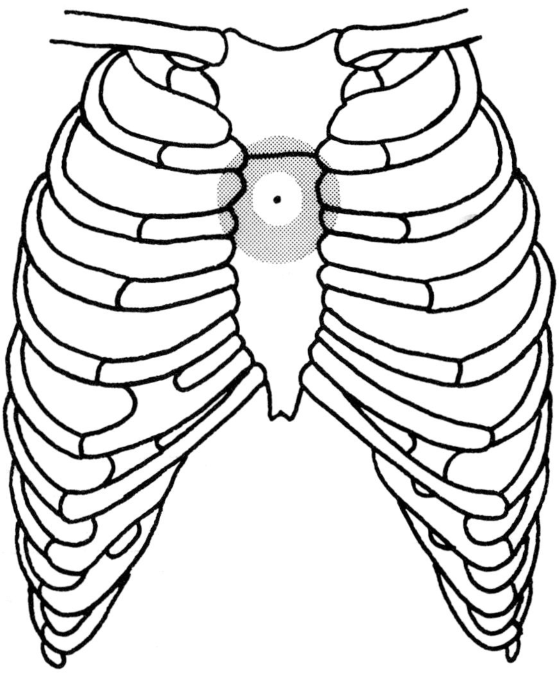

FIGURE 3. Location of site of sternal marrow puncture in second interspace.

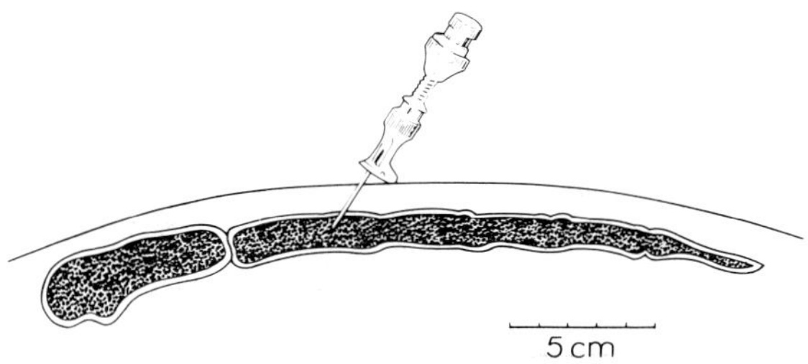

FIGURE 4. Section through sternum to show insertion of University of Illinois sternal puncture needle at 45° angle. The guard is set to control depth of puncture.

Other Sites

When there is localized bone pain, pressure tenderness, tumefaction, or roentgenological evidence of focal bone abnormality, the biopsy needle should be inserted at the site of the lesion.

Preparation of the Patient

Previous to bone marrow aspiration, needle biopsy, or surgical biopsy, the purpose and nature of the procedure should be explained to the patient, and written permission should be obtained from the adult patient. If the patient is a minor, permission is obtained from a parent or legal guardian. Inquiry should be made concerning sensitivity to local anesthetics.

The administration of preoperative sedatives to patients is optional. Sedation in preparation for needle aspiration or biopsy for younger children and for apprehensive

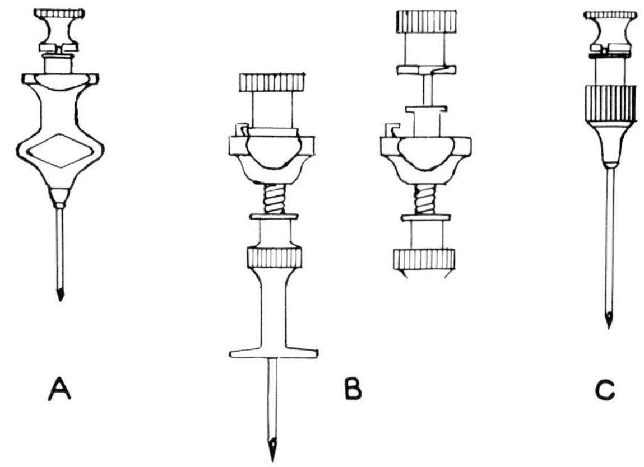

FIGURE 5. Types of marrow aspiration needles: A. Barker lumbar puncture needle filed to desired length and sharpened B. University of Illinois C. Osgood

adults is recommended, but if sedatives are given care must be taken that the patient is under observation at all times. Sedatives should not be employed for ambulatory patients responsible for their transportation or for those driving a car.

Marrow aspirations and needle biopsies are usually performed at the bedside of the patient or in a nearby examining room with the patient on the edge of the bed or on an examining table. There should be adequate light and a stand or small table upon which to place equipment and supplies.

Needles

Aspiration Needles

Recommended needles for marrow aspiration are the University of Illinois (Limarzi,)* Rosenthal,** Osgood,*** and Bierman† needles.

The University of Illinois needle* (Figure 5) was designed primarily for sternal puncture. This needle is too short for posterior iliac punctures, but it is suitable for anterior pelvic, spinous process, and tibial aspirations. This needle has a short bevel, a snugly fitting obturator that locks into place, a stout upper shaft, and a shoulder that facilitates a good grip. In addition there is an adjustable screw device to aid in controlling the depth of puncture. One complete turn of the guard corresponds with a change of distance of 1 mm. In operation the needle point is advanced until the surface of the bone is reached. The guard is then set for the desired distance of penetration through the cortex into cancellous bone. The recommended depth of entry into the marrow space of the sternum of adults is 3 to 4 mm. Distances of 5 to 10 mm are used for the iliac crest or spinous process. The needle is bored into the bone until the guard touches the skin.

The Rosenthal needle** (Figure 6) has a wide shank and a hub with a slot for a pin to maintain the obturator in a proper position in relation to the bevel of the needle point. The 18-gauge, 1 in. needle is preferred for sternal puncture and the stouter 16-gauge needle, 1 5/16 in. long, for other sites. It is recommended that an adjustable

* University of Illinois (16 gauge, V. Mueller and Co., Chamblee, Ga., 30341).

** Rosenthal (B-D 460LNR, 16G × 1 5/16 in., 18G × 1 in., Becton-Dickinson, Rutherford, N.J., 07070).

***Osgood (B-D 458LNR, 19G × ½ in, 18G × 1 in, 16G × 1 5/16 in, Becton-Dickinson, Rutherford, N.J., 07070).

† Bierman (Becton-Dickinson, Rutherford, N.J., 07070).

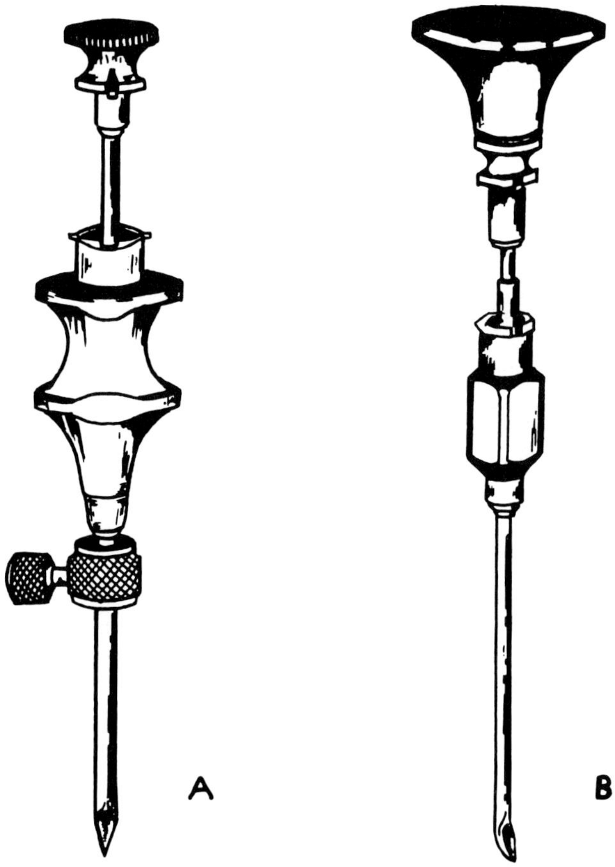

FIGURE 6. A. Rosenthal marrow aspiration needle with adjustable stop. B. Bierman marrow aspiration needle, Huber point.

stop‡ be employed when the sternum is used. A set of needles of the Rosenthal type can be prepared by filing off and sharpening 18- or 19-gauge lumbar puncture needles of the Barker type (Figure 5). The lengths should vary from 2 to 5 cm.

The simple and relatively inexpensive Osgood needle (Figure 5) with or without a guard, is preferred by many for sternal aspirations and for marrow punctures of children at all sites. The disadvantage of this needle is that the upper shaft does not have a large protruding rim or flange to aid in grasping while the needle point is forced through dense cortical bone.

The Bierman needle (Figure 6) has an obturator with a large flange at the top, which helps in pushing the needle point through calcified bone. The needle point has a lateral rather than a central opening (Huber point) that tends to prevent obstruction of the lumen by tissue fragments.

Biopsy Needles

The needle of choice for biopsy of the bone marrow is the Jamshidi[1] biopsy needle.*

‡ Adjustable stop (B-D 418S for needles 16 gauge or smaller, Becton-Dickinson, Rutherford, N.J., 07070).

* Jamshidi (Regular/Adult 4 in., 11 gauge; pediatric 3½ in., 13 gauge, 2 in., 13 gauge, Kormed, Inc, 2510 Northland Drive, St. Paul, Minnesota, 55120.)

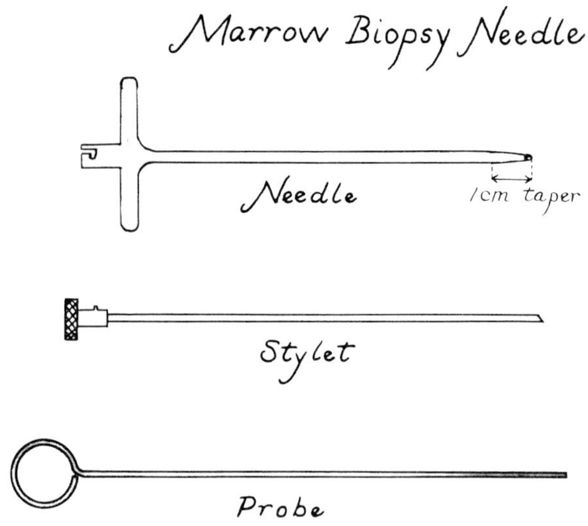

FIGURE 7. Jamshidi biopsy needle.

The pointed end of the obturator of this needle extends beyond the needle point, thus protecting the cutting tip while the point of the stylet is forced through hard cortical bone. The lumen of the distal end of the needle is tapered for a distance of 1 cm and is 2 mm in diameter, whereas the lumen in the upper shaft is 3 mm in diameter (Figure 7). The probe allows the trephined cylinder of marrow tissue to be removed with minimal compression and distortion.

The "regular adult" Jamshidi needle for biopsy of the posterior iliac crest of adults is 11 gauge and 4 in. in length. Smaller gauge and shorter needles are used for children and longer needles for obese patients.

Handles made of nylon rods can be prepared to fit over the needle hub and shoulder, thus making it possible to get a better grip, and to provide leverage while forcing the needle with a clockwise and counterclockwise motion through the calcified cortex.[2]

For those who are performing needle biopsies for the first time, it is recommended that initial punctures be made on cadavers.

Other Equipment and Supplies

The recommended sterile equipment and supplies are listed in Table 2, and nonsterile items are listed in Table 3. The recommended equipment and drugs that are to be included in an "Emergency Kit," which should always be available at the bedside for patients receiving anesthetic drugs and undergoing surgical procedures, are listed in Table 4.

Commercial kits for bone marrow aspirations and biopsies containing disposable equipment and supplies are useful for medical units where only occasional bone marrow procedures are performed, but for institutions where marrow examinations are performed frequently, the use of such sets limits the flexibility of techniques to be employed and unnecessarily increases the cost. Disposable puncture needles bend and break easily and are too expensive to throw away after a single use.

The tray for obtaining marrow specimens should contain several backup aspiration and biopsy needles so that any indicated procedure can be performed if unforeseen situations arise at the time of puncture. Biopsy needles are best autoclaved in a covered metal pan (Figure 8). Aspiration needles may be prepared by placement in large glass tubes with cotton at the bottom and a paper cover held in place by autoclave tape

Table 2
STERILE EQUIPMENT AND SUPPLIES, MARROW ASPIRATION, AND BIOPSY

Aspiration needle in large glass tube or covered pan
Jamshidi biopsy needle and hemostat in covered pad
2 Syringes 20 mℓ, disposable
2 Syringes, 6 mℓ, disposable
2 Needles, 21 gauge, 1 ½ in., disposable
2 Needles, 25 gauge, 5/8 in., disposable
Blade, Bard Parker #11, and surgical blade holder (disposable)
Iodine 3%
Alcohol swabs or 70% alcohol
Anesthetic in sterile rubber stoppered container
8 Gauze squares 3 × 3 in. (in separate wrapping)
Culture tubes
Adhesive bandage (or Band-Aid®)
2 Towels
Rubber gloves

Table 3
NONSTERILE EQUIPMENT FOR MARROW COLLECTION

Skin-marking pencil
1 Box glass slides (3 × 1 in.)
1 Box to hold smears to be processed
1 Box cover glasses, #1 (22 × 22 mm)
Modeling clay block
Paraffin-coated watch glass or Petri dish
Pasteur pipette or medicine dropper with rubber bulb
2 Wide-mouth bottles with cap containing 10% formalin or other fixative
1 Small vial containing glutaraldehyde (for electron microscopy, if indicated)
Disposal basin

Table 4
EMERGENCY KIT

Equipment

Airway (lifesaver tube)
Tourniquet
2 Tuberculin syringes, 1 mℓ with 25-gauge 5/8 in. needle attached
2 Syringes, 3 mℓ with 23-gauge 1-in. needle attached
Intravenous cannulas, 18 and 20 gauges
Solution administration set

Drugs (injectable)

Diphenyhydramine (Benadryl®) 1 mℓ ampule, 50 mg
Diazepam (Valium ®) 2 mℓ ampule, 10 mg
250 mℓ 5% dextrose and 0.9% sodium chloride, in plastic container

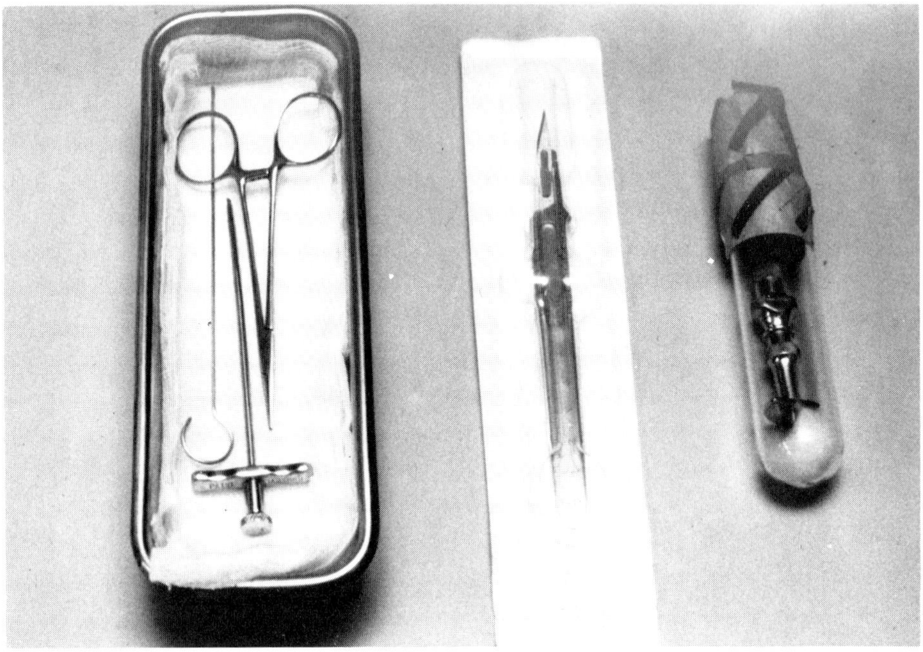

FIGURE 8. Left: Jamshidi biopsy needle and hemostat in sterile pan. Middle: Bard-Parker knife in sterile container. Right: Sterile glass tube containing Limarzi University of Illinois needle.

(Figure 8). The staff that is responsible for marrow punctures should also be responsible for the ordering, inspecting after each use, cleaning, sharpening, packaging, and sterilizing marrow needles so that blame cannot be placed on a third party or the supply room if the needles on the tray are unsatisfactory.

For cleansing the skin, Betadine®, Merthiolate®, or other topical antiseptic solutions may be substituted for iodine and alcohol.

The local anesthetic of choice is lidocaine hydrochloride. Untoward reactions to this drug are extremely rare. When reactions do occur, they usually take the form of agitation, tremors, or convulsive seizures. When there are central nervous system manifestations, the treatment recommended is the slow intravenous administration of diazepam. If there are signs of an allergic reaction, manifested by itching, urticara, difficulty in breathing, and signs of shock, the indicated drug is aqueous epinephrine, 0.3 to 0.5 mℓ subcutaneously followed by 0.1 to 0.2 mℓ at 10 to 15 min intervals if necessary. For follow-up treatment, 50 mg of diphenyhydramine may be given at 4-hr intervals.

Any patient may faint during an operative procedure, in which case the legs should be elevated and marrow puncture withheld until a normal state is achieved. If the patient develops a hyperventilation syndrome, reassurance and sedation are indicated. If the patient vomits or gags, he should be turned to a prone position to prevent pulmonary aspiration. If there is marked and persistent hypovolemic hypotension, intravenous fluids are indicated. For patients who may have respiratory difficulties, the maintenance of a clear airway is essential. Avoid unnecessary drugs.

Opinions differ about the fixative that is best to use for marrow tissue that is to be sectioned in preparation for staining. The authors recommend for general use neutral buffered 10% formalin. Other fixatives that may be used are Zenker's and sodium acetate-mercuric chloride-formalin mixture (B-5). (See histopathology texts for directions for preparing fixative solutions.) For electron micrographic sections, 5% glutaraldehyde is used.

Needle Aspiration

The operator should see that the patient is comfortable and that all equipment needed is available and convenient. The hands of the operator should be washed previous to the procedure.

The site of the intended puncture is determined by inspection and by palpation, and is marked with a skin-marking pencil or by an X—indentation of the skin made by the thumb nail. The skin is then cleansed in an expanding circle with 3% iodine followed by 70% alcohol using sterile swabs and a hemostat.

Approximately 4 mℓ of lidocaine hydrochloride or equivalent anesthetic solution is aspirated using a 21-gauge 1½ in. needle attached to a 5 mℓ syringe. The 21-gauge needle is then removed from the syringe and placed on a sterile towel or pan and a 25-gauge 5/8 in. hypodermic needle is substituted. A small amount of anesthetic solution is first injected intradermally raising a small bleb at the site of intended puncture. Following this the 21-gauge needle is reattached to the syringe, and the periosteum is infiltrated. Injection of large amounts of anesthetic solution into the subcutaneous fatty tissue serves no useful purpose in preventing pain, tends to obscure landmarks, and increases the chances of a systemic reaction.

Sterile gloves are not recommended for sternal punctures for they needlessly increase the complexity, the time required, and the expense. There is no more reason for using rubber gloves for aspiration of marrow from the sternum than for the aspiration of blood from a vein, provided the bare hands do not touch the cleansed area of skin or any part of the needle shaft. Sterile gloves are recommended when marrow is aspirated from sites other than the sternum, because palpation of the cleansed skin may be necessary, and both hands may be needed to support the shaft of the needle as it is pushed through dense cortical bone.

Sterile towels or drapes to isolate the operative field are optional. For sternal puncture it is recommended that a sterile towel be placed above the operative site, covering the neck and chin of the patient. For other puncture sites, one sterile towel is usually sufficient.

The aspiration needle, with obturator in place, is inserted through the skin and subcutaneous tissue until the point touches the bone. Using one hand to push the needle forward and the other hand to steady the needle hub and to control the depth and angle of puncture, the needle point is advanced with a twisting boring motion through the compact bony plate into the less resistant cancellous marrow. Pressure must be applied to the obturator head as well as the needle hub to prevent the stylet from "riding up" and causing the lumen of the needle to be obstructed.

There is usually a sensation of "give" as the needle passes through dense cortical bone, but in the presence of osteoporosis, the needle tip will slip into the medullary space without appreciable resistance. When the needle is embedded in marrow tissue, it will remain upright without manual support. The obturator is removed and its lower portion is protected from contamination by placement on the edge of the sterile tray or sterile towel. A plastic syringe or a 20 mℓ glass syringe with a tightly fitting barrel and a metal tip is inserted in the needle hub. The patient should be warned that there will be a brief pain as suction is applied so that he will not be alarmed and jerk away. The semiliquid marrow is vigorously pulled into the barrel of the syringe. Suction is discontinued as soon as marrow appears in the barrel of the syringe. The amount of aspirated material should be less than 1 mℓ. Aspirates having a larger volume are undesirably diluted with sinusoidal blood. Before the tip of the syringe is removed from the needle hub, the negative pressure within the syringe should be reduced to prevent spattering and distortion of cell membranes as the air rushes into the syringe.

The syringe, containing aspirated marrow, is removed and handed to the technical assistant who proceeds with the preparation of smears, spreading of marrow particles, and fixation of the marrow clot or spicules of cellular marrow.

The operator places the sterile stylet back into the lumen of the needle that remains in the medullary space. If the aspirated material contains visible fat and small marrow particles, the aspiration procedure is deemed satisfactory and the needle is withdrawn. If the marrow spreads do not appear greasy and if no cellular aggregates are visible, the position of the needle is slightly changed, the obturator is removed, and the tip of a dry and unused syringe is inserted into the needle hub and a second aspiration is attempted.

If culture of the marrow is indicated, marrow aspirate for this purpose should be obtained at this time.

Following collection of desired material, the needle is withdrawn, and the skin wound is covered with a sterile gauze square. Firm pressure is applied by the operator for several minutes. The skin wound is then covered with a Band-Aid® or small sterile dressing.

Occasionally it is not possible to aspirate bone marrow because the lumen of the distal end of the needle is plugged with trabecular bone or clot. Dry taps also may be due to faulty positioning of the needle or to replacement of the cellular marrow by fibrous tissue, calcific bone, granuloma, necrotic tissue, or metastatic malignant cells. A marked proliferation of cells as in stem cell leukemia or multiple myeloma may make the marrow so viscid and gelatinous and the cells so adherent to each other that they do not separate and flow into the needle when suction is applied. It is recommended that — in situations in which it is not possible to see marrow in the barrel of the syringe — the smallest amount of material at the tip of the needle should be spread on a slide, stained, and examined microscopically. This tiny bit of material may reveal cells in sufficient numbers to be satisfactory for microscopic examination, thus avoiding the necessity of performing an additional bone puncture.

In addition to making smears of bone marrow, it is essential that a smear be made of peripheral blood at the same time.

Processing of Aspirated Marrow

Immediately after collection, aspirated marrow is processed by a medical technologist or by a specially trained technical assistant. Smears and squash preparations of marrow particles are made on cover slips or slides.

To make smears on slides one small drop of aspirated marrow is placed near the end of three or more slides, and each drop is quickly spread before coagulation occurs. The spreader slide should have a smooth edge and should be held at an angle of approximately 30°. The errors most frequently made are the use of drops that are too large and an angle of the spreader slide that is too great, thus creating smears that are too thick. Spreads should be so thin that there is an area at least 1 cm long in the feather end of the smear in which the red cells are well separated. Smears of marrow on glass slides are identified by writing — with a lead pencil or sharp object directly on the thick end of the dried marrow films — the name of the patient and the date.

Many examiners prefer films of bone marrow on cover slips over slide preparations, because the cells in cover slip spreads are usually well separated, the nucleated cells are more evenly distributed, and mechanically traumatized cells and smudges are less frequent. The advantages to the examiner are offset by technical disadvantages. Dried films on cover slips are more difficult to label, to transport, and to stain than are smears on slides. Cover slips require mounting on slides before examination. The cover slip spreads for a given patient may be held upright in a clay block identified with the

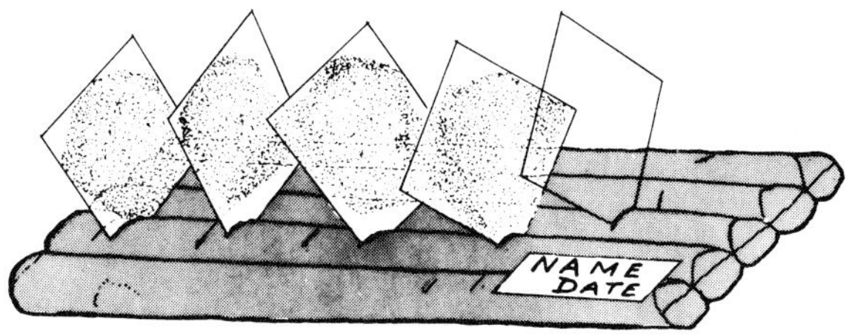

FIGURE 9. Films of marrow on cover slips supported in a clay block.

patient's name and date on the clay block (Figure 9) and carried back to the laboratory for final processing.

In addition to films of marrow on glass slides or on cover slips, squash spreads of marrow particles are also prepared. In order to make squash preparations, aggregates of soft and compressible marrow particles containing cells loosely held together by reticular fibers and by blood vessels are needed. They are obtained by placing a large drop of marrow aspirate on the end of a glass slide that is tilted, allowing the plasma and the free cells, mainly nonnucleated red cells, to separate and run downward. The cell conglomerates remain in the upper portion. One or several of these marrow particles is picked up on the corner of a slide and transferred to the surface of another slide, and another slide is placed on top of the marrow clump and compressed gently. The two slides are then pulled apart, causing the cells to spread out in a thin film. Similar spreads of marrow cells can be made using cover slips. Squash marrow spreads are less satisfactory than are thin smears for differential counts, but are of greater value than are thin smears for estimating cellularity, the number of megakaryocytes, and the presence or absence of islands of metastatic malignant cells.

Some physicians prefer to use anticoagulants such as EDTA or heparin to prevent fibrin formation in order to make multiple smears and to concentrate the marrow particles by centrifugation or by filtration. The addition of anticoagulants unnecessarily complicates the procedure because they interfere with critical staining and create artefacts.

Following the making of marrow spreads on slides or on cover slips, the plunger of the syringe containing the remaining marrow specimen is partially withdrawn. The syringe is held in an upright position until the marrow clots, following which the plunger is removed and the button or disc of clotted marrow and any residual clot in the barrel of the syringe is removed by an applicator stick or pipette, and placed in the fixative solution. Marrow clots, although simple to collect, to fix and to section, have the disadvantage of containing many nonnucleated red cells, a large amount of serum, and few marrow particles.

Various procedures have been devised to concentrate particles of marrow tissue. The most simple and practical method is to allow the residual marrow to clot in a watch glass or Petri dish, to drain off, by gravity, the serum and free cells, and remove them by means of a pipette or absorbent paper. Following this the marrow particles are aggregated in the retracted fibrin web and placed on a bit of lens paper. The edges of the lens paper are gathered together forming a sack that is placed in the fixing solution for sectioning and staining.

Particles of marrow aspirated by negative pressure from the medullary spaces through small needles are soft and semiliquid masses that seldom contain trabecular bone and therefore do not require decalcification.

Table 5
INDICATIONS FOR BIOPSY

Unsuccessful aspiration (dry tap)
Evaluation of cellularity in pancytopenias
Myeloproliferative diseases
Questionable lymphomas and other malignancies
Staging of known malignancies
Bone diseases
Granulomas
Amyloidosis
Lipid storage diseases
Follow-up after chemotherapy

Needle Biopsy

The advantage of core biopsies over tissue sections of marrow particles from aspirated material is that larger areas of marrow are available for examination, thus increasing the chance of finding focal lesions. Sections of trephined marrow reveal bony structures that are seldom present in aspirated particles. Core biopsies of bone marrow are of particular value in the various myeloproliferative syndromes, including polycythemia, essential thrombocythemia, and myelofibrosis, in order to evaluate the cellularity, the number of megakaryocytes, and the degree of fibrosis. Indications for needle biopsy are listed in Table 5.

In diseases of the blood and blood-forming organs, marrow biopsy is more likely to yield information of diagnostic value than biopsies of lymph nodes, liver, or spleen.

The examination of stained sections of core biopsies supplements, but does not replace, the scanning of marrow spreads and differential counts. Maximal information is obtained when cells are examined in thin smears as well as in sections of fixed tissues.

Selected references to scientific articles and monographs related to the techniques and interpretation of marrow biopsies are listed in the reference section.[3-12]

Biopsy Technique

After the site of puncture has been located and marked, the operative field cleansed, the local anesthetic injected, and the sterile towels or drapes placed, the operator puts on sterile gloves. A small incision is made with a surgical blade at the point of needle entry into the skin. The best results are obtained if marrow is first aspirated from the marrow space, using a small needle and if the material is processed as described above.

Next, the Jamshidi needle, with the obturator locked in place, is pushed through the site of skin incision and subcutaneous tissue to the surface of bone at an angle slightly different from that used for aspiration. Using a twisting motion and firm pressure, the point of the needle is bored through the compact cortex into the marrow space. The stylet is then removed. If aspirated material has not been previously obtained through a separate needle, it is obtained at this point by attaching a syringe to the biopsy needle, applying negative pressure, and aspirating a minimal amount of marrow for smears and squash preparations. Following this the core trephine specimen is obtained. The desired distance of penetration is controlled by placing one gloved index finger parallel with the biopsy needle shaft with the fingertip 2 to 3 cm above the skin surface. The needle is then advanced with a rotary motion until the end of the measuring finger touches the skin. The needle is then rotated for several complete turns to free the distal end of the marrow cylinder, following which, the needle is slowly withdrawn.

The marrow cylinder within the lumen of the needle is pushed from the hub end by means of a blunt probe inserted in the pointed end. The trephined core is placed in the proper fixative and sent to the histology laboratory for decalcification, sectioning, staining, mounting, and labeling.

Incisional (Surgical) Biopsy

Since the development of satisfactory biopsy needles and the use of the posterior crest of the ilium as a site for trephination, it is seldom necessary to resort to surgical biopsies. The major disadvantages of incisional biopsy are the necessity of operating room facilities, increased cost, and a surgical scar following the procedure. Incisional biopsies of the sternum can be performed under local anesthesia, but rib resection and surgical biopsies of bones other than the sternum require general anesthesia. A mastoid type of retractor aids in holding the incised skin, subcutaneous tissue, and periosteum from the operative site. Before cutting through cortical bone, the marrow should be aspirated and smears and squash preparations of marrow particles processed as described above.

A window, at least 1 cm in width, is cut through the cortical bone using a pointed surgical knife or a cork borer type of trephine, preferably with a sawtooth cutting edge. Following the removal and fixation of the block of tissue, including the cortex and attached trabecular bone marrow, bits of bone marrow are scooped out of the marrow cavity and placed on sterile gauze to allow the sinusoidal blood to drain away. Imprints of marrow particles are then made on glass slides.

Autopsy Sections

Unless smears of marrow are made immediately after death, making them for the purpose of cytologic studies of individual cells and for differential counts is a waste of time. Cytolysis occurs rapidly after death causing the cells, and particularly neutrophilic granulocytes, to be disrupted and smudged by the shearing forces involved in spreading cells on glass surfaces. Suspension of marrow cells in 5% bovine albumin or in serum from the cadaver is of aid in obtaining less disrupted cells for microscopic examination.

The sites of choice for obtaining blocks of marrow at the time of autopsy are the sternum, rib, and vertebral body. In diseases of the blood and blood-forming organs, it is preferable to obtain blocks from multiple sites, including the middle of the shaft of a long tubular bone such as the tibia. The surface of the bone from which blocks are to be chiselled or sawed should be dry to prevent hemolysis of red cells. When bones are sawed, bone dust is ground into the marrow spaces, creating artefacts that on microscopic examination may be falsely interpreted as necrosis. Bone dust in tissue sections can be avoided by cutting the block of decalcified bone at right angles to the sawed surface before the tissue is processed for final thin sectioning and staining.

Staining of Marrow Smears, Imprints, Tissue Sections

Wright Stain

Smears and imprints of marrow tissue, after drying thoroughly, are stained by the Wright procedure or by comparable methylene blue and eosin stains. Details about fixation and staining procedures may be obtained from textbooks of clinical pathology and/or hematology. The actual staining time must be determined in each laboratory for the particular batch of stain employed. The staining time is generally longer for marrow spreads than for peripheral blood smears.

Wright stain may be combined with dilute Giemsa stain as the diluting fluid in place of distilled water. Giemsa solution is diluted 1:50 with distilled water, which has a neutral pH. The combination of Wright stain plus diluted Giemsa solution is useful in salvaging smears in which cells are feebly stained.

It is recommended that smears be examined under low power after staining to detect whether the preparation is stained properly before mounting or adding oil to smear. If precipitated dye particles are present, add Wright stain to redissolve the precipitate and wash immediately.

Prussian Blue Stain for Iron

In order to detect aggregates of iron particles (siderotic granules), spreads or sections of marrow spicules are stained by the Perl Prussian blue procedure. Ionic iron reacts with ferrocyanide in an acid solution, forming blue precipitates of ferric ferrocyanide.

Blue-staining iron granules are located in the cytoplasm of tissue phagocytes and in the cytoplasm of nucleated red cells (sideroblasts). Siderotic granules in nucleated erythrocytes are best seen in thin smears examined under oil immersion. Stained iron in histiocytes is searched for in thicker portions of smears, in crush preparations, and in stained sections of marrow spicules. Sections of decalcified marrow tissue should not be used, for decalcification tends to decrease the amount of stainable iron. Control specimens known to be strongly positive for iron should always be examined to be sure that the stain is adequate.

Stainable iron is demonstrable in the bone marrow of healthy persons and in practically all anemias other than those due to iron deficiency, such as nutritional and blood loss anemias, anemias due to defective intestinal absorption and increased demand, loss of hemoglobin into the urine as in paroxysmal nocturnal hemoglobinuria, and bleeding into lung spaces (pulmonary hemosiderosis). Siderotic granules are demonstrable in megaloblastic anemias due to deficiencies in folic acid and/or B12. They are also seen in anemias associated with chronic infections, cachetic and wasting diseases, nephritis, lead poisoning, erythroleukemia, and other malignancies. Ineffective erythropoiesis in these latter conditions is due to the inability to utilize available iron rather than a lack of iron.

Iron stains are of greatest value in the differential diagnosis of hypochromic microcytic anemias. In true iron deficiencies, siderotic granules are markedly decreased or absent, whereas in thalassemias, sideroachrestic anemias, pyridoxine responsive anemia, and hereditary and acquired hemolytic anemias, stainable iron particles are increased. In sideroachrestic anemia the iron positive granules in the mitochondria tend to form a circle around the nucleus producing the so-called "ringed sideroblasts." Stainable iron is strikingly increased in hemochromatosis and in hemosiderosis.

Reticulum Stains

Stromal (connective tissue) elements in the bone marrow sections are indistinctly revealed by hematoxylin and eosin and by methylene blue and eosin (Romanowsky) stains. They are best demonstrated by silver impregnation methods and by trichrome stains. Special stains for reticulum and collagen are of aid in evaluating myelofibrosis, in distinguishing between sclerosing lesions and crush artefacts, and in differentiating between primary and metastatic malignancies. Native cells proliferating in the marrow tend to be individually enmeshed by reticular fibers, whereas cells foreign to the marrow, such as metastatic neuroblastoma or carcinoma cells, are surrounded as a group by fibers but not individually.

Other Stains

Cytochemical stains, such as Sudan Black B, peroxidase, trichrome, periodic acid-Schiff (PAS), specific and nonspecific esterases, and tartrate-resistant acid phosphotase may be used as indicated. Additional smears should be made at the time of the aspiration if these stains are to be performed. The reader is referred to hematology procedure manuals for specific directions for special stains.

Examination

Peripheral Blood

The first procedure is to examine a stained smear of peripheral blood and preferably a smear that was made at the same time the bone marrow material was obtained. A description of the morphology of the erythrocytes and the number and morphology of thrombocytes as well as differential count of leukocytes should accompany the bone marrow report. The comparison of the leukocyte differential count of the circulating blood with the count of marrow cells aids in the evaluation of the degree of dilution with sinusoidal blood. The presence of "blasts" and other immature cells in blood smears is much more significant than a slight increase in early cells in hematopoietic tissue.

Stained Marrow Smears, Squash Preparations, and Imprints

The second examination procedure is to grossly inspect every available stained spread of bone marrow to determine which are suitable for microscopic examination. Next, under low power or high dry magnification, thousands of cells are examined in multiple thick and thin areas of two or more of the best marrow spreads to evaluate cellularity, the number of fat cells, and the relationship of the various series of cell types to each other. While scanning, the less frequently occurring cells are noted.

Following the scanning procedure, a thin and well-stained area is selected, and a differential count of at least 200 and preferably 500 nucleated cells is performed.

To speed up the differential counts, two large, eight-cell counters are used. The punch key of each counter is labeled to correspond with the cell to be tallied. The operator notes periodically the number of cells counted on both instruments until the desired total count is reached. Percentages for each category are recorded on the final report form. A suggested report form is given in Figure 10. The numerous advantages of differential counts are summarized in Table 6.

Atypical and pathological cells that cannot be identified are grouped in separate categories under the heading of "Other Cells." In the final report atypical cells are described and their number stated.

In addition to the report of the percentages of the various nucleated cells, the ratio of white blood cells to nucleated red cells (WBC to Nuc RBC) should be recorded. It has been customary for many hematologists to relate the number of myelocytic cells to nucleated erythrocytes, the so-called "M to E ratio", but this method gives an erroneous impression when there is a marked increase in lymphocytes, monocytes, or plasmocytes, and a relative and absolute decrease in myelocytic cells.

Attention should be paid not only to abnormalities in the maturation of the various cell types, but also to degenerative changes and inclusions, crystals, and vacuoles in nuclei and in the cytoplasm.

While performing the differential count, one should note the characteristics of non-nucleated red cells and thrombocytes. Rouleaux formation of red cells and the relationship of leukocyte and tissue cells to each other (indentation, separation, attachment) are also observed. Other points to be noted include abnormal sizes and shapes of cells, abnormal lobulation of nuclei, mitotic figures, multiple nuclei, and cytoplasmic structures such as vacuoles, greenish-yellow, yellow-brown, or golden yellow hemosiderin, crystals, and phagocytized objects.

Megakaryocytes, like other large cells, are most numerous in thick spreads and at the feather edge of smears. The number of megakaryocytes is usually in the range of 5 to 20 per 1000 nucleated cells. Bcause of the uneven distribution in marrow spreads, it is best to evaluate their number in tissue sections. If there is a decrease in thrombocytes in the peripheral blood, a differential count of at least 25 consecutive megakary-

BONE MARROW

NAME__________ SEX___ AGE___ NUMBER__________

ADDRESS__________ REFERRING PHYSICIAN__________

SITE__________ DATE OF COLLECTION__________ OPERATOR__________

CLINICAL INFORMATION

ERYTHROCYTES-See peripheral blood report

MEGAKARYOCYTES

DIFFERENTIAL: Cells counted______ TISSUE SECTION (H AND E STAIN)

Normal	Percent
0-1 Stem cell	
1-5 Promyelocyte	
2-10 N Myelocyte	
5-15 N Metamyelocyte	
10-40 N Band	
10-30 N Segmented	
0-3 Eosinophil	
0-1 Basophil	
5-15 Lymphocyte	
0-1 Plasmocyte	
0-2 Monocyte	
Other cells	
0-1 Rubriblast	
1-4 Prorubricyte	
10-20 Rubricyte	
5-10 Metarubricyte	
2-5:1 WBC : Nuc RBC	

OTHER OBSERVATIONS

SUMMARY OF ABNORMALITIES

INTERPRETATION

________ Typed by   ________ Classification No.   ________ Examined by

FIGURE 10. Bone marrow report.

Table 6
ADVANTAGES OF DIFFERENTIAL COUNTS OF MARROW CELLS

Supplements scanning of marrow spreads and tissue sections
Favors a more critical appraisal of details of nuclear and cytoplasmic structures
Supplies quantitative (numerical) data of value in interpretation
- Leucocyte: nucleated red cell ratio
- Leucocytic series in relation to each other
- Maturation patterns

Furnishes base line information useful when successive examinations are indicated and which is of aid in:
- Establishing diagnosis
- Evaluating response to therapy
- Determining prognosis

If performed by professional assistant:
- Saves time for the histopathologist or hematologist making final report
- Spots cells for special examination and for photography
- Increases the range of scanning
- Stimulates interest and improves laboratory esprit
- Makes technical staff more critical and competent in examining peripheral blood smears
- Tends to encourage staff to make thinner and better marrow spreads

Provides referring physician with data upon which to base independent judgement
Provides the patient with greater return for his money

ocytes should be performed. These cells are classified as megakaryoblasts, promegakaryocytes, megakaryocytes, metamegakaryocytes, and naked nuclei.

Search should be made for islands of cells suggestive of malignancy and for etiologic agents such as *Histoplasma capsulatum*. Microscopic fields on stained slide smears containing unusual or atypical cells, which the examiner wishes to demonstrate to others or to photograph, may be circled with the point of a dissecting needle in the marrow film under lower power observation.

When examining marrow spreads, imprints, and tissue sections, attention should be given not only to cells but also to extracellular material. In plasma cell myeloma there may be cellular debris, and in hyperproteinemia there occasionally is a bluish background. With amyloidosis there are extracellular purplish and pink cloud-like homogeneous aggregates, which are darker in the central portion than at the margin. In tissue sections amyloid is manifested as hyaline deposits of purplish substance in walls of blood vessels as well as in intercellular spaces.

The reader is referred to excellent summaries by Nordenson,[13] Osgood and Seaman,[14] Leitner,[15] Rohr,[16] Zuelzer,[17] and Williams[18] for more detailed information about the history of marrow examinations, techniques, normal values, lesions observed in various diseases, and for a more complete bibliography. Differential values for peripheral blood and bone marrow according to various authors are listed in the *Biology Data Book*.[19] Reported differential counts of smears of marrow aspirates of humans[8,20-25] from modern textbooks of hematology are given in Tables 7 and 8.

Tissue Sections

Following the examination of peripheral blood and marrow smears, the next procedure is to examine stained sections of marrow particles and/or thin stained sections of trephined marrow cylinders. Marrow biopsies have the advantage over spreads of marrow cells in that they reveal fixed structures such as blood vessels, trabecular bone, lymphocytic nodules, and the pattern of the various cells in relation to each other. The anatomical structures to be examined and the abnormalities to be noted are listed in Table 9.

Tissue sections are inferior to smears for the identification of individual cells, but they are superior to smears in that they make it possible to evaluate the number of fixed and semifixed cells such as megakaryocytes, tissue phagocytes, osteoblasts, fibrocytes, and lipocytes. Histiologic sections are required in order to accurately determine the degree of cellularity, and to estimate the area occupied by fat cells compared with the space filled by blood cells and their progenitors (fat to cell ratio). Sections of marrow tissue confirm or refute the data obtained by differential counts, and in addition may reveal lesions such as necrosis, hemorrhage, islands of malignant cells, or granuloma.

Granulomas are small, granule-like, nodular and focal lesions that consist of cells grouped in a pattern, which is different from that of the surrounding cells. The term granuloma is sometimes used to describe nests of primary mestatic malignant cells in marrow tissue, and to designate groups of reactive cells that accumulate in focal areas in response to chemicals, physical agents, and/or antigenic factors.Most granulomas are manifestations of cellular responses to bacteria, fungi, viruses, protozoa, or other infectious agents. They consist of varying mixtures of reactive inflammatory cells that include neutrophils, eosinophils, monocytes, lymphocytes, plasmocytes, tissue phagocytes, histiocytes with prominent cytoplasm (epithelioid cells), and fibrocytes. Lymphocytes and plasmocytes tend to be most numerous at the periphery of the nodular areas. Multinuclear giant cells, fat cells, and cells containing crystals may be present. Nucleated red cells and megakaryocytes are absent. In tuberculous granuloma there

Table 7
BONE MARROW NORMAL VALUES

	Custer 1974	Dacie and Lewis 1970	Diggs 1971	Linman 1975	Miale 1972	Whitby and Britton 1969	Wintrobe 1974
Myeloblast	0.0—3.5	0.1—3.5	0.0—1.0	0.3—3.0	0.3—5.0	0.0—2.5	0.2—1.5
Promyelocyte	0.5—8.0	0.5—5.0	1.0—5.0	1.0—8.0	1.0—8.0	0.5—5.0	2.1—4.1
N. Myelocyte	7.0—34.6	5.0—20.0	2.0—10.0	7.0—20.0	5.0—19.0	2.0—8.0	8.2—15.7
N. Metamyelocyte	20.0—45.0	10.0—30.0	5.0—15.0	10.0—30.0	13.0—32.0	10.0—25.0	9.6—24.6
N. Band			10.0—40.0	15.0—35.0	15.0—30.0		9.5—15.3
N. Segmented	7.0—25.0	7.0—25.0	10.0—30.0		7.0—30.0	10.0—40.0	6.0—12.0
Eosinophil (all stages)	0.7—9.7	0.3—6.0	0.0—3.0	0.5—3.0	1.5—12.7	0.0—7.5	1.2—5.3
Basophil (all stages)	0.0—1.8	0.0—1.0	0.0—1.0	0.0—1.0	0.0—1.8	0.0—1.0	0.0—1.2
Lymphocyte	2.5—25.0	5.0—20.0	5.0—15.0	2.0—12.0	2.7—24.0	5.0—20.0	11.1—23.2
Plasmocyte	0.1—1.2	0.1—3.5	0.0—1.0	0.0—2.0	0.1—1.5	0.0—1.0	0.4—3.9
Monocyte	0.1—3.2	0.0—0.2	0.0—2.0	0.5—5.0	0.7—2.8	0.0—5.0	0.0—0.8
Other	0.3—2.6	0.1—2.0	—	0.2—1.0	0.2—2.0	—	0.0—0.9
Megakaryocyte	0.5—1.2	0.1—0.5	—	<0.01	0.03—0.4	—	0.0—0.4
Rubriblast	0.1—3.5	0.5—5.0	0.0—1.0	2.0—6.0	0.2—4.0	0.0—4.0	0.2—1.3
Prorubricyte	1.7—5.5	2.0—20.0	1.0—4.0		1.5—5.8	4.0—15.0	0.5—2.4
Rubricyte	5.0—20.0	2.0—20.0	10.0—20.0	12.0—20.0	5.0—26.4		17.9—29.2
Metarubricyte	5.0—23.8	2.0—10.0	5.0—10.0	6.0—10.0	1.6—21.0	7.0—19.0	0.4—4.6

Table 8
CHANGES IN DIFFERENTIAL COUNTS OF BONE MARROW WITH AGE

		Birth	1 Week	1 Week to 1 Year	1—4 Years	4—12 Years	Adult
Neutrophilic series	$\bar{x}$%[a]	54	65	37	50	52	57
	95% limits	31—77	21—79	22—52	32—68	35—69	39—79
Eosinophilic series	$\bar{x}$%[a]	3	3	3	6	3	3
	95% limits	1—5	1—5	1—5	2—10	1—5	1—5
Lymphocytic series	$\bar{x}$%[a]	6	13	36	22	18	17
	95% limits	2—10	7—19	18—54	8—36	12—28	10—24
Erythrocytic series	$\bar{x}$%[a]	34	15	17	19	21	20
	95% limits	18—50	5—25	7—27	11—27	11—31	10—30
M:E ratio	$\bar{x}$[a]	1.6	4.3	2.2	2.6	2.5	2.6

[a] The means (×) and 95% confidence limits in this table were calculated by combining data published by Osgood and Seaman, Sturgeon, Shapiro and Bassen, Veeneklaas and associates, and Diwany.

From Wintrobe, M. M., *Clinical Hematology,* 7th ed., Lea & Febiger, Phialdelphia, 1974, 71. With permission.

Table 9
ANATOMICAL STRUCTURES TO BE EVALUATED IN EXAMINATION OF TISSUE SECTIONS OF BONE MARROW

Bone structures
- Trabeculae
- Osteoblasts
- Osteoclasts

Blood vessels (arteries, arterioles, sinusoids)
- Lumen
- Wall
- Perivascular spaces

Cellular spaces
- Area occupied by fat cells in relation to blood cells and progenitors (fat to cell ratio)
- Megakaryocytes and other blood cells
- Lymph follicles
- Histiocytes
- Tissue basophils
- Pigment
- Fibrosis
- Necrosis
- Granulomas
- Giant cells
- Extracellular abnormalities
- Malignant cells
- Etiologic agents

may be central caseating necrosis, whereas necrosis is absent in granulomas associated with sarcoidosis.

Absence of demonstrable abnormalities in available stained sections does not exclude the possibility that there are lesions in other marrow areas; the observation of any form of deviation from normal is significant and should lead to further investigation.

Other Observations

The space in the report form under the heading of ''Other Observations'' (Figure 10) is reserved for the recording of miscellaneous information such as difficulty in puncture due to cortical density or unusual ease in penetration (osteoporosis), or of unusual experiences in obtaining aspirated material. This space is also used for recording characteristics revealed by special stains, and as a place to record the fact that material was collected for culture, electron microscopy, or other procedures.

Summary of Abnormalities

After recording the pertinent facts, the morphology of erythrocytes and megakaryocytes, the differential count of nucleated cells, the ratio of white blood cells to nucleated red cells, the degree of cellularity, and the anatomical characteristics of sections of marrow particles and/or biopsies, the next step is to summarize the observed abnormalities.

Interpretation

The physician who is responsible for the final report should have access to all known clinical facts, including previous treatment and abnormalities revealed by laboratory tests. His role is that of a medical consultant who is expected, not only to give an opinion, but also to furnish facts upon which the referring physician and others may base independent judgment.

Having summarized the abnormalities revealed by tissue sections, smears, and squash preparations, the final step for the consultant is to correlate these findings with clinical manifestations, the peripheral blood characteristics, and with the chemical, roentgenological, and other laboratory findings.

In some cases it is possible, on the basis of combined data, to make a definitive diagnosis or to exclude a disease that was clinically considered a possibility. Often the observed abnormalities are not specific for a given disease, but furnish valuable links in the chain of evidence that aid in differential diagnosis, prognosis, and management, and that furnish valuable indications for further study.

REFERENCES

1. **Jamshidi, K. and Swain, W. R.,** Bone marrow biopsy with unaltered architecture: a new biopsy device, *J. Lab. Clin. Med.*, 77, 335, 1971.
2. **Inwood, M. J.,** Jamshidi bone marrow needle modification, *J. Lab. Clin. Med.*, 86, 535, 1975.
3. **Bierman, L.,** A review of methods for aspiration and biopsy of bone marrow, *Am. J. Clin. Pathol.*, 23, 385, 1953.
4. **Silver, R. T.,** Bone marrow aspiration and biopsy, *Am. Acad. Gen. Pract.*, 31, 100, 1965.
5. **Burkhardt, T.,** *Bone Marrow and Bone Tissue*, Springer-Verlag, Basel, 1971.
6. **Schleicher, E. M.,** *Bone Marrow Morphology and Mechanics of Biopsy*, Charles C. Thomas, Springfield, Ill., 1973.
7. **Raich, P. C.,** Bone marrow needle biopsy: method and indications, *Wis. Med. J.*, 73, S155, 1974.
8. **Custer, R. P.,** *An Atlas of the Blood and Bone Marrow*, 2nd ed., W. B. Saunders, Philadelphia, 1974, 42, 537.
9. **Dutcher, T. B.,** Introduction to the interpretation of bone marrow sections, *Am. Soc. Clin. Pathol.*, 47-2-0200, 1, 1975.
10. **Dee, J. W., Valdivieso, M., and Drewinko, B.,** Comparison of the efficacies of closed trephine needle biopsy, aspirated paraffin-embedded clot section, and smear preparation in the diagnosis of bone marrow in involvement by lymphoma, *Am. J. Clin. Pathol.*, 65, 183, 1976.
11. **Block, M. H.,** *Text-Atlas of Hematology*, Lea & Febiger, Philadelphia, 1976.
12. **Rywlin, A.M.,** *Histopathology of Bone Marrow*, 1st ed., Cawley, L. P., Ed., Little, Brown, Boston, 1976.
13. **Nordenson, N. G.,** *Studies on Bone Marrow from Sternal Puncture*, Bortzels, Esselte, Stockholm, 1935.
14. **Osgood, E. E.and Seaman, A. V.,** The cellular composition of normal bone marrow as obtained by sternal puncture, *Physiol. Rev.*, 24, 46, 1944.
15. **Leitner, S. J.,** Bone marrow biopsy, in *Haematology in the Light of Sternal Puncture*, Britton, C. J. C. and Newman, L. E., Eds., Grune & Stratton, New York, 1949.
16. **Rohr, K.,** *Des Menschliche Kpochenmark*, Georg Thieme Verlag, Stuttgart, 1949, 94.
17. **Zuelzer, W. W.,** Normal and pathologic physiology of the bone marrow, *Am. J. Dis. Child.*, 77, 482, 1949.
18. **Williams, W. J.,** Examination of the bone marrow, in *Hematology*, 2nd ed., Williams, W.J., Beutler, E., Erslev, A. J., and Rundles, R. W., Eds., McGraw-Hill, New York, 1977, 25.
19. **Altman, P. L. and Dittmer, D. S.,** *Biology Data Book*, Vol. 3, 2nd ed., Federation of American Societies for Experimental Biology, Bethesda, 1974, 1862.
20. **Dacie, J. V. and Lewis, S. M.,** *Practical Haematology*, 4th ed., Churchill-Livingstone, London, 1970, 130.
21. **Diggs, L. W,** Hematological techniques, in *Textbook of Clinical Pathology*, Miller, S. E. and Waller, J. M., Eds., Williams & Wilkins, Baltimore, 1971, 37.
22. **Linman, J. W.,** *Hematology: Physiologic, Pathophysiologic, and Clinical Principles*, 1st ed., Macmillan, New York, 1975, 81.
23. **Miale, J. B.,** *Laboratory Medicine: Hematology*, 4th ed., C. V. Mosby, St. Louis, 1972, 327.
24. **Whitby, L. E. H. and Britton, C. J. C.,** *Disorders of the Blood*, 10th ed., Grune & Stratton, New York, 1969, 8.
25. **Wintrobe, M. M., et al.,** *Clinical Hematology*, 7th ed., Lea & Febiger, Philadelphia, 1974, 62.

MORPHOLOGY OF NORMAL BLOOD AND BONE MARROW CELLS: WRIGHT STAIN

L. W. Diggs and Ann Bell

The purpose of this chapter is to define the various types of normal blood cells in stained smears of peripheral blood and bone marrow. Definitions are based upon morphological characteristics of cells in thin dried smears stained by the Wright method as they appear when examined under oil immersion by light microscopy. The appearance of normal cells, as revealed by electron microscopy and by special stains and procedures, and the characteristics of abnormal cells associated with various diseases are given in other chapters in this handbook.

Opinions differ concerning the origin of free cells of the peripheral blood and fixed tissue cells of the blood-forming organs, the relation of the various cells to each other, and the capability and commitment of primitive cells to produce cells of different types. For the purpose of this presentation it is assumed that there are undifferentiated mesenchymal fixed tissue progenitor cells called "stem cells", which are multipotent. From these most primitive ancestral cells, the parent cells of each series of definitive cells are derived. The parent cell of each cell line is committed to produce cells with specific appearances and functions.

Within each family or clone the suffix "blast" is reserved for the most primitive cell of that series. The suffix "cyte" is used for the second and all later cells in the maturation sequence. The prefix "pro" is employed for cells during their second stage of maturation. In those developmental sequences in which there are more than three morphologically distinctive types, the prefix "meta" is used for the fourth cell type (Tables 1 and 2).

During their transition from immature to mature forms and later to senile and degenerative forms, blood cells of all types undergo progressive changes in their nuclear and cytoplasmic characteristics that are common to all cells (Figure 1).*

Table 1
TERMINOLOGY FOR BLOOD CELLS

Prefix	Suffix	Myelocytic series	Rubricytic series	Megakaryocytic series	Lymphocytic series
	— blast	Myeloblast	Rubriblast	Megakaryoblast	Lymphoblast
Pro —	— cyte	Promyelocyte	Prorubricyte	Promegakaryo-cyte	Prolymphocyte
	— cyte	Myelocyte	Rubricyte	Megakaryocyte	Lymphocyte
Meta —	— cyte	Metamyelocyte	Metarubricyte	Metamegakaryo-cyte	—

From Diggs, L. W., Sturm, D., and Bell, A., *Morphology of Human Blood Cells,* 4th ed., Abbott Laboratories, North Chicago, Ill., 1979. With permission.

Morphological Characteristics, General

Immature cells are large and become progressively smaller as they age (Figure 1). This is partially due to the fact that older and degenerate cells continually lose portions

* Color plates for Figures 1, 2, 3, 4, 5, 7, 8, 9, 10, and 14 are available in the 4th edition of *Morphology of Human Blood Cells* by Diggs, Sturm, and Bell and are printed and distributed by Abbott Laboratories, North Chicago, Illinois.

Table 2
BLOOD CELLS

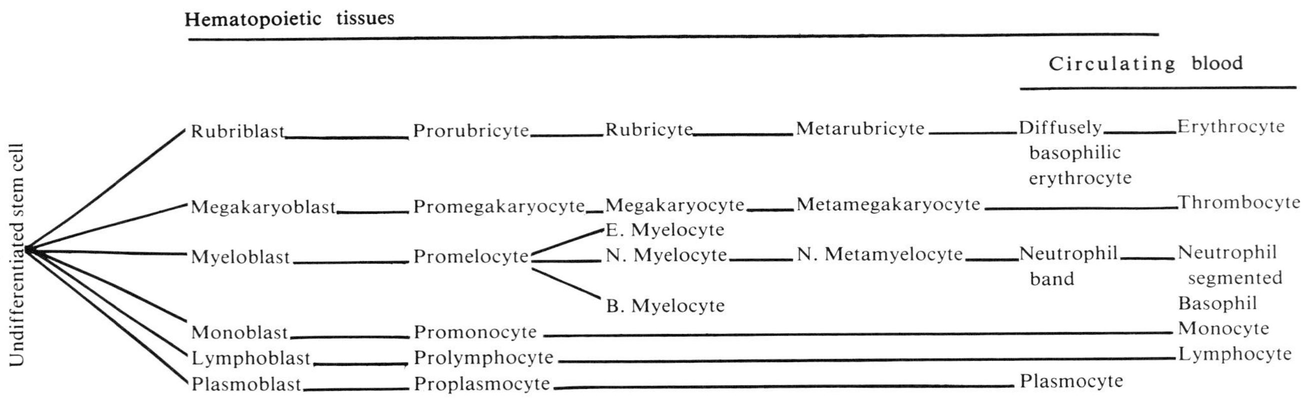

From Diggs, L. W., Sturm, D., and Bell, A., *Morphology of Human Blood Cells,* 4th ed., Abbott Laboratories, North Chicago, Ill., 1979. With permission.

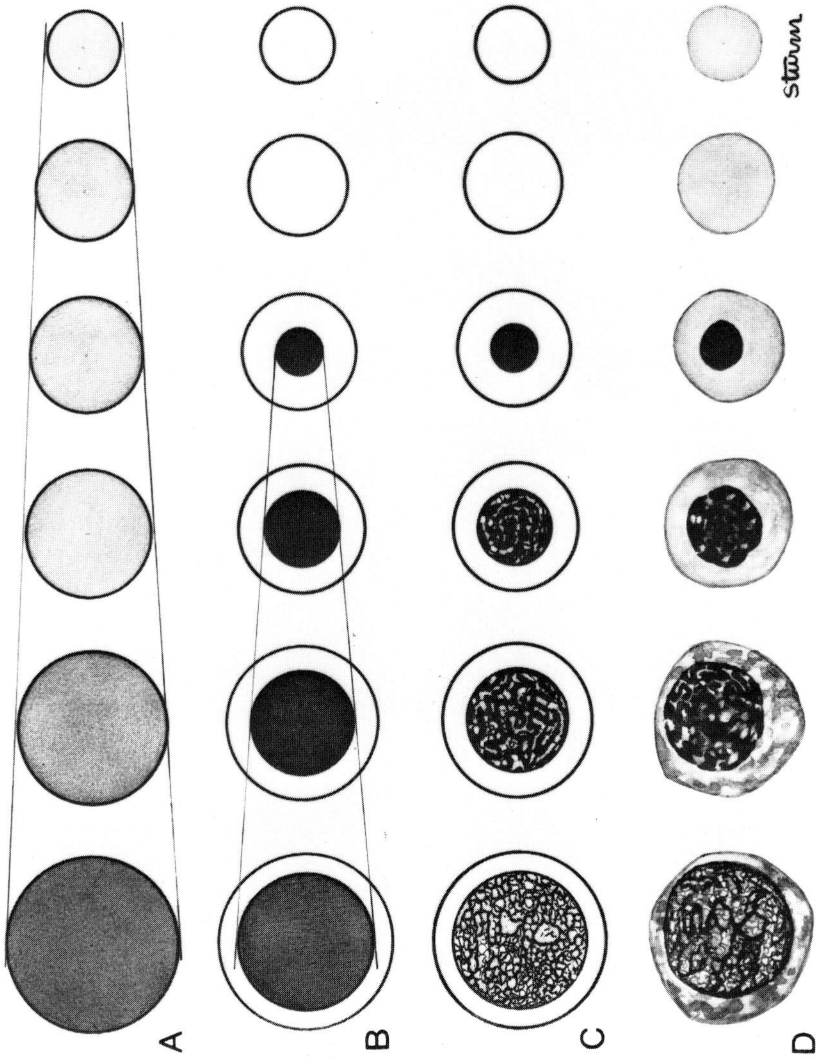

FIGURE 1. Maturation sequence, erythrocytic series. (A) Cell size, (B) nuclear size, (C) nuclear chromatin structure, (D) composite (left to right: rubriblast, prorubricyte, rubricyte, metarubricyte, diffusely basophilic erythrocyte, erythrocyte). (From Diggs, L. W., Sturm, D., and Bell, A., *Morphology of Human Blood Cells*, 4th ed., Abbott Laboratories, North Chicago, Ill., 1979. With permission.)

of their membranes and cytoplasm as they bang around in the turbulent blood stream and are pushed under arterial pressure through narrow vascular channels. Portions of cytoplasm may be pinched off by phagocytic cells. Megakaryocytes, during the later stages of their maturation, decrease in size due to the fragmentation of their marginal cytoplasm in the form of platelets. Cells also lose cytoplasm by the secretion of manufactured products and the excretion of waste. The nuclei of older nucleated red cells are extruded.

Immature cells as a class have larger nuclei in relation to cytoplasm than do older cells. The progressive decrease in the size of nuclei during the various stages of their maturation is due to the loss of nuclear material to the cytoplasm and to chemical dissolution of chromatin as the cells age. Nuclei are absent in mature erythrocytes and in thrombocytes.

The size of cells is influenced by factors other than their age. Variables include growth in preparation for mitosis, technical factors related to the making of smears, and the natural tendency for certain cells to flatten out or to round up as the smears dry.

During a given mitotic cycle the size of a given cell depends on the stage of growth that cell happens to be in at the time the smear is made. In preparation for mitosis, each cell doubles the amount of nuclear chromatin; the volume of the cell is approximately doubled. Cells that multiply rapidly with short growth periods between divisions and cells that have hereditary and acquired deficiencies and/or inadequate nutrients to support growth during the mitotic cycle tend to be small. Cells that have long growth periods between divisions and adequate nutrition tend to be large.

The diameters of the cells and of nuclei in smears of blood and marrow vary depending on the thickness of the film and the speed of drying. Cells that are thinly spread and rapidly dried tend to have greater diamters than those in thicker portions of the smear.

Monocytes tend to spread out on glass slides and have greater diameters than granulocytes and lymphocytes, which tend to round up when they are exposed to the air and foreign surfaces. It is obvious that size, as revealed by microscopic examination, is a most unreliable basis for cell classification and for the differential diagnosis of individual cells.

The color of the cytoplasm of primitive cells is predominantly blue due to the presence of RNA, which has an affinity for the blue or basic dyes. As the specific products within a cell are manufactured, the color of the cytoplasm becomes progressively lighter, less blue, and more red. Cells of the lymphocytic and plasmocytic series differ from other blood cell types in that the cytoplasm continues to stain blue in the later stages of maturation.

Immature cells with basophilic cytoplasm reveal a chromophobic zone adjacent to the nuclear margin and usually on the side of the nucleus where the cytoplasm is widest. In older cells with less intensely stained cytoplasm, the juxtanuclear light area is less evident.

Stem cells and blasts may reveal in their blue cytoplasm small and dust-like particles, but there are no distinct granules. In the cells that develop specific granules, the first granules to appear — the so-called "primary granules" — are dark and purple. The specific secondary granules that later develop are less dark, less blue, and more red. Granules of basophils maintain dark and predominantly blue hues in all stages of their maturation. The most distinct granules are found in mature eosinophils in which the granules are orange-red.

The nuclei of immature cells have round or oval shapes. Cells of the erythrocytic and plasmocytic series and fixed tissue cells continue to have round nuclei in all stages of their maturation. Older cells of the granulocytic, lymphocytic, and monocytic series reveal varying degrees of nuclear indentation in association with the development of amoeboid activity.

Immature nuclei, in contrast to the cytoplasm, are lightly stained and purplish-red. As the nuclei age, the color changes to dark blue.

The nuclear chromatin of early cells is fine and linear. As the nucleus matures, the chromatin strands degenerate and become thicker and more coarse. In older cells the chromatin becomes lumpy or clumped, and there is a tendency for the chromatin to aggregate near the nuclear margins. The last stages of degeneration are characterized by nuclei that are dense and darkly stained (pyknotic) (Figures 1 and 2).

Nucleoli are manifestations of youth, metabolic activity, and growth. Cells with demonstrable nucleoli are cells that are capable of mitosis and replication. Nucleoli are best seen in very thin smears. The usual number of nucleoli ranges from 1 to 4, and the diameter is in the 2 to 5 μ range. The structure is homogeneous and the color in the Wright stain is blue. Nucleoli are not enclosed by membranes, but they appear to have membranes because they tend to compress surrounding chromatin strands and therefore have dark boundaries.

Mitotic figures and cell division are signs of vigor that occur during the blast and intermediate stages of maturation. Replication ceases as the cells age and the nuclei undergo degenerative changes.

Phagocytosis of particulate matter is proof of the attainment of adult function. Other signs of maturity include blunt pseudopods, granules, and manufactured products in the cytoplasm and pyknotic nuclei. The mature cells in the peripheral blood are illustrated in Figure 3.

Under normal conditions the changes in size, shape, color, and structure of the nucleus and cytoplasm in a maturation sequence proceed in step with each other. In deficiency states and in various hereditary and acquired diseases, the maturation characteristics may be asynchronous. For instance, in iron deficiency anemia there is a defect in hemoglobin formation resulting in cells with mature nuclear structure that are smaller than normal, are irregular in shape, have less color and take a more blue stain than cells of the normal series. In B_{12} and folic acid deficiency, on the other hand, the cells may be well hemoglobinized and predominantly red whereas the nucleus may reveal immature characteristics. Whenever there is nonconformity in maturation characteristics, the most reliable criteria for identification is not the size, shape, or color of the cytoplasm or the color and shape of nuclei but the structure of the nuclear chromatin.

The separation of cell types in a maturation sequence and the definitions established for representative cells in each stage of development are arbitrary. There are differences of opinion about the number of stages that should be established and the morphological criteria that should be used for placing a cell in a given compartment. In all maturation sequences there are borderline or transitional cells that are difficult to classify. For hematologists who are examining smears of blood for their own information, classification is a personal matter. For reference laboratories, for the reporting of routine differential counts, and for proficiency testing, it is necessary to adopt ground rules for borderline cells.

The first rule is to consider the cell in relation to other cells and to evaluate the cell as a whole rather than to limit appraisal to a single characteristic such as color of the cytoplasm, size of the cell, or the shape of the nucleus. The other rule is to identify a doubtful transitional cell as the one that is more mature and that is numerically most likely to be correct. As an example, a cell that is intermediate between a metamyelocyte and a band leukocyte should be reported as a band; a cell that has morphological characteristics intermediate between a band and a segmented cell should be identified as segmented.

Blood Cells and Their Progenitors

Granulocytic Series

Granular leukocytes originate from morphologically undifferentiated committed precursor nongranular cells designated as "myeloblasts". The granules that appear in the later maturation stages, depending on their affiniy for the methylene blue and eosin dyes — which are constituents of the Wright's stain — are spoken of as basophilic, eosinophilic, or neutrophilic types (Figure 2).

Myeloblast

Myeloblasts (Figure 2) have irregular round or oval shapes. There may be blunt or pointed marginal tags. The diameter in stained smears is approximately two to three times that of nonnucleated red cells in the same microscopic field. The cytoplasm is dark blue, unevenly stained, and less darkly stained in the area adjacent to the nucleus than at the periphery. The intensity of the blue coloration is greater than in stem cells. There are no visible granules.

The nucleus is relatively large in relation to the cytoplasm and is round or oval with smooth margins. The nuclear chromatin is fine and linear and takes a relatively light purple-red stain. No portion of the nucleus is more darkly stained or more clumped than other portions. Several nucleoli usually are demonstrable as small, round, bluish homogeneous structures with a color resembling that of the cytoplasm.

Promyelocyte (Progranulocyte)

Promyelocytes as a class are slightly larger than the myeloblasts from which they derive. The nucleus is relatively large in relation to the cytoplasm. The shape of the cells is usually round or oval and the margins are smooth. They seldom are indented or compressed by adjacent cells. The color of the cytoplasm is blue with the intensity of color usually less than that in myeloblasts.

Progranulocytes contain varying numbers of granules that are intensely stained by the combined methylene and eosin stains, are dark purple, and may be visible over the nucleus. The nuclei are round. The chromatin strands are slightly more coarse than those of myeloblasts and are more unevenly stained. The color is purplish red. Nucleoli may or may not be visible.

Neutrophilic Myelocyte

Neutrophilic myelocytes as a class are round cells with smooth margins that are slightly smaller than promyelocytes and contain in their cytoplasm varying numbers of lightly stained pink and lavender neutrophilic granules intermingled with the more deeply stained basophilic (primary) granules. The secondary neutrophilic granules are identified in the less mature myelocytes and are first visible in a relatively light and reddish-pink area in the Golgi region adjacent to the nuclear margin ("dawn of neutrophilia"). In the older myelocytes the neutrophilic granules are evenly distributed, and the basophilic granules are less prominent.

As a rule the nuclei are round or oval, but the margins may be flattened on one side or slightly indented. Nuclear chromatin strands are of uneven thickness. Nucleoli are no longer visible.

Neutrophilic Metamyelocyte (Neutrophilic Juvenile)

The neutrophilic metamyelocyte differs from the neutrophilic myelocyte in that the nucleus has a kidney or bean shape. The extent of the indentation is less than half the width of the nucleus. Metamyelocytes as a class are slightly smaller, and the nuclear chromatin are more clumped and less linear than in typical myelocytes. The granules

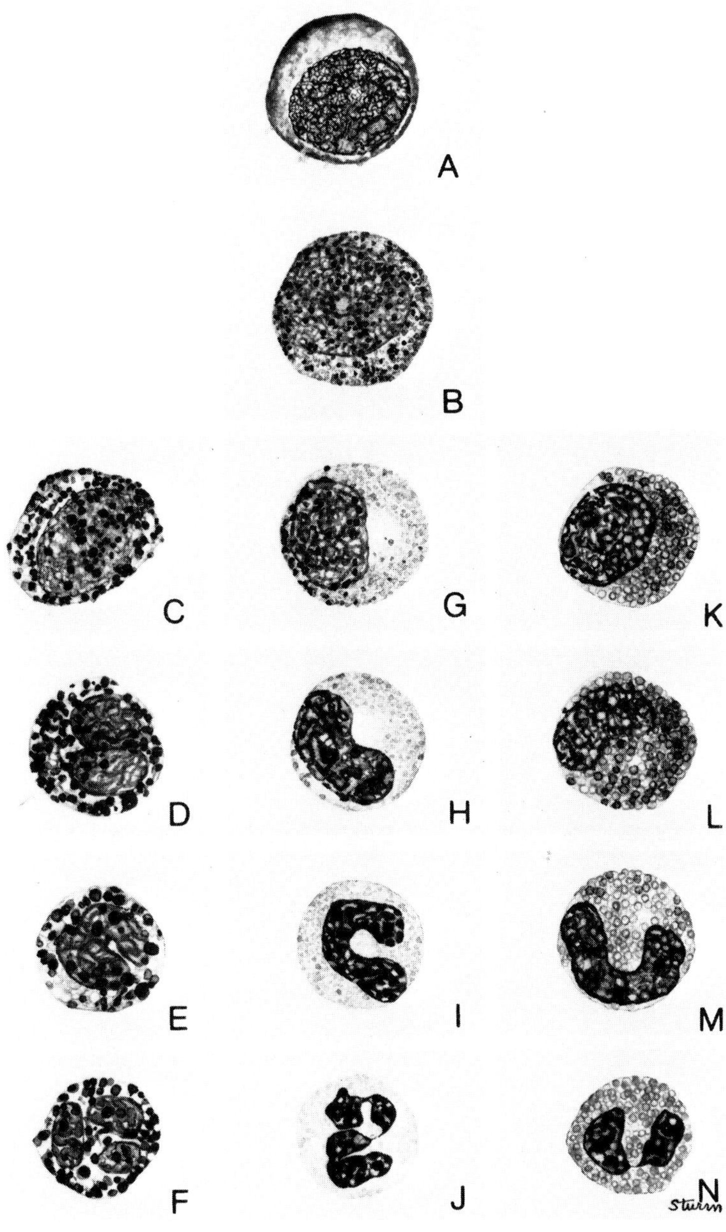

FIGURE 2. Myelocytic (granulocytic) maturation sequence. (A) Myeloblast, (B) promyelocyte (progranulocyte), (C) basophilic myelocyte, (D) basophilic metamyelocyte, (E) basophilic band, (F) basophilic segmented, (G) neutrophilic myelocyte, (H) neutrophilic metamyelocyte, (I) neutrophilic band, (J) neutrophilic segmented, (K) eosinophilic myelocyte, (L) eosinophilic metamyelocyte, (M) eosinophilic band, (N) eosinophilic segmented. (From Diggs, L. W., Sturm, D., and Bell, A., *Morphology of Human Blood Cells,* 4th ed., Abbott Laboratories, North Chicago, Ill., 1979. With permission.)

in the cytoplasm are numerous and evenly distributed. The majority of the granules have a light lavender pink color similar to that seen in the later band and segmented forms. There also remain a small number of primary darkly stained granules.

Barry College Library
Miami, Florida

Neutrophilic Band (Neutrophilic Stab, Nonsegmented, Nonfilamented)

Neutrophilic band cells are granular leukocytes intermediate between neutrophilic metamyelocytes and segmented neutrophils.

The typical band neutrophil is round and is approximately twice the width of erythrocytes in the same field. The cytoplasm takes a light pinkish stain and contains numerous distinct, fine, evenly distributed lavender granules and may contain a few purplish-red granules. The nucleus is deeply indented (more than half the width of the hypothetical round nucleus) and is in the shape of a curved link of sausage, a horseshoe, or bent stick with rounded ends. The margins of the connecting nuclear strand are parallel for an appreciable distance. The isthmus is wide enough to reveal chromatin material between the two sides at the most narrow portion. In smears of blood from healthy individuals the margins of nonfilamented neutrophils usually are smooth, without indentations, angulations, or protrusions. The nuclear chromatin of band neutrophils is irregularly clumped. Often there is a pyknotic mass at the opposite rounded ends of the nucleus. Based on these criteria the number of neutrophil bands in blood from a normal individual is less than 5%.

Neutrophilic Segmented Cell (Neutrophilic Filamented, Neutrophilic Polymorphonuclear, PMN)

Neutrophilic segmented leukocytes differ from band forms in that there are two or more lobes connected at some point by a narrow thread-like filament. The connecting link is so narrow that it appears as a single line. The margins of the various lobes of the nucleus are angular and indented. Nuclear appendages may be demonstrable. Marginal protrusions of the nuclei include projections with a broad base (sessile bodies), small finger-like processes, and small clubs with narrow stalks with chromophobic areas at the tip (tennis rackets). In smears of blood from females there are a few segmented cells that reveal darkly stained clubs (drumsticks), which are the specific sex chromatin structures.

Neutrophilic leukocytes intermediate between band and segmented cells are arbitrarily reported as segmented cells. The main difficulty in identifying transitional or borderline cells occurs when the lobules are touching or superimposed, making it impossible to see the connecting nuclear strands. If the margin of a given lobe extends as a continuous line connecting with the margin on the other side, the cell is reported as segmented, because the odds are great that the lobes are connected by a narrow strand rather than a wide band. Other factors that favor the identification of a given doubtful cell as a segmented cell include more than two lobulations, sharp nuclear marginal angulations, indentations, and appendages.

The majority of neutrophils in smears of blood from healthy individuals have two to four lobes. It is rare to find cells with five or more lobes.

Eosinophils (Eosinophilic Leukocytes)

It is generally accepted that eosinophilic cells with specific red-staining granules are derived from myeloblasts and promyelocytes, which are multipotent in the sense that they are committed to and produce cells with red or acidophilic granules (eosinophils) as well as cells with affinity for the blue dyes (basophils) and cells with pink or lavender granules (neutrophils) (Figure 2). In the most mature cells of all three of these cell lines, there are varying degrees of indentation, lobulation, and segmentation of the nuclei. Thus in the eosinophilic maturation sequence there are eosinophilic myelocytes, and eosinophilic metamyelocytes, band and segmented forms. So few eosinophils are usually observed that no useful clinical purpose is served by separating and reporting these cells according to their maturation shape, as is the custom with cells of the neutrophilic series.

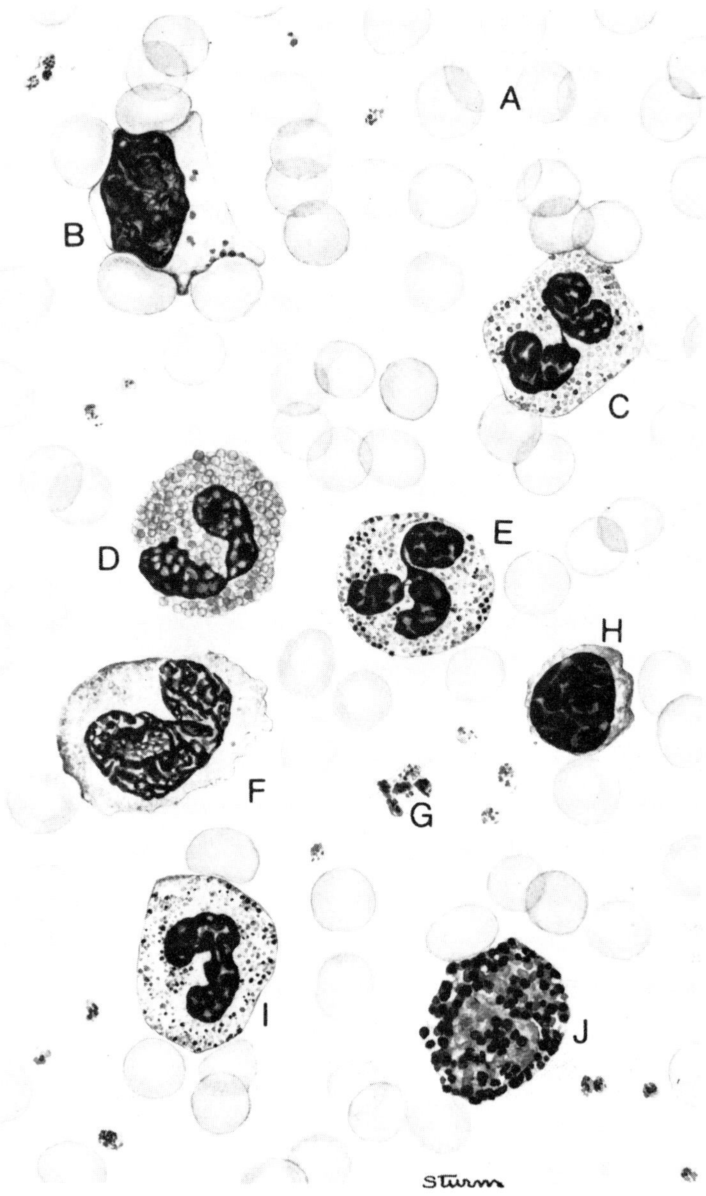

FIGURE 3. Cell types found in smears of peripheral blood from normal individuals. (A) Erythrocytes, (B) large lymphocyte with granules and deeply indented by adjacent erythrocytes, (C) neutrophilic segmented, (D) eosinophil, (E) neutrophilic segmented, (F) monocyte, (G) thrombocytes, (L) lymphocyte, (I) neutrophilic band, (J) basophil. The arrangement is arbitrary and the number of leukocytes in relation to erythrocytes and thrombocytes is greater than would occur in an actual microscopic field. (From Diggs, L. W., Sturm, D., and Bell, A., *Morphology of Human Blood Cells,* 4th ed., Abbott Laboratories, North Chicago, Ill., 1979. With permission.)

The size of mature eosinophils in the peripheral blood is approximately the same as neutrophils in the same microscopic fields. Eosinophils develop amoeboid activity slowly, and most of the nuclei are in the band or two-lobed stage. The granules are spherical, uniform in size, usually evenly distributed throughout the cytoplasm, and rarely overlie the nucleus (Figure 2). In good stains the granules are a bright orange-red with brownish tints. By focusing up and down, one can bring out highlights of individual granules or reveal them as perfect little circles. This spherical shape and the large size of the granules make it possible to differentiate eosinophils from neutrophils when the stain is unsatisfactory.

Basphils (Basophilic Leukocytes)

Basophils (Figure 2) like eosinophils and neutrophils may have round, indented, bands and segmented nuclei, but there are so few of these cells (usually less than 1%) in smears of blood from healthy individuals that all maturation stages are reported as a group rather than separated into maturation stages.

The size of basophilic leukocytes is approximately the same as the size of neutrophils. The background color of the cytoplasm is light pink. The granules of basophils are darkly stained, and the predominant or is blue. Individual granules, particularly those in the deeper layers of the cytoplasm surrounded by the pink cytoplasm, reveal various shades and tones of red and blue. Most of the granules are round. They vary in size and in number, are unevenly distributed, and often overlie and tend to obscure the lighter staining and relatively inconspicuous nuclei. Some of the granules appear to be surrounded by a chromophobic halo. The granules are water soluble and some of the granules may be washed out during the decoloration phase of the stain, leaving small globular chromophobic areas.

Basophilic ocytes have morphological characteristics similar to progranulocytes in that both have round and relatively immature nuclei and dark granules. Basophilic myelocytes are smaller than progranulocytes and have a more mature nuclear chromatin pattern and an absence of demonstrable nucleoli. In case of doubt it is recommended that the questionable cell be reported as a promyelocyte rather than as a basophilic myelocyte. Neutrophilic leukocytes may be darkly stained or reveal prominent bluish granules (so-called ''toxic granules''), which simulate the granules of basophils. When in doubt, interpret as a neutrophil, for this is most likely to be correct.

Lymphocytic Series

Lymphoblast

The size, shape, color, and structure of the nucleus and the cytoplasm of lymphoblasts are similar to those described under ''myeloblasts''. Nucleoli are usually demonstrable. Differentiation of lymphoblasts from other types of blasts is based on the source of the material and association with other cells rather than on distinctive morphological characteristics.

Prolymphocyte

Prolymphocytes differ from lymphoblasts in that the chromatin strands are thicker and more unevenly stained. Nucleoli may or may not be demonstrable.

Lymphocyte

The size of mature lymphocytes is variable (Figures 3, 4, and 5). In the thicker portions of the smear which dry slowly, lymphocytes tend to round up and to become more spherical. At the ends of the smears where the cells are flattened like pancakes, the diameters are wider, the nuclei are larger, and the nuclear chromatin is better visualized. The diameter of the nuclei of small lymphocytes is approximately the width of nonnucleated red cells. It is not clinically important to differentiate and to report lymphocytes according to their size on routine differential counts.

Most lymphocytes are round with smooth margins, but a few may reveal pointed

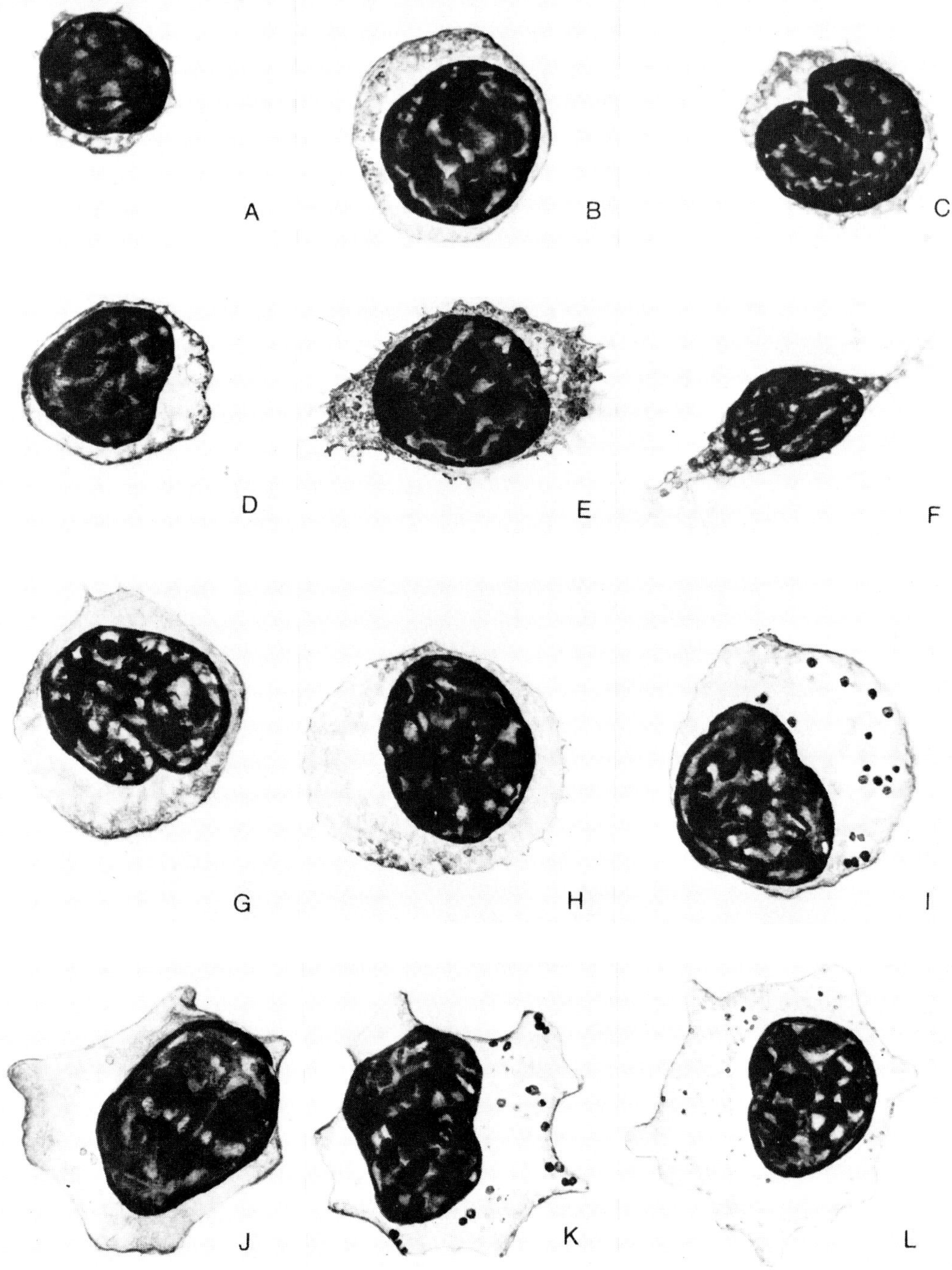

FIGURE 4. Mature lymphocyte variants, peripheral blood. (A) Small lymphocyte with bubbly cytoplasm and marginal pointed projections, (B) lymphocyte of intermediate size with perinuclear clear zone, (C) lymphocyte with indented nucleus, (D) lymphocyte, intermediate size with chromophobic areas in cytoplasm, (E) lymphocyte with hair-like cytoplasmic projections, typical nucleus, (F) spindle-shaped lymphocyte with indented nucleus, (G) large lymphocyte with indented nucleus and irregular shape, (H) large lymphocyte, (I) large lymphocyte with granules, (J) large lymphocyte, irregular shape, (K) large lymphocyte with granules and with cytoplasmic indentations caused by advacent erythrocytes, (L) large lymphocyte with a few granules. (From Diggs, L. W., Sturm, D., and Bell, A., *Morphology of Human Blood Cells,* 4th ed., Abbott Laboratories, North Chicago, Ill., 1979. With permission.)

and hair-like cytoplasmic protrusions. Other lymphocytes are spindle shaped, with tapering ends and with a few filaments extending outward from each end. In these elongated cells the nuclei are elliptical rather than round. Cells with fusiform shapes tend to have their long axes parallel like schools of swimming fish. Large lymphocytes are often surrounded and their cytoplasm indented by neighboring red cells producing holly-leaf and scalloped shapes.

The color of lymphocytes in all stages of their maturation is blue. The intensity of the blue is variable. The cytoplasm of the lymphocytes has a bubbly appearance due to chromophobic globules, but the majority of the lymphocytes have a homogeneous sky-blue appearance. Approximately a third of the larger lymphocytes in smears of blood from normal individuals have a few purplish-red granules. These granules are often surrounded by a small chromophobic halo.

The nuclei of lymphocytes are usually off center. Most of the nuclei are round with smooth margins, but they may be slightly indented. In malignancies of the lymphocytic system, nuclear clefts and divided nuclei may be demonstrable, but these forms are not seen in normal cells. Nuclei of mature lymphocytes are darkly stained and purplish-blue. The chromatin is aggregated at the margin of the nuclei. A perinuclear pale zone of cytoplasm is often demonstrable around the margin of the nucleus. This light area of cytoplasm surrounding the nuclear margin is due to deflection of light waves, which strike the dark nucleus and highlight the nongranular cytoplasm, producing a silver lining effect.

Some lymphocytes that have pyknotic nuclei and the morphological appearance of old and degenerate cells, when stimulated by mitogens or activated in vivo by antigens, possess the ability to de-differentiate and to revert back to stem cells. Rejuvenated (''anaplastic'',''transformed'',''transitional'') lymphocytes with blast-like (''blastoid'') morphological features are capable of mitosing and producing cells of various types, including cells of the plasmocytic series. Even though small cells with round and dark nuclei and narrow rims of nongranular bluish cytoplasm may have the theoretical potentiality of becoming multipotent progenitor cells, they should not be called ''stem cells'' until they have the morphological characteristics of undifferentiated cells. Cells are identified by what they look like now and not by what they might look like at some later date.

Plasmocytic Series

Plasmoblast

Plasmoblasts are morphologically similar to blasts of other cell lines. They are identified by association with a large number of identifiable plasmocytes, as in plasmocytic leukemia or in bone marrow smears of patients with classical multiple myeloma. Nucleoli usually are demonstrable.

Proplasmocyte

Proplasmocytes differ from plasmoblasts in that they are slightly more mature and have thicker and more aggregated nuclear chromatin and less distinct nucleoli.

Plasmocyte (Plasma Cell)

Plasmocytes in the circulating blood are round or oval cells with smooth margins (Figure 5). Plasmocytes in smears of bone marrow, like other fixed tissue cells that are mechanically traumatized at the time of aspiration, have irregular margins. Plasmocytes vary in size from cells comparable to mature neutrophils to cells that are two to three times the diameter of older granulocytes.

The cytoplasm is large in relation to the nucleus and is deeply basophilic. The dark

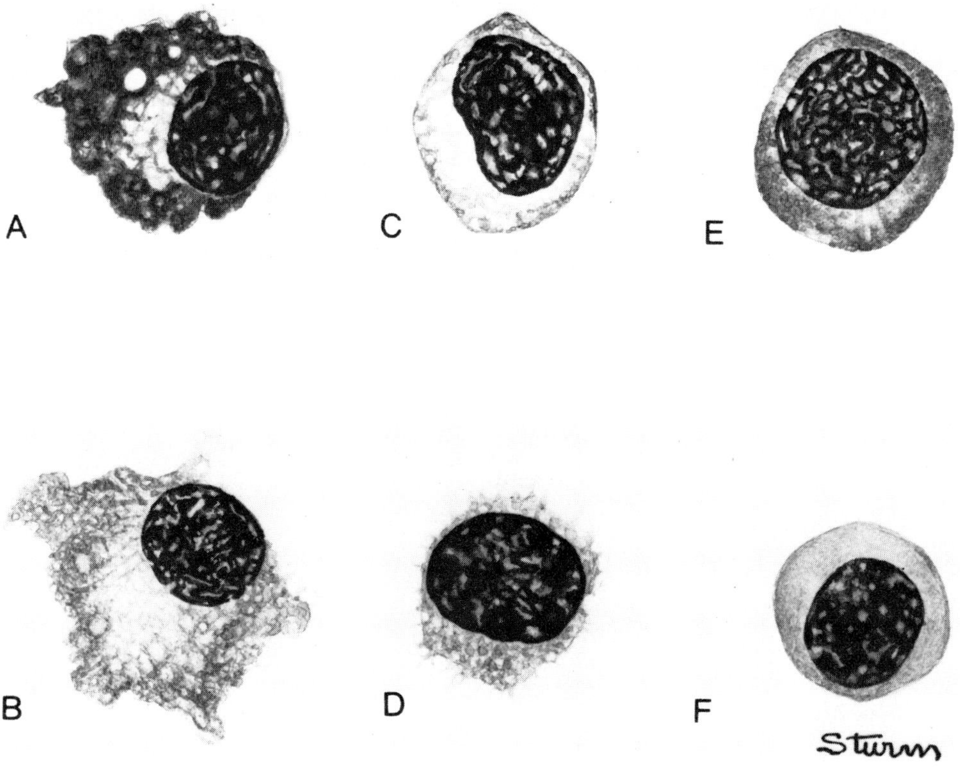

FIGURE 5. Plasmocytes left, lymphocytes middle, and nucleated red cells right. (A) Plasmocyte with eccentric nucleus, intensely staining cytoplasm, juxtanuclear clear zone, vacuoles, and irregular shape, (B) plasmocyte with irregular shape, eccentric nucleus, foamy and fibrillar cytoplasm, and light zone next to nucleus, (C) lymphocyte with slightly indented nucleus and unevenly stained cytoplasm, (D) lymphocyte with foamy cytoplasm and frayed (hair-like) cytoplasmic margins, (E) prorubricyte, (F) rubricyte. (From Diggs, L. W., Sturm, D., and Bell, A., *Morphology of Human Blood Cells.*, 2nd ed., Abbott Laboratories, North Chicago, Ill., 1970. With permission.)

blue color has a vivid and brilliant character. Terms that have been applied include ''pigeon blue'', ''cornflower blue'', or ''larkspur blue''. This velvety appearance with pinpoint highlights is thought to be due to numerous unstained mitochrondria surrounded by blue staining aggregates of RNA and by red staining immunoglobulin.

Plasmocytes are actively engaged in the synthesis of proteins (antibodies). Molecules of these proteins are usually dispersed throughout the cytoplasm, giving a fairly homogeneous appearance. In occasional plasmocytes the proteinaceous material is in the form of large aggregates, or pools, which stain bright red. In other cells the entire cytoplasm is fiery red. These cells are known as ''flame cells''. The red material may appear as globular bodies that usually are stained red (Russell bodies, eosinophilic bodies), but they may stain pastel shades of blue, yellow, and occasionally green. In some cells the globules are numerous and completely fill the cytoplasm (Mott, berry, morula, grape cells). The globular bodies in plasmocytes have the appearance of perfect circles as if drawn by a compass; when tightly packed together, they assume honeycomb-like hexagonal shapes (Figure 23). In some cells the secretory material is in the form of granules or elongated and pointed purple red crystals. In many plasmocytes there are occasional colorless spherical areas (vacuoles). Plasmocytes reveal a relatively light staining area adjacent to the nucleus. This juxtanuclear clear zone corresponds with the centrosome area. The cytoplasm in some cells has a fibrillar reticular structure.

The nucleus of plasmocytes is round and eccentrically located. The nuclear chromatin is lumpy. The dark chromatin masses tend to be aggregated near the nuclear margins.

Monocytic Series

Monocyte (Large Mononuclear, Mononuclear, Monocytic Leukocyte)

Mature cells of the monocytic series are larger than polymorphonuclear neutrophils (Figures 3 and 6). The cytoplasm of monocytes is usually three to four times wider than that of red cells in the same field. As a rule there is a large amount of cytoplasm in relation to the nucleus, and the cytoplasm is visible surrounding the nucleus.

The majority of monocytes have round or oval shapes with smooth margins. Others reveal cytoplasmic protrusions that are manifestations of their motility. These amoeboid and aggressive cells, instead of rounding up in films of blood as do lymphocytes and granulocytes, tend to spread out on the surface of the slides. Extended pseudopods are fixed in their outstretched position. Monocytic cells are less likely to be indented by adjacent cells than are large lymphocytes.

The color of the cytoplasm in mature monocytes in Wright-stained smears is dull gray-blue in contrast to that of neutrophils, which is brighter, lighter, and more pink. The juxtanuclear chromophobic zone is less distinct in monocytes than in lymphocytes and myelocytes.

Monocytes, like cells of the so-called granulocytic series, also contain granules. The granules vary in number, size, and color. Many monocytes have granules that are small, indistinct, and dust-like. The cytoplasm containing numerous small objects has a ground-glass appearance, in contrast to the cytoplasm of large lymphocytes, which is clear sky-blue. In other cells, distinct and darkly stained purplish granules in varying numbers are intermingled with granules that are reddish purple. The cytoplasmic marginal extensions (ectoplasm) do not contain granules. Pseudopods stain light blue and are transparent in contrast to the more opaque and granular inner cytoplasm (endoplasm). Small chromophobic globules (vacuoles) are often demonstrable in varying numbers in the cytoplasm.

Monocytes are capable of phagocytosis and may contain in their cytoplasm ingested particulate matter including whole blood cells, nuclear fragments, granules and crystals from other cells, pigmented masses, and various etiologic agents such as bacteria, fungi, and protozoa.

The nuclei of large mononuclear leukocytes may be round or oval, but as a rule are kidney or bean shaped. In occasional cells there are deep marginal indentations and band and segmented forms. Distinguishing features of monocytic cells that are not seen in cells of the myelocytic and lymphocytic series are nodular elevations and depressions which, when viewed from above, give a three-dimensional appearance of rounded hills and valleys, folds, or brain-like convolutions. The nucleus is predominantly red in contrast to the bluish-gray color of the cytoplasm. The nuclear strands tend to be evenly stained and less clumped than those of mature lymphocytes. There is also less tendency for the chromatin to be aggregated at the nuclear margins than in lymphocytes. The chromatin in some cells is coarse, and the linear strands are distinct.

Monocytes increase in size as they grow in the circulating blood and in the bone marrow and may be transformed into overgrown cells called "macrophages" (Figure 9). These cells, except for size, have the same morphological characteristics as described above for mature monocytes. Macrophages mainly reside in tissue spaces and are demonstrable in transudates and exudates, in serosal cavities, and in fluids from the gastrointestinal, genital, and respiratory tracts. They are too large to pass readily

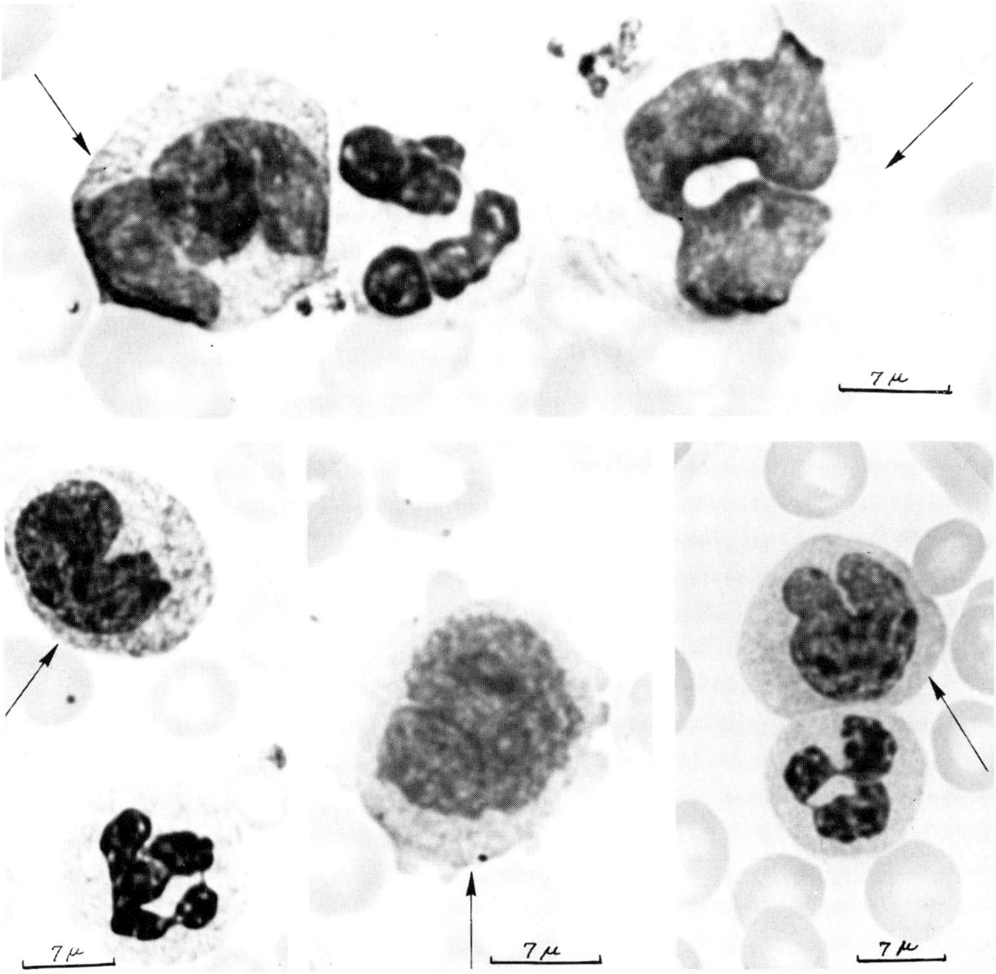

FIGURE 6. Monocytes (arrow). Other cells are neutrophilic segmented cells.

through the narrow lumens of terminal arterioles, capillaries, and arteriovenous shunts and are seldom seen in the smears of peripheral blood except in conditions in which there is marked proliferation of cells of the phagocytic system.

Monocytes and macrophages are closely related to fixed tissue histiocytes (phagocytic histiocytes). The main differences between monocytes, macrophages, and histiocytes are their motility and dwelling place. These three variants of closely related cells with similar scavenger functions are thought to be capable of reversible transformation from one to the other with or without first undergoing mitotic division.

Monoblast and Promonocyte

Primitive cells of the monocytic series are not identifiable as such in bone marrow and in peripheral blood smears except in malignancies of the cells of the phagocytic system as in monocytic leukemia, histiocytic leukemia, and malignant reticuloendotheliosis. The identification of early mononuclear cells is based mainly on the association of these cells with more mature monocytes having folded nuclei, blunt pseudopods, and vacuoles and phagocytic particles in their cytoplasm. Cells in monocytic

Table 3
SYNONYMS: NUCLEATED AND NONNUCLEATED RED CELLS

Rubriblast	Pronormoblast	Proerythroblast	
Prorubricyte	Basophilic normoblast	Basophilic Early	Erythroblast
Rubricyte	Polychromatophilic normoblast	Polychromatophilic Intermediate	Erythroblast
Metarubricyte	Orthochromatic normoblast	Acidophilic Oxyphilic Orthochromatic Late	Erythroblast
Diffusely basophilic erythrocyte	Reticulocyte	Proerythrocyte	
Erythrocyte	Erythrocyte	Erythrocyte	

malignancies are called monoblasts when the nuclear chromatin is fine and distinct, nucleoli are demonstrable, and there are no visible granules in the cytoplasm.

Erythrocytic Series

Rubriblast (Pronormoblast, Proerythroblast)

The size, shape, color, and structure of the cytoplasm and nuclei of the earliest rubriblasts are similar to myeloblasts (see above). In the slightly more mature variants of the rubriblasts — in which production of hemoglobin has begun — the blue color of the numerous ribosomes intermingles with the red color of the hemoglobin molecules and produces an intense purplish-blue color (Figure 1; Table 3).

Prorubricyte (Basophilic Normoblast, Early or Basophilic Erythroblast)

Prorubricytes are slightly smaller than rubriblasts, and their nuclear chromatin is more coarsely linear and clumped. The cytoplasm takes a predominantly basophilic stain. The nuclei are round, and the nuclear margins are smooth. There are no visible nucleoli and no identifiable structures in the cytoplasm of prorubricytes when examined by light microscopy (Figures 1 and 5).

Rubricyte (Polychromatophilic Normoblast, Polychromatophilic, or Intermediate Erythroblast)

Rubricytes are intermediate in size between prorubricytes and metarubricytes (Figures 1 and 5). The cells are round with smooth margins, and the color is homogeneous and reddish blue. The nuclei are round, centrally located, and stain dark blue. The chromatin material is coarsely linear and/or clumped.

Metarubricyte (Orthochromatic Normoblast; Eosinophilic, Oxyphilic, Orthochromatic, Late, Erythroblasts)

The cytoplasmic colors of metarubricytes are predominately red with various tints of blue (Figure 1). In some cells, the blue component is so slight that the color is similar to the color of nonnucleated mature erythrocytes, thus forming the basis for the adjectives "normochromic" and "orthochromic". The nucleus is pyknotic and reveals no residual linear structure. The nucleus often appears as a solid, dark blue, structureless, spherical mass.

Diffusely Basophilic Erythrocyte (Polychromatophilic Erythrocyte, Proerythrocyte)

Cells identified as "diffusely basophilic erythrocytes" are nonnucleated red cells intermediate between metarubricytes and mature erythrocytes (Figure 1). The cytoplasm contains residual RNA, which has an avidity for the basic or blue dye. The mixture of the blue stain with the red (acidophilic, eosin) coloration produces polychromatophilia. Diffusely basophilic cells, like their nucleated precursors, are spherical. They are slightly larger in diameter and volume than more mature discoid red cells.

Erythrocyte (Nonnucleated Red Cell, Discocyte)

The mature erythrocyte is a nonnucleated hemoglobin containing red cell that has a biconcave disc shape with round margins (Figures 1 and 3). The color in a good stain is orange-red. The thin central portion takes a lighter stain than the marginal area. An occasional red cell may have corrugated margins (crenated) or multiple pointed protrusions (burr cells). The size of erythrocytes varies from 6 to 8 μ with an average of approximately 7 μ.

Megakaryocytic Series and Thrombocytes

General

Cells of the megakaryocytic series differ from other blood cells in that the nucleus undergoes multiple mitotic divisions without a corresponding division of the cytoplasm. As a result, the older megakaryocytes are multinucleated giant cells. Some of them practically fill the oil immersion field. All of the nuclei undergo mitosis simultaneously producing 2, 4, 8, and, in rare instances, 16 and 32 nuclei in the same cell. The polyploid nuclei remain attached to each other and are superimposed, giving a multilobular appearance. As the cells age, the nuclear chromatin tends to remain linear rather than to aggregate in clumps. Nucleoli are demonstrable in the megakaryoblast stage and may or may not be visible in later stages.

The first granules to appear in the cytoplasm in the second or "pro" stage of maturation are adjacent to the nuclear margins. In later developmental stages, the granules are diffuse. Aggregates of granules bounded by membranes may appear at the periphery of the cells as differentiated platelets at any stage of maturation, but usually appear in the 4 to 8 nuclear stage. When nuclear and cytoplasmic maturation are asynchronous, it is recommended that the cell be identified by its cytoplasmic characteristics rather than by the structure of the nucleus. This is a departure from the usual rule, which holds that the chromatin structure of the nucleus is the most reliable criterion for identifying the maturation stage of a given cell.

Megakaryoblast

Megakaryoblasts are large, irregularly shaped cells with blunt pseudopods (Figure 7; Table 4). The cytoplasm is basophilic and unevenly stained. The cytoplasmic protrusions extending outward from the margin tend to stain more deeply blue than the cytoplasm adjacent to the nucleus and to contain chromophobic globules. There are no demonstrable granules. The nucleus is round or oval and takes a reddish stain. The chromatin has a granular appearance. Nucleoli are usually demonstrable.

Promegakaryocyte

Promegakaryocytes differ from megakaryoblasts in that bluish granules are demonstrable in the cytoplasm. Cytoplasmic marginal projections with rounded contours and containing colorless spherules are usually demonstrable. The cytoplasm and the ectoplasmic extensions are blue, with the extensions staining a lighter shade of blue. As a rule there are two nuclei during the promegakaryocyte stage of maturation (Figure 7).

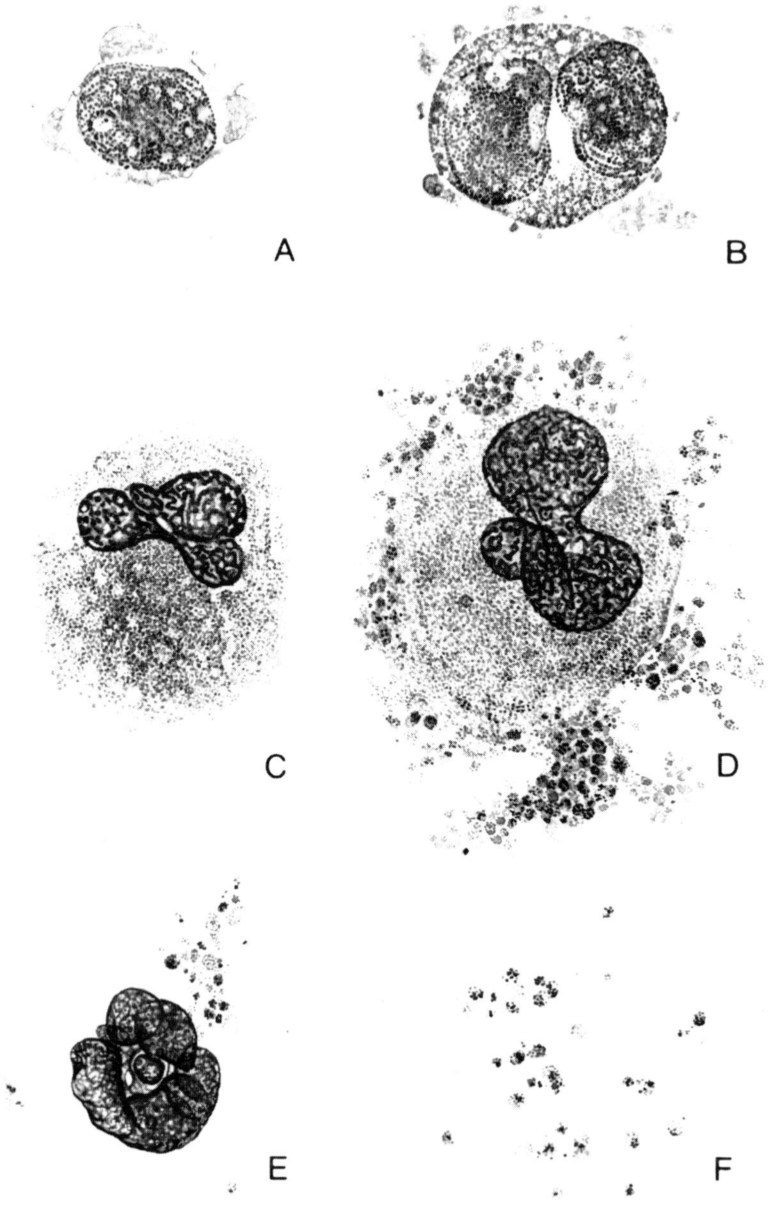

FIGURE 7. Megakaryocytic series. (A) Megakaryoblast, (B) promegakaryocyte, (C) megakaryocyte without thrombocytes, (D) metamegakaryocyte with thrombocytes, (E) metamegakaryocyte nucleus with attached thrombocytes, (F) thrombocytes. (From Diggs, L. W., Sturm, D., and Bell, A., *Morphology of Human Blood Cells,* 4th ed., Abbott Laboratories, North Chicago, Ill., 1979. With permission.)

Megakaryocyte (Megakaryocyte Without Thrombocyte)

Megakaryocytic cells in the third stage of maturation are large cells with relatively large amounts of cytoplasm and round shapes with fairly even margins (Figure 7). There are multiple connected nuclei. The chromatin pattern of these mature cells is coarsely linear with distinct spaces between chromatin strands. The cytoplasm contains numerous small, rather uniformly distributed granules that stain reddish-blue. Light staining areas may be demonstrable.

Table 4
MORPHOLOGICAL FEATURES OF CELLS OF THE MEGAKARYOCTIC SERIES

State of maturation	Cytoplasmic granules	Thrombocytes	Cytoplasmic tags	Nuclear characteristics
Megakaryoblast	Absent	Absent	Present	Single; fine chromatin structure; nucleoli
Promegakaryocyte	Few	Absent	Present	Double
Megakaryocyte	Numerous	Absent	Usually absent	Two or more nuclei
Metamegakaryocyte	Aggregated	Present	Absent	Four or more nuclei

From Diggs, L. W., Sturm, D., and Bell, A., *Morphology of Human Blood Cells,* 4th ed., Abbott Laboratories, North Chicago, Ill., 1979. With permission.

Metamegakaryocyte (Megakaryocyte With Thrombocytes)

Metamegakaryocytes in the fourth stage of maturation are characterized by irregular shapes and by the aggregation of granular cytoplasmic material into small masses, which are separated from each other by relatively clear bluish spaces or partitions (demarcation vesicles). Separated units of granular cytoplasm tend to aggregate near the periphery of the cytoplasm (Figure 7).

Megakaryocytes in the more advanced stages of maturation are slowly amoeboid. Portions of their cytoplasm protrude through the basement membrane and between the endothelial cells of the sinusoids of the bone marrow. From these cytoplasmic protrusions the differentiated, membrane-bound, and granular platelets separate and are swept into the flowing blood stream. Other megakaryocytes, escaping into the vascular channels of the marrow as intact cells, are transported by veins to the lungs, where they lodge in the terminal pulmonary arterioles. From these sites they continue to form and to liberate portions of their cytoplasm in the form of platelets. The naked nuclei that remain undergo degenerative changes or are phagocytized.

Thrombocyte (Platelet)

Thrombocytes are fragments of cytoplasm of megakaryocytes (Figures 3 and 7). The diameter of individual platelets in the blood of normal individuals varies from 1 to 4 micra.

In stained smears, thrombocytes are often aggregated in small clumps. Round, oval, and elliptical shapes with smooth margins are also observed. The cytoplasm stains light blue and contains varying numbers of small purplish granules which tend to aggregate in the center (granulomere) as contrasted with the nongranular marginal zone (hyalomere). Often there are multiple tentacle-like and hyaline marginal extensions.

Platelets often adhere to each other (Figure 3). Clumps of platelets are most numerous at the thin distal portions of blood smears. The number of platelets per oil immersion field in thin portions of the smear varies from 5 to 25. The number of platelets in the average oil immersion field multiplied by 20,000 gives the approximate number per cubic millimeter. No report of a blood smear is complete unless the platelet number is stated. Morphological abnormalities should be reported and described.

Fixed Tissue Cells of the Bone Marrow

Fixed tissue cells of all types originate from mesenchymal stem cells (hemohistioblasts). Like the cells of the peripheral blood, they undergo progressive maturation changes as they mature, but the changes in size and in nuclear shapes are less striking than in free blood cells. Between the most undifferentiated committed cells of a given tissue cell sequence and the definitive and functioning mature cells, there are intermediate forms, but tissue cells are so few and the morphological differences so subtle that no attempt is made to define "blast", "pro", and "meta" variants.

During the process of aspiration of bone marrow, the fixed tissue cells are forcefully ripped away from their moorings in the ground substance in which they are embedded and from the network of connective tissue fibers that intertwine around them. The result of mechanical trauma is that the margins of tissue cells are often tattered and torn and have a frayed appearance.

Fixed tissue cells are best seen in tissue sections and are scarce in spreads and imprints of marrow. Their frequency in marrow smears is not necessarily a true indication of their incidence.

Recognition of tissue cells in smears and imprints of bone marrow is important, because they may be falsely identified as malignant cells.

No attempt has been made to define or to illustrate cells under the heading of "reticulum cells" or "reticuloendothelial cells", for there is a lack of agreement about the meaning of these terms and their morphological characteristics.

The word "reticulum" and "reticular" are derived from the Latin word "rete" meaning "web" or "net". Anatomical pathologists and oncologists usually identify reticular cells as cells that produce reticular fibers having an affinity for silver ("argyrophilic fibers").

Many hematologists employ the phrase "reticulum cell" as a synonym for "stem cell", while others equate the "reticulum cells" with phagocytic histiocytes, the reticular or connective tissue component of the so-called "reticuloendothelial system".

Concepts about cells identified and reported as "reticuloendothelial cells" vary. "Reticuloendothelial cells" are usually thought of as cells that have an avidity for particulate matter. The cells of this ubiquitous system include all phagocytic cells, with the exception of granulocytic leukocytes. Some think of "reticuloendothelial cells" in an embryonic sense as primitive mesenchymal cells of the yolk sac. This concept equates "reticuloendothelial cells" with "stem cells". A third use of the term is that of a label for a convenient and face-saving trash basket to dump any atypical, irregularly shaped, and unidentified large cell.

Stem Cells (Hemohistioblasts)

Cells that are designated as hematopoietic "stem cells" are usually thought of in terms of their potentiality to produce cells of the blood and blood-forming organs. Morphologically they are differentiated from other cells by the characteristics that they lack rather than by the distinctive features that they reveal.

There is general agreement that stem cells are of mesenchymal origin, that they are fixed tissue cells, and that they are multipotent. It is also generally accepted that these cells grow and divide, producing daughter cells. Some of these retain the undifferentiated characteristics of their parent cells and are self-perpetuating. Others proceed to differentiate into specific types of free blood cells and fixed tissue cells.

Stem cells vary in size from the smallest lymphocytes to cells with diameters in the 20 to 40 μ range depending on their growth between divisions. The ratio of nuclear width to cytoplasmic width varies. Stem cells that usually are described and illustrated in hematological atlases are the larger forms. Like other fixed tissue cells including the "blast" cells of each cell line, the cytoplasmic shapes of stem cells of all sizes are irregular with tapering and blunt marginal protrusions (Figure 8).

The cytoplasm is blue. The color is less intense in the larger cells than in cells iden-

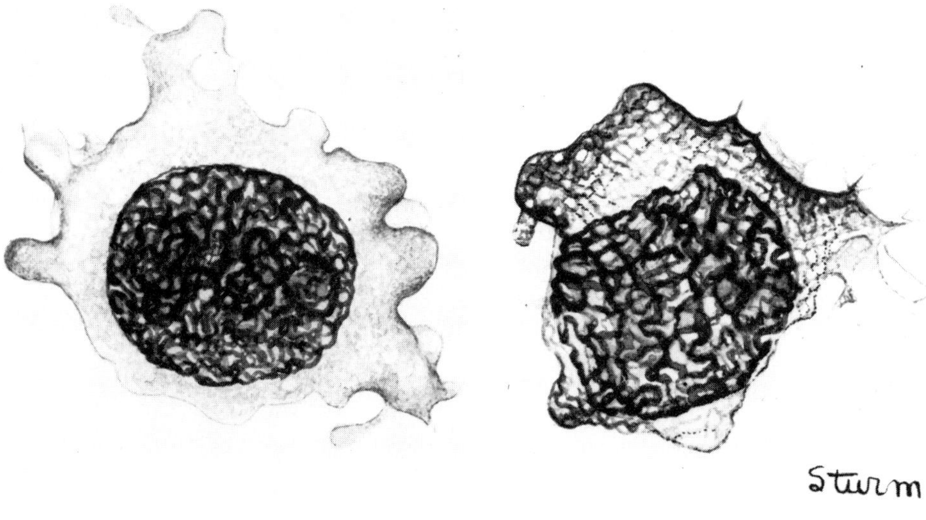

FIGURE 8. Stem cells. (From Diggs, L. W., Sturm, D., and Bell, A., *Morphology of Human Blood Cells*, 4th ed., Abbott Laboratories, North Chicago, Ill., 1979. With permission.)

tified as blast forms of definitive cell lines. In some stem cells the blue or basophilic stain is evenly distributed, giving a clear sky-blue appearance that in the older literature led to the designation of these cells as "lymphoid reticulum cells". In other stem cells, there is a network of delicate and slightly darker blue lines. Since the cytoplasm takes a light stain, the juxtanuclear chromophobic area (Golgi zone) is not as distinct in stem cells as in the slightly more mature blast cells that have larger amounts of cytoplasmic RNA and therefore stain a darker blue.

The cytoplasm of stem cells may contain a few small, dust-like purplish densities, but there are no distinct granules, chromophobic spherules (vacuoles), stained secretory globules, or phagocytized particles.

The nuclei of the larger forms of stem cells are usually wider than the nuclei in identifiable blood cells in the same field. The nucleus is round or oval and surrounded on all sides by cytoplasm. The chromatin is finely linear, and the strands are intertwined in a network pattern. Nucleoli, which vary in number from one to four, appear as spherical structureless areas that stain the same color as the cytoplasm (light blue).

Morphologically undifferentiated hematopoietic stem cells may be considered as "pro-blast" cells. The main difference between the two is the intensity of the blue color of the cytoplasm. This difference is subtle. The nuances of color produced by the stains and staining techniques used create so many variables that distinctions based on intensity of stain are of limited value. A person examining peripheral blood, a bone marrow smear, or tissue imprint who encounters an undifferentiated cell should tally that cell as a "stem cell" rather than a "myeloblast" or "blast" of any other cell series. In the final report, these cells are categorized as "stem cells" if their number is small. If the cells with primitive characteristics are numerous and there are transitional cells between the immature and the more mature forms, the questionable cells are reported as "blasts" of the line that predominates.

Histiocytes (Phagocytic Histiocytes, Tissue Macrophages)

The etymologic meaning of the word "histiocyte" is "tissue cell", but by long usage the cells called "histiocytes" are tissue cells that have the capability of phagocytosis.

Fixed tissue phagocytes are closely related to the phagocytic monocytes of the cir-

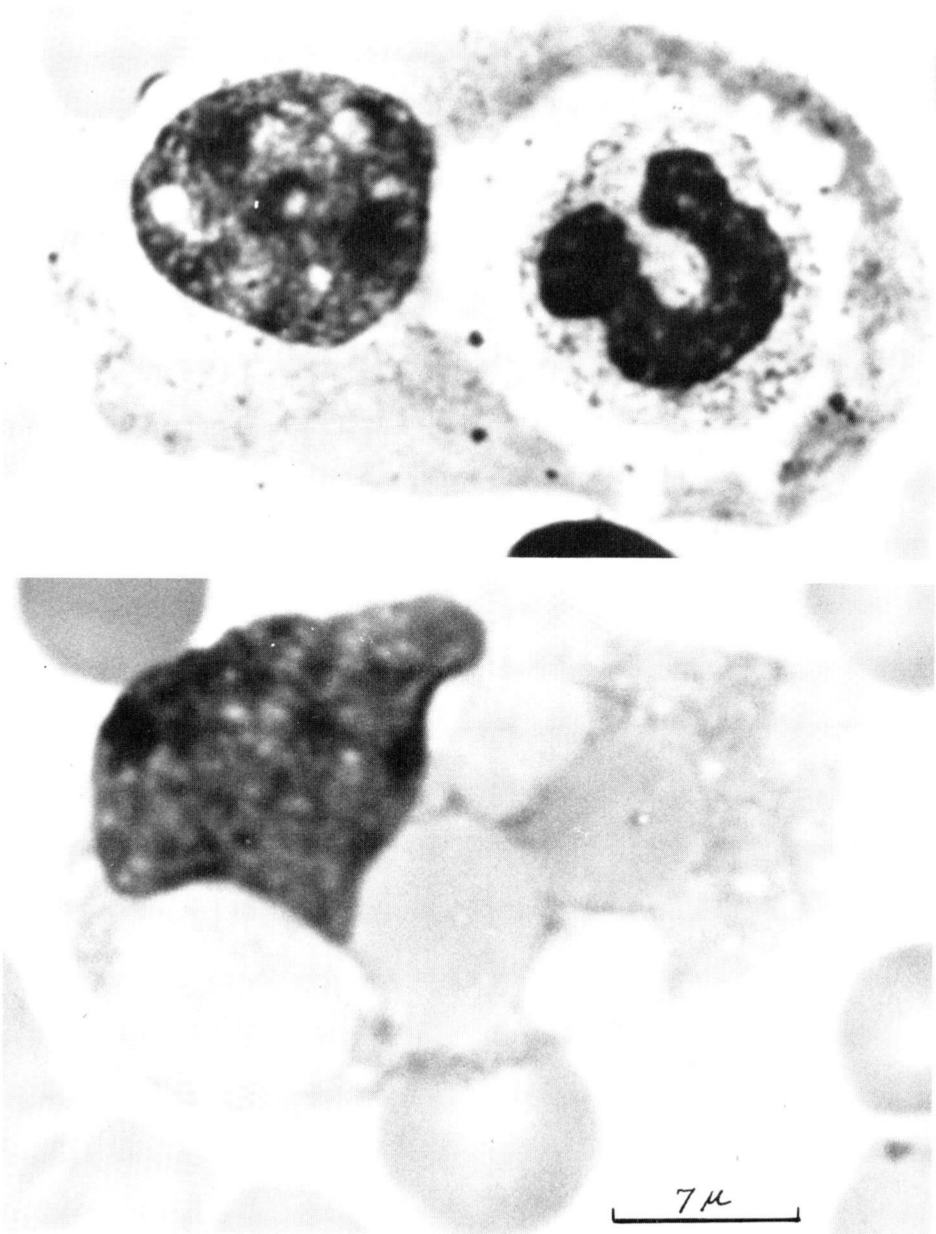

FIGURE 9. Upper: macrophage containing phagocytized neutrophilic leukocyte; lower: macrophage containing phagocytized erythrocytes.

culating blood and to the slowly moving cells of the tissue spaces, known as "macrophages" (Figure 9), which are considered to be overgrown monocytes. There is evidence that reverse transformations may occur between fixed tissue phagocytes, macrophages, and monocytes.

Histiocytes as a class are large. There is a large amount of cytoplasm in relation to the nucleus. These cells are often elongated and elliptical. As a rule the cytoplasmic margins are jagged, and there are tapering as well as blunt and rounded protrusions (Figure 10).

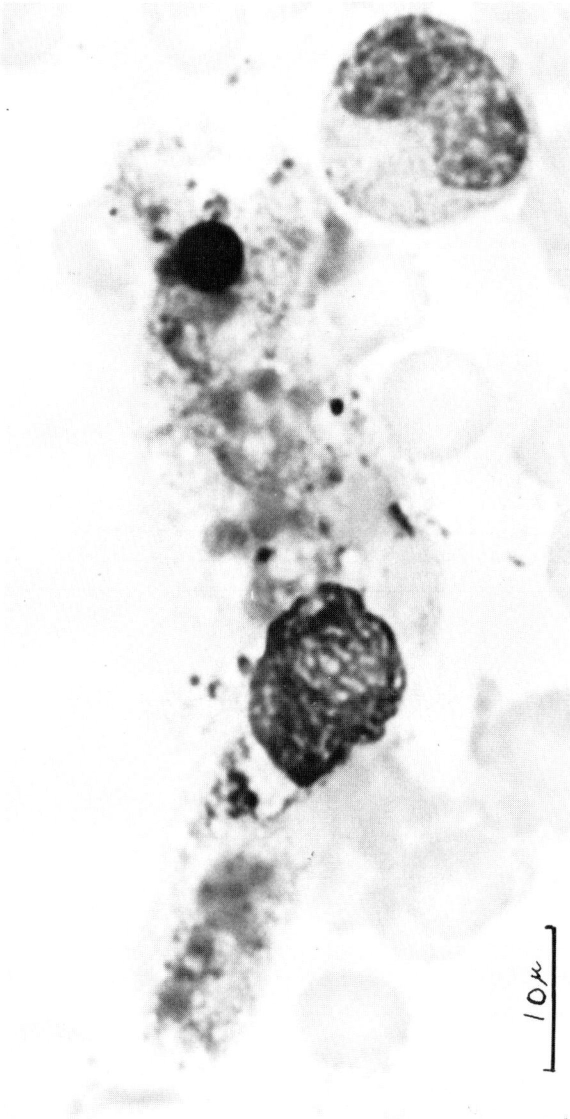

FIGURE 10. Histiocyte, a large elongated, irregularly shaped cell with vacuoles and phagocytized particles in cytoplasm. Smaller cell (right, lower) is a neutrophilic metamyelocyte.

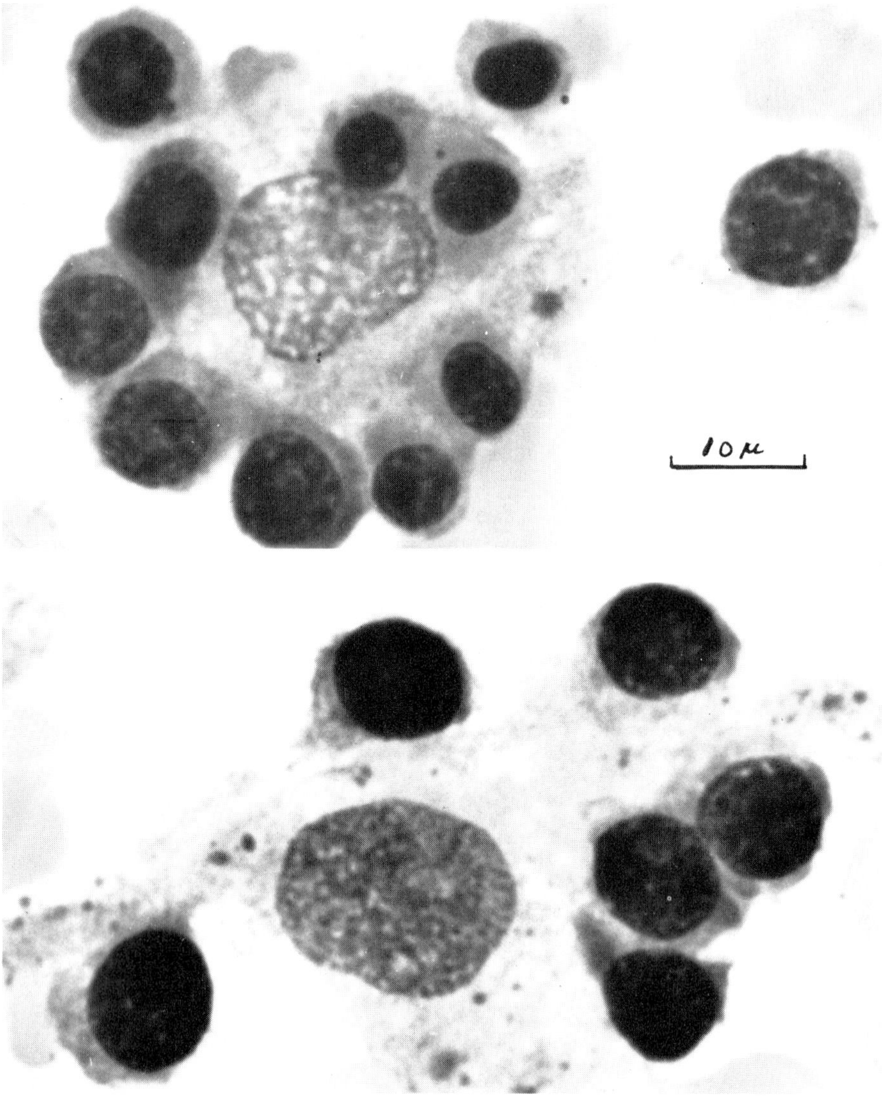

FIGURE 11. Nucleated red cells clustered around margin of histiocytes. (From Diggs, L. W., *Textbook of Clinical Pathology,* Miller, S. E. and Weller, J. M., Eds., Williams & Wilkins, Baltimore, © 1971, 84.

The cytoplasm stains light blue. Many of the cells reveal a delicate fibrillary structure. The cytoplasm often contains spherical chromophobic areas (vacuoles). There are varying numbers of granules that differ in size and in color. In addition to the granules, there may be phagocytized objects such as whole blood cells, nuclear fragments, parasites, bacteria, or pigment particles.

The nuclei of histiocytes, like the nuclei of all other fixed tissue cells, are round or oval, and the chromatin strands are distinct. Nucleoli are demonstrable when the cells are metabolically active and growing.

It is not possible, morphologically, to identify potentially phagocytic histiocytes from stem cells when they contain no demonstrable phagocytized material within their cytoplasm. Histiocytes with no visible particles in their cytoplasm occasionally may be identified by the fact that they are surrounded by clusters of nucleated red cells (Figure 11) or by lymphocytes and/or plasmocytes (Figure 12). It is presumed that such histio-

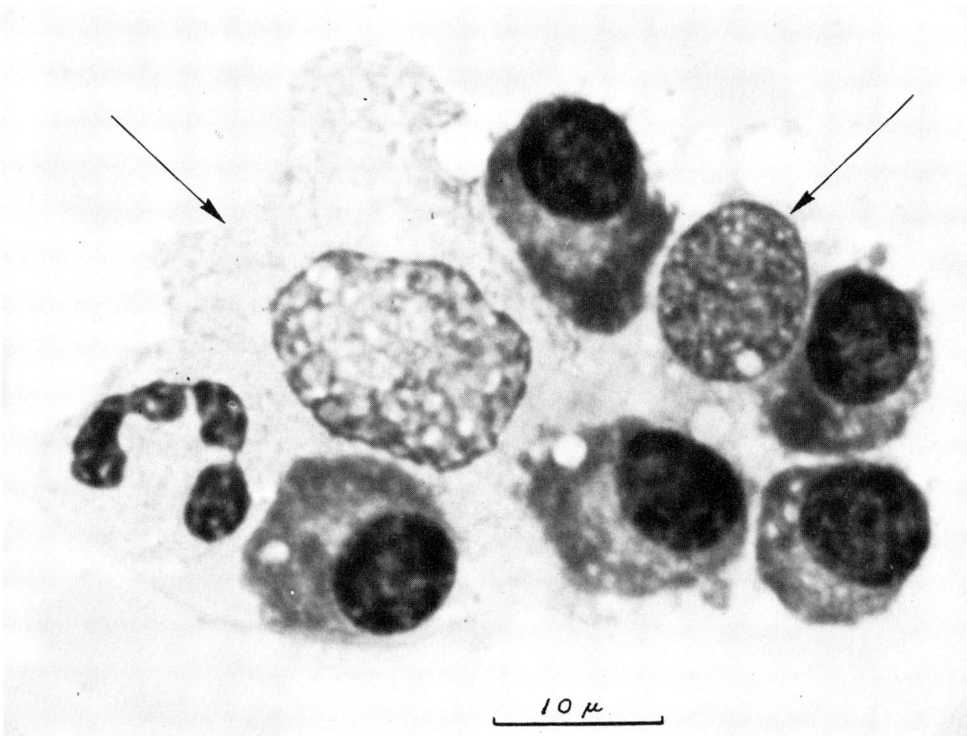

FIGURE 12. Plasmocytes in close proximity to margins of several histiocytes (arrows).

cytic cells contain invisible ingested material that is desired and needed by the satellite cells at their margins and that there is an exchange of material from the cytoplasm of histiocytes to other cells.

Tissue Granulocytes

Smears of material aspirated from the bone marrow of healthy individuals reveal small numbers of irregularly shaped fixed tissue cells that have granules in their cytoplasm similar to those observed in free blood cells. The relationship of tissue basophils to the basophilic granular cells of the peripheral blood and the relationship of tissue eosinophils and neutrophils to free blood cells with similar granules has not been clearly established. From a morphological standpoint the main difference is that of mobility.

Transitional cells between "stem cells" and tissue basophils, eosinophils, and neutrophils are demonstrable, but the "pro" and "blast" variants have not been sharply delineated.

Tissue Basophils (Mast Cells, Heparinocytes)

Tissue basophils as a class are larger than the free basophilic granulocytes of the peripheral blood (Figures 13 and 14). The more round or oval variants are approximately 2 to 4 times larger in diameter than the adjacent nonnucleated red cells. Many of the cells are elongated, narrow, and curved with tapering ends. There may be marginal cytoplasmic tags. The cytoplasm is obscured by numerous spherical granules of approximately the same size (0.2 to 0.4 μ). These granules are purplish and dark. The red and blue colors vary in intensity, but the predominant color is blue. Intensely basophilic granules often overlie the nucleus. Mechanically traumatized cells reveal

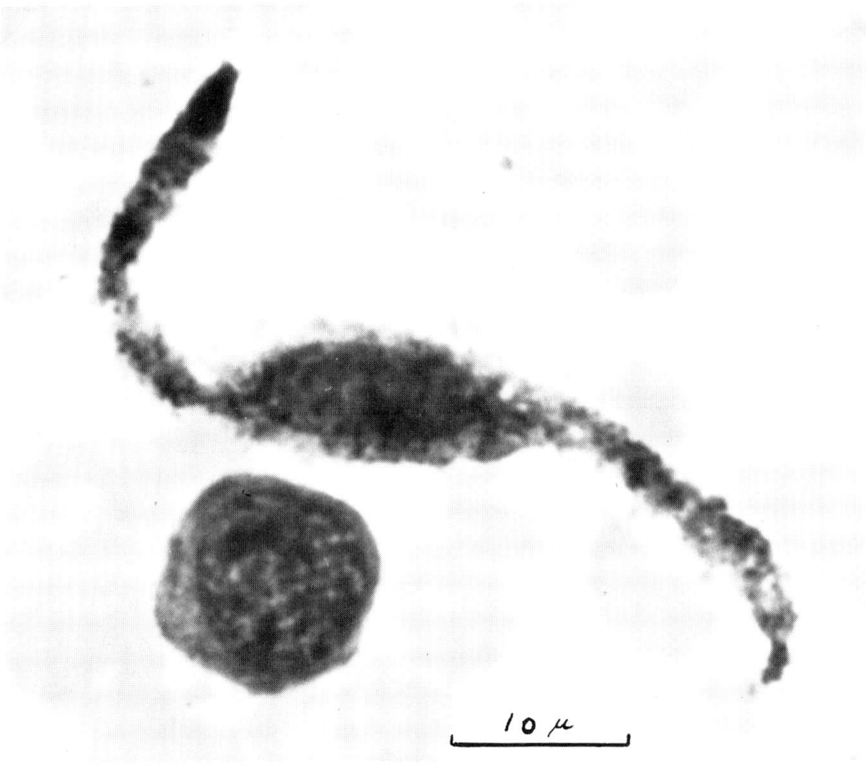

FIGURE 13. Tissue basophil (mast cell), elongated narrow cell with prominent dark granules. Cell (lower left), unidentified early cell.

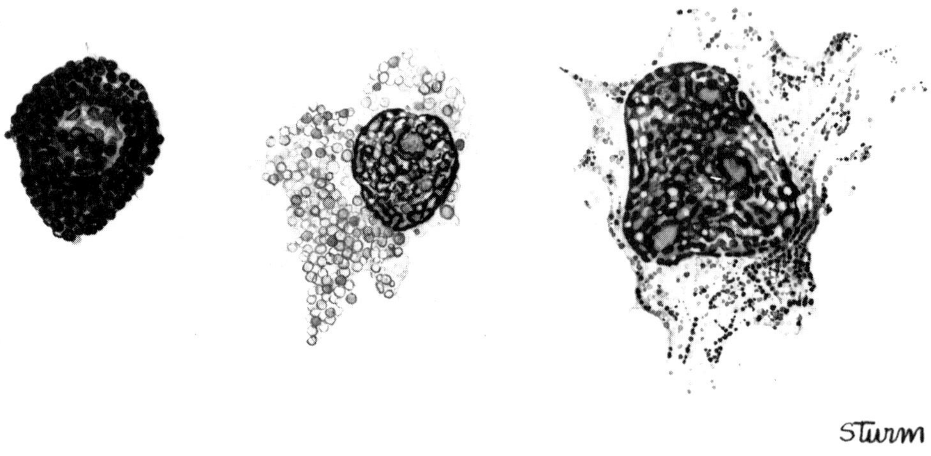

FIGURE 14. Tissue basophil (left), tissue eosinophil (center), tissue neutrophil (right). (From Diggs, L. W., Sturm, D., and Bell, A., *Morphology of Human Blood Cells,* 4th ed., Abbott Laboratories, North Chicago, Ill., 1979. With permission.)

spherical granules free in surrounding areas. In many cells there are chromophobic sperules (vacuoles), which probably are due to the washing out of water-soluble components during the staining process.

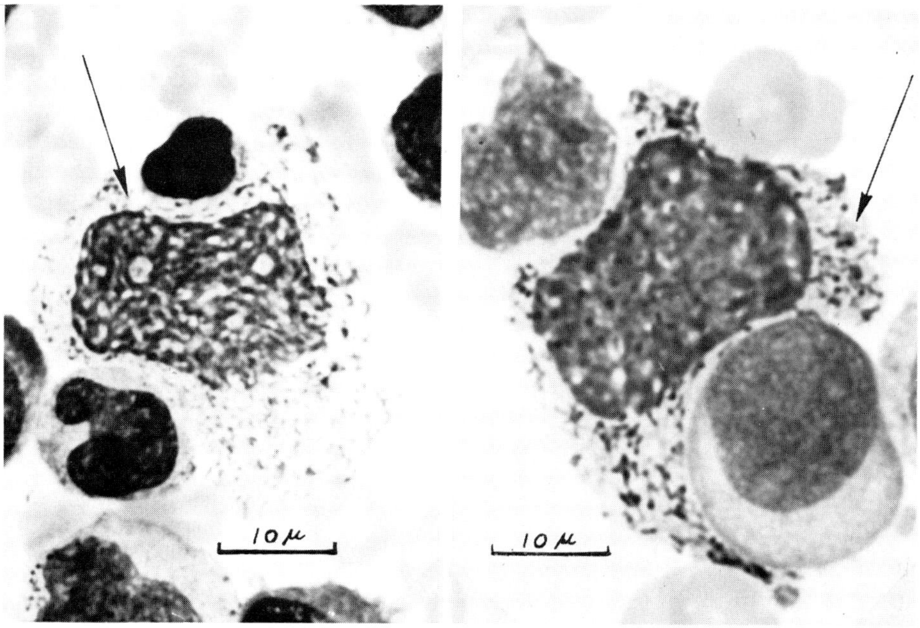

FIGURE 15. Tissue neutrophils (arrows).

The nuclei of tissue basophils are round, relatively small, and centrally located. They are light red. Nuclear chromatin structures are indistinct. There are no demonstrable nucleoli.

Tissue Eosinophils

Tissue eosinophils differ from the eosinophils of the peripheral blood in that they are larger, their margins are irregular, the nuclei are round, the chromatin strands are distinct, and nucleoli are usually visible (Figure 14). The primary granules, as in blood eosinophils, are purplish; the secondary granules are bright orange-red (eosinophilic). The granules are spherical, approximately the same size, numerous, and fairly evenly distributed.

Tissue Neutrophils (Ferrata Cells)

Tissue cells with neutrophilic granules are large cells with large nuclei and ample cytoplasm (Figures 14 and 15). The shape is irregular. There are multiple pointed cytoplasmic projections as well as blunt marginal protrusions. Tissue neutrophils are often indented by neighboring cells. They may be squeezed in between adjacent cells and sometimes seem to wrap around other cells.

The cytoplasm stains light blue and has a fine reticular structure. There are numerous granules with colors that range from pink or lavender to light purple. These granules are similar in color to the secondary granules of blood neutrophils. The granules vary in shape. Some are round, oval, or bacilliform, while others are elongated or curved or appear as beaded chains. The granules are unevenly distributed. In some areas they line up in parallel rows. There is no evidence of phagocytic activity. Vacuoles are rare.

The nuclei are round or oval and are usually centrally located. The nuclear chromatin is coarse and linear. One or several distinct nucleoli are usually demonstrable.

Tissue neutrophils have been interpreted by some hematologists as "hemohistioblasts", as "reticulum cells", and as "reticuloendothelial cells". Others have interpreted them as degenerated and traumatized progranulocytes or neutrophilic myelocytes and have denied their existence as morphological entities.

It is true that mechanically injured and squashed immature neutrophils with round nuclei, linear chromatin, nucleoli, and granules have characteristics similar to those of traumatized tissue neutrophils. In microscopic fields, where there is minimal cellular distortion and the cell margins are intact, there are distinct differences between fixed tissue neutrophils and blood neutrophils, just as there are differences between tissue basophils and blood basophils, and phagocytic histiocytes and amoeboid macrophages and monocytes. Tissue neutrophils as a class are larger than neutrophilic myelocytes. Their shape is irregular and there are tapering cytoplasmic extensions. Blood granulocytes tend to round up and to pull away from neighboring cells as they dry in stained smears, whereas tissue neutrophils are compressed by other cells. Histiocytic cells with finger and veil-like marginal protrusions tend to push neighboring erythrocytes and other cells away (Figure 16).

Bone Cells

Cells associated with bone formation are known as ''osteoblasts'', those involved in bone maintenance are called ''osteocytes'', and those associated with destruction and dissolution of calcified bone are identified as ''osteoclasts''.*

Osteoblasts

Osteoblasts synthesize and secrete intercellular substance (Figure 17). Deposition of calcium salt from the plasma within this bone matrix leads to the formation of calcific bone.

Osteoblasts in stained smears of bone marrow are large cells (25 to 30 μ) with a relatively large amount of cytoplasm. Most of the cells are narrow at one end and wide at the other, producing comet or tadpole shapes. The margins of the wider ends often reveal filamentous projections. The dark blue cytoplasm contains wavy fibrillar structures and multiple small, light-staining globules, producing a bubbly appearance. Within the cytoplasm there is a circular or oval chromophobic area, corresponding to the organelles of the Golgi zone. This relatively pale area may be adjacent to the nucleus, but is usually located out in the cytoplasm away from the nucleus.

The nucleus is round or oval and eccentrically located in the narrow end of the cell. The nuclei in some cells are partially extruded. The chromatin strands are similar to other fixed tissue cells in that they are linear and distinct. Nucleoli are usually demonstrable. Osteoblasts are not seen in smears of peripheral blood. They are best seen in tissue sections and are more numerous in marrow from infants than from adults and in diseases and conditions in which there is active bone formation.

Osteoblasts and plasmocytes in marrow smears have similar morphological characteristics in that both have irregular shapes, hyperbasophilic cytoplasm, secretory globules, and eccentric nuclei. Osteoblasts are larger than plasmocytes. The chromophobic area is usually at a distance from the nuclear margin rather than juxtanuclear (Figure 18). Osteoblasts often appear in clusters (Figure 19). Plasmocytes are usually separated from each other or may appear as cells grouped around the margin of a histiocytic cell (Figure 12).

* By usage the term ''osteoblast'' has been employed to identify mature bone marrow cells whose function is to form bone and not to indicate that the cells are ''blasts'' in the sense that they are undifferentiated progenitor cells. In keeping with the terminology used for other cells, the term ''osteocyte'' would be preferable to the term ''osteoblast.'' Unfortunately, by long usage, the term ''osteocyte'' has been applied to cells that are surrounded by bone matrix or that lie in Haversian canaliculi, encased by calcified bone.

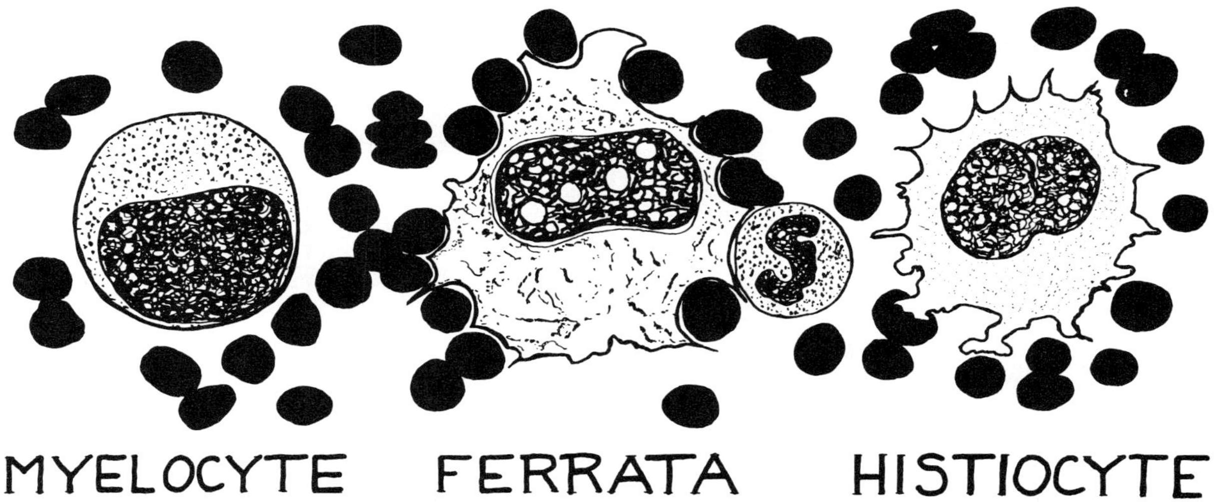

FIGURE 16. Relation of marrow cells to surrounding cells. Myelocytes tend to round up and to pull away from adjacent cells. Tissue neutrophils (Ferrata cells) are characteristically indented by neighboring cells. The veil-like ruffles and finger-like cytoplasmic projections of histiocytes tend to push adjacent cells away. (From Diggs, L. W., *Textbook of Clinical Pathology,* Miller, S. E. and Weller, J. M., Eds., Williams & Wilkins, Baltimore, © 1971, 155. With permission.)

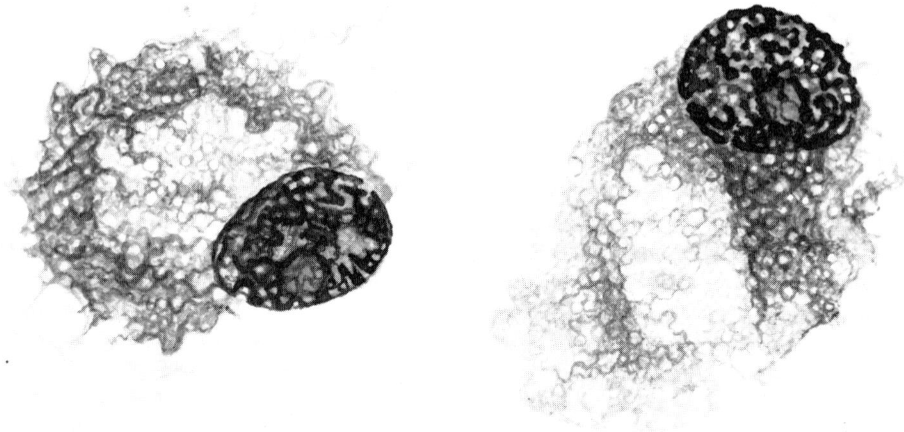

FIGURE 17. Osteoblasts. (From Diggs, L. W., *Textbook of Clinical Pathology,* Miller, S. E. and Weller, J. M., Eds., Williams & Wilkins, Baltimore, © 1971, 79.)

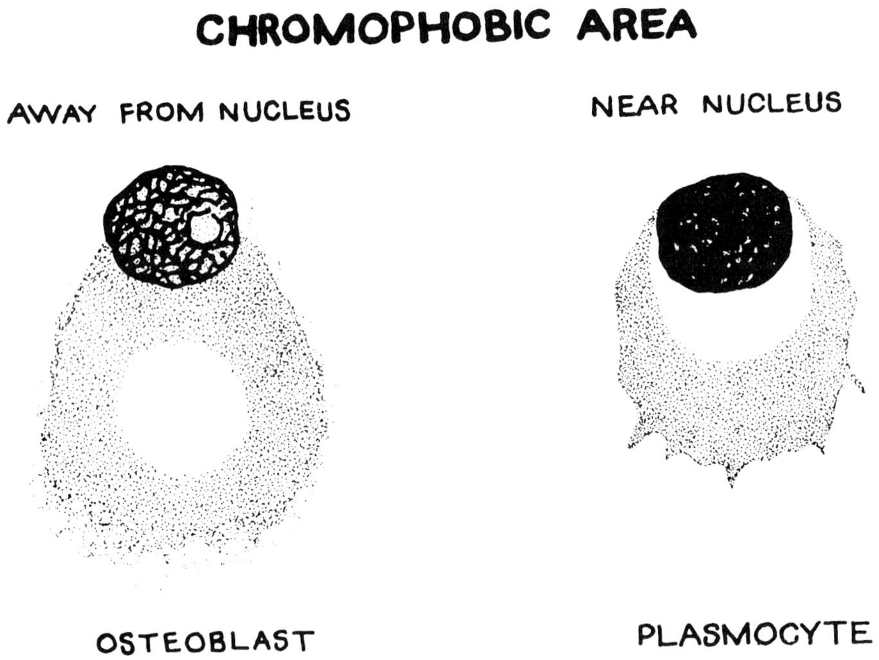

FIGURE 18. Drawing showing the position of the chromophobic area in the cytoplasm in a typical osteoblast and in a typical plasmocyte.

Islands of osteoblasts (Figure 19) simulate and may be mistaken for metastatic malignant cells. Malignant cells vary in size, shape, and structure. Their margins are often indistinct. Osteoblasts have well-defined margins, and the morphology of individual cells is approximately the same.

Osteoclasts (Polykaryocytes)

Osteoclasts are giant, multinucleated cells (Figure 20). Their shape is irregular. As a

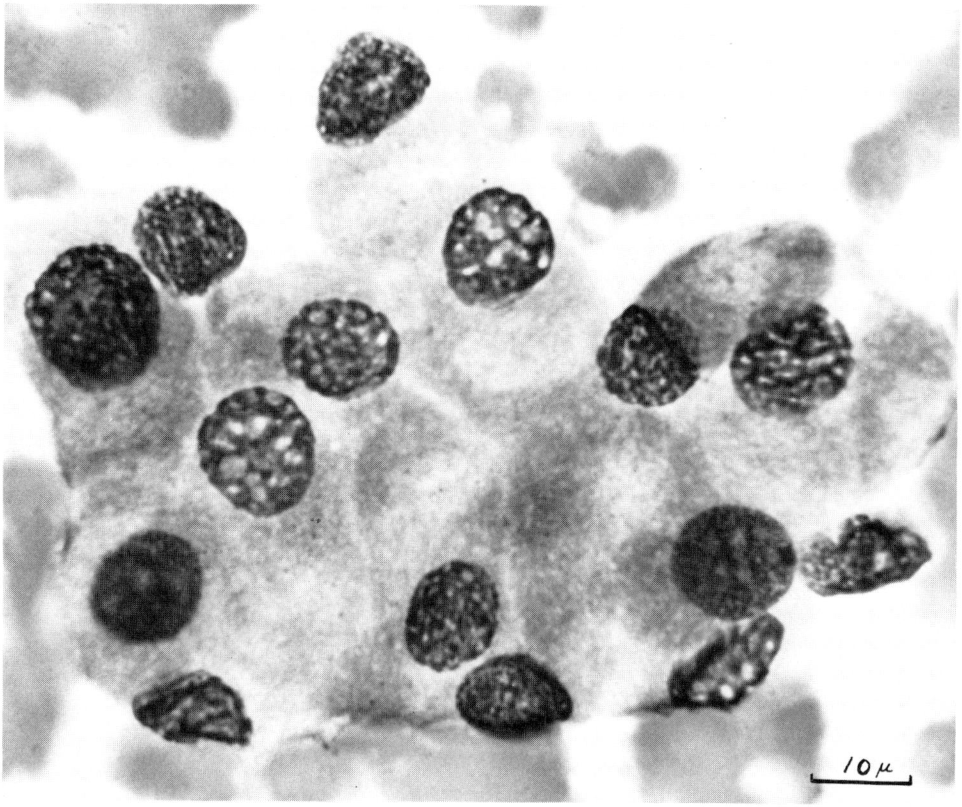

FIGURE 19. Cluster of osteoblasts.

rule these cells are elongated with tapering ends. The margins tend to be frayed. Some of the cells reveal transparent and pinkish-lavender ectoplasm. Others have a distinct ruffled or brush border that is characterized by finger-like processes and invaginations. The striated peripheral cytoplasm in some cells has a frothy or bubbly appearance. The cytoplasm is blue. The intensity of the blue is variable. In addition to indistinct bluish granules there may be small darkly stained blue-black fragments of phagocytized bone.

The number of nuclei is variable. The number may be even or odd and not necessarily a multiple of two as would be expected if the nuclei had been produced by mitotic division, assuming that all of the cells, as in megakaryocytes, undergo mitosis at the same time. The nuclei, in contrast to those megakaryocytes, are separate (Figure 21), and their margins are distinct. The nuclei are round or oval and are of approximately the same size (10 to 15 μ). The nuclear chromatic structure is usually coarsely linear. Nucleoli may or may not be visible.

The large size and multiple nuclei of osteoclasts is explained by the fusion of cells. Whether the cells that are fused are histiocytes, fibrocytes, or osteoblasts has not been clearly established. The ruffled borders, the evidence of endocytosis and phagocytosis of small particles, and the dissolution of calcified bone adjacent to the margins are morphological evidence that these cells are more closely related to phagocytic histiocytes than to cells that produce connective tissue fibers (fibrocytes) and bone matrix (osteoblasts).

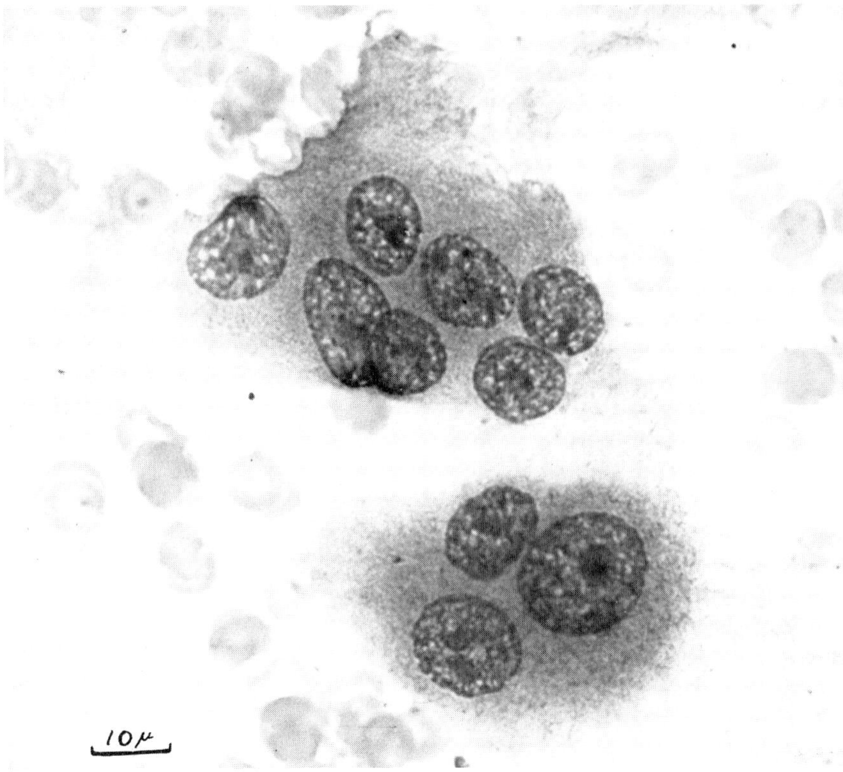

FIGURE 20. Osteoclasts.

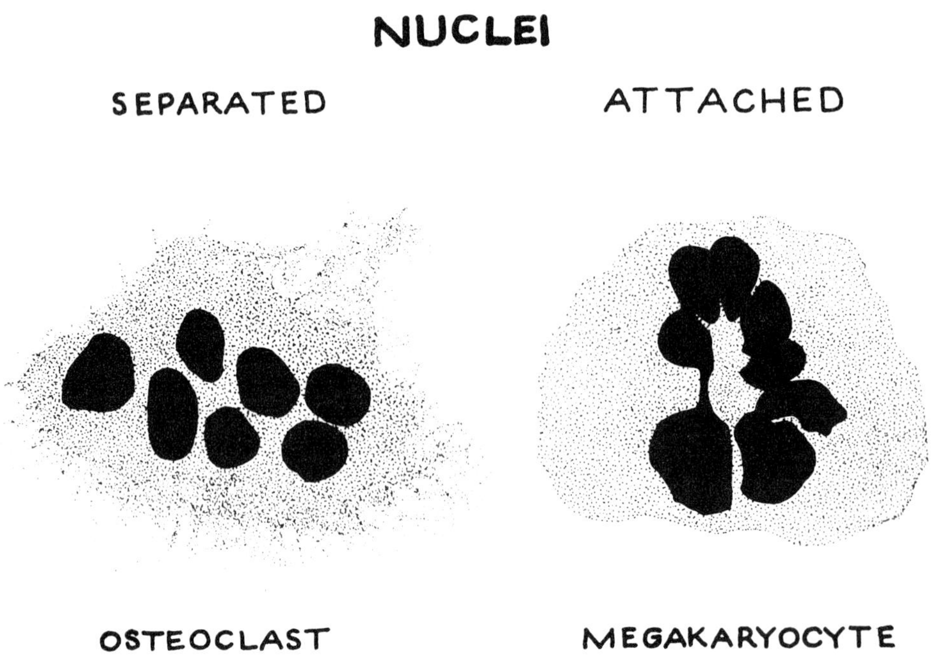

FIGURE 21. Drawing showing difference between multiple nuclei of megakaryocyte and osteoclast.

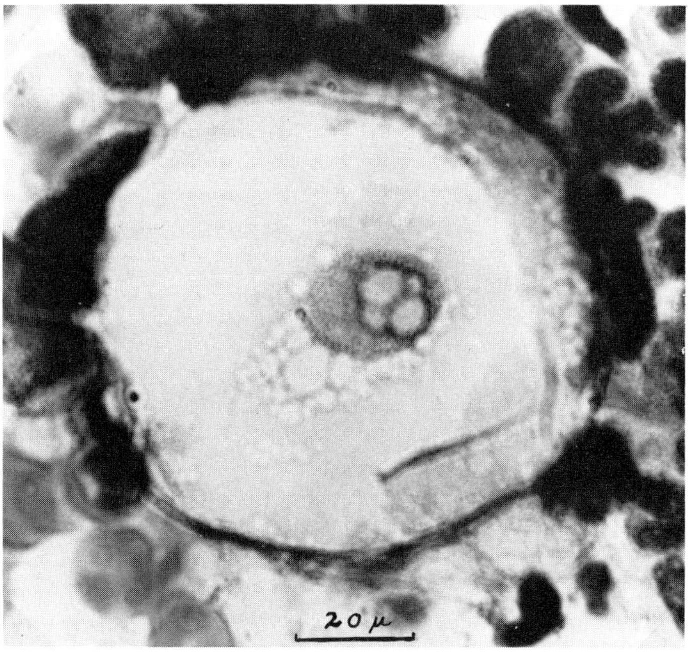

FIGURE 22. Fat cell.

Other Fixed Cells

Fat Cells (Lipocytes, Adipocytes)

Fat cells are seldom seen in thin smears of bone marrow, for they are ruptured in the process of spreading. When spread on a slide, the contained globules of fat tend to escape and leave the stroma and cell membranes as unidentifiable debris. In thicker portions of the marrow smears, individual fat cells (Figure 22) or groups of fat cells can be seen, surrounded by other marrow cells.

Mature fat cells are large round cells, comparable in size to megakaryocytes and osteoblasts. The small, round or oval nuclei are located eccentrically, presumably pushed to one side by the pressure of globules of fat in the cytoplasm. The chromatin structure of the nuclei is linear, and nucleoli are usually demonstrable (Figure 22).

The globules of fat in the cytoplasm are of varying size, are chromophobic, or stain a light blue or pink. The globules compress each other, producing irregular shapes. The lipid masses are separated in compartments by cytoplasmic material, which appears as delicate blue lines. The fixed character of the cells is revealed by multiple fibrils that extend outward from the cell margins and interlace with the fibers of fibrocytes.

Mesenchymal cells that manufacture fat are to be differentiated from secretory plasma cells with large aggregates of proteinaceous material in their cytoplasm. The secretory droplets in the grape or morula variants of plasma cells are spherical rather than irregular in shape and appear as perfect superimposed circles (Figure 23).

Endothelial Cells

Occasionally one sees in marrow smears fragments of small intact vascular channels, the lumens of which are bounded by elongated nongranular cells with oval nuclei (Fig-

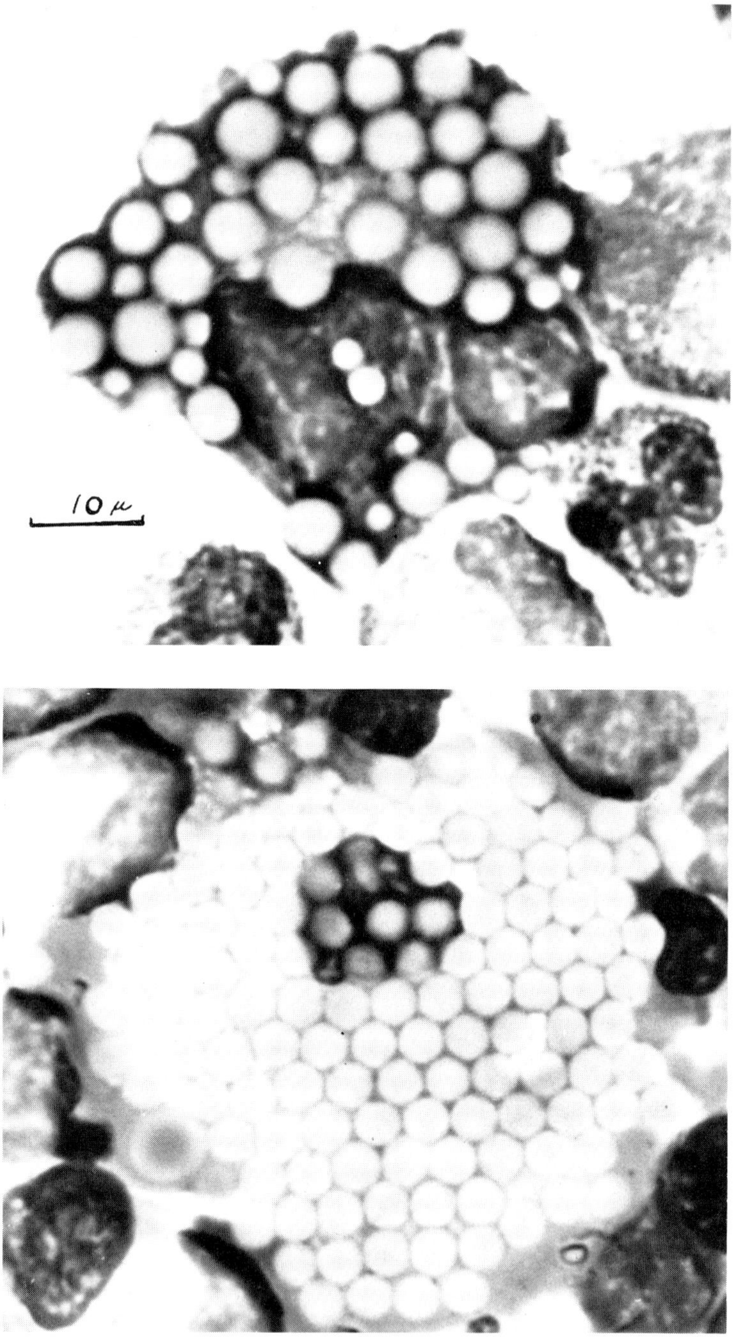

FIGURE 23. Plasmocytes with globular bodies.

ure 24). These cells are identified as endothelial cells by their organoid arrangement. Individual endothelial cells are not identifiable except by association with other cells.

Fibrocytes (Fibroblasts)

The connective tissue cells of the bone marrow and other blood-forming organs, identified as fibrocytes, are responsible for the formation of ground substance and

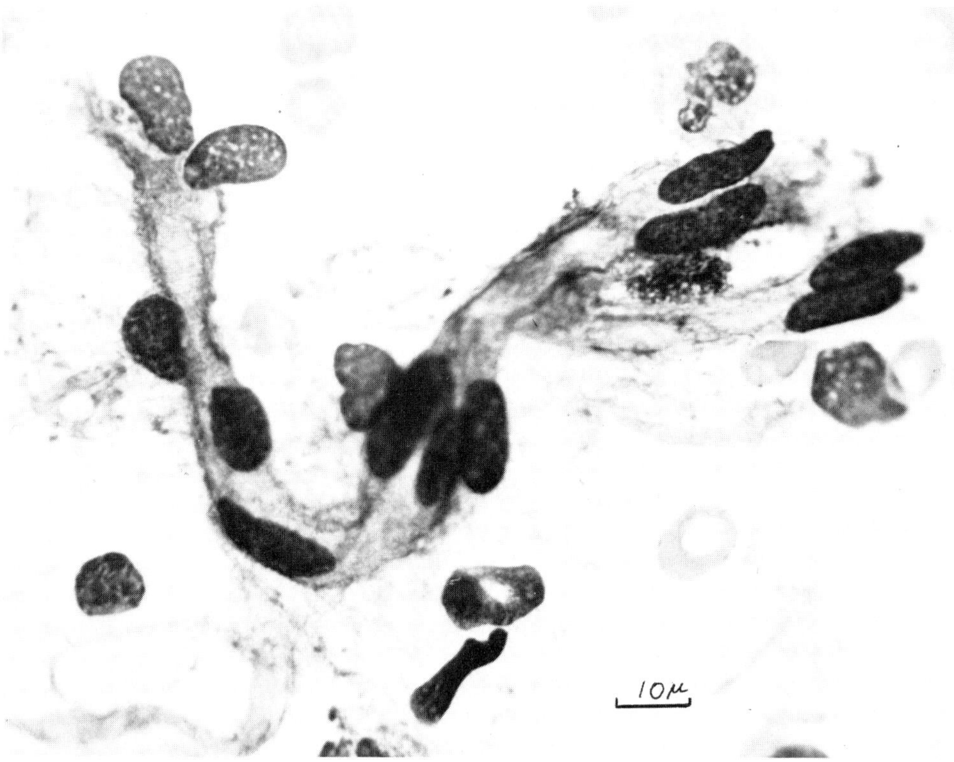

FIGURE 24. Endothelial cells.

connective tissue fibers. Fibrocytes are so firmly embedded in the ground substance or held so tightly in the web of reticular fibers that they are not seen, or at least not identified in bone marrow smears or imprints. They are readily demonstrated in tissue sections as elongated cells with tapering and often multiple and forked cytoplasmic extensions. The nuclei are relatively small, centrally located, and round, oval, or elliptical. The cytoplasm is lightly stained and often has a finely granular appearance.

Fibrocytes are not usually considered to be blood cells and no mention is made of them in most hematological texts. These cells, however, are of major importance in identifying numerous inflammatory, malignant, and other diseases of the blood-forming organs.

ROMANOWSKY AND RETICULOCYTE STAINS

P. N. Marshall

Romanowsky Stains

A Romanowsky stain may be defined as any stain comprising methylene blue and its products of oxidation (shown in Figure 1) and an eosin (eosin Y or B, shown in Figure 2). Romanowsky stains[1,2] have become firmly established as routine stains for hematological material, to the extent that blood cells are defined on the basis of their morphological appearance in Romanowsky-stained smears. In this section the composition, method of use, and properties of these stains are summarized; for a comprehensive treatment of these topics, the reader is referred to two recent reviews.[3,4]

Preparation of Stains

Materials Used

Methylene blue — Methylene blue is synthesized by Bernthsen's thiosulfate method.[5] The nominal dye is the sole major component of most commercial samples, although variable amounts of lower homologs (mainly azure B) and metallic salts contaminate most batches.[6-16] Pure methylene blue is required in at least one stain formulation.[17] For this purpose contaminating dyes may be removed from commercial samples by adsorption chromatography[15,16] or solvent extraction;[9,11,18] metallic salts may be removed by ion-exchange chromatography[15] or crystallization.[18]

Polychrome methylene blue — This generic term is used to describe any material produced by the oxidation of methylene blue. Generally, oxidation is accomplished by any of a number of procedures involving the use of chemical oxidants, extremes of pH, and elevated temperatures.[19-28] Historically, polychrome methylene blues have been divided into two classes. One class comprises products which, according to their originators, are complex mixtures of methylene blue and the products of oxidative demethylation and deamination shown in Figure 1, e.g., the polychrome methylene blue of Field.[19] The other class comprises products which are classically considered to be less heterogeneous, supposedly consisting largely, if not entirely, of single dyes, e.g., MacNeal's azure A.[24] With modern analytical techniques it has, however, been found that most products prepared by the oxidation of methylene blue are extremely heterogeneous mixtures.[29] Since the overwhelming majority of commercial products designated azure A, azure B, azure C, or methylene violet Bernthsen are prepared in this manner, the labeling of these various products will usually give little indication of their composition.[6,8,12,13,15,16] They are therefore best designated polychrome methylene blues and will be referred to as such throughout this chapter.

Since polychroming is difficult to control effectively on a commercial scale,[29] successive batches of dye obtained from the same supplier will probably vary in composition.[12,13] Commercial samples of methylene blue, in contrast to those of the azures and methylene violet Bernthsen, are prepared by synthesis; because of this they are, by and large, of reasonable purity (see above).

Azure B — Azure B is required in at least two stain formulations.[17,30] The dye may be obtained from polychrome methylene blue by chromatography.[15,16,31] Alternatively, it may be prepared by using a solvent extraction/crystallization procedure[18] or synthesized by an adaptation of Bernthsen's method.[9]

Eosin Y and eosin B — Eosin Y is manufactured by the direct bromination of fluorescein.[5] Commercial samples are somewhat variable mixtures of the nominal dye, 2′,4′,5′,-tribromofluorescein and fluorescein[13,32,33] (the structures of these compounds are given in Figure 2). Eosin B is prepared by treatment of 4′,5′,-dibromofluorescein

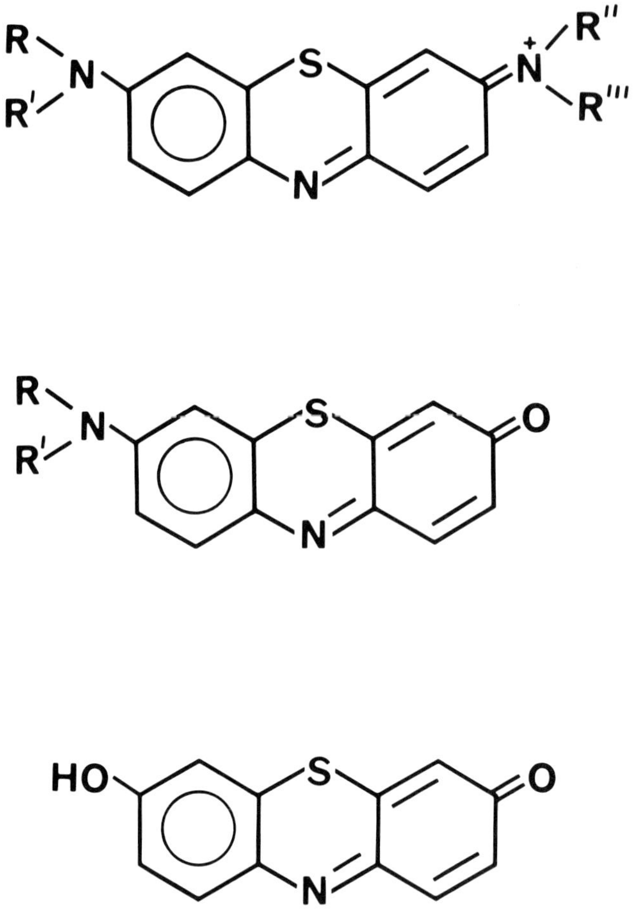

FIGURE 1. Structural formulae of methylene blue and its oxidation products.

Top: thionine series													
Methylene blue (CI 52015)	R	=	Me,	R′	=	Me,	R″	=	Me,	R‴	=	Me
Azure B (CI 52010)	R	=	Me,	R′	=	Me,	R″	=	Me,	R‴	=	H
Azure A (CI 52005)	R	=	Me,	R′	=	Me,	R″	=	H,	R‴	=	H
sym-dimethylthionine	R	=	Me,	R′	=	H,	R″	=	Me,	R‴	=	H
Azure C (CI 52002)	R	=	Me,	R′	=	H,	R″	=	H,	R‴	=	H
Thionine (CI 52000)	R	=	H,	R′	=	H,	R″	=	H,	R‴	=	H
Middle: thionoline series												
Methylene Violet Bernthsen	R	=	Me,	R′	=	Me						
Methyl thionoline	R	=	Me,	R′	=	H						
Thionoline	R	=	H,	R′	=	H						
Bottom: thionol												

with nitric and sulfuric acids.[5] Commercial samples of this dye are mixtures of the nominal compound and commercial eosin Y.[13]

Polychrome methylene blue eosinate — Polychrome methylene blue eosinates are salts in which the cations are methylene blue and its various products of oxidation, and the anion an eosin. The salts are obtained as precipitates whenever aqueous solutions of polychrome methylene blue and eosin are mixed.[34]

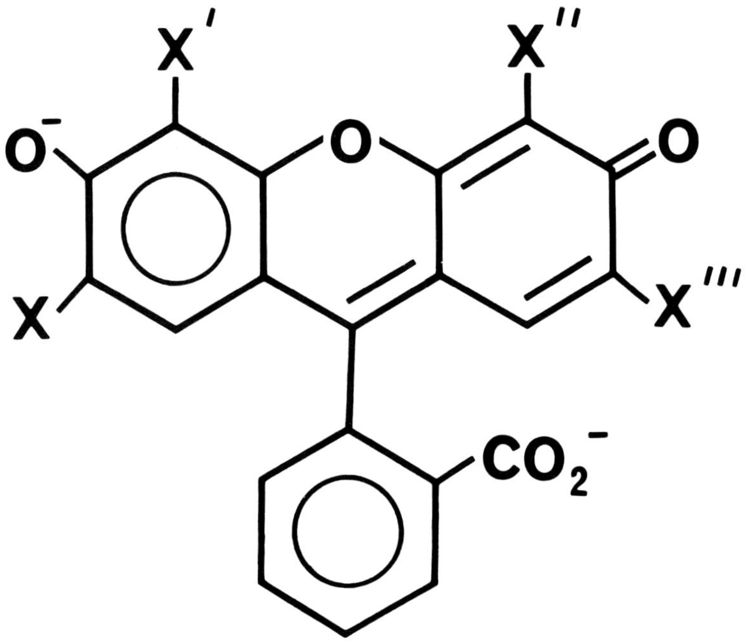

FIGURE 2. Structural formulae of fluorescein dyes.

Eosin Y (CI 45380)	X	= Br,	X′ = Br,	X″ = Br,	X‴ = Br
Eosin B (CI 45400)	X	= NO_2,	X′ = Br,	X″ = Br,	X‴ = NO_2
2′,4′,5′-tribromofluorescein	X	= Br,	X′ = Br,	X″ = Br,	X‴ = H
Fluorescein (CI 45350)	X	= H,	X′ = H,	X″ = H,	X‴ = H

Preparative Techniques

Although there are numerous techniques for the preparation of Romanowsky stains, all fall into one of four classes:

1. Stains prepared by mixing aqueous solutions of polychrome methylene blue and an eosin. These stains are extremely unstable, and for this reason are little used today. Stains of this class include those of Nocht[35] and Romanowsky.[2]
2. Stains prepared from polychrome methylene blue eosinate. Stock solutions are prepared by dissolving the eosinate in a suitable solvent, usually methanol or glycerol/methanol. The composition of some stains of this class, together with their method of use, is given in Table 1.
3. One-stage stains prepared by direct dissolution of polychrome methylene blue or specific thiazine dyes (i.e., without the preparation of an eosinate intermediate). The composition of some stains of this class, together with their method of use, is given in Table 2.
4. Two-stage stains. These require the preparation of two separate staining solutions which are used sequentially. One solution contains polychrome methylene blue; the other contains an eosin. Some examples are given in Table 3.

Properties of Stains

Scheme of Coloring

Successful Romanowsky stains produce the Romanowsky effect, the purple coloration of certain cell components being produced by the combined action of a thiazine dye and an eosin, but not by either dye acting alone. These cell components include

Table 1
THE COMPOSITION AND METHOD OF USE OF SOME ROMANOWSKY STAINS PREPARED FROM POLYCHROME METHYLENE BLUE EOSINATES

Composition		Method of use	Ref.
Polychrome methylene blue eosinate (B)[a]	0.15 g	Smears fixed "on slide"[b] with 1 vol of stain for 30 sec. Two vol of water then added and mixture left for 5 min. Stained smears rinsed in water for 1 min and air dried	Leishman[20]
Methanol	100 mℓ		
Methylene blue	0.1 g	Methanol-fixed smears stained for 45 min with mixture of stain and water (1:50 v/v), then rinsed in water and air dried	Roe et al.[34]
Methylene blue eosinate	0.2 g		
Polychrome methylene blue eosinate ("azure B eosinate")[c]	0.25 g		
Polychrome methylene blue eosinate ("azure A eosinate")	0.05 g		
Glycerol	50 mℓ		
Methanol	50 mℓ		
Polychrome methylene blue eosinate, four-fifths saturated solution in methanol	—	Smears fixed "on slide" with stain for 1 min. An unspecified volume of water then added and mixture left for 2—3 min. Smears rinsed in water and air dried	Wright[28]

[a] Eosinates prepared with eosin Y are simply termed "eosinates", those prepared with eosin B are indicated by (B).
[b] The term "on slide" refers to the practice of applying reagents as thin films to a horizontally positioned slide, as opposed to immersing the slide vertically in a larger volume of reagent.
[c] The originators' designation for the polychrome methylene blue is included in parentheses.

leukocyte nuclei and neutrophil granules, but no comprehensive list is yet available. The principal thiazine dye producing this effect is azure B,[17,30,38] but the effect may also be obtained with azure A.[39] The molecular processes involved in the Romanowsky effect are currently unknown. Successful stains impart characteristic colorations, typically blues and pinks, to other cell components. The general scheme of coloring is shown in Table 4.

Although many colored components are commonly present in Romanowsky stains, only azure B and an eosin are essential for acceptable results.[17,30,38] There is, however, some evidence that the addition of methylene blue to a mixture of these two dyes may enhance stain performance.[17,38]

Table 2
THE COMPOSITION AND METHOD OF USE OF SOME ROMANOWSKY STAINS PREPARED BY THE DIRECT DISSOLUTION OF COMPONENT DYES

Composition		Method of use	Ref.
Solution I			
Methylene blue	0.13 g	Smears fixed in methanol for 30 sec—1 min. Staining solution applied "on slide"[b] and washed off with water after 5—8 min. Smears air dried.	Kingsley[36]
Polychrome methylene blue ("azure A")[a]	0.02 g		
Glycerol			
Methanol	10 mℓ		
Phosphate buffer, pH 6.9	10 mℓ		
Water	30 mℓ		
	50 mℓ		
Solution II			
Polychrome methylene blue ("methylene violet Bernthsen")	0.026 g		
Eosin Y	0.09 g		
Acetone	70 mℓ		
Glycerol	10 mℓ		
Methanol	20 mℓ		
Mix equal volumes of Solutions I and II before use			
Methylene blue	0.1 g	Used as Leishman's stain	MacNeal[37]
Polychrome methylene blue ("methylene azure")	0.06 g		
Polychrome methylene blue ("methylene violet Bernthsen")	0.02 g		
Eosin Y	0.1 g		
Methanol	100 mℓ		
Methylene blue	0.045 g	Smears fixed in methanol for 5—10 min and then stained by immersion for 10 min in a mixture of stain (1 vol) and Sorensen's phosphate buffer, pH 6.8, 0.00132 *M* (5 vol.) Smears rinsed in buffer for 1 min and air dried	Marshall et al.[17]
Azure B	0.085 g		
Eosin Y, color acid	0.065 g		
Glycerol	50 mℓ		
Methanol	50 mℓ		
Solution A			
Azure B	0.4 g	Smears fixed "on slide" with stain (1 vol) for 4 min. Veronal acetate buffer, pH 6.5 (3 vol) then added and mixture left for 25 min. Smears rinsed in water and air dried	Wittekind et al.[30]
Methanol	100 mℓ		
Solution B			
Eosin Y	0.4 g		
Methanol	100 mℓ		
Solutions A and B mixed in proportion of 10:1 (v/v) before use			

[a] The originator's designation for the polychrome methylene blue is included in parentheses.
[b] The term "on slide" refers to the practice of applying reagents as thin films to a horizontally positioned slide, as opposed to immersing the slide vertically in a larger volume of reagent.

Table 3
THE COMPOSITION AND METHOD OF USE OF SOME TWO-STAGE ROMANOWSKY STAINS

Composition					
Solution A (or I)		Solution B (or II)		Method of use	Ref.
Methylene blue Polychrome methylene blue ("azure I")[a] Phosphate buffer, pH 6.6	0.16 g 0.1 g 100 mℓ	Eosin Y Phosphate buffer, pH 6.6	0.2 g 100 mℓ	Smears immersed in Solution A for 1 sec and rinsed in water; smears then immersed in Solution B for 1 sec, rinsed in water and air dried	Field[19]
Methylene blue Potassium dichromate Aqueous sulfuric acid (1% v/v) Water Solution boiled for 3 hr, cooled and 2 mℓ of aqueous potassium hydroxide (1% w/v) added	0.1 g 0.1 g 0.6 mℓ 100 mℓ	Eosin Y Water	0.2 g 100 mℓ	Smears fixed in methanol for 1 — 2 sec. Smears immersed in Solution I for 30 sec and rinsed in water. Smears then immersed in Solution II for 1 sec and rinsed. Immersion in Solution I repeated. Smears rinsed and air dried	Singh and Bhattacharji[26]

[a] The originator's designation for the polychrome methylene blue is included in parentheses.

Table 4
SCHEME OF COLORING OF SUCCESSFUL ROMANOWSKY STAIN

Nuclei	Purple	Granules	
Cytoplasms		Azurophil	Purple
Erythroblast	Dark blue	Basophil	Purple black
Erythrocyte	Pink	Eosinophil	Orange
Lymphocyte	Blue	Neutrophil	Purple
Metamyelocyte	Pink	Platelet	Purple
Monocyte	Grey blue	Primary	Red or purple
Myelocyte	Pink	Other inclusions	
Neutrophil	Pink	Auer body	Purple
Promyelocyte	Blue	Cabot ring	Purple
		Howell-Jolly body	Purple

Inconsistency in Performance

The major problem experienced with the vast majority of Romanowsky stains is batch-to-batch variation in performance; this problem is usually the result of variation in stain composition,[6-8,12-14,17,23,33,40-46] but factors such as biological variation between specimens and accidental variation in staining technique may also contribute. Variations in performance are inconvenient and are a potential source of diagnostic error.

Table 5
THIN-LAYER CHROMATOGRAPHIC METHODS FOR ROMANOWSKY STAINS AND THE DYES USED IN THEIR PREPARATION

Sorbent	Developing solvent	Ref.
Silica	Butan-1-ol: ethanol:acetic acid:water (50:20:10:20 v/v)	54
Silica	Butanol layer obtained by partitioning butan-1-ol (12 vol) against a mixture of 1% w/v aqueous ammonium chloride (5 vol) and 2% v/v aqueous formic acid (2 vol)	60

They may be largely prevented by the use of stains of constant composition.[12,17,30,47] The most convenient means of obtaining this type of stain is by the use of pure dyes. Two stains formulated with pure dyes are described in Table 2.

Stability

Two major factors determine the shelf life of stock solutions of Romanowsky stains.

Solvent — It has been found that the stain solvent has a marked influence on stability,[48] e.g., Lillie found that stains are more stable in a mixture of glycerol and methanol than in methanol alone.

Storage temperature — Stain stability decreases with increasing temperature,[49] e.g., Dean et al. found that their methanol-based stain was stable for at least 57 days when stored at 4°C, but degraded within a few days at 40°C.

Analysis of Stains

Analysis of Romanowsky stains and the dyes used in their preparation is an essential part of quality assurance. Many workers have used classical methods of organic chemistry (including elemental analysis and visible spectroscopy) for this purpose.[10,25,27,40-42,44-46,50-53] These techniques suffer from serious drawbacks when applied to the complex mixtures found in Romanowsky stains.[29,31,54] The only reliable techniques for the analysis of these mixtures are those which are separation based.[6,8,12,13,15,16,32,55-63] The most effective and rapid of these are thin-layer chromatography (tlc) and high performance liquid chromatography (hplc). Tlc is the technique of choice of semiquantitative analysis.[64] The apparatus is relatively inexpensive, readily available, and occupies little space. It is therefore very suitable for use in a hematology laboratory. Two well-documented tlc methods are available, and these are described in Table 5. Tlc data on the components of Romanowsky stains are given in Table 6. Hplc is the technique of choice for high-speed quantitative analysis.[64] Since the apparatus is costly and

Table 6
THIN-LAYER CHROMATOGRAPHIC DATA ON COLORED COMPONENTS OF ROMANOWSKY STAINS[a]

Component	Mean R_f, 1 SD (Number of measurements)	Color on dried chromatogram: In daylight	Color on dried chromatogram: In short-wave uv light
Methylene blue	0.06, 0.01 (24)	Blue	None
Azure B	0.11, 0.01 (24)	Blue	None
Unknown	0.15, 0.02 (15)	Blue	None
Azure A	0.19, 0.02 (23)	Blue	Red
Eosin B	0.22, 0.01 (15)	Magenta	Orange
sym-dimethylthionine	0.24, 0.02 (24)	Blue	Red
Azure C	0.25, 0.02 (24)	Blue	Red
Thionine	0.36, 0.02 (26)	Purple	Red
Methylene violet Bernthsen	0.47, 0.02 (25)	Blue	Red
Methyl thionoline	0.59, 0.03 (25)	Blue	Red
Eosin Y	0.60, 0.03 (24)	Red	Green yellow
Thionoline	0.65, 0.03 (25)	Purple	Red
Thionol	0.70, 0.03 (12)	Purple	Red
2′,4′,5′-tribromofluorescein	0.72, 0.02 (24)	Orange	Lime green
Fluorescein	0.79, 0.03 (25)	Yellow	Green yellow

[a] Technique of Marshall and Lewis.[60] Data from References 13 and 29.

not yet generally available, this technique is more suited for quality assurance in an industrial environment.

Colored components, although the most readily detected, are not the only components of Romanowsky stain powders and the dyes used in their preparation. Metal salts are also present, either as standardizing additives or manufacturing residues. It is convenient to estimate the total amount of metallic salts by ashing.[18,33,43] Assays of specific metals may be obtained by routine chemical methods.[7,14]

Stain components which exert a considerable influence on performance include the azures, methylene violet Bernthsen, eosin, and metallic salts.[39,41,43]

Reticulocyte Stains

The reticulocyte is the form of the immature erythrocyte produced by treatment of unfixed blood with cationic dyes or any other agents which precipitate ribonucleoprotein (RNP).[65-70] This precipitate has been variously termed granulofilamentous substance, reticulofilamentous substance, and reticulum.

Reticulocyte staining is an essential technique in diagnostic hematology, the number of reticulocytes in peripheral blood being a fairly accurate indication of erythropoietic activity. In this section some aspects of reticulocyte staining are described briefly. A detailed review of these topics has recently been published.[71]

Staining Techniques

Vital Staining

Correctly, this is the process of staining living cells. The term is commonly applied to reticulocyte staining, but is not strictly applicable. It has been demonstrated that treatment of blood with potassium cyanide before staining does not reduce the reticulocyte count,[72] and that cationic dyes kill immature erythrocytes at the concentrations used in reticulocyte stains.[65] In the context of reticulocyte staining, the term "vital staining" has therefore been extended to imply staining that occurs before fixation.[73]

In techniques such as Romanowsky staining, where fixation precedes or accompanies staining, immature erythrocytes are demonstrated not as reticulocytes but as polychromatic or stippled cells.[67,68,73-79]

Effect of Technique on Morphology

The granulofilamentous substance may take the form of a definite network, a number of fragments and rods, a few scattered dots, or diffuse fine granules. Its appearance is heavily dependent upon the degree of cell maturity, i.e., the quantity of RNP, and upon technical factors. These latter include the vital dye used,[70,79,80] its concentration,[68,74,81,82] mode of application,[73] staining time,[82] and the pH of the staining solution.[81,83]

Classification of Techniques

The following classification of reticulocyte staining techniques is essentially that of Osgood and Wilhelm.[72]

1. Techniques in which the blood specimen is applied to a dry film of dye on a slide or coverslip
   - Wet preparations: blood is applied to the film of dye and the preparation is sealed to prevent drying.[73,78,84]
   - Dry preparations: blood is applied to the film of dye and allowed to dry.[77,78]
2. Techniques in which a dye solution is mixed directly with the blood specimen
   - On-slide techniques: dye solution and blood are mixed on a slide before the production of dry (smear) or wet preparations.[74,82]
   - Incubation techniques: dye solution and blood are mixed in a suitable container (pipette, test tube, watch glass) before the production of dry or wet preparations.[85-88]

Evaluation of Techniques

Techniques involving wet preparations produce specimens which are generally too thick, making counting both slow and tedious.[72] Techniques involving dry preparations are inefficient; preparations tend to dry before staining is complete, and thus only a fraction of the immature erythrocytes are demonstrated as reticulocytes.[72,89,90] Techniques in which a dye solution is mixed directly with the blood specimen are widely held to be the most satisfactory, with little demonstrable difference between preparations obtained with on-slide or incubation techniques.[72]

Permanent Preparations

Permanent reticulocyte preparations are made by using a Romanowsky method to counterstain a vitally stained smear. During fixation and counterstaining the vital dye is totally or partially replaced by the cationic dyes present in the counterstain, but the morphology of the granulofilamentous substance is unaffected by these processes.[91]

Stains

Many cationic dyes have been used as reticulocyte stains. Several of these are listed in Table 7, but only the most important will be considered further.

Acridine Orange (Figure 3)

This dye readily combines with RNP (more specifically, ribonucleic acid) to produce a complex that emits a characteristic orange-red fluorescence in ultraviolet light.[103-105]

Table 7
SOME DYES USED FOR RETICULOCYTE STAINING

Dye (CI number)	Ref.
Acridine orange (46005)	65, 70, 80, 81, 84, 88
Acridine yellow (46025)	80, 92
Auramine O (41000)	93
Azure B (52010)	86
Brilliant cresyl blue (51010)	65, 67, 69, 70, 74, 77, 79, 87, 94—100
Janus green B (11050)	67, 69, 73, 79, 94
Methylene blue (52015)	65, 67, 73, 80, 94
Neutral red (50040)	65, 67, 70, 79, 80, 101
New methylene blue (52030)	65, 85, 102
Nile blue sulphate (51180)	65, 67, 69, 80, 98
Polychrome methylene blue (—)	79, 94, 98
Toluidine blue (52040)	67, 70, 80

Acridine orange has therefore been used as a reticulocyte stain.[81,84,88,106] Reticulocyte counts made by using preparations stained with this and certain other fluorescent dyes, are likely to be higher than those obtained after staining with absorbing dyes, since small particles of granulofilamentous substance are readily detected only after fluorescence methods.[84,88,93,106] Details of an acridine orange-staining procedure are given in Table 8.

Azure B (Figure 3)

Azure B was recently introduced as a reticulocyte stain by Marshall et al.[86] The results obtained with this dye are comparable to those obtained with brilliant cresyl blue or new methylene blue. The purification of azure B is well documented,[15,18,31] and the use of this dye in pure form therefore affords a convenient approach to the standardization of reticulocyte staining. A method in which azure B is used is given in Table 8.

Brilliant Cresyl Blue (Figure 3)

Brilliant cresyl blue is probably still the most widely used reticulocyte stain. Commercial samples of this dye are variable mixtures of numerous colored components and metallic salts.[86] The major disadvantage of brilliant cresyl blue is, therefore, batch-to-batch inconsistency in performance. These inconsistencies apply to the staining intensity of the granulofilamentous substance, the contrast between the granulofilamentous substance and the cell background, and with dry preparations, the density of an extraneous particulate dye deposit.[85,86,88,102] Details of the brilliant cresyl blue procedure are given in Table 8.

New Methylene Blue (Figure 3)

This dye was introduced as a reticulocyte stain by Brecher.[85] It was recommended as a substitute for brilliant cresyl blue, since the commercial product was then considered to be less variable in composition and thus afforded reproducible results. A recent study has failed to confirm this assertion, showing that the composition and performance of several commercial batches of new methylene blue varied greatly.[86]

Details of Brecher's method are shown in Table 8.

Table 8
METHODS FOR STAINING RETICULOCYTES

Composition of stain	Staining procedure	Results	Ref.
0.01% w/v acridine orange in 0.89% w/v aqueous sodium chloride	Blood (fresh or anticoagulated) diluted ? 10 × with stain in pipette. Contents of pipette shaken for 2 min and suspension applied to slide. Suspension coverslipped and preparation sealed with petrolatum	Granulofilamentous substance fluoresces orange red in uv light (wavelengths < 440 nm), the background appears dark	Vander et al.[88]
0.5—1.0% w/v azure B in citrate saline (1 vol of 3% w/v aqueous sodium citrate dihydrate and 4 vol of 0.9% w/v aqueous sodium chloride)	Two to four volumes of blood (anticoagulated with EDTA-K_2) are mixed with two to three volumes of stain in a test tube. The mixture is incubated at 37°C for 15—20 min. The cells are then resuspended and "wedge" smears are made	Granulofilamentous substance is stained deep blue, the background is stained blue green	Marshall et al.[86]
1% w/v brilliant cresyl blue in 0.89% w/v aqueous sodium chloride	Four volumes of fresh blood are mixed with three to four volumes of stain on a slide. The slide is stored for 20 min in a moist chamber, removed, and the cells are resuspended. "Wedge" smears are made	Granulofilamentous substance is stained deep blue, the background is stained blue green	Seip[100]
0.5% w/v new methylene blue in 1.6% w/v aqueous potassium oxalate	Equal volumes of blood (fresh or oxalated) and stain mixed on a slide, then drawn into a capillary pipette and left to stand for 10 min. Mixture then expelled onto slide and "wedge" smears are made	Granulofilamentous substance is stained deep blue, the background is stained blue green	Brecher[85]

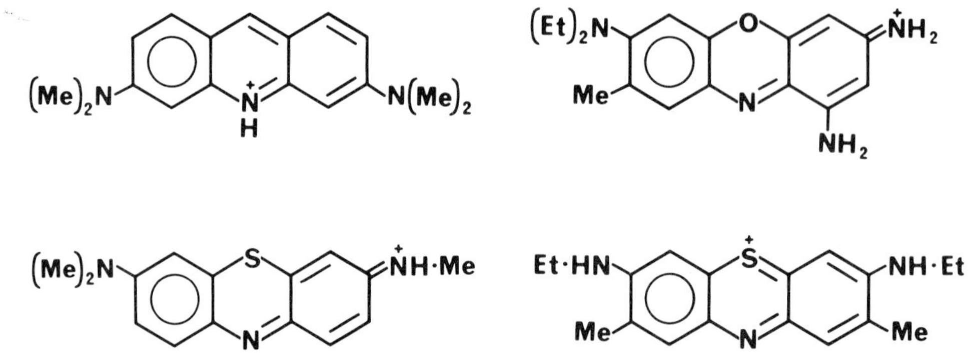

FIGURE 3. Structural formulae of dyes used in reticulocyte staining. Top left: acridine orange (CI 46005). Top right: brilliant cresyl blue (CI 51010). Bottom left: azure B (CI 52010). Bottom right: new methylene blue (CI 52030).

REFERENCES

1. **Malachowski, E.,** Zur Morphologie des Plasmodium malariae, *Zentralbl. Klin. Med.,* 12, 601, 1891.
2. **Romanowsky, D.,** Zur Frage der Parasitologie und Therapie der Malaria, *St. Petersburger Med. Wochenschr.,* 16, 297 and 307, 1891.
3. **Marshall, P. N.,** Romanowsky-type stains in haematology, *Histochem. J.,* 10, 1, 1978.
4. **Marshall, P. N.,** Romanowsky staining: state of the art and "ideal" techniques, in *College of American Pathologists 1977 Aspen Conference Proceedings,* College of American Pathologists, Skokie, 1979, Chap. 11.
5. **Venkataraman, K.,** *The Chemistry of Synthetic Dyes,* Vol. 2, Academic Press, New York, 1952, 747 and 792.
6. **Bellin, J. S. and Ronayne, M. E.,** Chromatographic analysis of photosensitizing dyes, *J. Chromatogr.,* 24, 131, 1966.
7. **Clemens, H. J. and Toepfer, K.,** Physikalische-chemische Eigenschaften von kommerziellen Thiazinfarbstoffen. II. Qualitative und quantitative Untersuchungen über die Verunreinigungen der Farbstoffe und das "Umlosën" zum Erhalt eines hohëren Reinheitsgrades, *Acta Histochem. Z. Histolog. Topochem.,* 31, 126, 1968.
8. **Dean, W. W., Lubrano, G. J., Heinsohn, H. G., and Stastny, M.,** The analysis of Romanowsky blood stains by high-performance liquid chromatography, *J. Chromatogr.,* 124, 287, 1976.
9. **Holmes, W.C.,** Subsidiary dyes in methylene blue, *Stain Technol.,* 2, 71, 1927.
10. **Holmes, W. C.,** The spectrophotometric evaluation of mixtures of methylene blue and trimethyl thionin, *Stain Technol.,* 3, 45, 1928.
11. **Lillie, R. D.,** Purification of the Thiazins and Spectra of Purified Dyes, Public Health Reports, Washington, Suppl. 178, 1944, 17.
12. **Lubrano, G. J., Dean, W. W., Heinsohn, H. G., and Stastny, M.,** The analysis of some commercial dyes and Romanowsky stains by high-performance liquid chromatography, *Stain Technol.,* 52, 13, 1977.
13. **Marshall, P. N. and Lewis, S. M.,** Batch variations in commercial dyes employed for Romanowsky-type staining: a thin-layer chromatographic study, *Stain Technol.,* 49, 351, 1974.
14. **Marshall, P. N. and Lewis, S. M.,** Metal contaminants in commercial thiazine dyes, *Stain Technol.,* 50, 143, 1975.
15. **Nerenberg, C. and Fisher, R.,** Purification of thionin, azure A, azure B, and methylene blue, *Stain Technol.,* 38, 75, 1963.
16. **Taylor, K. B.,** Chromatographic separation and isolation of metachromatic thiazine dyes, *J. Histochem. Cytochem.,* 8, 248, 1960.
17. **Marshall, P. N., Bentley, S. A., and Lewis, S. M.,** A standardized Romanowsky stain prepared from purified dyes, *J. Clin. Pathol.,* 28, 920, 1975.
18. **Marshall, P. N. and Lewis, S. M.,** The purification of methylene blue and azure B by solvent extraction and crystallization, *Stain Technol.,* 50, 375, 1975.

19. **Field, J. W.**, Further note on a method of staining malarial parasites in thick blood films, *Trans. R. Soc. Trop. Med. Hyg.*, 35, 35, 1941—1942.
20. **Leishman, W. B.**, Note on a simple and rapid method of producing Romanowsky staining in malarial and other blood films, *Br. Med. J.*, ii, 757, 1901.
21. **Lillie, R. D.**, Studies on polychrome methylene blue. II. Acid oxidation methods of polychroming, *Stain Technol.*, 17, 97, 1942.
22. **Lillie, R. D.**, Studies on polychrome methylene blue. III. Alkali methods of polychroming, *Stain Technol.*, 18, 1, 1943.
23. **Lillie, R. D.**, A Giemsa Stain of Quite Constant Composition and Performance, Made in the Laboratory From Eosin and Methylene Blue, Public Health Reports, Washington, 58, 1943, 449.
24. **MacNeal, W. J.**, Methylene violet and methylene azure A and B, *J. Infect. Dis.*, 36, 538, 1925.
25. **MacNeal, W. J. and Killian, J. A.**, Chemical studies on polychrome methylene blue, *J. Am. Chem. Soc.*, 48, 740, 1926.
26. **Singh, J. and Bhattacharji, L. M.**, Rapid staining of malarial parasites by a water soluble stain, *Indian Med. Gaz.*, 79, 102, 1944.
27. **Toepfer, K.**, Die Darstellung von Dimethylthionin (Azur A) für histochemische Reaktionen, *Acta Histochem. Z. Histolog. Topochem.*, 35, 195, 1970.
28. **Wright, J. H.**, A rapid method for the differential staining of blood films and malarial parasites, *J. Med. Res.*, 7, 138, 1902.
29. **Marshall, P. N.**, The composition of stains produced by the oxidation of methylene blue, *Histochem. J.*, 8, 431, 1976.
30. **Wittekind, D., Kretschmer, V., and Löhr, W.**, Kann Azur B-Eosin die May-Grünwald — Giemsa — Färbung ersetzen? *Blut*, 32, 71, 1976.
31. **Lohr, W., Grubhofer, N., Sohmer, I., and Wittekind, D.**, The azure dyes: their purification and physicochemical properties. II. Purification of azure B, *Stain Technol.*, 50, 149, 1975.
32. **Hanig, I. and Koch, L.**, Quantitative paper chromatography of D & C Red No. 21 (tetrabromofluorescein), *J. Assoc. Off. Agric. Chem.*, 46, 1010, 1963.
33. **Marshall, P. N., Bentley, S. A., and Lewis, S. M.**, A procedure for assaying commercial samples of eosin, *Stain Technol.*, 50, 107, 1975.
34. **Roe, M. A., Wilcox, A., and Lillie, R. D.**, Eosinates of the Azures and Methylene Blue in Preparation of a Satisfactory Giemsa Stain from Dyes of American Manufacture, Public Health Reports, Washington, 56, 1941, 1906.
35. Nocht, — Zur Farbung der Malariaparasiten, *Zentralbl. Bakt. Parasitkde, Infektionskr. Hyg. Abteilung I*, 24, 839, 1898.
36. **Kingsley, D. M.**, A new hematological stain. I. Constituents and methods of use. *Stain Technol.*, 10, 127, 1935.
37. **MacNeal, W. J.**, Tetrachrome blood stain: an economical and satisfactory imitation of Leishman's stain, *J. Am. Med. Assoc.*, 78, 1122, 1922.
38. **Marshall, P. N., Bentley, S. A., and Lewis, S. M.**, Standardization of Romanowsky stains. The relationship between stain composition and performance, *Scand. J. Haematol.*, 20, 206, 1978.
39. **Wittekind, D. and Löhr, W.**, Purification, standardization and quality control of Romanowsky dyes, in *Quality Control in Haematology. Symposium of the International Committee for Standardization in Haematology*, Lewis, S. M. and Coster, J. F., Eds., Academic Press, London, 1975, chap. 12.
40. **Lillie, R. D.**, Blood and malaria parasite staining with eosin azure methylene blue methods, *Am. J. Public Health*, 33, 948, 1943.
41. **Lillie, R. D.**, Factors influencing the Romanowsky staining of blood films and the role of methylene violet, *J. Lab. Clin. Med.*, 29, 1181, 1944.
42. **Lillie, R. D., and Roe, M. A.**, Studies on polychrome methylene blue. I. Eosinates, their spectra and staining capacity, *Stain Technol.*, 17, 57, 1942.
43. **Marshall, P. N., Bentley, S. A., and Lewis, S. M.**, An evaluation of some commercial Romanowsky stains, *J. Clin. Pathol.*, 28, 680, 1975.
44. **Saal, J. R.**, Giemsa stain for the diagnosis of bovine babesiosis. I. Staining properties of commercial samples and their component dyes, *J. Protozool.*, 11, 573, 1964.
45. **Scott, R. E. and French, R. W.**, Standardization of biological stains, *Mil. Surg.*, 55, 229 and 337, 1924.
46. **Toepfer, K.**, Analyse der May-Grunwald-Giemsafarbung als Beitrag zur Notwendigkeit des Arbeitens mit reinen, definierten Farbstoffen, *Verh. Dtsch. Ges. Innere Med.*, 78, 272, 1972.
47. **Gilliland, J. W., Rogers, C. H., and Sage, B. H.**, Blood stain for automatic differential analysis of leukocytes, *Clin. Lab. Prod.*, 3, 2, 1974.
48. **Lillie, R. D.**, The Deterioration of Romanowsky Stain Solutions in Various Organic Solvents, Public Health Reports, Washington, Suppl. 178, 1944, 1.
49. **Dean, W. W., Stastny, M., and Lubrano, G. J.**, The degradation of Romanowsky-type blood stains in methanol, *Stain Technol.*, 52, 35, 1977.

50. **Bernthsen, A.**, Studien in der Methylenblaugruppe, *Justus Leibigs Ann. Chem.*, 230, 137, 1885.
51. **Emery, A. J., Hazen, F. K., and Stotz, E.**, Spectrophotometric characteristics and assay of biological stains. III. The xanthenes, *Stain Technol.*, 25, 201, 1950.
52. **Stotz, E., Conn, H. J., Knapp, F. and Emery, A. J.**, Spectrophotometric characteristics and assay of biological stains, *Stain Technol.*, 25, 57, 1950.
53. **Toepfer, K.**, Die Thiazinfarbstoffe. Eigenschaften und Verhalten unter experimentellen Bedingungen, *Prog. Histochem. Cytochem.*, 1, 277, 1970.
54. **Löhr, W., Sohmer, I., and Wittekind, D.**, The azure dyes: their purification and physicochemical properties. I. Purification of azure A, *Stain Technol.*, 49, 359, 1974.
55. **Ball, J. and Jackson, D. S.**, Histological, chromatographic and spectrophotometric studies of toluidine blue, *Stain Technol.*, 28, 33, 1953.
56. **Graichen, C. and Molitor, J. C.**, Studies on coal-tar colors. XXII. 4,5-dibromofluorescein and related bromofluoresceins, *J. Assoc. Off. Agric. Chem.*, 42, 149, 1959.
57. **Horobin, R. W.**, Analysis and purification of biological stains by gel filtration, *Stain Technol.*, 46, 297, 1971.
58. **Horobin, R. W. and Murgatroyd, L. B.**, A comparison of rapid electrophoretic and chromatographic methods for the investigation of common histological dyes, *Histochemie*, 11, 141, 1967.
59. **Loach, K. W.**, Thin-layer chromatographic separation of methylene blue and related thiazine dyes, *J. Chromatogr.*, 60, 119, 1971.
60. **Marshall, P. N. and Lewis, S. M.**, A rapid thin-layer chromatographic system for Romanowsky blood stains, *Stain Technol.*, 49, 235, 1974.
61. **Persijn, J.-P.**, Improved solvents for paper chromatography of thiazine stains, *Stain Technol.*, 36, 27, 1961.
62. **Rahman, A. U., Sotorres, A. M., and Pasquare, N. J.**, Resolucion electroforetica y cromatographica de azul de toluidine y azur "A" en relocian a sus propiedades metachromaticas con heparina, *An. Asoc. Quim. Argent.*, 59, 111, 1971.
63. **Toepfer, K.**, Die Standardisierung von Thiazinfarbstoffen, *Acta Histochem. Z. Histolog. Topochem.*, Suppl. X, 215, 1971.
64. **Amos, R. and Perry, S. G.**, Liquid chromatography — columns or thin layers?, *J. Chromatogr.*, 83, 245, 1973.
65. **Bessis, M. and Breton-Gorius, J.**, Le réticulocyte. Colorations vitales et microscopie électronique, *Nouv. Rev. Fr. Hematol.*, 4, 77, 1964.
66. **Burt, N. S., Murray, R. G. E., and Rossiter, R. J.**, Nucleic acids of rabbit reticulocytes, *Blood*, 6, 906, 1951.
67. **Dustin, P.**, Contribution à l'étude histophysiologique et histochimique des globules rouges des Vertébres, *Arch. Biol. (Paris)*, 55, 285, 1944.
68. **Jensen, W. N., Moreno, G. D., and Bessis, M. C.**, An electron microscopic description of basophilic stippling in red cells, *Blood*, 25, 933, 1965.
69. **Seno, S., Yoshizawa, K., Nakamoto, T., and Kanda, S.**, A morphologic study of reticulocytes with special reference to the substantia granulo-filamentosa, *Folia Haematol. (Frankfurt)*, 2, 269, 1958.
70. **Staubesand, J., Wittekind, D., and Rentsch, G.**, Electronenmikroskopische Untersuchungen zum Feinbau der Reticulocyten. I. Mitteilung: Farbstoffabhängige Variationen in der Struktur der Substantia granulo-filamentosa, *Z. Zellforsch.*, 69, 344, 1966.
71. **Marshall, P. N.**, Reticulation, polychromasia and stippling of erythrocytes, *Microsc. Acta*, 81, 89, 1978.
72. **Osgood, E. E. and Wilhelm, M. M.**, Reticulocytes, *J. Lab. Clin. Med.*, 19, 1129, 1934.
73. **Davidson, L. S. P.**, The basophilic substance of the erythrocyte, *Edinburgh Med. J.* 37, 425, 1930.
74. **Brookfield, R. W.**, Blood changes occurring during the course of treatment of malignant disease by lead, with special reference to punctate basophilia and the platelets, *J. Pathol. Bacteriol.*, 31, 277, 1928.
75. **Brückner, H.**, Arbeiten über die basophile substanz in den jugendlichen roten Blutkörperchen. II. Uber die physikalisch-chemischen Eigenschaften der basophilen Substanz in den judendlichen Erythrocyten, *Archiv Hyg.*, 98, 95, 1927.
76. **Brückner, H. and Spatz, R.**, Über die Beurteilung des roten Blutbildes bei der Bleivergiftung unter Berücksichtigung verschiedener Darstellungsmethoden der polychromaten und basophil punktierten Erythrocyten, *Archiv Hyg.*, 97, 277, 1926.
77. **Davidson, S., McCrie, J. G., and Lovell Gulland, G.**, The treatment of pernicious anaemia with liver and liver extracts, *Lancet*, 214, 847, 1928.
78. **Hawes, J. B.**, A study of the reticulated red blood corpuscle by means of vital staining methods. Its relation to polychromatophilia and stippling, *Boston Med. Surg. J.*, 161, 493, 1909.
79. **Key, J. A.**, Studies on erythrocytes, with special reference to reticulum, polychromatophilia and mitochondria, *Arch. Intern. Med.*, 28, 511, 1921.

80. **Wittekind, D. and Rentsch, G.,** Farbabhangige Strukturvariationen der Substantia granulofilamentosa der Reticulozyten, *Blut,* 18, 13, 1968.

81. **Kosenow, W.,** Uber den Strukturwandel der basophilen Substanz junger Erythrozyten im Fluoreszenzmikroskop, *Acta haematol.,* 7, 360, 1952.

82. **Marcussen, P. V.,** The counting of reticulocytes, with special reference to the accuracy of the method, *Folia haematol. (Leipzig),* 61, 49, 1938.

83. **Gawrilow, R.,** Zur Lehre über die vitalfärbbare Substanz der Erythrozyten, *Folia Haematol. (Leipzig),* 38, 216, 1929.

84. **Marmont, A.,** Acridine orange fluorescence microscopy in haematology, in *Proc. 7th Congr. Eur. Soc. Haematol. London 1959,* Part 2, Bernard, J. and Disccombe, G., Eds., Karger, Basel, 1960, 361.

85. **Brecher, G.,** New methylene blue as a reticulocyte stain, *Am. J. Clin. Pathol.,* 19, 895, 1949.

86. **Marshall, P. N., Bentley, S. A., and Lewis, S. M.,** Purified azure B as a reticulocyte stain, *J. Clin. Pathol.,* 29, 1060, 1976.

87. **Robertson, O. H.,** The effects of experimental plethora on blood production, *J. Exp. Med.,* 26, 221, 1917.

88. **Vander, J. B., Harris, C. A., and Ellis, S. R.,** Reticulocyte counts by means of fluorescence microscopy, *J. Lab. Clin. Med.,* 62, 132, 1963.

89. **Trachtenberg, F.,** Retikulozytenstudien. I. Mitteilung: Zahl und Differenzierungsformel der Retikulozyten biem Normalen, *Folia Haematol. (Leipzig),* 46, 1, 1932.

90. **Whitby, L. E. H. and Britton, C. J. C.,** The relation of the stippled cell and the polychromatic cell to the reticulocyte, *Lancet,* 224, 1173, 1933.

91. **Nittis, S.,** The nature and the mechanism of staining of the erythrocytic reticulum, *Am. J. Med. Sci.,* 196, 177, 1938.

92. **Kosenow, W. and Mai, H.,** Über die Fluoreszenzmikroskopie der Blutzellen, *Z. Kinderheilk.,* 70, 552, 1952.

93. **Joossens, J. V. and Hendrickx, M.,** Une nouvelle méthode de numération des réticulocytes en microscopic de fluorescence, *Presse Med.,* 54, 536, 1946.

94. **Cunningham, T. D.,** A method for the permanent staining of reticulated red cells, *Arch. Intern. Med.,* 26, 405, 1920.

95. **Feissinger, N. and Laur, C.-M.,** Technique de préparation des hématies granuleuses ou réticulocytes, *Sang,* 4, 257, 1930.

96. **Heath, C. W. and Daland, G. A.,** The life of reticulocytes. Experiments on their maturation, *Arch. Intern. Med.,* 46, 533, 1930.

97. **Heath, C. W. and Daland, G. A.,** Staining of reticulocytes by brilliant cresyl blue. Influence of solutions of substances, *Arch. Intern. Med.,* 48, 133, 1931.

98. **Klima, R. and Rosegger, H.,** Untersuchungen über Färbbarkeit, Resistenz und Formeigenheiten der menschlichen Retikulocyten, *Folia haematol. (Leipzig),* 51, 414, 1934.

99. **Nizet, A.,** Recherches sur la physiopathologie des hematies I. Nouvelles techniques pour l'étude et la distinction des hematies granuleuses, *Acta Med. Scand.,* 117, 199, 1944.

100. **Seip, M.,** Reticulocyte studies. The liberation of red blood corpuscles from the bone marrow into the peripheral blood and the production of erythrocytes elucidated by reticulocyte investigations, *Acta Med. Scand.,* Suppl. 282, 146, 1953.

101. **Israel, O. and Pappenheim, A.,** Über die Entkernung der Saugethiererythroblasten, *Virchows Arch. Pathol. Anat. Physiol.,* 143, 419, 1896.

102. **Dacie, J. V. and Lewis, S. M.,** *Practical Haematology,* 5th ed., Churchill Livingstone, Edinburgh, 1975, 79.

103. **Armstrong, J. A.,** Histochemical differentiation of nucleic acids by means of induced fluorescence, *Exp. Cell Res.,* 11, 640, 1956.

104. **von Bertalanffy, L. and Bickis, I.,** Identification of cytoplasmic basophilia (ribonucleic acid) by fluorescence microscopy, *J. Histochem. Cytochem.,* 4, 481, 1956.

105. **Kasten, F. H.,** Cytochemical studies with acridine orange and the influence of dye contaminants in the staining of nucleic acids, *Int. Rev. Cytol.,* 21, 141, 1967.

106. **Thaer, A. A.,** Microfluorometric analysis of the reticulocyte population in peripheral blood of mammals, in *Cytology Automation. Proceedings of Second Tenovus Symposium, Cardiff 24th—25th October 1968,* Evans, D. M. D., Ed., Churchill, Livingstone, Edinburgh, 1970, 189.

AUTOMATION OF MORPHOLOGY IN HEMATOLOGY

J. W. Bacus

The use of new processing techniques to analyze and classify peripheral blood cells has developed rapidly in the last few years. This technology has now matured to the point where instruments are used routinely in clinical laboratories for automatic processing of blood specimens on a daily basis. This chapter provides: (1) a brief history of the development of these automated morphology systems, (2) a description of the physical principles of operation, including image digitization and pattern recognition classification techniques, and (3) a summary and evaluation of these automated systems. Other techniques also exist for performing substitute methods for morphology automation. Generally, these have involved flow methodology, enzyme staining, fluorescent light scattering, etc. These techniques have been adequately reviewed elsewhere[24-27,33] and will not be addressed here.

Brief History of the Development of Automated Morphology Systems

Table 1 lists some of the major research efforts, with a brief summary of the contributions each study has made to the development of some of our current automated morphology systems. This is not a complete list of all the research that has been performed in this area. A more comprehensive history of the development of automated morphology systems is contained in Reference 34.

The first automated classification results on blood cell images were obtained by Prewitt and Mendelsohn in 1966.[1] In this study a small select group of about 22 blood cell images — which were prepared according to a special staining procedure — were digitized, and features were extracted from the optical density histogram of each cell image. Analysis separated the cells into four classes: neutrophils, eosinophils, lymphocytes, and monocytes. A succession of research efforts[2-7] gradually increased the number of cell types that could be automatically classified. In a study by Ingram and Preston,[2] an on-line scanning microscope system was constructed for the classification of three categories of blood cells: monocytes, lymphocytes, and neutrophils. This apparatus located and classified the cells, and the results were compared with differential counts performed by technicians. A 100-cell differential count on this early prototype instrument took about 12 hr. Results from seven differential counts were reported.[2] In 1969, Young[3] published results of an automated classification of five cell classes, and in 1971, Bacus[5] published results extending classification algorithms to include all of the six major normal cell categories, including segmented and band neutrophils. Bacus also strongly advocated the confusion matrix method of analysis for the evaluation of machine classification accuracy, and compared the machine classifications with those of technologists on a cell-by-cell basis. It was after these first four studies[1-3,5] that most of the instrument developments were initiated, leading to the automated differential counters that exist today.

Concurrently with the development of these automated differential counters, other research was also taking place. For example, in 1974, Brenner et al.[13] extended the number of cell types classified in a research environment to 17. During the early 1970s a number of groups started exploring methods of using digital image-processing technology to analyze red blood cells. Initially, Green[15] and Bentley and Lewis[16] simply measured size, density, and shape of normal red blood cells or single populations of red cells. Later, Bacus[17] and Bentley and Lewis[18] developed techniques to extend this methodology to automatically identify subcategories of normal and abnormal red cells. In 1977, Bacus and Weens[19] extended these classification strategies to the analysis of

Table 1
RESEARCH RELATED TO THE DEVELOPMENT OF AUTOMATED MORPHOLOGY

Summary	Ref.
4 Cell types, optical density histogram for features	1
3 Cell types, Golay logic	2
5 Cell types, color	4
6—9 Cell types, comparison of cell classification errors made by machines and by morphologists	6
17 Cell types	13
Size, density, and shape measures on normal blood cells	15, 16
Classification of abnormal red cells	17, 18
Automated RBC morphology related to anemia diagnosis	19
Abnormal lymphocytes, B and T lymphocytes, nuclear texture measurements	20, 22

specimens with clearly defined anemias and compared the results with those obtained with normal specimens. In this same time frame, work continued on abnormal types of white blood cells. Necheles et al.[20] studied lymphocytes and acute leukemia and used simple nuclear and cell area descriptors to predict the duration of remission in leukemic patients. Bartels et al.[21-23] have used measurements of nuclear size, density, and texture to study the distinction between B and T lymphocytes.

Principles of Image Processing and Pattern Recognition Systems

Image Digitization

Figure 1 represents four processing stages in the quantification, analysis, and classification of single cell images. These operations comprise the major conceptual steps in the automated processing of blood smears and in the description of cell morphologies; each will be discussed in turn.

The acquisition of the digital image is the first step in the quantification of morphology. The microscope generates an optical image that is an intensity mapping, in the image plane, of the optical density of the object of interest. Figure 2 shows the digitization process. An optical image of a blood cell is indicated (A), with one scan line of an electro-optical conversion device indicated across the image. The resulting analog signal relates to the optical density of the image (C). This analog signal has been quantized into grey levels (D). Repeated lines scanned at small incremental levels result in a two-dimensional matrix (B). This can be conveniently stored in a digital computer as a two-dimensional array of numbers, with the smaller numbers relating to low optical densities and higher numbers, or grey levels, relating to higher optical densities.

There are several methods of digitization, the choice of which depends upon matching the advantages and disadvantages of the particular method to the solution of the

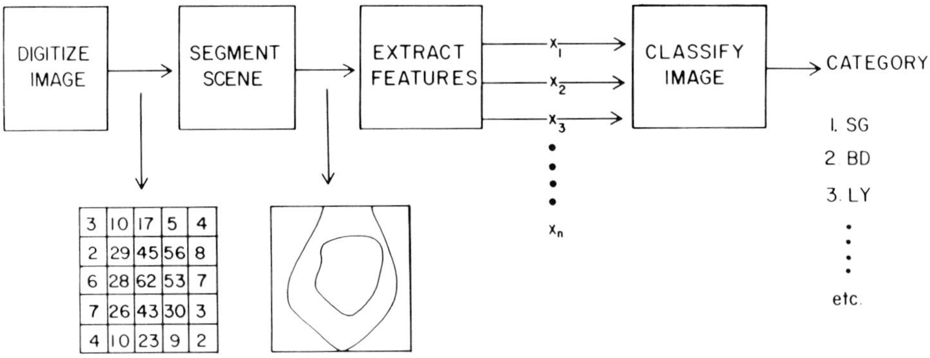

FIGURE 1. Four processing steps in the quantification, analysis, and classification of individual blood cell images.

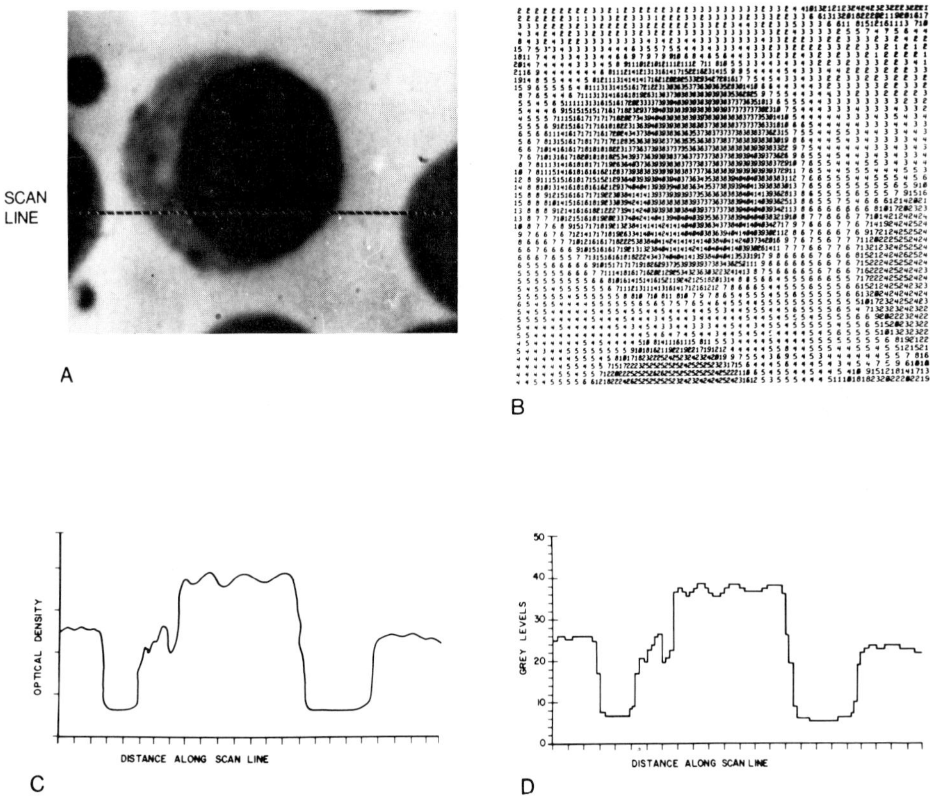

FIGURE 2. Image digitization process. (A) Optical image of a blood cell. (B) Two-dimensional matrix. (C) Optical density. (D) Grey levels.

instrument requirements.[35-37] For example, four methods are: (1) flying spot scanning, (2) rotating mirror systems, (3) image array devices, and (4) television digitization. In the cathode ray tube (CRT) flying spot scanner method, a computer or some other logic controls a D/A converter to position an illumination point on a CRT faceplate. A front optical system maps that point onto a point in the specimen — in the object plane — and a back optical system collects the light in the object plane for analog conversion in a photomultiplier tube. The output of the photomultiplier tube is in turn sampled by analogue to digital conversion circuitry, and the resultant digital values are stored in an array as indicated in Figure 1. A second photomultiplier tube can be used to monitor the incident light to correct for uneven illumination from the CRT phosphor, and to obtain a base-line signal for the conversion of the transmitted light to optical density measurements. Advantages of this type of system are extremely reliable determinations of the optical density in the object plane, wide variation of spatial resolution, and the possibility of utilizing either a continuous raster scan or a random access mode. The disadvantages include the restrictions imposed by the spectral characteristics of the various CRT phosphors, and restrictive configurations of the system relating to the interactive human visual observations in the object plane.

The rotating mirror type of flying spot scanner incorporates a fixed source of illumination, such as a tungsten source or an arc lamp. Otherwise, the principles involved are the same as for a CRT flying spot system. This modification overcomes the restriction of range of spectral illumination in the CRT system, but a disadvantage is the necessary introduction of mechanical scanning devices to scan the object plane.

Image sensing arrays have recently been developed and have been incorporated into the television type of video cameras that can either be run by television sync generators or directly controlled by computer or other logic. Advantages of these arrays are their small physical size and their compatibility with television equipment while still providing the photocell type of recording characteristics. Disadvantages include the lack of wide spectral sensitivity, especially in the blue and uv regions.

Image digitization can be obtained directly from television signals by sampling at fixed rates with an A/D converter into a computer. Advantages of this are the wide variety and low cost of video hardware, and the general applicability to the sampling of any optical image. The main disadvantage is that optical densities in the object plane are not measured accurately without the incorporation of specialized circuitry.

Scene Segmentation

After the digitized image is stored in computer memory, the next step is to automatically isolate, in terms of finding boundaries or regions, morphological areas of interest in the scene. This can be accomplished by outlining the nucleus region, the cytoplasm region, background areas, touching red cells, etc. Common techniques involve monochromatic optical density, or grey level histograms,[1] bivariate color-density distributions,[42] boundary and edge-finding algorithms,[38] or combinations of the above.[41] Since blood stains encountered in practice are often bispectral, many automated approaches have used color information to obtain the scene segmentation.[4,40,42,43] Multispectral approaches have also been used in bone marrow analysis.[39] Obviously, if this step is not performed properly, features such as area, size, color, etc. (which will be described in the next section) will not be measured correctly. For red cell analysis, scene segmentation is most easily accomplished by setting a clipping level, using illumination only at 418 nm. This works well if the scene is evenly illuminated with no shading.

The evaluation and comparison of scene analysis procedures have been largely subjective or inferential, i.e., accomplished by showing photographs of "improved" results. Recently, a quantitative error measure useful in the comparison of scene analysis techniques has been developed that may help to alleviate some of the previous problems in evaluating the differences between various methods.[44]

Feature Measurement

Although the methods of measurement vary greatly in the various research efforts and in the instruments that have been developed, a common set of features has gradually evolved. In general, these relate to conceptual entities such as nuclear size, nu-

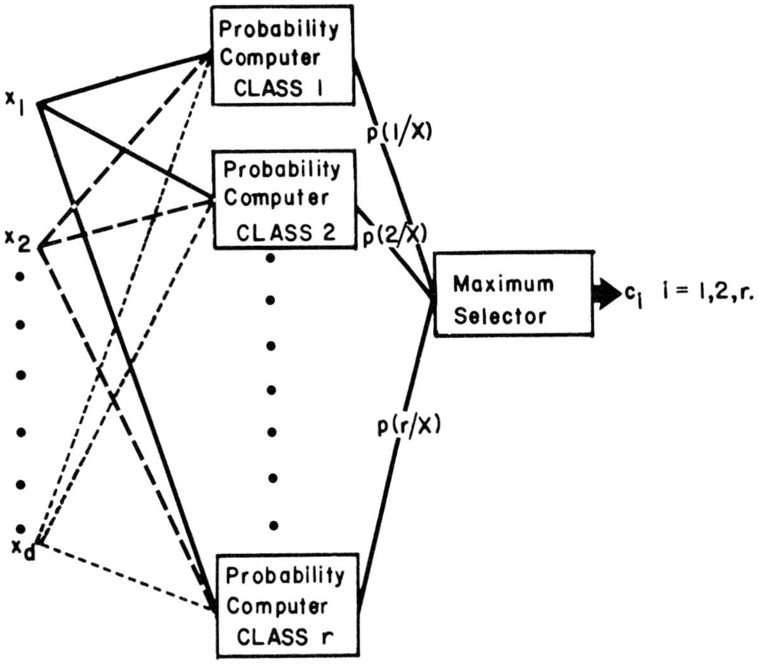

FIGURE 3. The use of the feature vector, as an input in a statistical classifier to compute the probability that the cell described belongs in any one of the various specified categories.

clear density, cytoplasm size, cytoplasm color, various nuclear shape measurements, and, in some cases, nuclear texture.[6,13] Red blood cell measurements have been made of size, shape, central pallor, and optical density as related to hemoglobin content on an individual cell basis.[15,19]

Variations in the feature measurements primarily result from differences in image digitization and scene segmentation. This results in different configurations of the image in computer memory. Also, differences in spectral configurations of the instrumentation and in staining technique significantly alter feature measurements. For example, the measurement of color can be defined in many ways. It obviously depends on the stain used, the spectral thruput of the entire system, the number of color measurements made, and the mathematical definition of color used. Similarly, there can be many different definitions of shape, although the definition of circularity as — the perimeter squared of an object divided by the area — is in common use. No standard definition of texture has, as yet, evolved.

Cell Classification

As described in the last section, a number of features are generally measured on each cell image as it stays in the "digital aperture" of a pattern recognition system. These measurements can then be thought of as a feature vector, which represents this image in an n-dimensional measurement space. There are two major methods of cell classification that utilize this information. One relates to creating a mathematical model in the n-dimensional space, such as a multivariate Gausian model, which describes the clusters of measurement values as they characteristically relate to each cell category.[45,46] In this case, the measurements from each cell would be passed into a series of probability calculators as indicated in Figure 3, which would calculate the probability that the cell belonged to any one of a specified number of categories. The computation resulting in the highest probability would signify which was the most probable class, based upon the measurements given. Much of the research work and implementation of existing systems use this type of classification technique.

Another major method of classification is to use decision logic, that is, to consider one or multiple sets of features at each stage in the logic. A system of white blood cell classification based on this technique has been proposed,[12] and a system of red blood cell classification[19] also illustrates this technique well.

Clinical Evaluation of Systems

Four commercial systems currently exist that automatically perform the white blood cell differential count. These are: (1) DIFF 3, (2) ADC® 500,[43] (3) HEMATRAK®,[10] and (4) LARC®.[54,55] The evaluation of these systems in the clinical setting has proved to be a very difficult process. The principal problem relates to the separation of the statistical error inherent in counting[47] from the automatic machine classification errors on individual cells, as compared to the classification errors of the trained technologist,[7] and defining an appropriate comparison metric useful for these analyses. The HEMATRAK® and the LARC®, which were introduced in the early 1970s, have been used in more clinical studies than the other systems. Principal studies have been reported for the LARC®,[48,49] for the HEMATRAK®,[30-32] and for the DIFF 3.[50] The ADC® 500[43] has only recently been announced and has not yet been thoroughly evaluated.

With regard to cell classification accuracy, a summary of the evidence would indicate that on a cell-by-cell basis, the instruments are performing at about a 90 to 95% accuracy level on neutrophils, eosinophils, and lymphocytes, as compared to technologist accuracies of approximately 99%.[7] Monocytes seem to be somewhat less accurately classified, probably less than 90% for most instruments, as compared to the technologist 95% level. Basophils are difficult to evaluate because of their low percentage of occurrence, but the automated instruments are probably also somewhat less than 90% accurate on these cells, as compared to the greater-than-99% accuracy for technologists. In general, the state-of-the-art for classification of the normal cells is at a point where most of the errors that occur relate to fluctuations in staining cells and artifactual distortions of cells in preparations. For example, if a machine misses a smudge cell that can barely be identified by a human as a neutrophil, should this be counted as a mistake?

Classification errors for segmented and band neutrophils should be evaluated by using operating characteristic curve techniques. The two instruments that have provided data to assess these classifications[51,52] have indicated that the classification errors are at points on the curve where there are few errors for segmented neutrophils — approximately 3% and high errors for band neutrophils — approximately 35%. Clearly, this is an area where improvements should be made, and there is some active research in this area.[53] The principal problem seems to be overlapping and touching nucleus portions, as indicated by Mui, Fu, and Bacus.[28]

Thus the current automated instruments are not quite as accurate as the best human classifiers for normal cells. As is well known, however, there are large random errors in the manual differential count, which come from many sources. One of the advantages of automated techniques is that they are reproducible and are not subject to these large random errors. For example, in practice, there are many untrained technologists who have higher errors than those referred to above for manual methods. Another important consideration is that because the statistical errors associated with manual counts are so much higher than the classification errors described above, comparable performance levels, with higher precision and greater thruput can be obtained with the automated equipment. Studies have definitely shown that reproducibility is greater with the automated differential counters than with the manual techniques.[48] The accuracy of classification of abnormal cells has not been documented thoroughly.

REFERENCES

1. **Prewitt, J. M. S. and Mendelsohn, M. L.**, The analysis of cell images, *Ann. N.Y. Acad. Sci.*, 128, 1035, 1966.
2. **Ingram, M. L. and Preston, K., Jr.**, Automatic analysis of blood cells, *Sci. Am.*, 223, 72, 1970.
3. **Young, I. T.**, Automated Leukocyte Recognition, Ph.D. thesis, Massachusetts Institute of Technology, Cambridge, 1969.
4. **Young, I. T.**, The classification of white blood cells, *IEEE Trans. Biomed. Eng.*, 19, 291, 1972.
5. **Bacus, J. W.**, An Automated Classification of the Peripheral Blood Leukocytes by Means of Digital Image Processing, Ph.D. thesis, University of Illinois Medical Center, Urbana, 1971.
6. **Bacus, J. W. and Gose, E. E.**, Leukocyte pattern recognition, *IEEE Trans. Syst. Man Cybern.*, 2, 513, 1972.
7. **Bacus, J. W.**, The observer error in peripheral blood cell classification, *Am. J. Clin. Pathol.*, 59, 223, 1973.
8. **Bacus, J. W. and Trobaugh, F. E., Jr.**, An Automated Classification of Peripheral Blood Cells by Means of Digital Image Processing. I. Theory of Operation. II. Development and Testing of a Working Laboratory Model, presented before XIV Int. Congr. of Hematol., Sao Paulo, Brazil, Abstr. 47 and 48, July 1972.
9. **Bacus, J. W.**, Design and Performance of an Automated Leukocyte Classifier, IEEE catalog number 74CH0885-4C, in Proc. 2nd Int. Jt. Conf. Pattern Recognition, 1974, 374.
10. **Miller, M. N.**, Design and clinical results of Hematrak®, an automated differential counter, *IEEE Trans. Biomed. Eng.*, BME-23, 400, 1976.
11. **Ornstein, L. and Ansley, H. R.**, Spectral matching of classical cytochemistry to automated cytology, *J. Histochem. Cytochem.*, 22, 453, 1974.
12. **Tycko, D. H., Anbalagan, S., Liu, H. C., and Ornstein, L.**, Automatic leukocyte classification using cytochemically stained smears, *J. Histochem. Cytochem.*, 24, 178, 1976.
13. **Brenner, J. F., Gelsema, E. S., Necheles, T. F., Neurath, P. W., Selles, W. D., and Vastola, E.**, Automated classification of normal and abnormal leukocytes, *J. Histochem. Cytochem.*, 22, 697, 1974.
14. **Eden, M.**, Image processing techniques in relation to studies of red cell shape, in *Red Cell Shape*, Bessis, M., Weed, R. I., and Leblong, P. F., Eds., Springer-Verlag, New York, 1973, 141.
15. **Green, J. E.**, Computer Methods for Erythrocyte Analysis, IEEE catalog no. 70CS1C, in Proc. Symp. Feature Extraction and Selection in Pattern Recognition, Argonne, Ill., October 1970, 100.
16. **Bentley, S. A. and Lewis, S. M.**, The use of an image analyzing computer for the quantitation of red cell morphological characteristics, *Br. J. Haematol.*, 29, 81, 1975.
17. **Bacus, J. W., Belanger, M. G., Aggarwal, R. K., and Trobaugh, F. E., Jr.**, Image processing for automated erythrocyte classification, *J. Histochem. Cytochem.*, 24, 195, 1976.
18. **Bentley, S. A. and Lewis, S. M.**, The morphological classification of red cells using an image analyzing computer, *Br. J. Haematol.*, 32, 205, 1976.
19. **Bacus, J. W. and Weens, J. H.**, An automated method of differential red blood cell classification with application to the diagnosis of anemia, *J. Histochem. Cytochem.*, 25, 614, 1977.
20. **Necheles, T. F., Brenner, J. F., Bonacoss, I., Fristensky, R., and Neurath, P. W.**, The computer-assisted morphological classification of acute leukemia. I. Preliminary results, *Biomedicine*, 25, 241, 1976.
21. **Olson, G., Wied, G. L., and Bartels, P. H.**, Differentiation of chicken thymic and bursel lymphocytes by cell image analysis, *Acta Cytol.*, 17, 454, 1973.
22. **Bartels, P. H., Olson, G. B., Layton, J. M., Anderson, R. E., and Wied, G. L.**, Computer discrimination of T and B lymphocytes, *Acta Cytol.*, 19, 53, 1975.
23. **Anderson, R. E., Olson, G. B., Shonk, D., Howarth, J. L., Wied, G. L., and Bartels, P. H.**, Computer analysis of defined populations of lymphocytes irradiated in vitro. I. Evaluation of murine thoracic duct lymphocytes, *Acta Cytol.* 19, 126, 1975.
24. **Saunders, A. M.**, Development of automation of differential leukocyte counts by use of cytochemistry, *Clin. Chem.*, 18, 783, 1972.

25. **Mansberg, H. P., Saunders, A. M., and Groner, W.**, The HEMALOG D white cell differential system, *J. Histochem. Cytochem.*, 22, 711, 1974.
26. **Curbelo, W., Schildkraut, E. R., Hirschteld, T., Webb, R. H., Block, M. J., and Shapiro, H. M.**, A generalized machine for automated flow cytology system design, *J. Histochem. Cytochem.*, 24, 388, 1976.
27. **Shapiro, H. M., Schildkraut, E. R., Curbello, R., Laird, W. C., Turner, R. B., and Hirschfeld, T.**, Combined blood cell counting and classification with fluorochrome stains and flow instrumentation, *J. Histochem. Cytochem.*, 24, 396, 1976.
28. **Mui, J. K., Fu, K. S., and Bacus, J. W.**, Automated classification of blood cell neutrophils, *J. Histochem. Cytochem.*, 25, 633, 1977.
29. **Koepke, J. A.**, A delineation of performance criteria for the differentiation of leukocytes, *Am. J. Clin. Pathol.*, 68, 202, 1977.
30. **Dutcher, T. F., Benzel, J. E., Egan, J. J., Hart, D. J., and Christopher, E. A.**, I. Instrument description and reproducibility studies, *Am. J. Clin. Pathol.*, 62, 525, 1974.
31. **Benzel, J. E., Egan, J. J., Hart, D. J., and Christopher, E. A.**, II. Normal cell identification, *Am. J. Clin. Pathol.*, 62, 530, 1974.
32. **Egan, J. J., Benzel, J. E., Hart, D. J., and Christopher, E. A.**, III. Detection of abnormal cells, *Am. J. Clin. Pathol.*, 62, 537, 1974.
33. **Anon.**, *Advances in Automated Analysis, Technicon International Congress 1976*, Vol. 1, Mediad, Tarrytown, New York, 1977, 294.
34. **Bacus, J. W.**, The development of automated differential systems, *Pathologist*, 33, 127, 1979.
35. **Mendelsohn, M. L., Mayall, B. H., Prewitt, J. M. S., Bostrom, R. C., and Holcomb, W. G.**, Digital transformations and computer analysis of microscopic images, in *Advances in Optical and Electron Microscopy*, Cosslett, V. E., Ed., Academic Press, New York, 1968, 77.
36. **Biberman, L. M. and Nudelman, S.**, *Photoelectric Imaging Devices*, Vol. 1, Optical Physics and Engineering Series, Plenum Press, New York, 1971.
37. **Biberman, L. M. and Nudelman, S.**, *Photoelectric Imaging Devices*, Vol. 2, Plenum Press, New York, 1971.
38. **Brenner, J. F., Necheles, T. F., Bonacossa, I. A., Fristensky, R., Weintraub, B. A., and Neurath, P. W.**, Scene segmentation techniques for the analysis of routine bone marrow smears from acute lymphoblastic leukemia patients, *J. Histochem. Cytochem.*, 25, 601, 1977.
39. **Aus, H. M., Ruter, A., TerMuelen, V., Bunzer, U., and Nurnberger, R.**, Bone marrow cell scene segmentation by computer-aided color cytophotometry, *J. Histochem. Cytochem.*, 25, 662, 1977.
40. **Mui, J. K., Bacus, J. W., and Fu, K. S.**, A Scene Segmentation Technique for Microscopic Cell Images, IEEE catalogue no. 76CH1170-OC, in Proceedings of Symposium, Computer-Aided Diagnosis of Medical Images, November 1976, 99.
41. **Prewitt, J. M. S.**, Object enhancement and extraction, in *Picture Processing and Psychopictorics*, Lipkin, B. S. and Rosenfeld, A., Eds., Academic Press, New York, 1970, 75.
42. **Bacus, J. W.**, A whitening transformation for two-color blood cell images, *Pattern Recognition*, 8, 53, 1976.
43. **Green, J. E.**, Parallel Processing in a Pattern Recognition Based Image Processing System: the Abbott ADC-500 Differential Counter, IEEE publication no. 78CH1318-5C, in Proceedings IEEE Pattern Recognition and Image Processing, June 1978, 492.
44. **Yasnoff, Y. A., Mui, J. K., and Bacus, J. W.**, Error measures for scene segmentation, *Pattern Recognition*, 9, 217, 1977.
45. **Fukunaga, K.**, *Introduction to Statistical Pattern Recognition*, Academic Press, New York, 1972.
46. **Sebestyen, G. S.**, *Decision Making Processes in Pattern Recognition*, Macmillan, New York, 1970.
47. **Barnett, C. W.**, The unavoidable error in the differential count of the leukocytes of the blood, *J. Clin. Invest.*, 12, 77, 1933.
48. **Trobaugh, F. E., Jr. and Bacus, J. W.**, Design and performance of the LARC automated leukocyte classifier, in *The Differential Leukocyte Count*, Koepke, J., Ed., College of American Pathologists, Skokie, Ill., 1979.
49. **Arkin, C. F., Sherry, M. A., Gough, A. G., and Copeland, B. E.**, An automatic leukocyte analyzer, validity of its results, *Am. J. Clin. Pathol.*, 67, 159, 1977.
50. **Gilmer, P.**, Perkin Elmer DIFF 3 Clinical Trials, in *The Differential Leukocyte Count*, Koepke, J., Ed., College of American Pathologists, Skokie, Ill., 1979.
51. **Trobaugh, F. E., Jr. and Bacus, J. W.**, Evaluation of the Performance of the LARC™ Automated Leukocyte Differential Counter in Regular Use, presented at the 16th Int. Congr. of Hematol., Kyoto, Japan, September 1976.
52. **Niitani, K.**, Evaluation of Hematrak Automatic Counter, presented at the 16th Int. Congr. Of Hematol., Kyoto, Japan, September 1976.

53. **Mui, J. K., Fu, K. S., and Bacus, J. W.,** Feature Selection in Automated Classification of Blood Cell Neutrophils, IEEE publication no. 78CH1318-5C, in Proceedings IEEE Pattern Recognition and Image Processing, June 1978, 486.
54. **Bacus, J. W.,** Design and Performance of an Automated Leukocyte Classifier, IEEE catalog no. 74CH0885-4C, in Proc. 2nd Int. Jt. Conf. on Pattern Recognition, 1974, 374.
55. **Megla, G. K.,** The LARC automatic white blood cell analyzer, *Acta Cytol.,* 17, 3, 1973.

Identification and Enumeration of Blood Cells

IDENTIFICATION AND ENUMERATION OF BLOOD CELLS

A. Richardson Jones and Alex M. Saunders

Traditional Cell Counting

The invention of the first practical microscope by Antonie van Leeuwenhoek in the 17th century allowed the cellular composition of blood to be recognized for the first time and led to an appreciation of the potential significance of quantification of the formed elements which had been made visible. Leeuwenhoek himself attempted to measure the size of chicken erythrocytes[1] and to enumerate them under the microscope after drawing them into a glass capillary of known dimensions.

During the following years steady progress was made in optical technology leading to the development, in the 19th century, of the familiar ruled hemacytometer chamber. There are many variations of the basic hemacytometer design, most involving the pattern of the ruled area of the chamber. The most widely used design is the "improved" Neubauer chamber which has a total ruled area of 9 mm^2, each square millimeter being divided into 25 smaller squares. The central square millimeter is further subdivided into 16 squares and is the area over which erythrocytes are enumerated, while the four corner one millimeter squares are used for leukocyte counting. Hemacytometers in which the ruled lines appear to be brightly illuminated are to be preferred for their help in reducing visual fatigue. Detailed descriptions of the improved Neubauer and other hemacytometers are to be found in all reference books dealing with laboratory diagnostic procedures.

The hemacytometer method for enumerating erythrocytes and leukocytes, while finding little use in the routine laboratory, may have value as a reference method. For example, it may be used adjunctively with electronic methods to generate the assigned values of whole blood reference controls or may be used as a method of last appeal if an unusual difficulty is encountered in the use of an automatic blood counting device. For this reason, a summary of the limitations and sources of error of the hemacytometer count is given here. For a more detailed discussion of chamber count errors, consult Daland.[2]

The differences among the methods for enumerating erythrocytes and leukocytes in the counting chamber lie in the composition of the diluting fluids, the dilution ratio of the blood, and the area of the chamber counted. The diluting fluid for leukocytes (typically 2% acetic acid) hemolyses the erythrocytes while leaving the leukocytes intact and visible under the microscope. A simple stain, such as Gentian Violet, may be added to enhance the visibility of the leukocyte nuclei.

The diluting fluid for erythrocyte counting preserves both red and white cells. Although leukocytes are thus present in the counting chamber together with erythrocytes, they contribute little error because of their numerical ratio to erythrocytes (1:1000) and because they can usually be identified morphologically.

Methods of enumerating erythrocytes and leukocytes in peripheral blood, whether by the hemacytometer or an electronic counter, share the following limitations:

- Failure to ensure that the sample is adequately representative of the blood of the subject. Typical errors are the use of excessive congestion in drawing a venous blood specimen or the failure to establish a free flow of blood when sampling from the capillary bed. Adherence to Standards TSH3 and PSH4 for blood specimen collection published by the National Committee for Clinical Laboratory Standards is recommended.[3,4]

- If a container is used to transport the specimen to the laboratory, serious errors can arise from incorrect choice of anticoagulant, inadequate mixing immediately prior to pipetting the specimen, or from hemolysis due to the use of an overvigorous mixing technique. Refer to NCCLS Standard TSH5 for a full description of precautions to be taken in transporting specimens.[5]
- Poor choice or improper use of the pipet, or diluter, used to prepare the measured sample from the specimen. Any pipet or diluter used for this purpose should be calibrated or adjusted to the highest standards of which the laboratory is capable.
- Improper choice of diluting fluid, including errors made in its preparation, and inadequate mixing of sample and diluent can cause error, either by damage to the cells or by nonuniform distribution of cells in the diluent.

Hemacytometer counting methods add the following sources of error to those already listed.

- Dimensional inaccuracy of the chamber
- Improper seating of the cover glass
- Loss of flatness of the cover glass
- Improper filling of the chamber
- Insufficient settling of the cells
- Statistical errors of counting too few cells
- Nucleated red cells counted as leukocytes
- Leukocytes counted as erythrocytes

The effect of dimensional errors and the effect of the error of distribution are inescapable but can be minimized. There are simple techniques for calibrating pipets by weighing mercury contained in them or delivered from them, but the dimensions of a hemacytometer chamber cannot be readily determined. Attempts to measure the ruled area with a micrometer eyepiece and to measure the depth of the chamber by critically focusing the microscope are of no value and may give misleading results. The most practical approach to compensating dimensional errors in the chamber lies in the use of several hemacytometers each of which is separately and repeatedly filled and counted. The average value of repeated counts in each chamber will provide some indication of chamber-to-chamber discrepancies.

The error of cell distribution within the chamber is similar to the sampling error described by Poisson for rice grains scattered randomly over a ruled surface. Berkson et al.[6] give a definitive analysis of the imprecision of cell counting associated with random distribution within the chamber. Daland[2] teaches the management of multiple chamber counts and recommends the use of the following formula:

$$CV = \sqrt{\frac{8464}{n_b} + \frac{21}{n_c} + \frac{22}{n_p}}$$

where n_b is the total number of cells counted in n_c chambers, n_c is the number of chambers examined, and n_p is the number of individual dilutions made from the specimen and counted.

Mattern et al.[7] described a systematic bias in chamber filling which can cause a significant loss of accuracy.

Automated Cell Counting — Background

The single-chamber, single pipet cell count has an unacceptably high error (at least

± 500,000 for a "normal" red cell count of 5,000,000 per cubic milimeter), and improvement of counting statistics by counting a larger number of cells is time-consuming, tedious, and costly. The imprecision and inaccuracy of the single-filled hemacytometer red cell count led to its virtual abandonment for routine hematologic diagnosis during the 1950s. Detection of disorders affecting erythrocytes was generally made by hemoglobinometry, measurement of packed cell volume by centrifugation, and inspection of the stained slide. Chamber counts of leukocytes remained in general use for want of a satisfactory alternative.

The diagnostic value of erythrocyte parameters such as mean corpuscular hemoglobin (MCH) and mean corpuscular volume (MCV) was limited by the poor precision of the chamber count. This led to attempts to apply new developments in electronic and opto-electronic technology to the automation of blood cell counting.

The first of these devices attempted to automate the hemacytometer count and to reduce imprecision by increasing the number of cells counted. The human eye was replaced by a sensitive photodetector (multiplier phototube) which viewed the image of the counting chamber projected through a small aperture. A motor-driven mechanical stage moved the counting chamber in a precisely controlled pattern so that a known area of the chamber was scanned. Cells falling on the edge of the scanning raster were dealt with by the method of Wolff.[8] Two counters based on these principles enjoyed a brief commercial life. These were the Casella and the Jaco-Jones automatic blood cell counters, but none have survived to this day. For a useful review of the theory and practice of this class of counter, see Lagercrantz.[9]

The mechanical scanning approach suffered extreme problems in maintaining focus of the microscope optics and in achieving sufficiently good optical contrast between the cell and the background (signal to noise ratio). Several attempts were made to overcome the focusing problem by using the flying spot microscope described by Roberts and Young.[10] Cell counters based on the flying spot principle were made in various laboratories, but none became widely used. More recently, a flying spot scanner has been implemented in a commercial differential leukocyte classifier.

Attempts were made to use a television camera in place of the human observer and one such instrument was offered for sale by RCA without any commercial success. One simple instrument attempted to estimate the concentration of red cells by photoelectric measurement of the turbidity of a diluted suspension of blood. The apparent turbidity of such a suspension is influenced, not only by the number of cells present, but by the average size of the cells and by the amount of hemoglobin. This instrument attempted to solve this problem by simultaneously measuring hemoglobin concentration colorimetrically and average red cell diameter diffractometrically. These data were applied to a nomogram to correct the turbidity reading.

Frommer[11] devised a cell counter in which a dilute cell suspension flowed through a flat chamber at the focus of a microscope whose viewing area was restricted by a narrow slit. A photodetector recorded the presence or absence of a cell, and pulse-shaping and integrating circuits caused the passage of cells to produce a steady signal, the magnitude of which was proportional to the ratio between the length of time the slit was occupied by a cell and the length of time no cell was present, hence to the concentration of cells flowing through the system. The influence of cell size was minimized by "idealizing" the pulses generated by the cells passing the slit.

It is possible that one or more of the scanning-type counters, or the Frommer counter, would have become accepted by the scientific community had it not been for the invention of two particle-counting systems which were based on causing cells to flow, substantially individually, in a stream through a precisely defined detector zone. Although these two systems were "flow-through" systems, there was no other resemblance between them. One system, devised by Wallace Coulter[12,13] causes a known

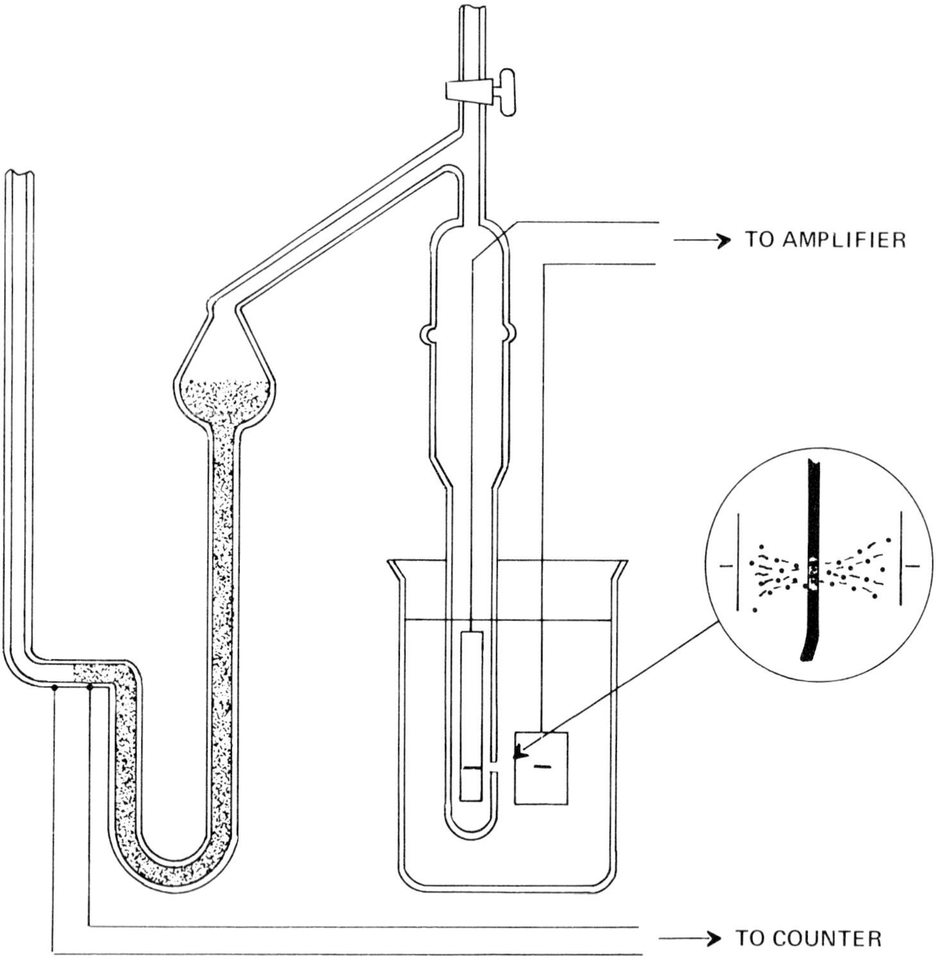

FIGURE 1. Schematic arrangement of an electronic impedence detector.

volume of cells suspended in a conductive diluent to pass through a small aperture. The presence of a cell within the boundaries of the aperture, by displacing its own volume of diluent, caused a change of electrical impedance across the aperture, the magnitude of which was closely proportional to the volume of the cell.

The other flow system is an extension of Frommer's, insomuch as cells are made to pass a narrow slit while suspended in dilute liquid. Simplified optical devices, which take advantage of strong light-scattering phenomena in an otherwise dark field are coupled to photomultipliers. A single pulse of light defines a single cell. Several such devices have come into commercial distribution and have been improved by addition of fluidic controls or by using lasers for the light source.

Although not blood cell counters, two related devices deserve brief mention. The first of these is the whole blood impedance meter. This device was based on the supposition that the net impedance of a column of blood is proportional to the volumetric ratio of red cells to plasma. Unfortunately, the supposition proved to be invalid. The second is the Waterfield halometer. This device makes use of the fact that a dried blood film behaves as a transmission diffraction grating. That is, a light beam projected through the film will give rise to a spectral halo, the dispersion angle of which is proportional to the modal diameter of the cells in the film. Unfortunately, the halo becomes ill-defined when marked anisocytosis is present.

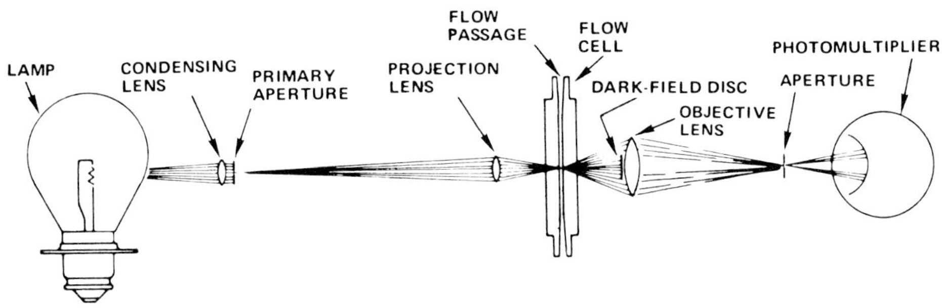

FIGURE 2. Schematic arrangement of an optical detector system.

Automated Cell Counting — Methods

In this section an attempt will be made to describe and evaluate the conceptual aspects of the most widely used types of cell counting devices. No attempt will be made to give detailed structural descriptions of the commercial forms of cell counters which are currently on the market, since any such description would be diminished in value by design changes made from time to time to existing commercial instruments and by the arrival of new contenders for the marketplace. Readers wishing detailed descriptions of commercially available instruments are advised to request such information directly from the manufacturer. A list of the major manufacturers of automatic blood counters is appended to this chapter.

There are two principal types of automatic cell counting instruments in use at the present time: (a) instruments based on the detection and measurement of changes in electronic impedance produced by a cell traversing a small aperture (the Coulter Principle) and (b) instruments based on the measurement of the optical characteristics of cells directed past one or more optical detectors by a laminar flow system.[14]

Since the great majority of cell counts are made by electronic impedance counters, these will be discussed in greater detail than optical detector counters.

Electronic Impedance Counters

This type of counter makes use of the fact that erythrocytes (and other cells) are essentially nonconductors of electricity. If suspended in a conductive liquid, they function as discrete insulators. When a dilute suspension of cells is drawn through a small cylindrical aperture, the passage of each individual cell momentarily increases the resistance (or impedance) of the electrical path between two submerged electrodes, located one on either side of the aperture.

Inherent in the electronic impedance system, in addition to particle counting, is the proportionality between cell volume and the amplitude of the electrical pulse produced by the passage of the cell through the aperture. The effective impedance between the electrodes is virtually entirely due to the impedance offered by the volume of conductive liquid within the boundaries of the aperture. The displacement of some of this liquid by the presence of a cell, or other particle, will raise the impedance of the conductive pathway by an amount proportional to the volume of liquid displaced. Theoretical analysis of the behavior of particles within an aperture (abundantly confirmed by actual observation) shows that the height of the electrical pulse produced by the cell is the parameter which most nearly exhibits proportionality to the cell volume.[15-18] The importance of this aspect of the impedance detector counter can hardly be overstressed, for it permits the selective counting of cells within very narrow size-distribution ranges by electronic selection of the pulses they generate.

As we have shown in our discussion of the hemacytometer, even simple and straightforward counting methods are beset by difficulties and limitations. The impedance detector counter is no exception to this: a discussion of the limitations and the ways in which such limitations can be successfully minimized is given in the following section. Many of the comments apply with equal force to optical detector systems.

Effect of Diluent

In a counting system which is highly sensitive to the volume of the individual particles being counted, it is clear that the conductive liquid in which the particles or cells are suspended shall have the minimum influence on their biological integrity and, hence, on their size. Although this requirement is important for accurate counting of any type of cell, it is a critical requirement for counting red cells, because some form of selection or discrimination must be made as to the magnitude of the electrical pulses to be identified with the cells being counted. If no discrimination were made, the count would contain a substantial contribution from particles smaller than the smallest erythrocyte. Of less concern when counting erythrocytes (but of great importance when counting other cells) is the establishment of some constraint on the upper size limit of cell-generated pulses.

Most instruments have provision for the appropriate pulse height range to be selected, but such adjustments are based on the presumption that the cells will not be distorted in such a manner as to cause them to fall outside the selected size range. For example, the exposure of erythrocytes to a hypertonic conductive liquid will cause shrinkage of the cells to an extent which makes a substantial proportion of them produce electrical pulses below the selected lower limit of the counting range. Alternatively, if the conductive liquid is hypo-osmotic for erythrocytes, the cells will become tumescent by absorbing water and will generate pulses which are inappropriately large. In counters which have an upper pulse height selection adjustment, such pulses may be excluded from the count.

Therefore, the conductive liquid must be iso-osmotic for the cells being counted in order that they may retain their characteristic size and shape during the counting process. Quite subtle alterations in the composition of the conductive liquid may cause changes in the apparent volume of erythrocytes. This holds for optical detectors also, because scattered light is also proportional to size of erythrocyte.

Another effect of the conductive liquid is its influence on the deformability of cells. Some blood cells such as leukocytes and platelets are relatively rigid whereas the erythrocyte, presumably due to its bag-like structure, is readily deformed under the hydrodynamic stresses to which it is exposed during its passage through the aperture. This phenomenon causes a slight, but significant, effect on the apparent size of the cell, with resulting effect on pulse height.

A further problem encountered in the design of the conductive liquid is the fact that bacteriostatic or fungicidal agents, the addition of which is necessary to keep the solution "clean", confer a slight but undesirable rigidity on erythrocytes exposed to it. A case in point is the use and subsequent discontinuance of sodium azide as a preservative in cell counting diluents. The original use of this substance was based on its high level of acceptance as a preservative in many biological reagents. Fresh red cells suspended in azide-containing diluent acquired a degree of rigidity that made them closely resemble the stabilized red cell suspensions which were used as reference controls. Thus, at least in terms of apparent erythrocyte size distribution and mean corpuscular volume, little if any discrepancy was observed between whole blood specimens and reference control material.

After it was shown to be capable of generating an explosion hazard when left in prolonged contact with metallic drain pipes, most manufacturers discontinued the use of sodium azide as a bacteriostatic agent in cell counting diluents. The result of this has been the observation of occasional discrepancies between the mean corpuscular volumes of fresh blood specimens and those of reference controls. It is to be hoped that this problem will be diminished through the availability of reference controls containing erythrocytes which, in spite of being preserved, have a size and deformability equivalent to the erythrocytes in fresh blood. Bessis and co-workers[19,20] have described the potential diagnostic significance of erythrocyte deformability and have suggested instrumentation for its measurement.

In addition to the requirement that the conductive liquid maintain the cells as close as possible to their natural size, shape, and mechanical deformability, it should not contain particles which might contribute to the count. Diluents used for platelet counting are particularly critical in this regard since exclusion of the particulate material from commercial solutions becomes difficult for particles in the platelet size range.

The electrical conductivity of cell-counting diluents may have a significant effect on the performance of some types of impedance detector counters or no effect on other types, depending on the design of the circuit which senses the resistance change caused by a particle within the aperture. This consideration will be discussed later.

The diluents used for leukocyte counting in the electronic impedance counter must have the capability of destroying erythrocytes without significantly affecting leukocytes and must do this rapidly enough to satisfy the short processing times used in the fully automatic, multiparameter cell counters. Lytic agents which have been found satisfactory include saponin and quarternary amines.

The Coincidence Error

A stable suspension of blood cells or other particles does not have its individual particles separated from each other by uniform distances. In fact the probability with which a given number of particles occupies a given volume of suspension is a three-dimensional version of the familiar Poisson distribution referred to in the section on hemacytometer chamber counts. This means that, for a given cell concentration, there will be a predictable frequency with which some particles are sufficiently close together to be simultaneously within the boundaries of the aperture. When two or more particles occupy the aperture simultaneously the sensing circuit will only respond as though a single particle were present, and one member of the doublet will be "lost" from the total count. Counts lost in this manner are referred to as the coincidence error or coincidence loss.

There also exists the possibility that adjacent pulses produced by closely spaced (but not spatially coincident) cells may be presented to the amplifying circuit more quickly than it is able to respond. This unusual circumstance can also lead to a failure to detect and count the second member of a pair of particles.

Clearly, both spatial and electronic coincidence error can be minimized by diluting the specimen to a degree which makes the probability of two or more cells occupying the aperture simultaneously vanishingly small. However, this is done at the expense of reducing the total number of cells counted in a given volume of suspension, thus compromising the precision of the count. The coincidence error can also be reduced by using an aperture with smaller contained volume. This leads to an increased likelihood of blockage and to an increase in the hydrodynamic forces needed to force the cell suspension through the aperture or, if the pressure drop across this small aperture is kept within reasonable limits, there will be an increase in the amount of time required to pass a given volume of suspension through it.

Electronic impedance counters designed for counting erythrocytes and leukocytes use apertures with a diameter of 100 μm and a length of 100 μm. A 50,000-fold dilution of the blood specimen passes through such an aperture in reasonable time and allows both good counting statistics and a predictable coincidence error for erythrocytes. The

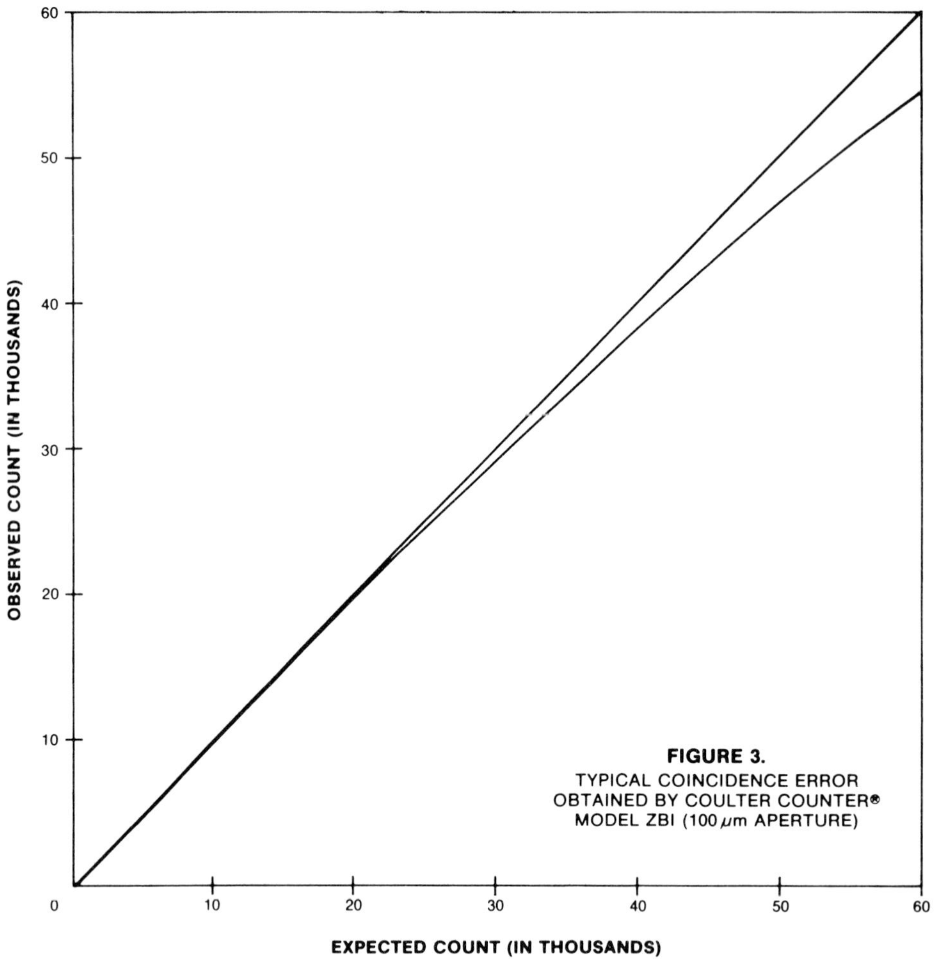

FIGURE 3. Typical coincidence error obtained by Coulter Counter® Model ZBI (100 μm aperture).

coincidence error is corrected in the simplest types of counter by using a factor derived from a table furnished with the instrument. More sophisticated counters employ an analog compensating circuit or calculate the corrected count value by means of a built-in microcomputer.

The full analysis of the interrelationships of all the factors contributing to the coincidence loss is complex, even if simplified versions of aperture geometry, current-density distribution, particle shape and size, electrical pulse shape, and hydrodynamic forces within the aperture are used. The ultimate test of the validity of any coincidence-correcting method lies in its ability to provide a convincing straight-line extrapolation when applied to the counts obtained from a series of progressive dilutions of the same cell-containing material. A simple experiment may be performed by counting dilutions of blood ranging from 500,000-fold to 50,000-fold and plotting the observed counts against the dilution factor, subtracting any background count due to the diluent and making repeated counts at the greater dilutions in order to obtain good counting statistics. Extrapolation of a straight line from assumed zero intercept through the most dilute count values will reveal an apparent count-shortage in the less dilute count values as shown in Figure 3. From these data it is possible to derive a correction factor table over the range of count values for which the instrument is to be used. If this experiment is performed on instruments which have built-in coincidence-correction circuits it will provide a statement of the span and efficiency of these circuits. This topic is further explored in connection with the discussion of instrument calibration.

The correction of coincidence is important not only in simple enumeration of cells, but for providing accurate data for parameters such as mean corpuscular volume, mean corpuscular hemoglobin, and for computation of mean corpuscular hemoglobin concentration.

Aperture Characteristics

It has been stated that the electronic impedance counter uses the displacement of conductive fluid by a particle to generate an electrical pulse, the magnitude of which is nearly proportional to the volume of the particle. The overall sensitivity of this type of counting system depends not only on the absolute volume of liquid displaced from the aperture but on the relative volumes of particle and conductive liquid contained within the aperture boundaries. Thus the larger the contained volume of the aperture, the smaller the proportionate change of resistance produced by a given size of particle. The smaller the contained volume of the aperture, the larger the proportionate change of resistance by the particle.

General-purpose counters are capable of being fitted with a variety of aperture sizes and they also have provision to adjust aperture current, pulse amplification factor, and pulse height limits within which the counting circuit will be triggered. The correct procedures for selecting and adjusting these parameters are contained in the Operator's Reference Manual provided with each instrument. Once the correct adjustments have been made, it is essential that the aperture be maintained in a scrupulously clean condition. Any "build up" within the boundaries of the aperture will lead to an apparent increase in the sensitivity of the counting circuit. Because of the importance of maintaining a clean aperture, counters of the electronic impedance type should always be equipped with some type of direct-view or projection microscope for visually monitoring the appearance of the aperture. In addition, there should be an oscilloscope which displays the pulses generated by the cells passing through the aperture together with a display of the minimum and maximum pulse heights between which the counting circuit will be triggered. Even relatively inexperienced operators can readily detect alterations in the oscilloscope pattern produced by partial aperture blockage. Some counters are equipped with a device which gives an audible signal once every thousand counted pulses. Partial blockage of an aperture during a count will result in a readily detectable change of cadence in this audible signal.

Dedicated-purpose blood counters, such as the Coulter Counter® Model S Series, as well as having visual and cathode-ray tube monitors, have addressed the question of aperture integrity by passing the cell suspension simultaneously through three parallel but independent apertures. At the conclusion of the counting process, the counts obtained from the three apertures are compared. If statistically significant discrepancy is observed among the counts, the count which is in disagreement is discarded and the reported value is derived from data provided by the two apertures which are in agreement. This maneuver, which is referred to by the manufacturer as "voting", leads to a reduction in the total number of cells counted to only two-thirds of the number that would be counted if all three apertures were functioning normally. This results in a slight but barely significant increase in the coefficient of variation of the system. The operator's attention is drawn to the fact that a vote-out has occurred, and that the cause of this should be investigated and corrected before continuing to use the instrument.

The Sensing Circuit

There are a variety of circuits which are capable of detecting a change in a resistive pathway. The simplest of these measures the change in current carried by the aperture when a constant voltage is applied across it. Another method is to make the aperture the electrical equivalent of one arm of a Wheatstone Bridge and measure the change of imbalance of the bridge caused by the presence of a particle within the aperture. These and similar resistance measurement methods have the serious disadvantage of being sensitive to the conductivity of the conducting liquid. Thus, in addition to requiring extremely close tolerances to be placed on the chemical composition of diluting and lysing reagents, these arrangements are sensitive to temperature change. Sufficiently close control of these parameters might be feasible in instruments which are intended only to count, but accurate volume measurements are not reliable under these conditions. It is therefore important to know the degree to which an electronic impedance instrument is sensitive to the effects of diluent conductivity. All counters manufactured by Coulter Electronics, Inc. with the exception of the original Model A, are virtually immune to the effect of diluent conductivity. This is achieved by furnishing the electrical energy which passes through the aperture from a closely regulated constant-current source, and by using as a detection means an amplifier with zero input impedance. For an explanation as to why such a system is independent of the conductance of the pathway between the current source and the detector input, the reader should refer to a standard work on operational amplifier design and application.[21]

An important characteristic of the electronic impedance principle is that the shape of the electrical pulse produced by a particle passing through the aperture is affected in some degree by the pathway taken by the particle in its approach to the aperture — whether or not it travels through the aperture near the axis and whether it leaves the posterior boundary of the aperture in a straight or a curved pathway.[22]

Several attempts have been made to induce particles to follow an optimum pathway through the aperture.[23] These methods, in principle, attempt to introduce a fluid stream containing the sample into the center of the main body of diluent which is moving through the aperture. One version of this arrangement is described by Schulz and Thom[24] and is used in the Coulter Counter Model TF®. This system generates a short sheath-flow segment in the vicinity of the aperture, an arrangement which markedly increases the ability of the aperture to resolve small differences of particle volume in a heterogenous sample.

Optical Cell Counters

Although two distinct methods of light-scattering measurement and of light-loss measurement are employed in a variety of flow-through optical counters, it is difficult, at times, to separate these two phenomena, and even the manufacturers do not always make clear distinctions as to which one of these is employed.

Equally important to the actual optical device is the fluidic control design as it influences both the precision with which a final dilution is accomplished and the volume of fluid which is to be counted in each sample. This volume must be equivalent to that of a reference by which the instrument is calibrated. Reagents are also important in the optical counting devices because they strongly influence the optical signal. The chief ways in which this signal is influenced are by changing the quality of the cells under examination, for example, by a process of formaldehyde fixation and by surrounding the cell with more or less refractile media in an attempt to increase or decrease the refractility of certain components in the cell suspension.

As can be expected, the prototype systems designed by most manufacturers strongly resemble microscopes used in clinical laboratories: indeed, the starting point in many systems was the simple replacement of the well-known flat microscope slide in the specimen plane of an ordinary microscope with a more-or-less tubular device through which the cell suspensions flowed under simple fluidic control. During the development all but the essential components were stripped away and modifications were made in order to match more closely the requirements of electronic measurements made by photomultipliers or simple photodiodes in comparison to observations made by the human eye. Nevertheless, the chief components of the well-known microscope remain intact in the commercial fluidic cell counters. These components are

1. Light source
2. Lens for concentrating light on the specimen plane
3. Field aperture used to limit the view field in the specimen plane
4. A light limiting aperture used to control stray light

Beyond the specimen plane the similarity among different systems is not so clear. Some systems have eliminated objective lenses and replaced them with large photo-measuring devices placed critically in the light path. Other commercial devices continue to use light-collecting objective lenses beyond the specimen and to focus light by means of further lenses onto light-measuring devices which are either photomultiplier tubes or photodiodes.

For the purpose of measuring light-scattering phenomena the system must be so arranged that a bright light focused on the specimen plane is not all transmitted to the measuring device unless a refractile object is in the view volume. The usual arrangement for visual microscopy is to put an opaque object in the light path in such a way that a hollow cone of light is focused onto the specimen plane. As the rays of this hollow cone diverge beyond the specimen plane, their angle is wider than the angle of the collecting lens or objective: hence, only light which is refracted into the objective by a specimen will be seen by an observer. However, the hollow cone of light design is wasteful of light, and therefore produces a less powerful signal than other possibilities. An improved design in the late 60s placed the dark field aperture beyond the specimen plane and objective in such a position that it completely occluded the original light as controlled by the light-limiting aperture. Light refracted by a specimen generally went to the side of this opaque disc and was refocused on a photomultiplier tube by a relay lens just beyond the opaque disc. In general, devices which used this narrow-forward-angle scattering design are able to resolve differences in size of objects quite well, because intensity of light scattering is related very strongly to the cross-sectional area presented by the object at the instant when it crosses the light path. Hence, by the use of proper electronic comparators a series of thresholds can be so devised that small and larger objects are separately counted. It is quite usual with optical flow devices to permit the operator to set the thresholds that seem most appropriate on the day on which the work is being done.

The actual view volume in light-scattering devices varies with the manufacturer and instrument. For example, the Technicon SMA 4® and Technicon Hemalog 8® have view volumes limited by a field aperture of 10×100 μm, while the third dimension is limited by the depth of focus of the system objective. This latter is supposed to be between 7 and 12 μm. Hence, the total view volume is in the order of 1×10^4 μm^3. These instruments operate without a sheath-flow principle and the only limitation on the fluidic flow cell is that laminar-flow principles be obeyed. By this is meant that the optical axis must transsect the most central portion of the stream where the stream is moving most rapidly.

In contrast, the Hemalog D®, also made by Technicon, as well as the Ortho HEMAC® system, use a sheath-stream principle described further below which also limits the portion of view volume in which cells may be located. In the Hemalog D®, for example, the light slit has dimensions of 20×100 μm, but the sample stream within the sheath is only 60 μm in diameter. The total view volume, therefore, is 5.6×10^4 μm^3. The principle of sheath flow with a central sample stream was devised by Crosland-Taylor.[14] Its main advantage in present-day instruments comes from the fact that the sample stream is completely enclosed within the optic. This permits more precise measurement of each particle passing the view volume, because it ensures that the whole object is visible to the measuring devices. In contrast, those devices in which a slit is superimposed on a wide flowing specimen stream stand a chance of particles being in part inside and in part outside the view volume. Hence, it is more difficult to provide reproducible thresholds in these devices, and this makes them less useful for multiparametric measurement and counting.

The electrical signals produced by the photodetectors in response to the presence of a cell in an optical sensing system have the form of pulses, the heights of which are proportional to the magnitude of the parameter being measured. These electrical pulses are passed on to shaping and counting circuits or rejected as being spurious by electronic subsystems which are generally similar to those found in electronic impedance counters.

Calibration of Automated Cell Counters

Although the various types of automated blood cell counters differ substantially in the principles used for the detection of cells, they otherwise possess sufficient similarity to permit some general statements to be made about their calibration.

All automatic counters in use today are of the flow-through type. That is, a known volume of a suitably diluted blood specimen is caused to flow past a cell detector which produces electrical signals in response to the passage of cells. The sum of these electrical signals for the volume of suspension which passes the detector is presented to the operator by some form of digital display, meter reading, or hard copy.

The counting process comprises the following clearly defined stages, the accuracy of each combining to determine the accuracy of the entire counting system.

1. Blood sample dilutor
2. Suspension metering system
3. Particle detector
4. Particle discriminator
5. Display scaling factor

Blood Sample Dilutor

The dilution process may take place separately from the counting process and be performed by conventional volumetric pipets and flasks or, more commonly, by some type of automatic dilution apparatus. Fully automatic cell counters such as the SMA 4®, SMA 7®, and Hemalog D® manufactured by Technicon Instrument Corporation and the Model S®, Model S Senior®, and Model S-Plus® manufactured by Coulter Electronics, Inc., have integral dilutor systems that are not amenable to calibration independently from the whole system.

External dilutors should be calibrated in terms of the procedure they are to be used for. Thus a calibration method for a dilutor used for the preparation of red-cell suspensions should employ blood as the test medium and cell-counting diluent as the diluting agent. Procedures based on direct gravimetric measurement of sample and diluent volumes, while apparently sophisticated, do not give satisfactory results.

It is recommended that a number of separate reference dilutions of fresh whole blood be prepared in Class A glassware and that each of these dilutions be counted in replicate in the automatic cell counter. The mean and two standard deviations of these data will provide a value and confidence limits for the reference method.

Multiple automatic dilutions of the same whole-blood specimen are then made in the automatic dilutor and are then counted without altering the counter controls. The mean and standard deviation of these data are compared with those of the manual dilution data set.

Whether or not a significant difference is found between the two data sets, consider the possibility that the automatic dilutor may, because of high stream velocity, cause loss of red cells by mechanical hemolysis. Only if this interference can be excluded or accurately estimated should the dilutor be adjusted, or a calibration factor assigned to it.

The calibration method for dilutors for white cell counting involves the additional consideration of the effectiveness of the hemolytic or refractile agent used to allow the instrument to identify the white cells. Otherwise the principles described for calibration of red-cell dilutors should be followed.

Suspension Metering System

The volume of cell suspension which is inspected by the detector system of an automatic cell counter is usually controlled by either a displacement pump (e.g., mercury manometer) or by controlling the time the liquid flows at a carefully controlled velocity past the detector. The former method is readily calibrated by measurement of the displacement of liquid in the system by attaching a filled micrometer burette which, in turn, has been calibrated gravimetrically. The control of the counted volume by timed flow does not, unfortunately, lend itself to calibration by methods which are separate and distinct from the counting process itself. This is also true of the peristaltic pumping technique employed in the Technicon family of cell counters.

Particle Detector

Calibration of the detector consists of two parts: firstly, an estimate of the nonlinearity of the detector caused by the presence within its geometric boundary of more than one cell simultaneously; and secondly, an estimate of the error introduced by the pass band of the detector circuitry in preventing the complete separation of electrical pulses caused by cells passing through the detector in rapid succession.

Helleman[25] has presented an analysis of these conditions and has proposed a method for estimating coincidence error by making counts at two differing cell concentrations.

We consider Helleman's solution, elegant though it is, to be too restricted to answer the practical problems of detector calibration for the variety of detectors and amplifiers (including optical detectors) in use today. The purpose of detector calibration is to answer the question "If n particles traverse the detector, will n electrical pulses be generated?" The theory of particle detectors, confirmed by experience, requires a negative answer to this question and further requires that the relationship between "particles in and signals out" be exponential and, therefore, not capable of being expressed as a simple numerical calibration factor. The situation is further complicated by the fact that some types of counter are furnished with circuitry which substantially corrects the nonlinearity of the detector response.

Practical detector calibration consists of constructing a performance graph which has, on its abscissa, the relative expected count and, on its ordinate, the relative observed count. This is done by making a series of precise 10% dilutions of a normal fresh whole blood, in its own plasma, over the range of 100 to 10% of the original specimen. These preparations are counted after being diluted in the standard manner, and the data is graphed as indicated. The graph will be curvilinear for instruments without coincidence-correction circuitry and virtually linear for instruments which provide coincidence correction. From the graph a detector calibration (or "correction") factor can be derived for every observed count value. This factor takes both spatial and temporal coincidence into effect. As a rough guide to the expected magnitude of this factor, a Coulter Counter® without coincidence correction circuitry and with aperture dimensions 100 μm diameter by 100 μm length will show approximately a 13% discrepancy between expected and observed red cell counts for "normal" blood diluted 1:50,000.

In addition to the need to estimate nonlinear response, particle detectors must be optimally adjusted for sensitivity. Optical detectors require strict adherence to manufacturer's recommended settings for light source intensity, focusing, and alignment. Photodetectors must be properly positioned, particularly when forward light-scattering intensity is measured.

Electronic impedance detectors need no mechanical adjustment but require the correct setting of aperture current and amplifier gain in order to achieve a range of pulse heights appropriate to size range of particles being counted and the physical dimensions of the aperture in use. Fully automated, multiparameter electronic impedance counters such as the Coulter Counter® Model S have aperture current and amplifier gain controls which are not readily adjustable, but the simpler counters are provided with a wide range of adjustment.

Particle Discrimination

Optical detector systems rely, in some degree, upon histochemical differentiation of cells, prior to their passage through the detector. A practical histochemical system of cell differentiation is described by Saunders.[26]

Both optical detectors and electronic impedance detectors perform the final identification of cells by selecting for counting only those pulses falling within a narrowly defined amplitude range. Electronic impedance detectors rely entirely on pulse amplitude for the recognition of cell classes.

The circuit which selects pulses on the basis of amplitude is known as a pulse height discriminator. The level at which a pulse is rejected as being too small is known as the lower threshold, while the level at which a pulse is blocked as being too large is known as the upper threshold.

The importance of the lower threshold is easily seen. When red cells are being counted it permits the separation of pulses into two categories: those which are larger than the smallest red cell, and therefore to be counted, and those which are smaller than the smallest red cell, and therefore to be rejected. Blood rarely contains significant numbers of particles larger than the largest type of red cell. Thus, in erythrocyte counting, the upper threshold of the discriminator does not play an important role in the cell selection process.

When counting platelets the upper threshold setting of the discriminator becomes important in electronic impedance counters. Except for marked megathrombocytemia, platelets larger than 36 to 40 μm^3 are rarely encountered. Any cell larger than this is likely to belong to the erythrocyte or leukocyte families and is to be excluded from the count.

The multiparameter automatic counters have factory set upper and lower thresholds but the general-purpose, single channel type of counter requires that the manufacturer's recommended setting for upper and lower threshold controls for different counting procedures be strictly observed.

Display Scaling Factor

The methods used to display the result of a count fall into two categories. The exact number of pulses passed through the pulse height discriminator may be shown on conventional digital display, or the display may be a meter, a strip chart recorder, or printer which gives a number proportional to the number of cells which have passed through the particle detector system. The distinction between the two types of display systems is important because the proportional type of display makes it necessary to calibrate the instrument with some form of calibrator suspension and does not allow the counter to be used as a primary measuring device.

Display systems which give a one-for-one count display do not need to be calibrated but it is advisable to perform a periodic check to ensure that the counter is capable of accepting pulses which are separated by the shortest time interval likely to be generated by the detector and discriminator systems.

Proportional displays must be adjusted in order to make the displayed cell count conform to the actual cell concentration of the specimen. The procedures for doing this on various commercial cell counters are described in the Operator's Reference Manuals furnished with the instruments. Care should always be taken that the degree of adjustment necessary to achieve accurate scaling of the display does not result in the scaling control being set at either end of the adjustment limits. If this is found to be the case, there is a high probability that the adjustment is, in fact, compensating for improper operation of one of the systems previously described.

Calibrator Materials

The preceding description of the calibration requirements of automated blood cell counters has indicated that the final calibration of certain types of cell counters cannot be achieved by calibration of their individual subsystems. It depends on the operator adjusting the instrument to make it display the "correct" result when it is presented with a blood specimen or surrogate, the values of whose parameters are accurately known. This is a situation which parallels the calibration of automated chemical analyzers but is complicated by the fact that the technical difficulties of manufacturing a calibrator for blood counters are considerably greater than its chemical counterpart. In spite of these difficulties, which are principally those of achieving adequate stability of the blood cell parameters over a reasonable shelf life, some calibrator suspensions are in commercial distribution. An alternative to the use of a manufactured calibrator is the calibration of a number of fresh blood specimens from normal individuals by "reference" measurement techniques. These specimens are then measured by the automated instrument. If there is a discrepancy between the two sets of values, the instrument is adjusted to agree with the reference method.

The principal advantage of using fresh blood specimens to transfer values is that the short elapsed time between the two sets of measurements ensures the blood cells will not have undergone any significant deterioration. It is not necessary to use preservatives or additives which might introduce artifacts into the measuring system. The disadvantages of the fresh blood calibration system are the relatively large number of measurements of each parameter which are necessary to ensure good sampling statistics and the fact that the accuracy of the final calibration of the automated instrument is only as good as the accuracy of the reference methods.

Reference methods commonly used are

- The microhematocrit method for the determination of packed cell volume (PCV). This method is known to be precise and accurate[27] but it does not measure the "true" packed cell volume since approximately 3% of the volume of the centrifuged red cells consists of entrained plasma.[28] Electronic impedance or optical measurements of mean corpuscular volume do not include trapped plasma and therefore, it is customary to correct the observed packed cell volume for this. A reference method has been proposed which includes an isotope dilution technique as a means of accurately measuring the plasma entrained in centrifuged cells, but its complexity will probably preclude its acceptance in the routine hematologic laboratory.[29]

- Hemoglobin measurement is generally made by the cyanmethemoglobin (hemiglobin cyanide) method. The procedure described by van Assendelft et al.[30] should be followed as closely as possible.
- The erythrocyte count is most frequently carried out on one of the "simple" electronic impedance counters. Counters of this type are relatively easy to maintain in good working order with their subsystems calibrated to manufacturer's limits as defined in the preceding section. The use of counting chambers has been discussed earlier and, providing that a multiple-chamber, multiple-count method is carefully followed, this would be a satisfactory if somewhat tedious alternative to the use of a properly adjusted electronic impedance counter.
- The choice of procedure used for the reference leukocyte count lies between the carefully performed counting chamber procedure and the use of a properly adjusted electronic impedance counter. The former method offers the advantage of high specificity, the counted cells being easily recognized under the microscope as leukocytes, particularly when a nuclear stain is added to the diluting fluid. The electronic impedance counter offers the advantage of high precision but may suffer in specificity when compared to the chamber count because the electronic impedance counter detects those particles, larger in volume than 36 μm^3, which remain after the red cells have been hemolyzed. Experience indicates that this method of defining leukocytes is satisfactory for normal blood but that it may have limitations in pathological conditions.
- There does not appear to be a single, generally accepted, reference method for platelet counting. Methods using electronic impedance detector counters such as the Coulter Counter® Thrombocounter or the J. T. Baker MK-4/HC find favor over the chamber counting methods because of the better precision they offer.

Quality Control in Automated Cell Counting

In order to insure a high level of confidence in the accuracy of the information generated by automated cell counting instruments, it is necessary to perform an ongoing, systematic assessment of instrument performance by testing it with reference control material. Participation in some form of quality control program is mandatory for those clinical laboratories regulated by U.S. law.

Quality control procedures for automatic blood counters may use either assayed or unassayed reference control material. The former is typically a commercial product; the latter is prepared in the laboratory.

The principle purpose of a quality control program is to assess both short- and long-term stability of the measurement system. The effectiveness of this process depends upon the stability of the reference control material. Bull et al.[31] have described a method of using fresh blood samples from normal subjects and have shown that the red cell parameters from a group of 20 normal people show remarkable uniformity and stability. This method does not provide information about the accuracy of the cell counting system; nor can it be used for quality control of white blood cell and platelet counting instruments, since these formed elements do not possess the subject-to-subject nor the day-to-day stability shown by red blood cells.

Reference control material with assigned values for formed element parameters and hemoglobin has usually undergone a stabilization process in order for the product to have a useful shelf life. It cannot, therefore, be expected to behave in the same way as fresh blood. For instance, the stabilization process may effect the packing characteristics of the red cells, rendering the material unsuitable as a control for centrifugal packed cell volume measurements. The white cell moiety is usually a surrogate made from preserved red cells of either human or animal origin. Thus neither the size distribution nor morphological characteristics of the "white cells" in this type of reference control material are equivalent to those found in fresh blood. Because of these and other limitations, careful attention must be paid to precautions and limitations of use stated by the manufacturer in the package insert which accompanies the product. One important constraint which must always be observed is whether or not the product may be used as a calibrator or whether its use is restricted to quality control purposes.

Performance Characteristics of Automated Cell Counters

The multiplicity of types of automated cell counters and the general paucity of definitive published information regarding their performance suggested that any discussion of the expected performance of these devices should be restricted to those which are considered to be state-of-the-art by their manufacturers.

A practical guide to the performance of widely used automated cell counters is to be found in the regularly published results of the check sample survey program conducted by the College of American Pathologists. These data are obtained under impartial, blind-test conditions and reflect the actual performance of the measurement systems under real-life laboratory conditions.

Since 1976 manufacturers of in vitro diagnostic products have been required to provide users with extensive information. This includes, in the case of a dedicated-purpose device such as an automated blood cell counter, a statement of the performance characteristics of the device including limitations of use and sources of error. The Technicon 8/90 hematology analyzer and the Coulter Counter® Model S Plus have been taken as examples of automated cell counters whose performance characteristics are required to be published under the Labeling Regulations (21 CFR 809). These two instruments are also substantially equivalent to each other as to the range of parameters measured.

Performance characteristics describe the following variables:

Precision — This is a statement of the observed variability of instrument performance when replicate measurements are made of a single blood specimen. When the measurements are made in a continuous series the observation is referred to as "in run" precision. When the replicate measurements are divided into sets, each set being separated by a time interval during which the instrument is shut down or in stand by, the precision statement is run-to-run or day-to-day. Precision is stated as the standard deviation of the data at a stated level. In order to provide effective evaluation of the instrument's performance under actual clinical laboratory conditions, it is desirable to measure precision at the high and low values of the parameter as well as within the normal range.

Accuracy — The values obtained by the instrument are compared to values obtained by a reference method over as wide a range of values as possible. It is preferred to use actual clinical material rather than simulated ranges prepared by dilution or concentration of normal specimens. The correlation between the instrument and the reference method is expressed by the method of least squares, the slope, or bias, between the two methods, and the value of the intercept.

Linearity — The relationship between the test instrument and the reference method is expected to be a linear one and the range over which the desired straight-line relationship exists must be stated.

Drift — Some instruments, particularly those which rely on analog rather than digital measurement systems, may exhibit a slow and systematic change of output with time. This change may be a change of calibration slope or it may be a progressively increasing departure from a zero intercept. The degree and extent of drift, if present, will usually be the factor which determines the frequency of recalibration of the system.

The following tables of results and the explanatory text have been reproduced from the Operator's Reference Manual for the Coulter Counter® Model S Plus and from the product labeling for the Technicon Hemalog 8/90 hematology analyzer with the permission of the respective companies.

Technicon 8/90 System Definitions

Precision

Precision is defined as the degree of variability among repeated independent measurements of reference material. The precision of the Technicon 8/90 system was studied over a period of time using replicate samples of reference material. Within-run precision refers to the reproducibility of the method when samples are reanalyzed within a short time interval. Day-to-day precision extends the within-run estimates to include run-to-run variability in test results over a period of several days.

Accuracy and Linearity

The accuracy and linearity of the Technicon 8/90 system were determined by correlation with the Hemalog 8 system. Prepared mixtures of plasma and red blood cells were formulated to span the entire range of measurement.

Drift

The drift of the Technicon 8/90 system is expressed as the total change in concentration over the period of time required to sample 40 specimens (one recalibration cycle). The change in concentration is due to a baseline shift that is linear with time. Drift was studied using replicate samples of reference materials.

Hemoglobin

Precision

The precision data for this method are as follows:

Precision Study

Hemoglobin concentration g/dℓ	Within-run precision SD	Within-run precision CV%	Day-to-day precision SD	Day-to-day precision CV%
13.0	0.05	0.4	0.09	0.7

Accuracy

The accuracy data for this method are as follows:

$y = 0.98x - 0.1$
$s_{y.x} = 0.08$
$n = 12$
$r = 0.999$

Linearity

There is no significant nonlinearity over the range 0.6 g/dℓ to 20.0 g/dℓ

Drift

The average drift within a recalibration cycle (40 specimens) is −0.2 g/dℓ.

Table 1
PRECISION STUDY

Test	Level	Units	Within-run precision (SD)	Within-run precision (CV%)	Day-to-day precision (SD)	Day-to-day precision (CV%)
Platelets (+ WBC)[a]	258.3	$\times 10^3$ cells/mm^3	6.50	2.5	—	—
WBC	6.8	$\times 10^3$ cells/mm^3	0.10	1.4	0.10	1.4
RBC	3.9	$\times 10^6$ cells/mm^3	0.03	0.8	0.07	1.8
MCV	97.4	μm^3	1.03	1.1	1.97	2.0
MCH	31.9	pg	0.26	0.8	0.47	1.5
MCHC	32.7	90	0.20	0.6	0.72	2.2

[a] Precision data for the platelet (+ WBC) channel were determined from the drift study.

Packed Cell Volume

Precision

The precision data for this method are as follows:

PCV level %	Within-run precision SD	Within-run precision CV%	Day-to-day precision SD	Day-to-day precision CV%
38.0	0.3	0.8	1.1	2.9

Accuracy

The accuracy data for this method are as follows:

$y = 0.94x + 2.8$
$s_{yx} = 2.2$
$n = 24$
$r = 0.993$

Linearity

There is no significant nonlinearity over the range 20 PCV% to 60 PCV%.

Drift

The average drift within a recalibration cycle (40 specimens) is 0.0%.

Cellular Parameters

Precision

The precision data for the platelets (+ WBC), WBC, RBC determinations, and the calculated indices are summarized in Table 1.

Accuracy

The accuracy data for the platelet (+ WBC), WBC, and RBC methods are as follows:

Platelet (+ WBC)

$y = 1.004x + 10.5$
$s_{yx} = 13.3$
$n = 10$
$r = 0.999$

Table 2
LINEARITY STUDY

Test	Linearity range
Platelet (+WBC)	66×10^3 cells/mm^3 to 800×10^3 cells/mm^3
WBC	3.0×10^3 cells/mm^3 to 40×10^3 cells/mm^3
RBC	0.0×10^6 cells/mm^3 to 6.0×10^6 cells/mm^3

WBC

$y = 0.97x - 0.2$
$s_{yx} = 1.02$
$n = 11$
$r = 0.997$

RBC

$y = 0.95x + 0.09$
$s_{yx} = 0.45$
$n = 26$
$r = 0.984$

Linearity

The linearity data for the platelet (+WBC), WBC, and RBC methods are summarized in Table 2.

Drift

The average drift for the platelet (+WBC) method within a recalibration cycle (40 specimens) is 1.2×10^3 cells/mm^3.

There is no detectable drift for the WBC, RBC, MCV, MCH, and MCHC methods within a recalibration cycle (40 specimens).

Coulter Counter® Model S Plus

Performance Characteritics

General — Performance characteristics provided only apply to an instrument that has been properly maintained as indicated in this manual using ISOTON® II, LYSE S® II, ISOTERGE® II, and 4C® PLUS Normal. Techniques for preparing prediluted samples vary from operator to operator, creating the potential for human error. For this reason, performance characteristics cannot be stated for the prediluted-sample mode.

Precision — Precision is specified at 1 SD based on 31 determinations of the same sample and verified by numerous data sets in various locations. The three computed parameters on the Model S-Plus, that is, Hct, MCH, and MCHC, are digitally calculated and have no adjustment. The precision of these parameters is affected by the precision of the measured parameters involved in the calculation. These computations are accurate to one least significant digit on the print-out form (Table 3).

Accuracy — Accuracy is defined as the 95% confidence limits for maximum percentage error between a best-fit line drawn through multiple points and a theoretical line indicating zero deviation from the reference method. The accuracy indicated can be obtained over the range stated only when enough samples are run for valid statistics. Background counts are subtracted from both methods.

Table 3
PRECISION

Parameter	Precision
WBC	Less than 00.2 × 10^3 cells/mm^3 at 10.0 × 10^3 cells/mm^3
RBC	Less than 0.05 × 10^6 cells/mm^3 at 5.00 × 10^6 cells/mm^3
Hgb	Less than 0.18 g/dℓ at 15.0 g/dℓ
MCV	Less than 1.0 μm^3 at 90.0 μm^3
RDW	Less than 0.35 at 10.0 RDW units
PLT	Less than 2.0 × 10^3 cells/mm^3 at 030. × 10^3 cells/mm^3
	Less than 10. × 10^3 cells/mm^3 at 300. × 10^3 cells/mm^3

Table 4
ACCURACY

Parameter	Accuracy (%)	Range
WBC	2	00.5 to 99.9 × 10^3 cells/mm^3
RBC	1	1.00 to 7.00 × 10^6 cells/mm^3
Hgb	1	03.0 to 30.0 g/dℓ
Hct	2	10.0 to 70.0%
MCV	2	50.0 to 200.0 μm^3
RDW	5	05.0 to 20.0 RDW units
PLT	5	030. to 700. × 10^3 cells/mm^3

Table 4 describes the accuracy of the Model S-Plus over the range specified. Measurements from multiple blood samples are compared with the reference method described and apply when the Model S-Plus is calibrated in accordance with this manual.

Accuracy has been determined by comparing average readings obtained from Model S-Plus systems vs. those obtained from established reference instruments using blood samples obtained from normal and hospitalized populations. The comparison used to establish the accuracy of specific parameters is described below.

WBC and RBC

Semiautomatic Coulter Counter® RBC and WBC measurements were performed using duplicate 1:500 dilutions in ISOTON® II with ZAP-OGLOBIN® II for WBC. All samples were counted on a Coulter Counter® Model ZBI with a 100-μm aperture adjusted according to the Operator's Reference Manual. Coincidence correction is in accordance with published tables.

Hgb

Hemoglobin measurements were performed using duplicate dilution of samples in modified Drabkin's reagent. The resulting solution was allowed to stand for 15 min and was then read on a Beckman® DK2 Spectrophotometer at 540 nm. Measurements were calibrated against the known extinction coefficient of hemiglobin cyanide at 540 nm.

Hct

Microhematocrit measurements were performed in triplicate on a microhematocrit centrifuge. The microhematocrit centrifuge was operated at 10,000 x g for 5 min. Results of the microhematocrits were corrected for 3% trapped plasma by multiplying the answer by 0.97.

MCV

MCV measurements were performed by dividing the microhematocrit measurements described above by the RBC measurements made on the Coulter Counter® Model ZBI with a 100-μm aperture. The resulting value for MCV was multiplied by 10.0 to give the final answer in cubic micrometers.

RDW

The red cell distribution width index was determined using the Coulter Channelyzer® Model C-1000, attached to a Coulter Counter® Model ZBI equipped with 50/60-μm aperture with edit. This system was calibrated to the known MCV of fresh human blood samples. A 1:50,000 dilution of the blood sample in ISOTON® II was presented to the instrument, and the red count of the suspension was determined as the particle count over the range of 36 to 360 μm^3. The lower threshold setting was gradually increased until the red count had decreased to 80% of its original value and the corresponding volume of the resulting threshold setting was tabulated as the 80th percentile. The threshold was decreased further until the count reached 20% of the original count; the volume corresponding to the resulting threshold setting was tabulated as the 20th percentile volume. The red cell distribution width index (RDW) is calculated from the following relationship.

$$\text{RDW} = \frac{(\text{20th} - \text{80th}) \text{ percentile volume}}{(\text{20th} + \text{80th}) \text{ percentile volume}} \times 100 \times 0.66$$

The K factor (constant) of 0.66 is a normalizing factor used to convert all RDW measurements (which average approximately 15.1 when the factor is not used) to a convenient value of approximately 10.0.

PLT

Comparison platelet counts were performed using duplicate samples of each specimen, sedimented using the Coulter Thrombo-Fuge®, and the resulting platelet-rich plasma was diluted using ISOTON® II. The diluted platelet suspension was counted using a Coulter Counter® Model ZBI with a standard 70-μm aperture set at 2.5 and 25 μm^3 (referenced to latex spheres). A Coulter Channelyzer® Model C-1000 was connected to verify normal distributions and valleys at the threshold settings. The ZBI platelet counts were corrected for coincidence by use of the coincidence correction chart in the Model ZBI Operator's Reference Manual, and then converted to whole blood platelet counts.

Other Flow Counters

Two extensions of optical cell counting are included here for the sake of completeness. Both have been applied to commercial practice. One is a device for single cell processing and sorting; the other is the differential leukocyte counter (Hemalog D) previously mentioned which also uses flow detection techniques.

Both Becton-Dickinson and Coulter Electronics have developed particle separators based on the original technique of Fulwyler. Liquid containing particles flows past a sensing device which may be optical or electronic. Beyond the sensor the liquid stream is projected into air, but is broken into minute droplets by the action of a high-fre-

Table 5
COMPARISON OF WBC COUNTS ON HEMALOG D AND COULTER S OF 22 VOLUNTEERS OVER 6 DAYS[a]

	Day 1	Day 2	Day 3	Day 4	Day 5	Day 6
Mean of WBC counts	7.10	8.24	7.18	7.26	6.43	7.00
Mean of difference hemalog D-Coulter S	1.75	2.38	−0.37	0.36	−0.55	−0.19
Mean of difference duplicate on hemalog D	−0.01	0.09	−0.08	0.63	−0.49	0.49

[a] Samples were submitted to a well-known commercial laboratory under two fictitious names on 6 different days over a period of 3 months. All counts × 1000 cells per mm^3.

quency crystal vibrator. As the particles leave the orifice, a charge may be placed on specific droplets, thus enabling large charged plates to deflect these droplets which are received in a catch basin separate from the main stream. Particles or cells with various characteristics are sorted into a series of catch basins. The main use of this device is in immunologic research[32] where viable cells are sorted, for example by use of immune-specific fluorescent stains, and are later used for biological experiments. It may be considered as a means of purifying cell types for subsequent experiment.

Hemalog D, developed by Technicon Instrument Corporation, uses specific cytochemical techniques to identify the various cell types in human blood.[33] These techniques are automated so that dilutions, addition of reagents, and metering of sample into the sensor are continuously done without operator interaction. The detector device is optical, having both light-scattering and light-absorption sensors. By a combination of signals from the two sensors and the use of judicious thresholds, a classification of leukocytes is implemented. The advantage of the technique is in improved precision of the test. However, some degree of monitoring to insure correlation to microscopic methods of clasification is required. This can be considered a disadvantage compared to automated pattern recognition methods of differential leukocyte counting.

Performance

Some cautions must be given on overall performance of counting devices using flow techniques. In the following tables and discussions, this caution is expressed in the form of published data and one unpublished illustrative experiment on white blood cell counting. The experiment may or may not represent the worst case of real-life situations, since the values were actually reported from a commercial laboratory on days when other patient work was also reported. The results were not surprising when the statistical expectations are analyzed.

Day-to-Day

Table 5 provides results of an experiment which illustrates the difficuty of judging instrument performance. Samples were submitted to a well-known commercial laboratory. Duplicate test tubes with fictitious names assigned were sent for each of 22 volunteers on 6 days. Two samples, 3 hr apart, were sent and analyzed in different batches, but the results of the time samples were averaged.

Both tubes were analyzed by the Hemalog D for reproducibility. The first tube was

Table 6
MEASURE OF AGREEMENT BETWEEN CHAMBER COUNTS AND COULTER COUNTER (MODEL A) COUNTS, USING IDENTICAL DILUTIONS[a]

	Chamber count	Coulter count
Mean	7.5	7.6
SD±	2.6	2.7
Correlation coefficient	0.978	
Number of patients	41	

[a] Computed from data of Akeroyd et al.[35]

also analyzed by the Coulter S. The purpose of examining data in this way was to illustrate the potential variation due to calibration settings and thresholding.

Note that on 4 of the 6 days mean difference of the two instruments was within the same range as reproducibility of one instrument. However, on 2 other days, there was a gross discrepancy. If either set of results had been reported alone, there would have been no suspicion of this difference, which is in great part due to daily calibration. Note that correctness of one or other instrument is not at issue.

The usual reproducibility of each instrument is stated by the manufactuer to be between ±3 and 5% within 1 day's operation. Since calibration requires operation of the instrument, it follows that reproducibility of calibration also has a coefficient of variation of ± 3 to 5%. Thus each instrument may be 6 to 10% high or low and still be within the 95th percentile of its operating range. When the two instruments are at opposite ends of calibration error, there may be as much as a 20% consistent difference of all reports for the whole day.[34]

The use of control materials with established values would prevent such inconsistencies in daily values.

Accuracy

The best published study on agreement with manual counts of any instrument is by Akeroyd.[35] By peforming sufficient replicates of each sample to eliminate questions of reproducibility, extremely good agreement between instrument and chamber count was established. However, it should be noted that this experiment tested only the counting ability of the Coulter instrument, because the identical dilutions were used in both techniques. Table 6 is a recalculation of results on Table 1 of Akeroyd,[35] in which the very high counts (which overly influence results) were eliminated. Thus the final accuracy of a result strongly depends on the automated dilution and the instrument calibration. Although no published account exists of optical counters evaluated independenly of their dilution techniques, the author has had similar experience with the Hemalog D flow cell and optics prototypes.[36]

Precision

Table 7 summarizes published reports of precision of the various automated instruments. The difference between "duplicate" and "routine" values for Coulter Model A is that the former repeats the count only, whereas the latter repeats the dilution as well. That is, both samples are treated as new unknowns in the routine laboratory. A similar degradation in reproducibility was observed for Hemalog D when comparing

Table 7
REPRODUCIBILITY OF AUTOMATED WBC COUNTERS

Instrument	C.V. (±)	Source
SMA 4	6%	Green
Coulter Model A	2.3% (Duplicate)	Feichtmeir
	6.1% (Routine)	Feichtmeir
Hemalog 8	2.5%	Thom
Coulter Model S		
Hemalog D	2.5%	Statland
	4.1%	Saunders (unpublished)
Celloscope 401	1.6% (Cetrimide)	Lappin
	3.5% (Saponin)	

experimental results (2 to 5%) to blind-coded routine requests sent to a clinical laboratory.

Results on the Celloscope 401 are included as representative of an electronic counter not manufactured by Coulter Electronics Company. Note that various stromatolysing reagents yield different reproducibility.

Normal Range

A complete set of normal Hematologic ranges as determined by Coulter Model S has recently been published[37] for both males and females and for age groups from newborns to ages above 80 years. Similar values are available for the Hemalog 8.

Conclusion

Traditional and automated white blood cell counting methods are critically examined. Sources of error are identified, and references are given for ranges of normal values.

APPENDIX I

Method of Cross-Calibration of Two Automated White Blood Cell Counting Instruments

Step 1. Perform thresholding procedure on both instruments according to manufacturer's instructions.

Step 2. Perform calibration on the primary instrument using manufacturer's reference material

Step 3. Obtain a normal blood sample of sufficient volume to perform 12 runs on automated instruments;
i.e., 5 for primary instrument
6 for secondary instrument
1 for spare or waste

Step 4. Obtain 5 separate counts from the reference sample on the primary instrument. Calculate average of 5 results.

$$[\Sigma x/n = \bar{x}]$$

Step 5. Calibrate secondary instrument using the reference sample and the average of 5 runs on the primary sample.

Step 6. Using the same reference sample, obtain 5 separate counts on the secondary instrument. Calculate the average of these 5 results.

$$[\Sigma y/n = \bar{y}]$$

Step 7. Compare the average of the primary to the average of the secondary instrument.

$$[\bar{y} - \bar{x} = \bar{\Delta}]$$

Step 8. The difference of two averages ($\bar{\Delta}$) must be less than 10% of the grand average of two instruments.

$$100 \times \bar{\Delta} / \frac{\bar{x} + \bar{y}}{2} < 10\%$$

Step 9. If the difference is outside the 10% limit, start over at Step 3.

APPENDIX II

Summary of Automated and Semiautomated Cell Counting Instruments Available in Commerce as of Mid-1979S

Manufacturer/location	Product name and parameters measured
Clay Adams (Division of Bector Dickinson) 209 Webro Road Parsippany, NJ 07054	HA4, Ultra-Logic 800, Ultra-Flow 100; 8 parameter CBC and whole blood platelets
Coulter Electronics, Inc. 590 W. 20th. Street Hialeah, Florida 33010	Hemo-W; 2 parameter DN, ZBI, ZF; 3 and 4 parameter S, S Sr., S Plus; full automation S Plus; whole blood platelets
Hycel Division 7920 Westpark Drive Houston, TX 77063	700,300/500, HPC 103; platelets, RBC, WBC, HCT on 103,
Labex Norwood	Rebuilt Coulter and General Science
Modolus Norwood	Rebuilt Coulter and General Science
J. T. Baker Diagnostics 2266 Avenue A Bethlehem, PA 18017	JTB 500, JTB 700, MK4/HC; platelets, distribute General Science
Mallinckrodt 1644 Locust Avenue Bohemia, NY 11717	RBC, WBC, HCT, adjustable threshold
Ortho Instrumments Westwood, MA 02090	7 parameter HEMAC 4000; 8 parameter ELT-8 with whole blood platelets
Royco (Division of Hycel) 141 Jefferson Drive Menlo Park, CA 94025	920A, 720A(Hgb), Cell Crit IV and X; RBC, WBC, MCV, Hgb, Hct
Technicon 511 Benedict Avenue Tarrytown, NY 10591	Model 8/90; RBC, WBC, MCV, Hgb, MCH, MCHC, platelets
TOA (Division of Kasho U.S.A. 1025 Grandview Drive South San Francisco, CA 94080	Sysmex#110, Sysmex#108, Sysmex#100; PL 110 for platelets, RBC, WBC

REFERENCES

1. **Schierbeek, A.**, Inleiding tot *De Van Leeuwenhoek — brief van 9 oktober 1676*, Utigave Gist-en iritusfabrieken, Delft, 1676.
2. **Daland, G. A.**, *Syllabus of Laboratory Examinations in Clinical Diagnosis*, Harvard University Press, Cambridge, Mass., 1961.
3. *Standard Procedures for the Collection of Diagnostic Blood Specimens by Venipuncture*, National Committee for Clinical Laboratory Standards, Villa Nova, Pa.
4. *Standard Procedures for the Collection of Diagnostic Blood Specimens by Skin Puncture*, National Committee for Clinical Laboratory Standards , Villa Nova, Pa.
5. *Standard Procedures for the Storage and Transport of Diagnostic Hematological, Biochemical and Serological Body Fluid Specimens*, National Committee for Clinical Laboratory Standards, Villa Nova, Pa.
6. **Berkson, J., Magath, R. B., and Hurn, M.**, The error of estimate of the blood cell count as made with the hemacytometer, *Am. J. Physiol*, 128, 309, 1940.
7. **Mattern, C. F., Brackett, F. S., and Olson, B. J.**, Determination of number and size of particles by electrical gating: blood cells, *J. Appl. Physiol.*, 10, 56—70, 1957.
8. **Wolff, H. S.**, An apparatus for counting small particles in random distribution with special reference to red blood corpuscles, *Nature (London)*, 165, 967, 1950.
9. **Lagercrantz, C.**, On the theory of counting individual microscopic cells by photoelectric scanning. An improved counting apparatus, *Acta Physiol. Scand.*, 26, Suppl. 92, 1952.
10. **Young, J. Z. and Roberts, F.**, A flying spot microscope, *Nature (London)*, 167, 231, 1951.
11. **Frommer, P. L.**, An automatic "counter" for blood cells, *Ann. N.Y. Acad. Sci.*, 99, 233—241, 1962.
12. **Coulter, W. H.**, *High Speed Automatic Blood Cell Counter and Cell Size Analyzer*, National Electronics Conference, Chicago, Ill., 1956.
13. **Coulter, W. H.**, *Means for Counting Particles Suspended in a Fluid*, U.S. Patent, 656,508,1953.
14. **Crosland-Taylor, P. J.**, A device for counting small particles suspended in a fluid through a tube, *Nature (London)*, 171, 37, 1953.
15. **Eckhoff, R. K.**, An experimental indication of the volume proportional response of the Coulter Counter for irregularly shaped particles, *J. Sci. Inst.*, 44, 648—649, 1967.
16. **Grover, N. B., Naaman, J., Ben-asson, S., and Doljanski, F.**, Electrical sizing of particles in suspens. III. Rigid spheroids and red blood cells, *Biophys. J.*, 12, 1099—1116, 1972.
17. **Waterman, C. S., Atkinson, E. E., Wilkins, B., Fischer, C. L., and Kimsey, S. L.**, Improved measurement of erythrocyte volume distribution by aperture-counter signal analysis, *Clin. Chem.*, 21, 1201—1211, 1975.
18. **Kachel, V. and Ruhenstroth-Bauer, G.**, Methodik und Ergebissne Optiseher Formfactorunter-suchungen bei der Zellvolumenmessung nach Coulter, *Micros. Acta*, 75, 419—423, 1976.
19. **Bessis, M. and Mohanda, N.**, A diffractometric method for the measurement of cellular deformability, *Blood Cells*, 1, 307, 1975.
20. **Bessis, M. and Mohandas, N.**, Deformability of normal, shape-altered and pathological red cells, *Blood Cells*, 1, 315, 1975.
21. **Deboo, G. J. and Burrous, C. N.**, *Integrated Circuits and Semiconductor Devices: Theory and Application*, McGraw-Hill, New York, 1971, 147—213.
22. **Adams, R. B. and Gregg, E. C.**, Pulse shapes from particles traversing Coulter orifice fields, *Phys. Med. Biol.*, 17, 830-841, 1972.
23. **Shuler, M. L., Aris, R., and Tsuchiya, H. M.**, Hydrodynamic focusing and electronic cell-sizing techniques, *Appl. Microbiol.*, 24, 384-388, 1972.
24. **Schulz, J. and Thom, R.**, Electrical sizing and counting of platelets in whole blood, *Med. Biol. Eng.*, 11, 447—454, 1973.
25. **Helleman, P. W.**, *The Coulter Electronic Particle Counter: Aspects and Views in Counting and Sizing of Eythrocytes*, Zetwertk: N. W. Fototekst, Nieuw Loosdrecht, Druk: Koninklijke Drukkerij C. C. Callenbac, N. V. Nijkerk, The Netherlands, 1972.
26. **Saunders, A. M.**, The automation of cytochemical methods for automated cytophotometers, *J. Histochem. Cytochem.*, 25, 1001—1012, 1977.
27. **McGovern, J. J., Jones, A. R., and Steinberg, A. G.**, The hematocrit of capillary blood, *N. Engl. J. Med.*, 253, 308, 1955.
28. **England, J. M., Walford, D. M., and Waters, D. A. W.**, Re-assessment of the reliability of the haematocrit, *Br. J. Haematol.*, 23, 247, 1972.
29. **England, J. M.**, *Recommendations for Reference Methods for the Determination of Packed Cell Volumes of Blood*, International Committee for Standardization in Hematology, World Health Organization, Geneva, 1978.

30. **van Assendelft, O. W., Buursma, A., Holtz, A. H., van Kampen, E. J., and Zijlstra, W. G.,** Quality control in haemoglobinometry with special reference to the stability of haemiglobincyanide reference solutions, *Clin. Chim. Acta,* 70, 161-169, 1976.
31. **Bull, B. S., Elashoff, R. M., Heilbron, D. C., and Coperus, J.,** A Study of various estimators for the derivation of quality control procedures from patient erythrocyte indices, *Am. J. Clin. Pathol.,* 61 (No. 4), 473—481, 1974.
32. **Hulett, H. R., Donner, W. A., Sweet, R. G., and Herzenberg, L. A.,** Development and application of a rapid cell sorter, *Clin. Chem.,* 19, 813, 1973; Stovel, R. T. and Sweet, R. G., Individual cell Sorting, *J. Histochem. Cytochem.,* 27, 284—288, 1978.
33. **Saunders, A. M.,** The automation of cytochemical methods for automated cytophotometers, *J. Histochem.,* 25, 1001—1012, 1977.
34. **Saunders, A. M.,** unpublished.
35. **Akeroyd, J. H., Gibbs, M. B., Vivano, S., and Robinette, R. W.,** On counting leukocytes by electronic means, *Am. J. Clin. Pathol.,* 31, 188, 1959.
36. **Saunders, A. M.,** unpublished.
37. **Simmons, A.,** Establishment of normal hematologic values using the Hemalog™, *Am. J. Med. Technol.,* 40, 321, 1974.

The Red Cell

THE RED CELL

Emin Kansu and Allan J. Erslev

Production

Site of Erythrocyte Production

Red cell formation has been observed in the yolk sac outside the embryo after about 3 weeks of gestation (Figure 1).[1] During this yolk sac phase, the erythrocytes are nucleated and contain embryonic hemoglobins, ε_4 (Gower 1) and $\alpha_2\varepsilon_2$ (Gower 2).[2] A few weeks later, red cell production moves to the liver, and erythrocytes, subsequently produced from liver, spleen, and bone marrow, are nonnucleated and contain fetal hemoglobin ($\alpha_2\,\gamma_2$). Bone cavities form during the fifth fetal month, but are first used primarily for the production of granulocytes. The liver is the chief site of red cell production during fetal life. The spleen plays a brief role between the third and seventh month, after which time the bone marrow cavities slowly get involved in erythropoiesis. Shortly after a child is born, red cell production takes place almost exclusively in the bone cavities, and splenic and hepatic hematopoiesis ceases. Hemoglobin A ($\alpha_2\,\beta_2$) gradually replaces fetal hemoglobin in the circulating erythrocytes until the normal adult level of Hemoglobin A (98%) is reached when an infant is about 6 months of age.[4]

In the normal adult, blood cell formation is the prerogative of bone marrow cavities. These cavities grow in volume throughout life because of progressive bone reabsorption, and available space soon outstrips the spatial needs of the immature blood cells for normal proliferation. As early as 2 to 4 years of age, fat cells emerge in order to take up excessive space. The bone marrow becomes increasingly fatty, with almost complete replacement of hematopoietic cells in the marrow of peripheral bones at the age of 20. At that time, even the cavities of central flat bones contain about 50% fat. The preference during adult life of central bone marrow cavities for blood production may be related to higher temperature and better vascularity in the cavities.[5] However, it also has been suggested that peripheral bone marrow cavities are programmed for an eventual fatty involution.[6] Further fatty infiltration continues throughout life because of bone resorption and, in old age, also because of a slight decrease in the circulating red cell mass and in the number of immature cells needed to maintain such a mass.[7]

Bone marrow tissue obtained by aspiration appears as a random mixture of cells of various lines and various maturities. However, the bone marrow structure is far from random. It is a highly organized tissue scaffolded by reticular cells and anchored on a spoke-like vascular system (Figure 2).[8] Arterioles provide blood that slowly percolates through cords of immature cells until it reenters the vascular system through pores in central sinusoidal walls (Figure 3). The sinusoids consist of a fenestrated basement membrane, partially covered on the inside by endothelial cells and on the outside by branching structural reticular cells (Figure 4).[9] The reticular cells cover the fenestrations in the basement membrane and may play a role in regulating entry of hematopoietic cells through the sinusoidal wall.[10] They branch out and provide a mesh work in which hematopoietic cells lie nested. They can control the volume of the hematopoietic space, either acutely by becoming more or less hydrated and gelatinous, or chronically by becoming fatty. Although in the past reticular cells were believed to be phagocytic and part of the reticuloendothelial system, the current concept of their function is that they are merely supporting cells without phagocytic or immunologic properties.

The hematopoietic cells lie in cords or wedges between the vascular sinuses in the

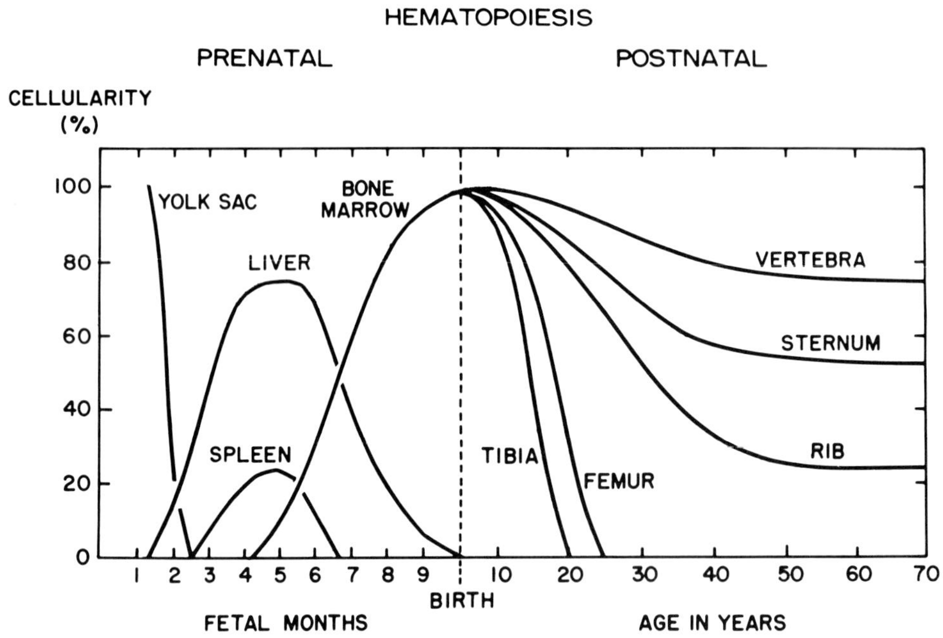

FIGURE 1. Expansion and regression of hematopoietic tissue during fetal and adult life. (From Erslev, A. J. and Weiss, L., *Hematology*, 2nd ed., Williams, W. J., Beutler, E., Erslev, A. J., and Rundles, R. W., Eds. McGraw-Hill, New York, 1977, 57. With permission.

mesh work created by reticular cells. The erythroblasts lie closely against the outside surface of the vascular sinuses in distinct clusters, so-called erythroid islands (Figure 5).[11] These consist of a number of erythroblasts lying in small nests on the surface of a single macrophage (Figure 6). The macrophage sends out extensive slender membranes that envelop each of the erythroblasts and provide a close physical metabolic relationship (Figure 7). Undoubtedly, the macrophage provides nutrients to the erythroblasts and removes both the unused intracellular elements in the erythroblasts, such as sideroblastic particles, and the finally extruded pyknotic nucleus. Eventually, the erythroblasts will lose some of the stickiness that keeps them attached to the macrophages and will attempt to squeeze through the pores of the basement membrane into the venous sinusoids (Figure 8). The loss of stickiness may be explained by a loss of transferrin receptors,[12] and the denucleation appears to be caused primarily by the pitting action as the erythroblasts attempt to squeeze through a narrow pore (Figure 9).[13]

In regard to the other marrow elements, megakaryocytes also lie directly on the vascular wall. When mature, the cytoplasm peels off and enters the sinuses in long ribbons made up of individual platelets. Granulocytes differentiate deeper in the hematopoietic cords away from the vascular sinuses. They are presumably more motile and, when mature enough, will enter the vascular sinuses. Nerve cells are present in abundance and seem to be responsive to intramedullary pressure. Pressure-related nerve signals could adjust vascular perfusion and cellular release to changes in growth pressure within the hematopoietic compartments.[14]

Erythrocyte Maturation Sequence

The morphology of the developing erythroblasts has been closely correlated with the biochemical events that underlie blast transformation of small mononuclear stem cells to proerythroblasts and their subsequent multiplication, maturation, and enucleation.

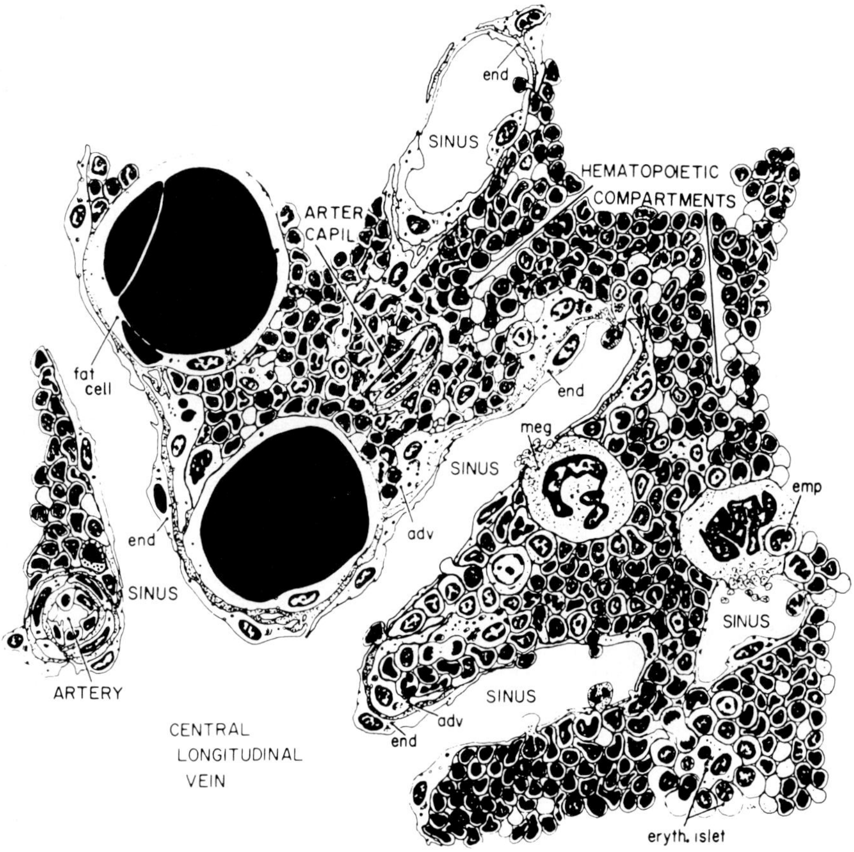

FIGURE 2. Bone marrow schematic view of cross section near central longitudinal vein. The sinuses are cut along their long axis, the vein, in cross section. A portion of the nutrient artery (Art) is present as is an arterial capillary. Hematopoietic cells lie between the sinuses constituting the hematopoietic compartment. Where hematopoiesis is relatively quiet the wall of the sinus and of the central longitudinal vein is trilaminar consisting of endothelium (end), a basement membrane, and adventitial cell (adv). The adventitial cell may become voluminous, encroaching upon the hematopoietic space and thereby displacing hematopoietic cells. The increased volume of the adventitial cell may be due to a gelatinous change wherein its cytoplasm becomes rarefied, presumably due to hydration. If this change is widespread, the marrow may become grossly white and gelatinous. A second and more common basis for large bulk of adventitial cells is fatty change, where they become fat cells. Contrariwise, when hematopoiesis is active, the hematopoietic compartment is large and packed with myelocytes, erythroblasts,and megakaryocytes. The sinus wall becomes thin, reduced to an endothelial layer alone as the adventitial cells are displaced or lifted from the wall by infiltrating hematopoietic cells. Apertures appear in the endothelium, moreover, as maturing hematopoietic cells cross the sinus wall and enter the sinus lumen. Megakarocytes characteristically lie against the outside of the sinus wall, discharging platelets into the lumen through an aperture. Occasionally the cytoplasm of megakarocytes is entered by other cell types which remain visible and later leave the megakarocyte. The phenomenon is known as emperipolesis (emp). Erythroblasts tend to be present in clusters near the sinus wall. Erythroblastic islets may be present. Granulocytes usually develope mear the center of the hematopoietic space. Lymphocytes occur throughout the marrow. Macrophages are common, and mast cells, plasma cells, and other connective tissue cells are also present. (From Weiss, L and Greeps, R. O., *Histology,* 4th ed., McGraw-Hill, 1974. With permission.)

Such correlations have transformed the basically static light microscopy to a dynamic science, and the recent addition of transmission and reflecting electron microscopy has enormously enhanced our understanding of cellular structure and function.

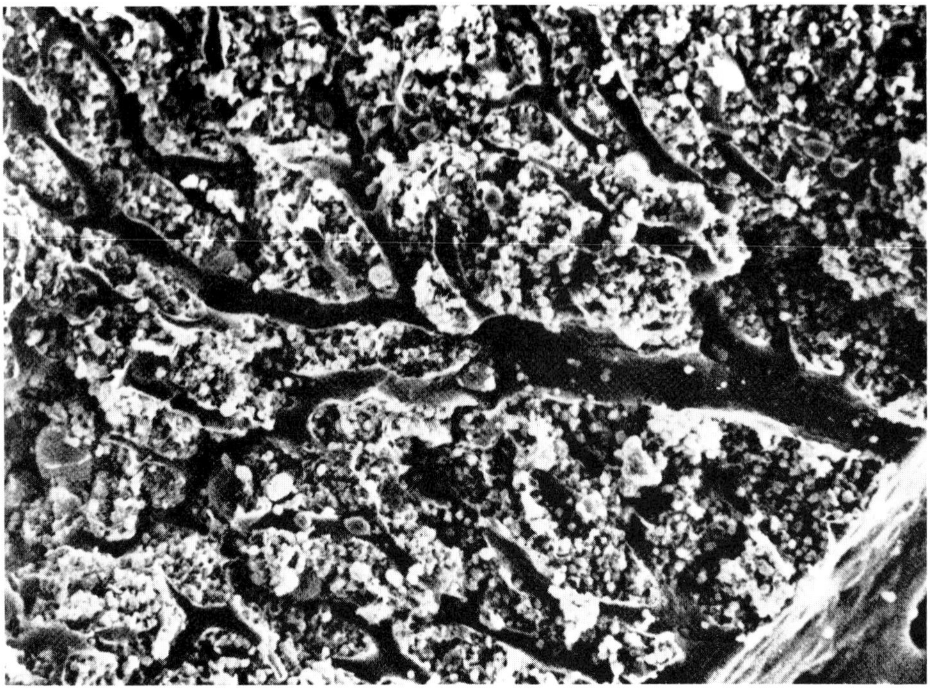

FIGURE 3. The venous vessels of the bone marrow appear here in an arborizing pattern: smaller venous sinuses converge into large venous sinuses. The central longitudinal vein lies in the lower right hand corner. The orifices in its wall represent the entrance of its tributary venous sinuses. (From Weiss, L., *Anat. Rec.*, 186, 161, 1976. With permission.)

The Erythropoietic Stem Cell

The immediate precursor cell of the morphologically recognizable erythroblasts has been referred to as an erythropoietin-responsive or erythropoietin-committed stem cell, or as an erythroid colony-forming unit (CFU-E). Like other stem cells, it is believed to be a small mononuclear cell indistinguishable from lymphocytes (Figure 10a). However, it is specifically programmed to be triggered by erythropoietin into DNA synthesis and blast transformation.[16]

Proerythroblast

The product of this blast transformation is an irregular oval cell 20 to 25 μm in diameter. It often shows evidence of ameboid motions by displaying "dog-eared" cytoplasmic extensions. The nucleus is perfectly round and relatively large, and contains finely dispersed chromatin with one or several nucleoli. It is clearly separated from the deep blue cytoplasm by a distinct nuclear membrane. The intense cytoplasmic basophilia is caused by numerous polyribosomes and other acid organelles. However, the cytoplasm is devoid of visible granules when stained with the usual Romanovsky stains (Figure 10b). The cell actively incorporates iron for subsequent hemoglobin synthesis and, at high magnification with the electron microscope (at least 100,000 times), ferritin molecules can be seen dispersed in the cytoplasm.

Basophilic Erythroblast

Concomitant to, but not dependent on, the first mitotic division, the basophilic erythroblast emerges. This cell is similar to the pronormoblast but is smaller in size and generally measures from 16 to 18 μm in diameter. As the cell matures, the size of the

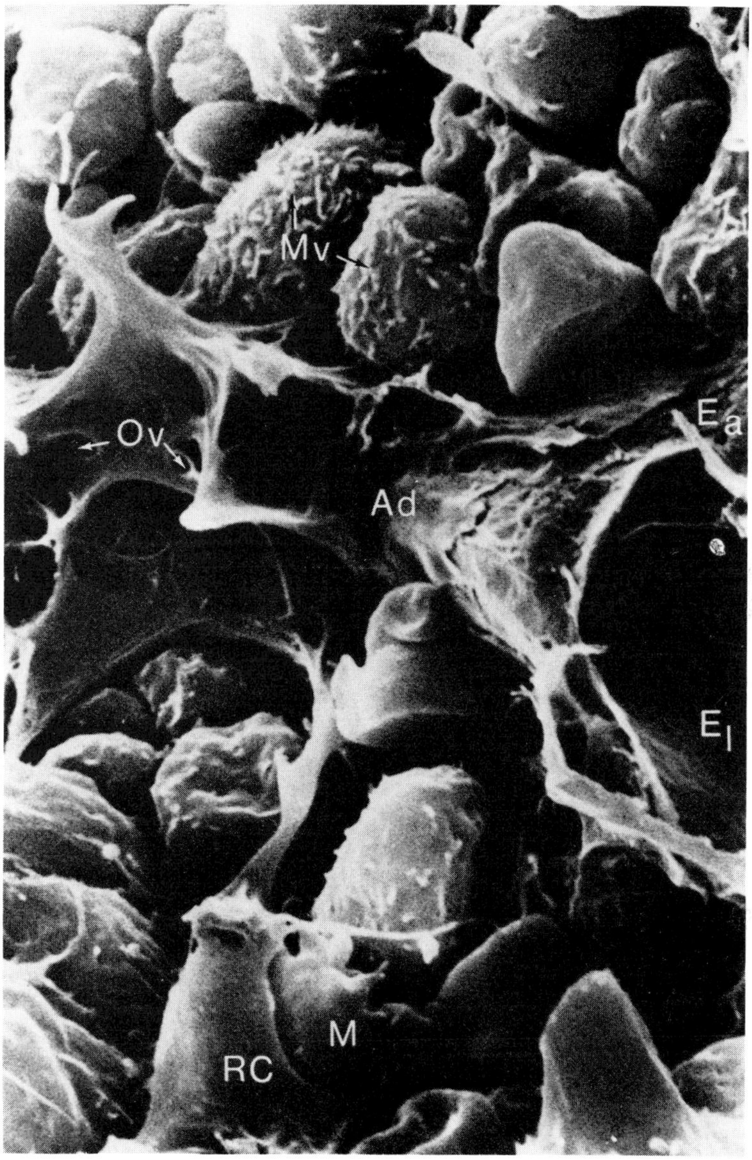

FIGURE 4. A vascular sinus crosses the field from left to right, coming out toward the surface; its lumen is exposed at the right hand margin of the field. Both the luminal (E_L) and the adventitial (E_A) surfaces of the endothelium can be seen. The broad cytoplasmic expanse of an adventitial reticular cell (Ad) covers much of the outside surface of the vascular sinus and branches richly, far out into the hematopoietic compartment. Its processes pass between, and closely surround, hematopoietic cells. At one place, reticular cell cytoplasm (RC) almost completely surrounds a myelocyte (M). The oval fenestrae (Ov) in the broad reticular cell processes are typical. Several cells bearing microvilli (Mv) lie close against the adventitial surface of the sinus at its upper aspect. These microvilli may well have developed preparatory to transmural passage of these cells. Many hematopoietic cells have been removed in this preparation, due to the loosening effects of perfusion. (From Weiss, L., *Anat. Rec.*, 186, 161, 1976. With permission.)

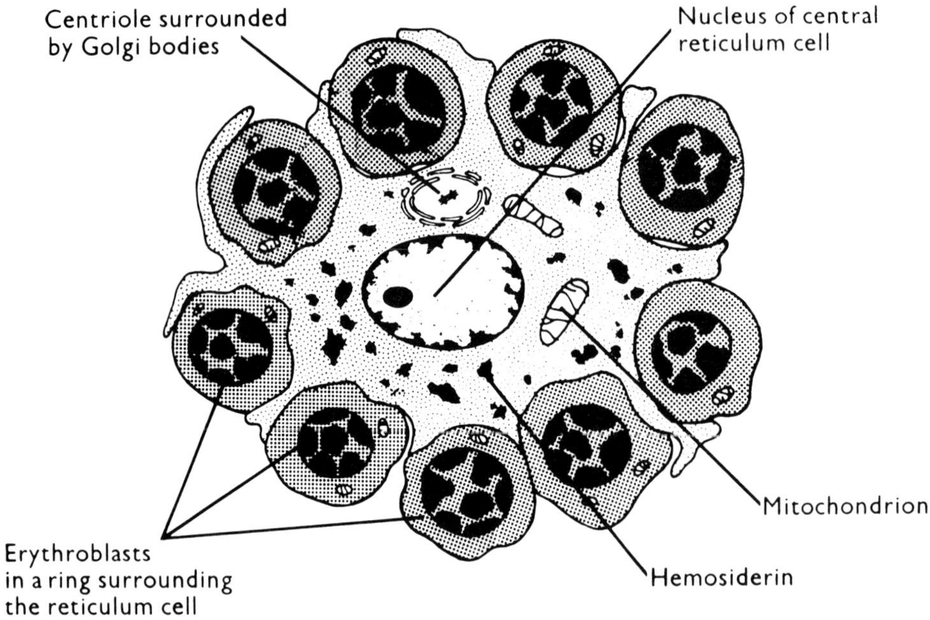

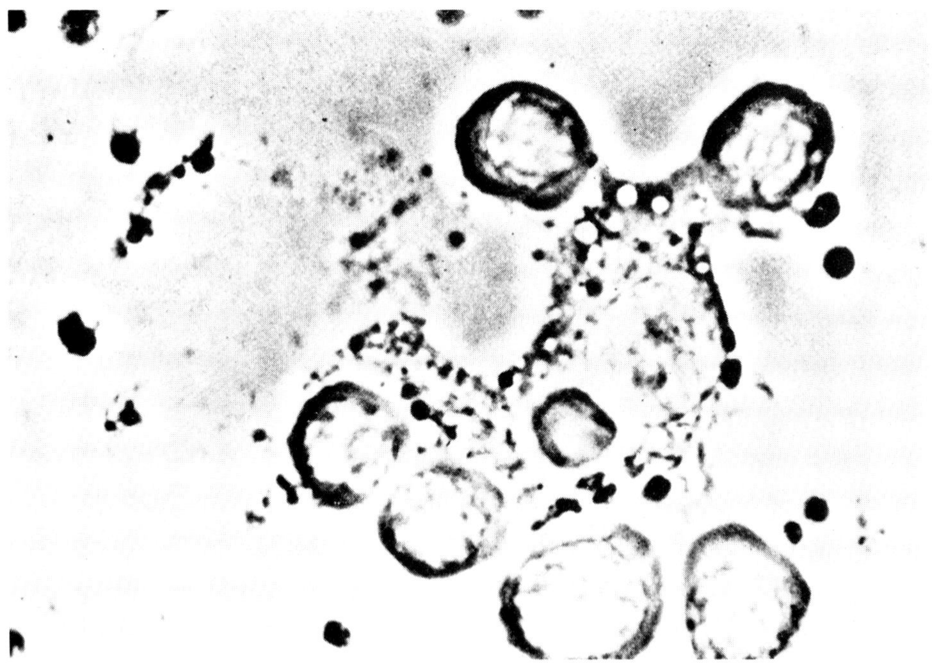

FIGURE 5. (A) The erythroblastic island is composed of a central reticulum cell and surrounding normoblasts at various stages of development. The reticulum cell contains stores of iron in the form of ferritin. It is closely related to its surrounding normoblasts, often enclosing them with active pseudopodic movement. It ingests and destroys the ejected normoblast nucleus and engulfs aged or damaged erythrocytes, conserving their iron as ferritin. (B) Erythroblastic island in the living state, seen in the phase contrast microscope. (From Lessin, L. S. and Bessis, M., *Hematology,* 2nd ed., Williams, W. J., Beutler, E., Erslev, A. J., and Rundles, R. W., Eds., McGraw-Hill, New York, 1977, 103. With permission.)

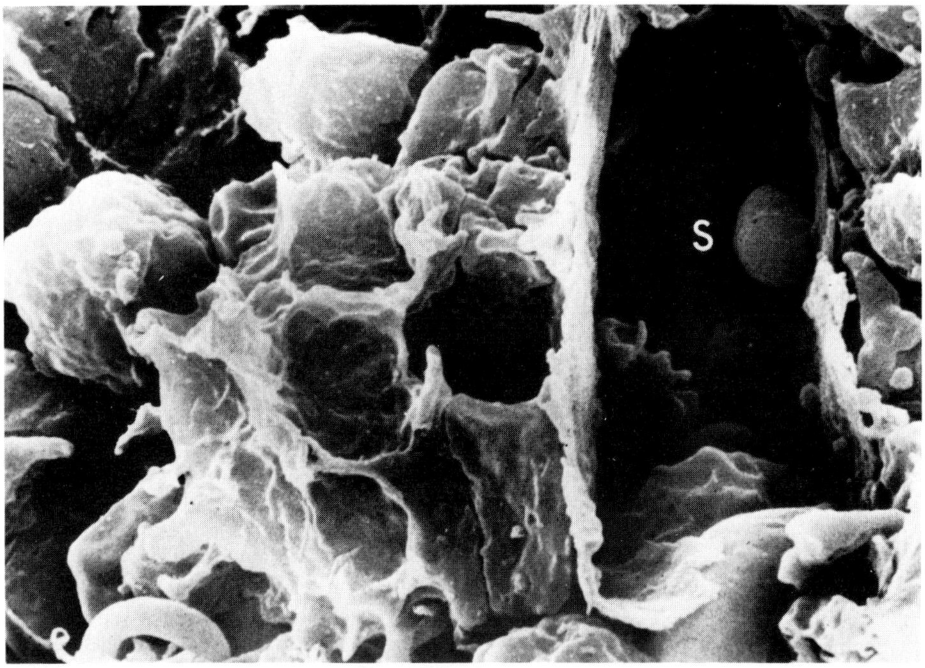

FIGURE 6. A macrophage, likely the central cell in an erythroblastic islet, is applied to the outside surface of a venous sinus (S). The macrophage bears indentations on its surface, representing sites where erythroblasts had lain. (From Weiss, L., *Anat. Rec.*, 186, 161 1976. With permission.)

nucleus decreases rapidly, and as a result the cytoplasmic border becomes relatively larger. The nucleus at this stage shows coarse, granular chromatin masses, often arranged in clock-face fashion, and is without visible nucleoli (Figure 10c). The cytoplasm stains a uniform dark blue due to the presence of polyribosomes. An emerging perinuclear halo and a juxtanuclear clear zone reflect the presence of a Golgi apparatus involved in the assembly of hemoglobin molecules. Mitochondria are very abundant, and microtubules can be seen around the centrioles in the cytoplasm.

Polychromatophilic Erythroblast

At the time of the second mitotic division in the erythropoietic series, the hemoglobin concentration in the cytoplasm has increased enough to give the cell a dirty greenish coloration. This so-called polychromatophilic erythroblast is smaller than its basophilic precursor, measuring approximately 12 to 15 μm in diameter. As maturation and hemoglobin synthesis progress, the nucleus becomes further reduced in size, and the chromatin gets more condensed (Figure 10d). The electron microscope reveals increased nuclear clumping of chromatin and decreased concentration of cytoplasmic polyribosomes. Iron-containing siderosomes can now be identified within the cytoplasm.[17]

Orthochromatic Erythroblast

The final mitotic division of the erythroblast produces the smallest of the series, varying from 10 to 15 μm in diameter. Its pyknotic dense nucleus occupies one fourth of the cell area (Figure 10e). The mitochondria are reduced in number and size, and some of them show signs degeneration. Polyribosomes are present, but in decreasing numbers. At this stage the nucleus is expelled, carrying with it a thin portion of cytoplasm. The expelled nucleus is phagocytized by the macrophages, and the remainder of the cell seals up and forms a nonnucleated reticulocyte.

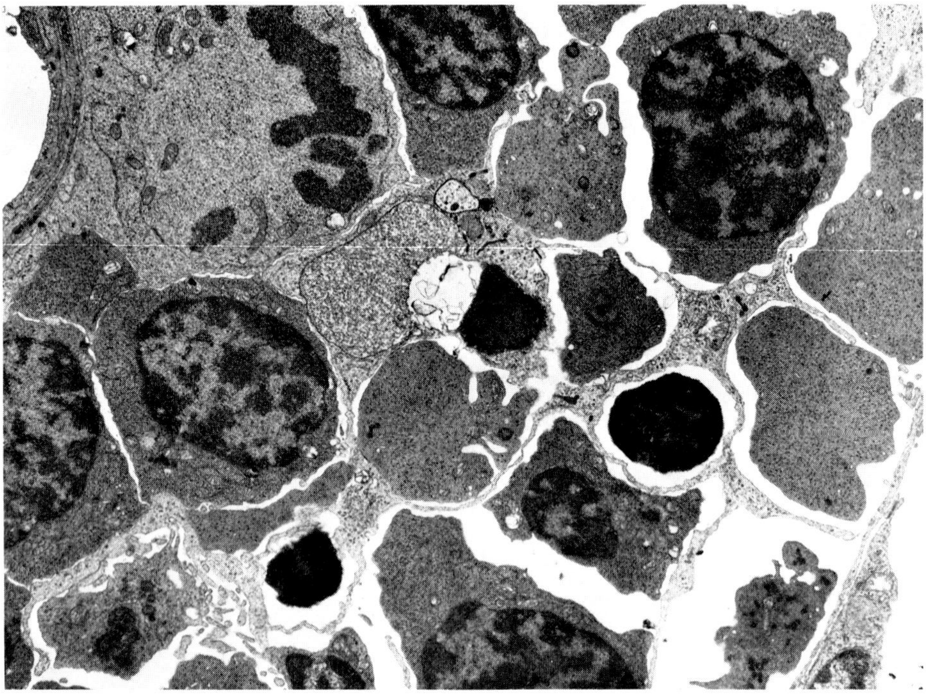

A

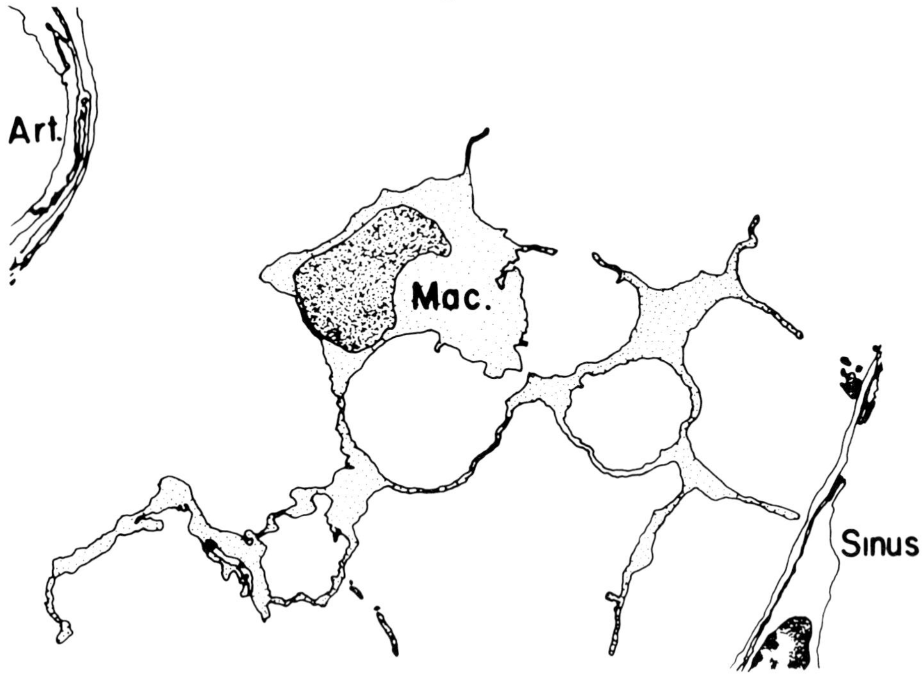

B

FIGURE 7. As seen in the photograph (A) and, more distinctly, from the tracing (B), a single macrophage (Mac) extends long, slender, branching processes which enclose erythroblasts in different degrees of maturation. This is the central macrophage in an erythroblast islet. The islet lies between an arterial vessel in the upper left corner (ART) and a venous sinus (SINUS) in the lower right corner. Note the degree of cell separation after perfusion. This degree of cell separation is valuable in loosening hematopoietic cells so that they fall out of the tissue and reveal the macrophages and reticular cells. (From Weiss, L., *Anat. Rec.*, 186, 161, 1976. With permission.)

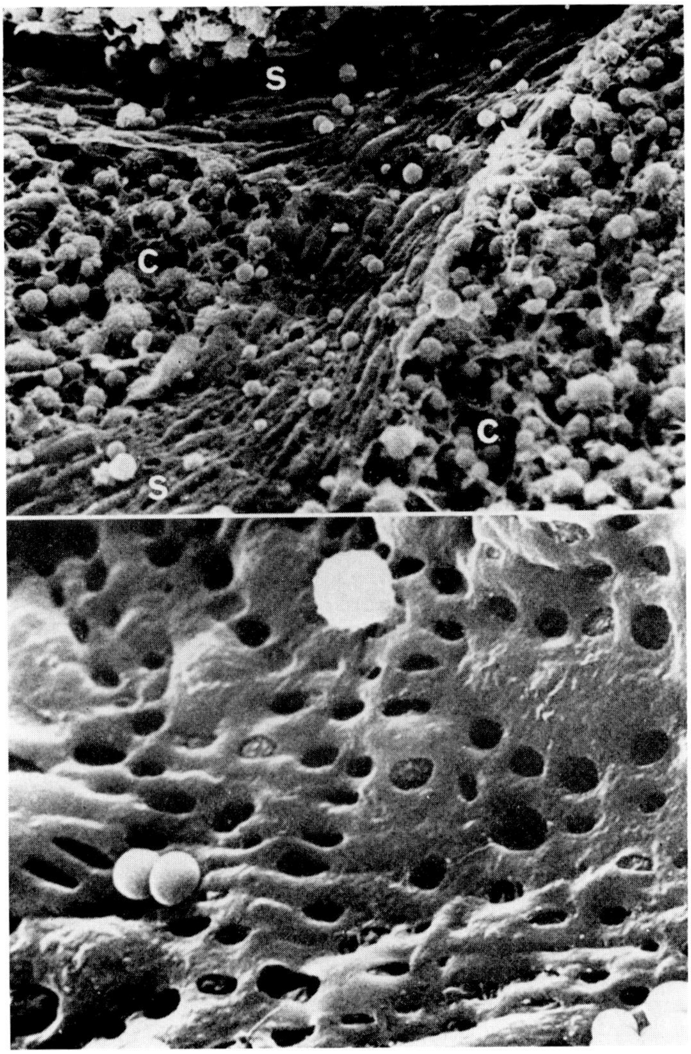

FIGURE 8. The inside surface of venous sinuses (s) (a). The erythroblasts are in the process of squeezing through the pores of the basement membrane into the venous sinusoids. (From LeBlond, P. F., *Nouv, Rev. Fr. Hematol.*, 13, 771, 1973. With permission.)

Reticulocyte

The reticulocyte is larger than the average erythrocytes and has a slightly grayish-red appearance (polychromasia) because of the presence of a small number of ribosomes, mitochondria, and remnants of Golgi apparatus (Figure 10f). Supravital staining with oxydant dyes like brilliant cresyl blue or methylene blue will produce precipitation and aggregation of ribosomes and other organelles and will result in the formation of deep blue-staining reticular material characteristic of the reticulocyte. The cell matures over a period of 2 to 4 days, with a loss of cellular membrane, cytoplasmic fluid, and unneeded organelles.

Erythrocyte

The final product of this maturation of reticulocytes is the formation of mature biconcave or uniconcave, disc-shaped, circulating erythrocytes. Erythrocytes are

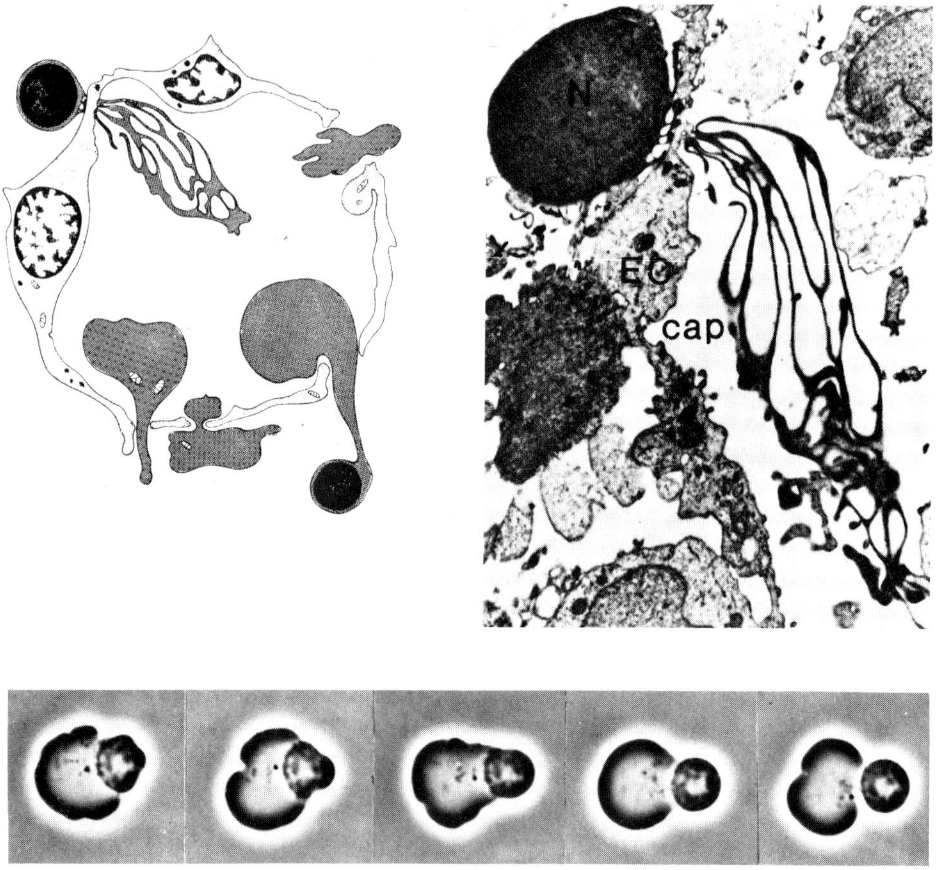

FIGURE 9. Reticulocytes undergoing their characteristic movements are passing between endothelial cells of the capillary. On the right, an electron microphotograph illustrates the ejection of the normoblast nucleus (N), and diapedesis of the resultant reticulocyte across the endothelial cell (EC) into the sinusoidal capillary space (cap). Portions of a film from phase contrast microcinematography show the ejection by an orthochromatic normoblast of its nucleus (lower panel). (From Bessis, M., *Living Blood Cells and their Ultrastructure*, Springer-Verlag, New York, 1973, 139. With permission.)

stained bright pink with Romanowsky stains and display a relatively pale middle third (Figure 10g). A normal mature erythrocyte contains about 300 million hemoglobin molecules, constituting 33% of its total cytoplasmic mass (MCHC). It has a diameter of 7.5 to 8.3 μm, an average thickness of 1.7 μm, and a volume of about 83 fl (MCV). The surface area is approximately 140 μm^2. Mature cells in man are soft and malleable, capable of passing through capillaries with diameters a mere fraction of their own. As the cell ages it becomes more rigid, until finally its decreased malleability leads to retention in a reticuloendothelial filter bed and destruction there. The survival of this denucleated cell for about 120 days, despite rapid circulation through narrow passages, unfavorable water, electrolyte gradients, and high ambient oxygen tension, is due to the structure of the red cell membrane. It provides malleability, self-healing after injuries, insulation from the circulating plasma contents, and selective uptake and secretion of metabolic compounds. It is composed of a lipid bilayer, with the polar hydrophilic ends of the phospholipid molecules pointing towards the extracellular and intracellular fluids, and the nonpolar hydrophobic fatty acid chains directed towards the center. Cholesterol molecules are inserted between the phospholipid molecules in both halves of the bilayer.[18] This structure provides excellent insulation, since the al-

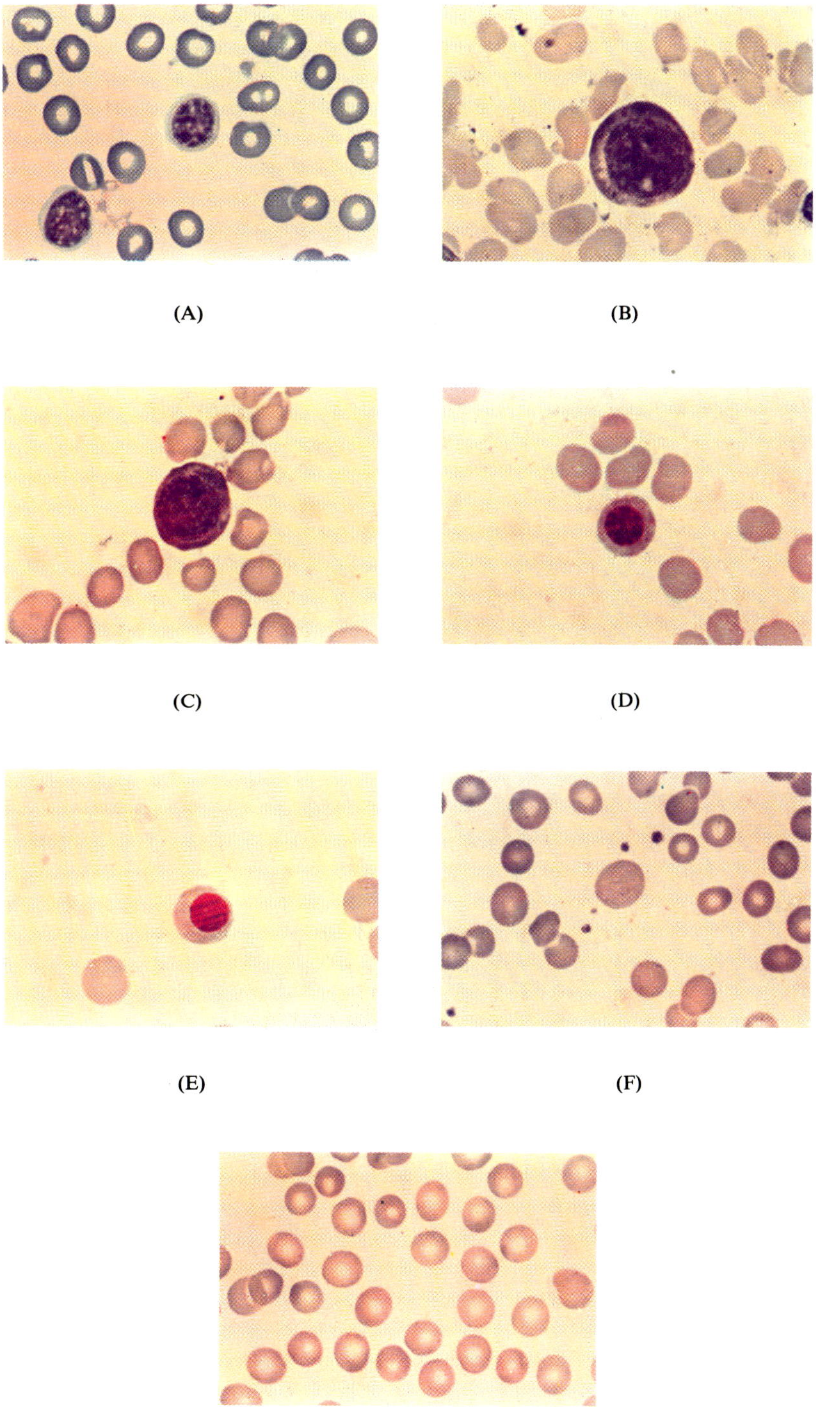

(A) (B) (C) (D) (E) (F) (G)

FIGURE 10. Erythrocyte maturation sequence: (A) Stem cell (B) Proerythroblast (C) Basophilic erythroblast (D) Polychromatophilic erythroblast (E) Orthochromatic erythroblast (F) Reticulocyte, and (G) Erythrocytes (All magnifications × 750-oil immersion.)

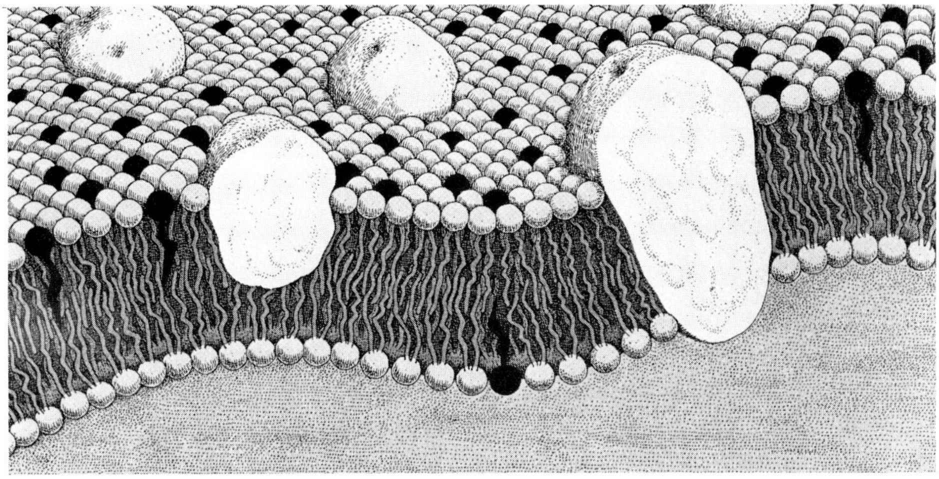

FIGURE 11. In the current model of a cell membrane, lipid molecules are arranged in a bilayer, their hydrophilic ends protruding from the membrane and their hydrophopic "tails" directed towards the center. Cholesterol molecules (black) are positioned in either bilayer. Embedded in this lipid matrix, and sometimes extending through it, are proteins which make up the membrane's "active sites". (Huehns, E. R. and Shooter, E. M., Review article, human haemoglobins, *J. Med. Genet.*, 2, 48, 1965. With permission.)

ternative hydrophilic and hydrophobic layers are almost completely impenetrable for most macromolecules and micromolecules. Inserted in this lipid structure are red cell membrane proteins which, as suggested by Singer, are globular and positioned according to their polar charges[19] (Figure 11). The hydrophobic ends of these protein molecules are embedded in the hydrophobic center of the lipid bilayer, whereas hydrophilic ends are ringed with hydrophilic lipid heads at the inner or outer surface.[20] The ultrastructure of red cell membrane can be visualized by the freeze-etching technique, which reveals a split bilayer pocked with particles, some penetrating the bilayer and others only reaching through one half of it[21,22] (Figure 12). This structure confirms the validity of the Singer model.

The protein molecules of the red cell membrane can be isolated and identified by routine protein separation procedures.[23,24] The possible arrangement of the isolated major erythrocyte membrane proteins is shown in Figure 13. Some proteins, so-called glycophorins, pass all the way through the lipid bilayer and may be positionedin groups, providing channels between the cytoplasm and the surrounding plasma. Such transmembraneous proteins appear to be attached to a meshwork of proteins, so-called spectrins, positioned at the internal aspect of the membrane.[25] These proteins probably provide stability to the semifluid membrane. Furthermore, by anchoring transmembraneous protein molecules, they may be responsible for the fact that intact erythrocytes in the adult do not exhibit the so-called "capping phenomenon". In other mammalian cells, the transmembraneous proteins can move freely in the lipid membrane and may move to one end (cap) of the cell when exposed to labeled cross-reacting, antiprotein antibodies.[11] On the outside, transmembraneous and more superficial proteins serve as anchors on which branching monosaccharide chains provide cells with their specific receptors and specific antigenic identity.[26]

Humoral Control of Red Cell Production

The circulating red cell mass is carefully maintained at a size optimal for its primary mission of transporting oxygen from lungs to tissues. As with all homeostatic controls,

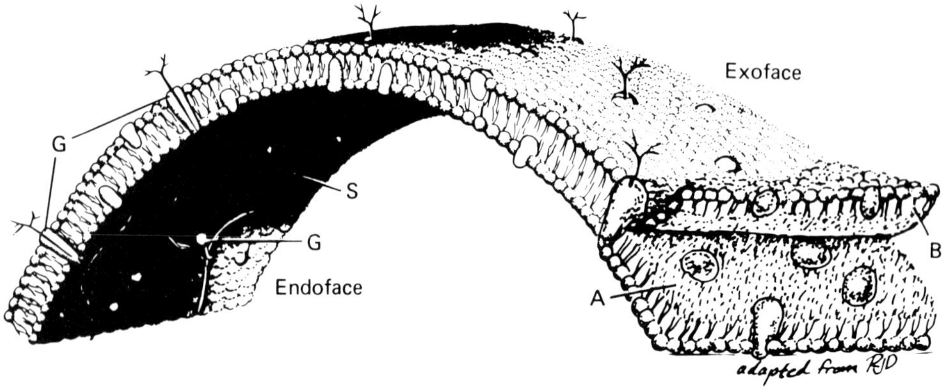

FIGURE 12. Diagrammatic model of a portion of the red cell membrane, depicting the lipid bilayer and the relative position of the membrane protein components of the bilayer. Glycophorin (G) molecules traverse the membrane with a projection from the external surface (exoface). On the internal surface (endoface), the spectrin network is shown as submembrane filaments attached to the internal aspect of the glycophorin protein. At the right, a portion of membrane is cleaved, as in the freeze-etching process, to reveal the A surface below and the B surface above. (From Lessin, L. S. and Bessis, M., *Hematology*, 2nd ed., Williams, W. J., Beutler, E., Erslev, A. J., and Rundles, R. W., Eds., McGraw-Hill, New York, 1977. With permission.)

this maintenance is accomplished by a feedback loop between a sensor and an adjustor[27] (Figure 14). The sensor of the size of the red cell mass is undoubtedly set to monitor oxygen in the tissues.[28,29] Theoretically, it could also monitor other parameters relating to the red cell mass such as volume, viscosity, or breakdown products. However, the red cell mass is designed almost exclusively for the purpose of transporting oxygen, and all experimental and clinical observations are in accord with the concept that oxygen availability is the parameter that triggers the red cell mass sensor. This sensor, in turn, controls the production or release of a humoral mediator or hormone named erythropoietin, capable of transmitting signals to the adjustor.[30]

The adjustor is the erythroid tissue in the bone marrow. It responds to the signals mediated by erythropoietin, and it can adjust the rate of red cell production and thereby the size of the red cell mass over a wide range.[31] This basic feedback mechanism is capable not only of maintaining a constant optimal level of red cells in circulating blood, but also of adjusting it to acute or chronic changes in oxygen demand or oxygen supply.

The kidney is generally accepted as the location for the oxygen sensor,[32] although only crude erythropoietin preparations have been studied to date. Isolated renal hypoxia will lead to the generation of erythropoietin, whereas isolated kidney injury will reduce erythropoietin production. Bilateral nephrectomy, however, will not eliminate erythropoietin production because of the presence in the circulation of small amounts of erythropoietin derived from an extrarenal source. During fetal life, extrarenal erythropoietin is the major source of circulating erythropoietin[33] and presumably is made by the reticuloendothelial system[34] or, more likely, by the liver.[35,36] However, this extrarenal component decreases rapidly at time of birth, and in the adult 90 to 95% of the circulating erythropoietin is generated via a renal oxygen sensor. The exact intrarenal location of the oxygen sensor has not yet been determined. The medulla, with its borderline low oxygen tension, would be a reasonable location for a device designed to monitor tissue oxygen supply. Furthermore, renal cysts may contain large amounts of erythropoietin, most likely derived from the tubular endothelial lining of the cyst wall.[37] On the other hand, a cortical location of the oxygen sensor would place it in close proximity to the juxtaglomerular apparatus, a device often linked to erythropoi-

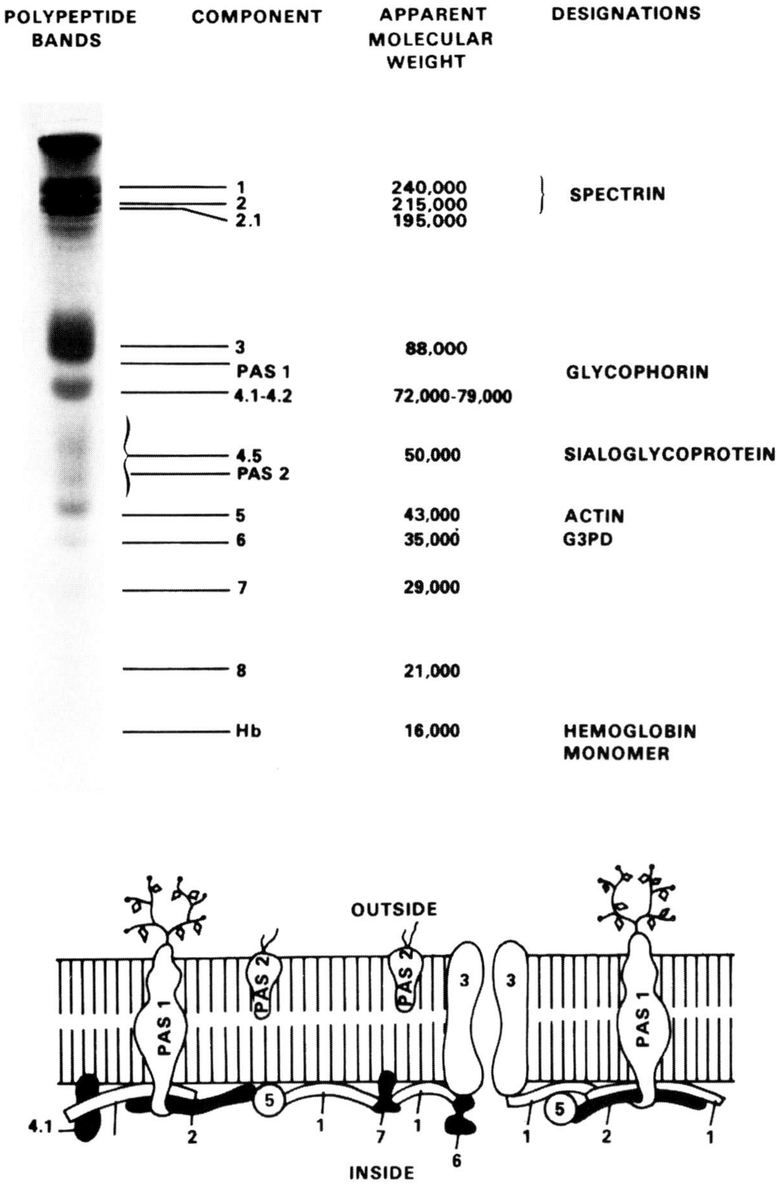

FIGURE 13. Electrophoretogram of the protein of human red cell membrane separated in a sodium dodecylsulfate-polyacrylamide gel and stained with Coomassie brilliant blue. Below is a schematic representation of the insertion of these polypeptides in the lipid bilayer of the human red cell membrane. The numerical designation for the major polypeptides is adopted from Fairbanks et al[23]. PAS-1, or Glycophorin, is the transmembraneous protein which bears the oligosaccharides and charged sialic acid groups at the external membrane surface. At the internal surface it presumably makes contact with spectrin components 1 and 2. These spectrin components form a continuous meshwork on the internal aspect of the membrane and interact with component 5, actin. Component 3 is a large molecular weight transmembraneous protein, that may contain a central aqueous core and serve in transmembraneous transport of cations and other substances. Component 6 represents glyceraldehyde-3-phosphate dehydrogenase, an enzymatic component present on the internal membrane surface. (From Lessin, L. S. and Bessis, M., *Hematology*, 2nd. Ed., Williams, W. J., Beutler, E., Erslev, A. J., and Rundles, R. W., Eds., McGraw-Hill, New York, 1977, 103. With permission.)

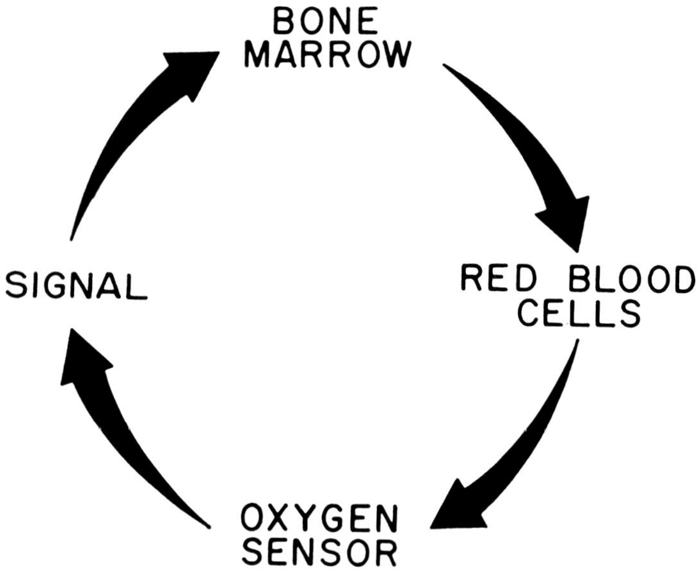

FIGURE 14. The basic feedback loop which links red cell production to the tissue oxygen tension of oxygen.

etin production.[38] Furthermore, fluorescent antibodies to erythropoietin tend to locate in the cortical glomeruli.[39] Because of the low A-V oxygen difference in cortical blood, the venous blood would have a high saturation with oxygen, which would place it at the flat part on the oxygen dissociation curve. Here a small difference in oxygen saturation would cause a large change in oxygen tension, an attractive feature for an oxygen-sensing device.

Although it would seem reasonable that the site of erythropoietin production would be located in close proximity to the oxygen sensor, most of the attempts to extract erythropoietin from kidney have been futile. This failure has led to the hypothesis that erythropoietin is not made by the kidney, but rather that the oxygen sensor in the kidney generates an enzyme capable of activating an inactive plasma pro-erythropoietin produced elsewhere, presumably in the liver.[40] However, it has been shown that an isolated kidney, perfused with a plasma-free medium, is capable of synthesizing and releasing erythropoietin.[41] This observation makes it most likely that erythropoietin is produced by the kidney, and that the inability to isolate erythropoietin from the kidney is due to the presence of a renal erythropoietin inhibitor[42] or perhaps a complete lack of storage capacity. However, the exact mechanism of biogenesis of erythropoietin remains quite controversial.

The mediating hormone, erythropoietin, is a glycoprotein with a molecular weight of about 40,000 and a half-life in rats and rabbits of a few hours.[43] In man the half-life has been claimed to be considerably longer, but conclusive data are not available. Small amounts are cleared in the urine, whereas the major catabolism is believed to be in the liver. This glycoprotein is a weak antigen, but antibodies produced have shown definite species differences in the erythropoietin molecules.[44] Immunoassays are being developed, but currently the only reliable assay is a bioassay performed in mice rendered polycythemic in order to eliminate endogenous erythropoietin.[45] Erythropoietic response to injected erythropoietin is measured in these animals by measuring the red cell utilization of injected radioactive ion (Figure 15). At least four mice have to be used for each assay — as indication of the crudeness of this test. Nevertheless, it is

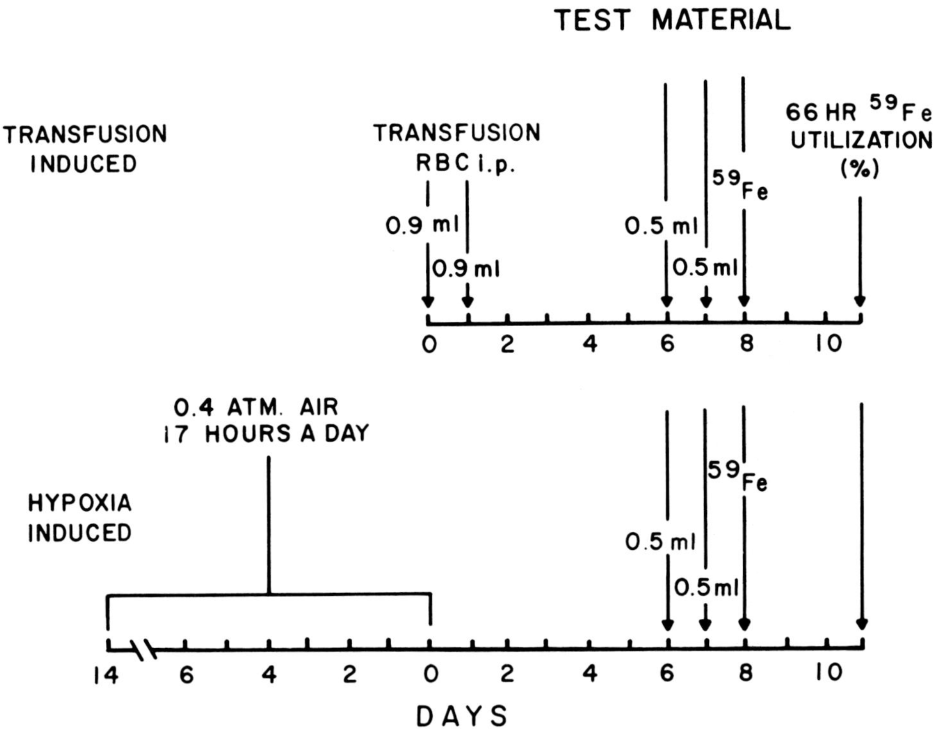

FIGURE 15. Assay procedure for erythropoietin in mice rendered anemic by hypertransfusion, or by exposure to hypoxia.

useful and fairly reproducible (Figure 16). The amount of erythropoietin present in plasma with normal levels of hemoglobin is extremely small (about 10 milliunits/mℓ), but it increases rapidly to thousands of milliunits/mℓ in severe anemic hypoxia (Figure 17). Although the renal clearance is small, the total amount of erythropoietin present in a 24-hr urine specimen may be considerable, and assays of concentrated urines can be clinically useful (Figure 17). As is also evident from Figure 17, the relationship between hemoglobin concentration and erythropoietin titer is not represented by a sharp band, but rather by a diffuse area. This is due not only to the crudeness of the assay, but also to the fact that the oxygen sensor, and therefore the erythropoietin production, is responsive to many other factors in addition to hemoglobin concentration. Ambient oxygen pressure, pulmonary function, hemoglobin oxygen affinity, cardiac output, blood volume, and renal blood flow all influence oxygen transport to the kidney and are all involved in affecting erythropoietin production (Figure 18).

In the bone marrow, the site of action of erythropoietin appears to be a small number of mononucleated, undifferentiated cells designated as erythropoietin-sensitive or erythropoietin-committed stem cells.[28] These cells are derived from multipotential or pluripotential stem cells that are capable of differentiating in many directions, but under most conditions are dormant and inactive.[46] They are called into action by local factors triggered by cell depletion, and if this depletion involves the erythroid system, the multipotential stem cells will differentiate to unipotential erythropoietin-sensitive stem cells. These cells will proliferate and replace themselves for a long period of time, but if exposed to erythropoietin they will undergo blast transformation and become pronormoblasts. This differentiating action is still somewhat mysterious, perhaps because relatively crude preparations of erythropoietin have been used. It is assumed that

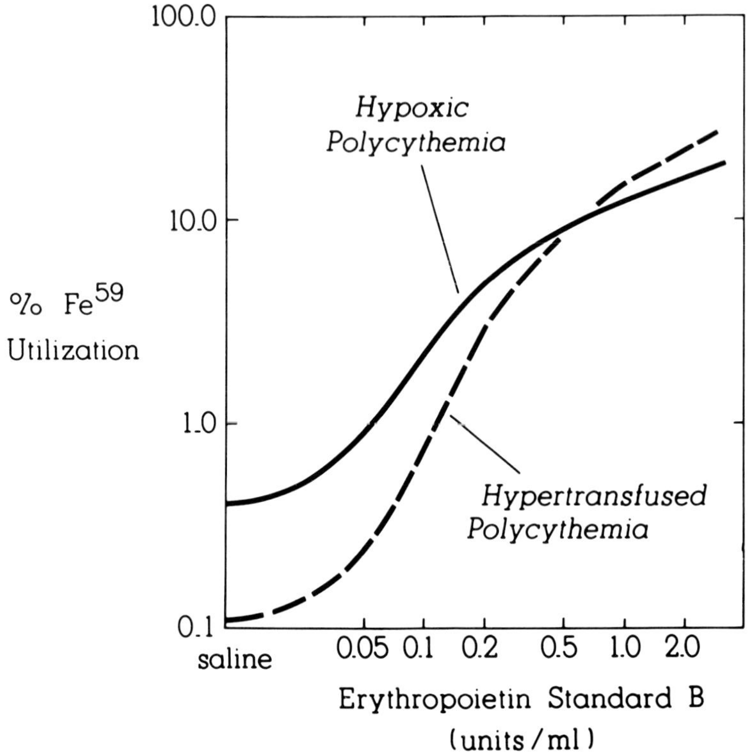

FIGURE 16. Dose-response curve of standard reference human urinary erythropoietin in mice rendered polycythemic by hypertransfusion, or by exposure to hypoxia.

there are receptors on the stem cell surface for erythropoietin, and that either erythropoietin enters the cell or that erythropoietin will initiate an intracellular chain effect involving adenyl cyclase and cyclic AMP or GMP.[47,48] The final result is the generation of a species of RNA that induces a mitotic division, hemoglobin initiation, or both. Whether or not erythropoietin affects the subsequent maturation of the newly differentiated pronormoblasts has not been resolved. However, it is not necessary for the orderly transformation of pronormoblasts to mature red blood cells. Erythropoietin has been claimed to have an effect on the release of reticulocytes through the basement membrane of the venous sinuses in the bone marrow.[49] It has been shown that high erythropoietin content will cause a short intramedullary transit time of nucleated red cells and an early release.[50] However, this release could also be due to the crowding of an increased number of erythroid cells in rigid bone marrow compartments.

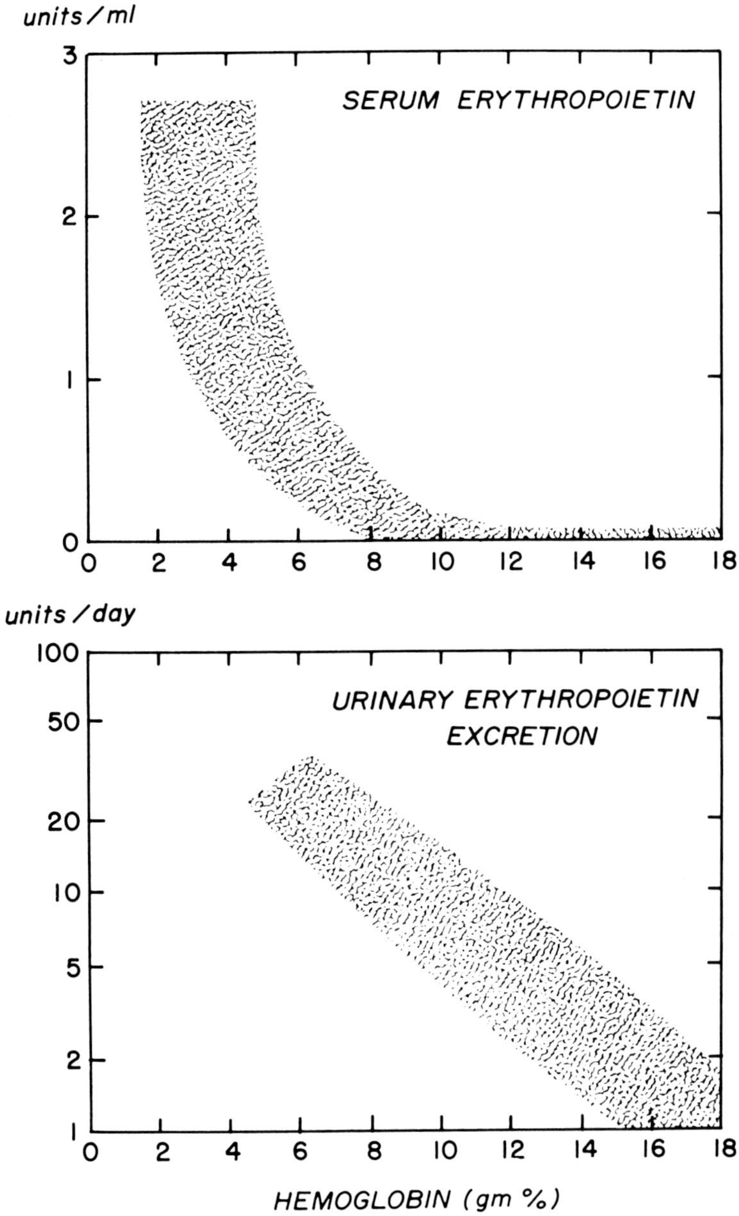

FIGURE 17. The relationship between hemoglobin and the content of erythropoietin in plasma (upper panel), and the 24-hr excretion of erythropoietin in urine (lower panel).

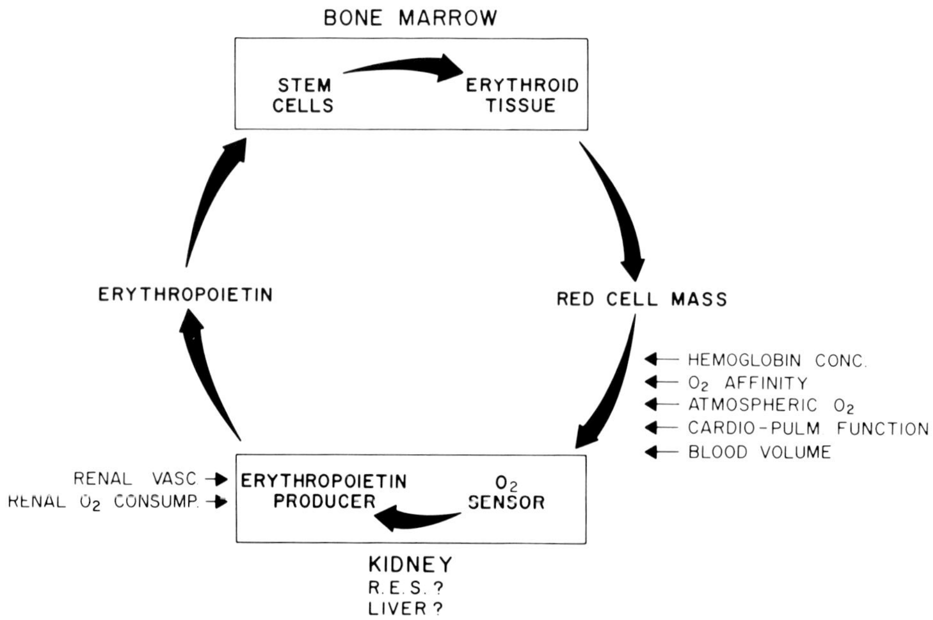

FIGURE 18. Current concept of feedback loop maintaining the red cell mass at an optimal size.

REFERENCES

1. **Bloom, W. and Bartelmez, G. W.,** Hemopoiesis in young human embryos, *Am. J. Anat.*, 67, 21, 1940.
2. **Hecht, F.,** Predominance of hemoglobin Gower I in early human embryonic development, *Science*, 152, 31, 1966.
3. **Hudson, G.,** Bone marrow volume in the human foetus and newborn, *Br. J. Haematol.*, 11, 446, 1965.
4. **Huehns, E. R. and Shooter, E. M.,** Review article: human haemoglobins, *J. Med. Genet.*, 2, 48, 1965.
5. **Huggins, L. and Blockson, B. H.,** Changes in outlying bone marrow accompanying a local increase of temperature within physiologic limits, *J. Exp. Med.*, 64, 253, 1956.
6. **Crosby, W. H.,** Experience with injured and implanted bone marrow: relation of function to structure, in *Hematopoietic Cellular Proliferation*, Stohlman, F., Jr., Ed., Grune & Stratton, New York, 1970, 87.
7. **Smith, J. S. and Whitelaw, D. M.,** Hemoglobin values in the elderly, *Can. Med. Assoc. J.*, 105, 816, 1971.
8. **Weiss, L.** in *Regulation of Hematopoiesis*, Vol. 1, Gordon, A. S., Ed., Appleton-Century-Crofts, New York, 1970.
9. **Weiss, L.,** The hematopoietic microenvironment of the bone marrow: an ultrastructural study of the stroma in rats, *Anat. Rec.*, 186, 161, 1976.
10. **LeBlond, P. F., Chamberlain, J. K., and Weed, R. I.,** Scanning electron microscopy of erythropoietin-stimulated bone marrow, *Blood Cells*, 1, 639, 1975.
11. **Lessin, L. S. and Bessis, M.,** Morphology of the erythron, in *Hematology*, 2nd ed., Williams, W. J., Beutler, E., Erslev, A. J., and Rundles, R. W., Eds., McGraw-Hill, New York, 1977, 103.
12. **Jandl, J. H.,** Agglutination and sequestration on immature red cells, *J. Lab. Clin. Med.*, 55, 663, 1960.
13. **Bessis, M.,** *Living Blood Cells and their Ultrastructure*, Springer-Verlag, New York, 1973, 139
14. **Erslev, A. J. and Weiss, L.,** Structure and function of the bone marrow, in *Hematology, 2nd ed.*, Williams, W. J., Beutler, E., Erslev, A. J., and Rundles, R. W., Eds., McGraw-Hill, New York, 1977, 57.

15. **LeBlond, P. F.**, A scanning electron microscopic study of the transmural passage of blood cells in spleen and bone marrow sinusoids of the rat, *Nouv. Rev. Fr. Hematol.*, 13, 771, 1973.
16. **Erslev, A. J.**, Production of erythrocytes, in *Hematology*, 2nd ed., Williams, W. J., Beutler, E., Erslev, A. J., and Rundles, R. W., Eds., McGraw-Hill, New York, 1977, 203.
17. **Bessis, M.**, *Living Blood Cells and Their Ultrastructure*, Springer-Verlag, New York, 1973, 119.
18. **Singer, S. J. and Nicolson, G. L.**, The fluid mosaic model of the structure of cell membranes, *Science*, 175, 720, 1972.
19. **Singer, S. J.**, Architecture and topography of biologic membranes, *Hosp. Pract.*, 8, 81, 1973.
20. **Singer, S. J.**, The molecular organization of membranes, *Ann. Rev. Biochem.*, 43, 805, 1974.
21. **Lessin, L. S. and Bessis, M.**, Morphology of the erythron, in *Hematology*, 2nd ed., Wlliams, W. J., Beutler, E., Erslev, A. J., and Rundles, R. W., Eds., McGraw-Hill, New York, 1977, 103.
22. **Weinstein, R. S. and McNutt, N. S.**, Ultrastructure of red cell membrane, *Semin. Hematol.*, 7, 259, 1970.
23. **Fairbanks, G., Steck, T. L., and Wallach, D. F. H.**, Electrophoretic analysis of the major polypeptides of the human erythrocyte membrane, *Biochemistry*, 10, 2606, 1971.
24. **Steck, T. L.**, The organization of proteins in the human red blood cell membrane, a review, *J. Cell Biol.*, 62, 1, 1974.
25. **Marchesi, V. T. and Furthmayr, H.**, The red cell membrane, *Ann. Rev. Biochem.*, 45, 667, 1976.
26. **Singer, S. J.**, Molecular biology of cellular membranes with applications to immunology, *Adv. Immunol.*, 19, 1, 1974.
27. **Erslev, A. J.**, Feedback circuits in the control of stem cell differentiation, *Am. J. Pathol.*, 65, 629, 1971.
28. **Erslev, A. J.**, Production of erythrocytes, in *Hematology*, 2nd ed., Williams, W. J., Beutler, E., Erslev, A. J., and Rundles, R. W., Eds., McGraw-Hill, New York, 1977, 203.
29. **Nathan, D. G.**, Regulation of erythropoiesis, *N. Engl. J. Med.*, 296, 685, 1977.
30. **Erslev, A. J.**, The role of erythropoietin in the control of red cell production, *Medicine*, 43, 661, 1964.
31. **Crosby, W. H. and Akeroyd, J. H.**, The limit of hemoglobin synthesis in hereditary hemolytic anemia, *Am. J. Med.*, 13, 273, 1952.
32. **Fisher, J. W., Busuttil, R., Rodgers, G. M., Mujovic, V., Paulo, L., Fink, G., and George, W. J.**, The kidney and erythropoietin production: a review, in *Erythropoiesis*, Nakao, K., Fisher, J. W., and Takaku, F., University Park Press, Tokyo, 1975, 315.
33. **Zanjani, E., Peterson, E. N., Gordon, A. S., and Wasserman, L. R.**, Erythropoietin production in the fetus: role of the kidney and maternal anemia, *J. Lab. Clin. Med.*, 83, 281, 1974.
34. **Peschle, C., Marone, G., Genovese, A., Rappaport, J. A., and Condorelli, M.**, Increased erythropoietin production in anephric rats with hyperplasia of the reticuloendothelial system induced by colloidal carbon or zymosan, *Blood*, 47, 325, 1976.
35. **Schooley, J. C. and Mahlmann, L. J.**, Extrarenal erythropoietin production by the liver in the weanling rat, *Proc. Soc. Exp. Biol. Med.*, 145, 1081, 1974.
36. **Fried, W.**, The liver as the source of extrarenal erythropoietin production, *Blood*, 40, 671, 1972.
37. **Thorling, E. B.**, Paraneoplastic erythrocytosis and inappropriate erythropoietin production, a review, *Scand. J. Haematol.*, Suppl. 17, 1, 1972.
38. **Demopoulos, H. B., Highman, B., Altland, P. D., Gerving, M. A., and Kaley, G.**, Effect of high altitudes on granular juxtaglomerular cells and their possible role in erythropoietin production, *Am. J. Pathol.*, 46, 497, 1965.
39. **Busuttil, R. W., Roh, B. L., and Fisher, J. W.**, Cytological localization of erythropoietin in the human kidney using the fluorescent antibody technique, *Proc. Soc. Exp. Biol. Med.*, 137, 327, 1971.
40. **Gordon, A. S. and Zanjani, E. D.**, Humoral control of hematopoiesis, *Adv. Intern. Med.*, 18, 39, 1972.
41. **Erslev, A. J.**, Renal biogenesis of erythropoietin, *Am. J. Med.*, 58, 25, 1975.
42. **Kazal, L. A., Erslev, A. J., and Miller, O. P.**, The renal erythropoietin inhibitor, in *Leukemia and Aplastic Anemia*, Il Pensiero Scientifico, Rome, 1975, 181.
43. **Goldwasser, E.**, The purification and properties of erythropoietin: a critical review, in *Erythropoiesis*, Nakao, K., Fisher, J. W., and Takaku, F., University Park Press, Tokyo, 1975, 75.
44. **Rioux, E. and Erslev, A. J.**, Immunologic studies of a partially purified sheep erythropoietin, *J. Immunol.*, 101, 6, 1968.
45. **Erslev, A. J.**, Erythropoietin assay, in *Hematology*, 2nd ed., Williams, W. J., Beutler, E., Erslev, A. J. and Rundles, R. W., Eds., McGraw-Hill, New York, 1977, 1616.
46. **Lajtha, L. G.**, Haemopoietic stem cells, *Br. J. Haematol.*, 29, 529, 1975.
47. **Piantadosi, C. A., Dickerman, H. W., and Spivak, J. L.**, Sequential activation of splenic nuclear RNA polymerases by erythropoietin, *J. Clin. Invest.*, 57, 20, 1976.

48. **Graber, S. E., Bomboy, J. D., Salmon, W. D., and Krantz, S. B.,** Effect of erythropoietin preparations on cyclic AMP and cyclic GMP levels in rat fetal liver cell cultures, *J. Lab. Clin. Med.*, 90, 162, 1977.
49. **LeBlond, P. F., Chamberlain, J. K., and Weed, R. I.,** Scannng electron microscopy of erythropoietin stimulated bone marrow, *Blood Cells*, 1, 639, 1975.
50. **Papayannopoulou, T. and Finch, C. A.,** Radioiron measurements of red cell maturation, *Blood Cells*, 1, 535, 1975.

The White Cell

THE LEUKOCYTE: MORPHOGENESIS AND ULTRASTRUCTURE

Richard D. Brunning and Janet L. Parkin

The leukocytes in the peripheral blood are subdivided into five primary morphologic types: the neutrophils, eosinophils, basophils, monocytes, and lymphocytes. The neutrophils, eosinophils, and basophils are collectively referred to as granulocytes because of the presence in their cytoplasm of granules which have morphologic and tinctorial characteristics unique for each of these cell types. The granulocytes and the monocytes have their origin in the bone marrow where their proliferation, maturation, and development occur under the influence of a factor or factors which are not well understood.[1-3]

The blood phase of the granulocytes and monocytes is brief and represents the passage of cells from their site of origin in the bone marrow to the extravascular tissues where their primary function of participating in the body's defense mechanisms occurs. The half life of the neutrophil in the blood is approximately 6 to 7 hr.[3] The greatest portion of the neutrophil life span of approximately 10 to 14 days is in the bone marrow where maturation and development occur. The tissue phase of the neutrophil life cycle lasts approximately 4 to 5 days.

The primary role of the neutrophil is the phagocytosis and destruction of microorganisms.[4,5] The blood monocyte is a phagocytic cell that appears to be the major source of the macrophages which accumulate at inflammatory sites.[6] The manner in which the eosinophils and basophils function is less certain. The eosinophil granules contain cationic protein, and eosinophils are increased in allergic inflammation. The basophil granules contain heparin and histamine. The basophils are involved in hypersensitivity reactions.

The major sites of lymphopoiesis are widely distributed throughout the body: lymph nodes, Peyer's patches, and spleen. The lymphocytes participate in the body's defense mechanisms by their role in cellular and humoral mediated immunity.[9]

Granulocytes

The neutrophils, eosinophils, and basophils appear to originate from a common bone marrow precursor cell, the myeloblast, and progress through parallel developmental stages. The myeloblast is derived from a morphologically unidentifiable precursor or stem cell which is shared with the erythroid, megakaryocyte, and monocyte series as evidenced by the detection of the Philadelphia (Ph) chromosome in these cell lines in chronic myelogenous leukemia.[10-12] Whether this precursor cell is derived from a stem cell which is shared with the lymphoid cell line is speculative, although available evidence suggests that leukemic, lymphoid-appearing cells may possess the Philadelphia chromosome.[13-16]

On the basis of evolving nuclear and cytoplasmic characteristics, the sequential steps in granulocyte development have been designated as promyelocyte, myelocyte, metamyelocyte, and segmented stages (Figure 1*).[17,18] A step intermediate between the myelocyte and segmented stages, referred to as the band stage, is used by several observers; this designation has utility only in the neutrophil series. The myeloblast, promyelocyte, and myelocyte stages of development are characterized by proliferation and maturation; mitotic activity ceases with the myelocyte stage,[3] and the metamyelocyte and segmented stages are characterized only by differentiation and maturation as

* All figures follow text.

reflected in changes in nuclear configuration and chromatin pattern. Only mature or segmented cells of the three types of granulocytes and a small number of band forms of the neutrophil series are found in the peripheral blood of normal individuals.

Granulocyte development in the bone marrow is most characteristically exemplified by the neutrophil series (Figure 2).[19] The general cytoplasmic and nuclear features of neutrophil development are essentially similar for the basophil and eosinophil series. The morphologically identifiable precursor cell of these three cell lines, the myeloblast, has a moderate amount of agranular, basophilic cytoplasm. The nucleus, which is round or oval in outline, has a delicate chromatin pattern and prominent nucleoli, generally two to four in number. The promyelocyte stage of development commences with the appearance of azurophilic granules in the cytoplasm. During this stage, the promyelocyte continues to exhibit nucleoli and cytoplasmic basophilia. The myelocyte stage is marked by the appearance of specific (neutrophil) granules in the cytoplasm, progressive loss of cytoplasmic basophilia, disappearance of nucleoli, and coarsening of the nuclear chromatin. With subsequent maturation from the metamyelocyte to segmented neutrophil stage, the nucleus undergoes progressive changes in configuration which result in a multilobulated nucleus. The changes in the nucleus and cytoplasm are accompanied by a progressive decrease in cell size from the promyelocyte to the mature cell. Because the developmental sequence is a continuum, many cells will be in transition from one stage to the next. The primary nuclear and cytoplasmic characteristics of the various developmental stages in the neutrophil series as seen in Romanowsky stained smears are summarized in Table 1.

The ultrastructural characteristics of the developing neutrophil series in man have been described by several investigators.[19-23] The salient features of these studies are summarized in Table 2. The nuclear and cytoplasmic changes noted in light microscopy are reflected in the electron microscopic studies. Ultrastructurally, the earliest identifiable cell in the granulocyte series, the myeloblast, is approximately 10 μm in diameter; it has a moderate amount of cytoplasm which contains abundant free polyribosomes and mitochrondria (Figure 3). The nuclear chromatin is finely dispersed with minimal condensation at the nuclear margin. In appropriate planes of section, nucleoli are prominent.

The neutrophil promyelocyte is the largest cell in the developmental series and measures approximately 15 μm in diameter (Figure 4). The moderately abundant cytoplasm contains a large Golgi and moderate amounts of slightly dilated, rough endoplasmic reticulum. The prominent identifying feature of the promyelocyte stage is the production of electron-dense granules from the concave surface of the Golgi.[19] These granules, which correspond to the azurophilic granules of the promyelocyte in Romanowsky stained smears, are round or elliptical and measure approximately 500 nm. As studied by ultrastructural cytochemistry, these granules are peroxidase positive (Figure 5). The nucleus of the promyeloctye displays more chromatin condensation than the myeloblast nucleus. As in the myeloblast, nucleoli may be identified.

The myelocyte stage of the neutrophil is marked by the onset of production of specific granules. These granules are also referred to as neutrophil or secondary granules; they are peroxidase negative and arise from the convex surface of the prominent Golgi. The specific granules are smaller and less dense than the azurophil granules and are round, approximately 200 nm in diameter, or ellipsoid, 130 × 1000 nm. Occasionally, the specific granules are dumbbell shaped. According to Bainton et al.[19] the secretory phase of granulocyte development, as characterized by granule production, ceases with the myelocyte stage. Maturation in metamyelocytes and segmented neutrophils is characterized by progressive nuclear chromatin clumping and nuclear lobulation.

The mature forms of the three granulocyte lines — the neutrophil, eosinophil, and basophil — are readily distinguished in Romanowsky stained smears by their distinc-

Table 1
CHARACTERISTICS OF NEUTROPHIL DEVELOPMENT IN ROMANOWSKY STAINED BONE MARROW SMEARS

	Myeloblast	Promyelocyte	Myelocyte	Metamyelocyte	Band	Segmented neutrophil
Size	(10—18μ)	(12—20μ)	(10—18μ)	(10—18μ)	(10—16μ)	(10—14μ)
			Cytoplasm			
Amount	Moderate amount	Nuclear cytoplasmic ratio less than in myeloblast	Decreasing nuclear cytoplasmic ratio	—	—	—
Color	Moderate to intensely basophilic	Moderately basophilic	Slightly basophilic	Light—no basophilia	Light	Light
Granules	None	Azurophilic-blue to purple	Azurophilic and specific	Azurophilic and specific	Azurophilic and specific	Azurophilic and specific
			Nucleus			
Configuration	Round to oval	Round to oval	Round to oval to slightly flattened on one side, may be slightly eccentric in location	Indented (indentation is less than ½ of the diameter of the hypothetical circumference of the nucleus)	Indentation is greater than 50% of the diameter of circle circumscribed by the nucleus; convex and concave surfaces have appreciable length of parallel sides; no filaments	Segmented with filaments connecting two or more lobes
Chromatin structure	Delicate	Fine	Slightly coarse	Coarse-clumped	Clumped	Clumped
Nucleoli	Prominent usually 2—4	Present	Indistinct or absent	None	None	None

Table 2
ULTRASTRUCTURAL CHARACTERISTICS OF NEUTROPHIL DEVELOPMENT

	Myeloblast	Promyelocyte	Myelocyte	Metamyelocyte	Segmented neutrophil
Size	($\sim10\mu$)	($\sim15\mu$)	($\sim10\mu$)	(~10—14μ)	(~10—14μ)
Nucleus	High nuclear cytoplasmic ratio; finely dispersed chromatin with slight condensation at margin; prominent nucleoli	Round to slightly indented, dispersed chromatin, prominent nucleoli	Indented nucleus, slight clumping of chromatin with peripheral condensation	Indented, clumped chromatin	Lobulated nucleus, clumped nuclear chromatin
Cytoplasm	No granules, abundant ribosomes and mitochondria, few strands of rough endoplasmic reticulum	Large number of round and elliptical electron-dense granules (peroxidase positive); prominent Golgi, moderate amount of rough endoplasmic reticulum	Two granule populations, dense granules (primary, azurophil, nonspecific) which are peroxidase positive and less dense specific (secondary, neutrophil) — spherical, ellipsoid, and dumbbell-shaped (peroxidase negative); prominent Golgi	Two granule populations, azurophil and specific; less prominent, inactive Golgi	Two granule populations: specific $\sim70\%$ azurophilic $\sim30\%$ glycogen particles

tive granule populations (Figure 1). The cytochemical characteristics[24] and morphologic features of the mature forms of these three cell types as seen in Romanowsky stained smears are summarized in Table 3.

Ultrastructurally the mature neutrophil (Figure 6) is characterized by marked clumping and margination of the nuclear chromatin, the absence of nucleoli, and lobulation of the nucleus. The Golgi is small and ribosomes are sparse. Glycogen particles may be numerous. Granules are abundant and consist of at least two types: the nonspecific (azurophil or primary) which were produced during the promyelocyte stage comprise approximately 30% of the population, and the specific or neutrophil which arose in the myelocyte stage make up 70% of the granules. The specific or peroxidase-negative granules are less electron dense than the peroxidase-positive granules, appear as spheres, rods, or dumbbell-shaped structures and are generally smaller than the azurophil or peroxidase positive granules (Figure 7). With different methods of fixation and staining, the distinction between the two granule types may be accentuated or diminished.[21] A third population of distinct granules has been proposed by some investigators.[21,23]

The mature eosinophil under electron microscopy (Figure 8) is characterized by the presence of large, round, electron-dense granules which generally contain a central crystalline structure that may show a distinct periodicity; the crystalline core is surrounded by a less dense matrix. The nucleus shows marked clumping, and nucleoli are not found. Immature eosinophils contain granules which may be homogeneously dense and which do not contain a central crystalline structure (Figure 9). Scott and Horn proposed an origin of the eosinophil granules in cytoplasmic vacuoles that may be derived from the rough endoplasmic reticulum.[25] They suggested that the granules in the mature eosinophil evolve from the immature granules produced in the earlier stages of development. Bainton and Farquhar,[26] based on ultrastructural study of granule development in the eosinophils of rabbits and rats, concluded that eosinophil granules arise from the Golgi, similar to neutrophil granulogenesis. They concluded that granule development in eosinophils was analagous to neutrophil granule development with the production of a primary granule population in the promyelocyte stage of development and the production of specific granules during the myelocyte stage.

Ultrastructurally, the granules of the mature basophil (Figure 10) are composed of a membrane that encloses small dense particles which are of uniform size in any one granule, but which may show considerable size variation in different granules of the same cell.[27] Some of the granules may contain myelin figures. As in the eosinophil and neutrophil, glycogen particles may be numerous.

Monocytes

The derivation of the monocyte was the focus of controversy for several years. Recent evidence from cell kinetic studies,[28] bone marrow culture,[29] cytochemistry,[30,31] and ultrastructural study[32] points to the bone marrow as the site of origin of the monocyte. The bone marrow precursors of the monocyte, the monoblast, and the promonocyte are difficult to identify in the marrow of normal individuals and are found in abundance only in leukemic processes of the monocyte system. Whether monocytic leukemia simulates normal monocytopoiesis remains to be clarified, as does the relationship of the monoblast to the myeloblast. Accordingly, caution must be used in extrapolating features of monocytogenesis observed in patients with leukemic conditions to normal monocytopoiesis.

As observed in Romanowsky stained smears in leukemic situations,[33] the monoblast (Figure 11) is large, approximately 18 μm in diameter, and has abundant blue-grey cytoplasm which may contain very delicate, reddish granulation. Cytoplasmic projec-

Table 3
FEATURES OF NONLYMPHOCYTIC CELLS IN BLOOD SMEARS

	Mature neutrophil	Mature eosinophil	Mature basophil	Mature monocyte
Size	(10—14μ)	(10—15μ)	(10—14μ)	(12—30μ)
Cytoplasm	Numerous small pink orange to pink granules; slightly acidophilic cytoplasm	Large, bright orange to reddish orange spherical granules; slightly basophilic cytoplasm	Large granules, blue to purple in color; granules frequently washed out; frequently overlie nucleus; slightly acidophilic cytoplasm	Scattered azurophilic granules; slightly basophilic to gray cytoplasm
Nucleus	2—5 lobes; clumped chromatin	Majority bilobed; clumped chromatin	3—4 lobes; clumped chromatin	Round, indented or horseshoe shaped; coarsely striated nuclear chromatin
Cytochemical reactivity	Myeloperoxidase (cyanide sensitive), Sudan black B, alkaline phosphase, chloracetate esterase, acid phosphatase, alkaline phosphatase	Myeloperoxidase (cyanide resistant)	Toluidine blue O, myeloperoxidase ±	Nonspecific esterase; variable slight positivity with myeloperoxidase and Sudan black B

tions or pseudopod formation may be prominent. The oval or round nucleus has a reticular chromatin pattern and usually one or two prominent nucleoli. The identification of this cell as a monoblast rests on its reactivity for nonspecific esterase.[34] Ultrastructurally, as in light microscopy, there is considerable morphologic heterogenity to the cells which may be considered "monoblasts", and a description of the ultrastructure of the monoblast represents a composite of a morphologic spectrum. The leukemic monoblast (Figure 12) has abundant cytoplasm which may manifest an irregular or uniform distribution around the nucleus. There are numerous free ribosomes, mitochrondria, and short strands of rough endoplasmic reticulum. Electron-dense granules and fibrillar arrays may be present, frequently in a juxtanuclear location. Nuclei are round or oval and have a finely dispersed chromatin; in some monoblasts the chromatin is extremely fine with essentially no evidence of clumping. Nucleoli are prominent.

The promonocyte is the form intermediate between the monoblast and the differentiated monocyte. The morphologic limits of this stage are arbitrarily defined, and, like the monoblast, it is found with frequency only in monocytic leukemia.[35] The promonocyte in Romanowsky stained smears is a large cell with abundant cytoplasm which may contain dust-like to fine azurophilic granules. Unlike the monoblast, the nucleus of the promonocyte shows variable degrees of nuclear contortion and indentation which identify it with the monocyte series (Figure 11). At times, the nuclear contortion is somewhat cerebriform in appearance. The promonocyte, similar to the monoblast, reacts positively for nonspecific esterase. The nuclear chromatin is somewhat more coarse than in the monoblast; nucleoli can usually be identified. Ultrastructurally, the promonocyte shows lobulation of the nucleus (Figure 13) which has slightly more con-

Table 4
FUNCTION AND LOCATION OF T AND B LYMPHOCYTES[38]

	T cells	B cells
Function	Initiation of delayed hypersensitivity reactions Initiation of solid tissue allograft rejection Initiation of graft vs. host reactions Elaboration of lymphokines Defense against facultative intracellular bacterial and rickettsial pathogens, fungi, and many viruses Responsive to phytohemagglutinin or allogeneic cell stimulation in vitro ? Immunosurveillance against cancer	Synthesis and secretion of immunoglobulins and specific antibodies (IgM, IgG, IgA, IgD, IgE) Progenitor of plasma cells Primary defense against high grade encapsulated bacterial pathogens Detoxification of certain proteins, polypeptides, and other toxins Neutralization of viruses (especially secretory IgA in respiratory tract and gut) Interference with absorption of foreign proteins from respiratory tract and gut
Location	Blood (65 to 80% of blood lymphocytes) Lymph node: deep cortical areas (paracortex) Spleen: perivascular areas of the white pulp (perivascular lymphocyte sheath)	Blood (15 to 25% of blood lymphocytes) Lymph node: germinal centers (lymphoid follicles, pyroninophilic cells) and medullary cords (secretory lymphocytes and plasma cells) Spleen: lymphoid follicles of white pulp and red pulp cords (chief site of splenic antibody production)

densation of the nuclear chromatin than the monoblast. However, even at this stage, the nuclear chromatin may be very finely dispersed. The cytoplasm contains dense granules, ribosomes, and numerous strands of rough endoplasmic reticulum. There frequently are arrays of microfibrils in a paranuclear location.

The mature monocyte in the blood of normal individuals is an extremely polymorphous cell in routine smears (Figure 11). It is the largest cell in normal blood and has abundant cytoplasm which is grey to grey-blue in color. The cytoplasm contains a small number of scattered azurophilic granules. The nucleus may exhibit considerable variation in shape; round, oval, horseshoe-shaped, and contorted nuclei may be noted. The nuclear chromatin has the appearance of coarse strands. Somewhat indistinct nucleoli may be identified in the nuclei of some monocytes in well-prepared smears. The monocyte reacts with the nonspecific esterase technique utilizing various substrates.[34] Scattered peroxidase-positive granules may be demonstrated in monocytes.

On electron microscopy, the mature monocyte is characterized by abundant cytoplasm which contains numerous small, dense granules and a prominent Golgi (Figure 14). Bundles of microfilaments, frequently in a paranuclear location, may be present. Numerous vesicles are frequently noted. The nucleus is indented, and the chromatin shows peripheral condensation. Nucleoli are frequently identified, but are not prominent.

Ultrastructural cytochemistry has demonstrated two distinct phases of monocyte development in the marrow of normal individuals based on granule development.[32] Immature monocytes or promonocytes have peroxidase reactivity in all of their granules; mature monocytes contain a mixture of peroxidase-positive and peroxidase-negative granules. The immature monocyte, therefore, appears to be engaged in the production of granules which are peroxidase positive, and mature monocytes produce granules which are peroxidase negative.

Lymphocytes

The prevailing concept of the lymphocyte system is that functionally it is comprised of two separate but interacting components: the B lymphocytes and T lymphoocytes.[9,36,37] The origin of the B lymphocytes in humans is uncertain but may be the bone marrow and/or the Peyer's patches; these cells participate in humoral-mediated immunity, i.e., they synthesize immunoglobulin. The T lymphocytes, which have an association with the thymus gland and differentiate under the influence of thymic hormone, are responsible for cell-mediated immunity. Both B and T lymphocytes coexist, albeit in different anatomic areas, in normal lymph node tissue.[38] Despite the functional and geographic differences (Table 4), B and T lymphocytes are presumably derived from a common stem cell[39] which may originate in the bone marrow.[38,40]

The distinction between B and T lymphocytes presently rests on membrane surface markers.[40-42] Several markers have been identified for these two cell systems. The most widely used defining characteristic of the B cell is the presence of high density membrane surface immunoglobulin; the T cells are identified by the presence on their membrane surface of binding sites for sheep erythrocytes. Generally accepted membrane surface markers for the B and T cell systems are shown in Table 5. When high density surface immunoglobulin is used as a marker for B cells and spontaneous rosette formation with sheep erythrocytes is used as a marker for T cells, peripheral blood from normal individuals contains approximately 10 to 30% B lymphocytes and 25 to 80% T lymphocytes, depending on the conditions of incubation.[40] In animal studies, the B lymphocyte is a relatively short-lived cell, having a life span of approximately 2 weeks; the majority of T lymphocytes are relatively long-lived cells with life spans of months and possibly years.[43]

Table 5
MARKERS OF HUMAN PERIPHERAL BLOOD LYMPHOCYTES[40]

	B cells	T cells
Surface Ig	+	−
Human B lymphocyte antigen (HBLA)	+	−
Sheep erythrocyte receptors (E rosette)	−	+
Human T lymphocyte antigen (HTLA)	−	+
Fc receptors (aggregated IgG or EA rosette)	+	−
Complement receptors (EAC rosette)	+	−

Unlike normal myelopoiesis there is no comparable spectrum of morphologic development which can be described for normal lymphocytopoiesis. Size or cytologic characteristics cannot be used as indicators of age or developmental potential. It has been established that small lymphocytes have the capacity to transform to large blast-like cells under external influences such as antigenic stimulation and that they retain the potential to revert to smaller cells.[44,45] As a result, the lymphocytes in normal individuals should be viewed as a system of cells with a wide range of morphologic and biologic characteristics.

The lymphoblast, unlike the myeloblast which is found in the bone marrow of normal individuals, is found in the blood and bone marrow only in cases of acute lymphocytic leukemia or lymphoblastic lymphoma.[46,47] A somewhat more mature-appearing cell, the prolymphocyte, is also found in increased numbers in forms of acute lymphocytic leukemia. Cells resembling lymphoblasts may be found in small numbers in imprints of lymph nodes from normal individuals.[46] Cells resembling prolymphocytes are present in abundant number in normal lymph node imprints. Morphologically similar cells are found in the marrow of normal individuals; they are most abundant in the marrow of infants and young children.[48] What relation these lymphoid cells in normal individuals have to the lymphoblasts and prolymphocytes of acute lymphocytic leukemia is uncertain. There is no substantial evidence to indicate that lymphocytopoiesis in acute lymphocytic leukemia recapitulates normal lymphocytogenesis. The large blast-like lymphoid cells which occur in patients without leukemia processes and are morphologically distinct from the lymphoblasts in acute lymphocytic leukemia probably represent examples of transformed or antigenically stimulated lymphocytes.

The lymphoblast of acute lymphocytic leukemia is a relatively large cell with a fine nuclear chromatin pattern, one to three nucleoli, and a moderate rim of lightly basophilic cytoplasm (Figure 15). The prolymphocyte is a smaller cell which appears to be intermediate in maturity to the lymphoblast and mature lymphocyte. The nucleus of this cell has a coarser chromatin pattern than the lymphoblast, nucleoli which are somewhat indistinct, and sparse, slightly basophilic cytoplasm. On ultrastructural examination, the lymphoblast has no distinctive characteristics. The cytoplasm contains scattered ribosomes, almost no rough endoplasmic reticulum, and a few large mitochrondria (Figure 16). The nucleus may be round, oval, or indented. The nuclear chromatin shows some condensation at the nuclear margin and scattered clumping. Nucleoli are frequently prominent.

The peripheral blood lymphocytes from normal individuals exhibit considerable heterogeneity in size, nuclear pattern, and amount of cytoplasm. Historically the lymphocytes have been separated on the basis of size into small, medium, and large types. The small lymphocytes range from 6 to 9μ, the medium from 9 to 12μ, and the large from 12 to 14μ. No functional characteristics can be attributed to a lymphocyte on the basis of size, and this separation should be viewed solely as a morphologic convenience.

The small lymphocyte is generally characterized by an intensely hyperchromatic, blue purple nucleus which may be round, ovoid, or indented (Figure 15). Unusually, the nuclear chromatin is less intensely hyperchromatic. Nucleoli may occasionally be identified. The cytoplasm is very sparse and at times may only be noted in the area of nuclear indentation. A minority of these lymphocytes will contain a small number of azurophilic granules.

The medium and large lymphocytes are marked by a lighter staining of the nucleus than is characteristic of the small lymphocyte. The nucleus is usually round or ovoid in outline, and the chromatin is smooth in appearance; in Romanowsky stained preparations, the nucleus stains somewhat purplish. The moderate rim of cytoplasm is clear to slightly basophilic and may contain coarse azurophilic granules (Figure 17).

Ultrastructurally, the small lymphocyte has a sparse to moderate amount of cytoplasm which contains a paucity of structures (Figure 18).[49] The Golgi is small, rough endoplasmic reticulum is generally absent, and the ribosomes are single and small. The nucleus may be round, oval, or indented. The nuclear chromatin is distributed in heavy chromatin clumps. Nucleoli may be identified in some small lymphocytes, but they are not unusually prominent and have the same electron density as the chromatin clumps. The medium to large lymphocytes have a moderate to abundant amount of cytoplasm. A low percentage of these cells contains various types of dense granules which apparently correspond to the azurophilic granules of light microscopy. Approximately 5 to 10% of the lymphocytes from normal individuals contain dense granular structures which consist of bundles of parallel tubular arrays (Figure 19).[50]

The large, atypical hyperbasophilic lymphocyte which is found in the peripheral blood of individuals with a variety of viral infections or immune reactions has ultrastructural features which are intermediate to those of plasma cells and lymphocytes (Figure 20). The abundant cytoplasm contains several strands of rough endoplasmic reticulum and numerous monoribosomes and polyribosomes. The nuclear chromatin is slightly to moderately dispersed. In appropriate planes of section, nucleoli may be prominent.

Plasma Cells

The plasma cell, the primary source of the immunoglobulins, is the quintessential immunocyte of the B cell component of the immune system. It is widely distributed throughout the body and is found in bone marrow, lymph nodes, spleen, thymus, and intestinal tract. Plasma cells comprise up to 1% of the nucleated marrow cells in normal individuals. Two theories for the origin of the plasma cells are extent, a lymphocytic origin[45,52] or a derivation from reticulum cells;[46,53] it is possible that plasma cells may evolve from both pathways.[51]

The most immature identifiable cell of the plasma cell line is the plasmoblast. It is a relatively large cell, approximately 15 to 25 μm in diameter, which has a moderate amount of intensely basophilic cytoplasm (Figure 21). The nucleus, which may be centrally located or slightly eccentric, has a coarsely reticular chromatin pattern. With maturation, there is progressive clumping of the nuclear chromatin and loss of distinct nucleoli. Intermediate stages of development have been referred to as proplasmocytes.[17] The size of the mature plasma cell varies from 10 to 20 μm in diameter. The nucleus, which shows marked chromatin clumping, is eccentric in position (Figure 21). Nucleoli are not generally evident. The cytoplasm is intensely basophilic except for the paranuclear "hof". The cytoplasm of the plasma cell may contain inclusions of varying tinctorial qualities, size, and shape. A commonly encountered cytoplasmic structure is the Russell body, which is a hyalin, spherule-like structure with a light blue to yellow color in Romanowsky stained smears. These inclusions may occur singly or in large numbers.

Ultrastructurally, the outstanding feature of the plasma cell is the prominent lamellae of rough endoplasmic reticulum which are arranged in parallel configurations (Figure 22). The lamellae contain a slightly electron-dense, amorphous, flocculent substance which may represent synthesized immunoglobulin.[54,55] Occasionally, the endoplasmic reticulum contains round, densely osmiophilic structures which correspond to the Russell bodies of light microscopy (Figure 23).[56] The prominent juxtanuclear Golgi is responsible for the clear or "hof" area as seen in the plasma cell in Romanowsky stained smears. Mitochrondria which are round or elongate may be numerous. The nucleus shows peripheral chromatin clumping. Nucleoli are not usually evident in the mature plasma cell.

Mast Cells

The mast cell or tissue basophil is found in connective tissue throughout the body. Mast cells may be present in very low numbers in normal bone marrow. The number of mast cells in the marrow is increased in a wide range of disorders including mastocytosis, macroglobulinemia, and liver disease. On Romanowsky stained bone marrow smears the mast cell ranges from 10 to 25 μm in diameter. The nucleus is generally round and centrally located. The cytoplasm contains numerous, round, relatively uniform-in-size basophilic granules. In some instances, the granules may be so numerous as to obscure the nuclear margin. Similar to the basophil, the granules in the mast cell stain metachromatically with the toluidine blue O stain. The outline of the cell may be round, oval, or elongate, depending on the type of preparation. Ultrastructurally, the striking feature is the presence of numerous dense granules in the cytoplasm (Figure 24). The granules are large but exhibit some variation in size, shape, and electron density. The nuclear chromatin shows marked clumping.

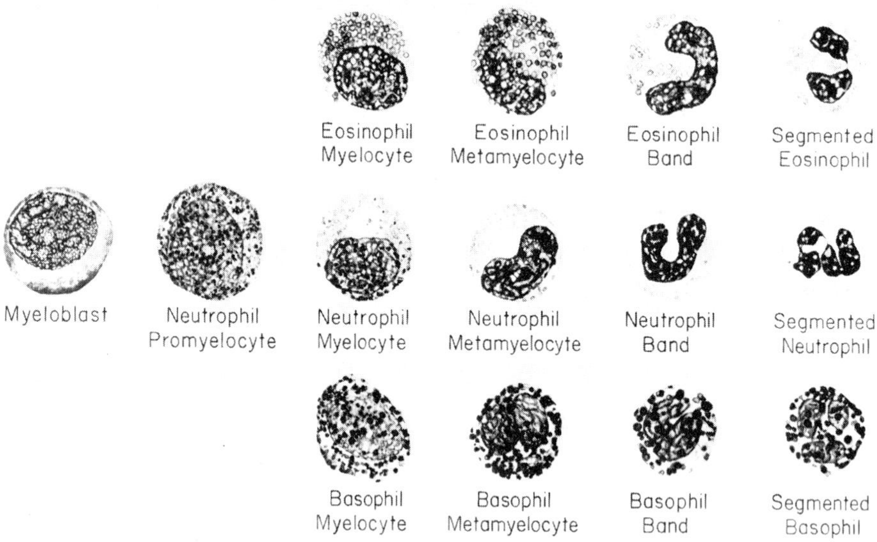

FIGURE 1. Normal granulopoiesis. The neutrophils, eosinophils, and basophils arise from a common precursor, the myeloblast, and progress through parallel developmental stages (Modified from Diggs, L. W., Sturm, D., and Bell, A., *The Morphology of Human Blood Cells,* W. B. Saunders, Philadelphia, 1956. Reproduced with the permission of the authors and W. B. Saunders.)

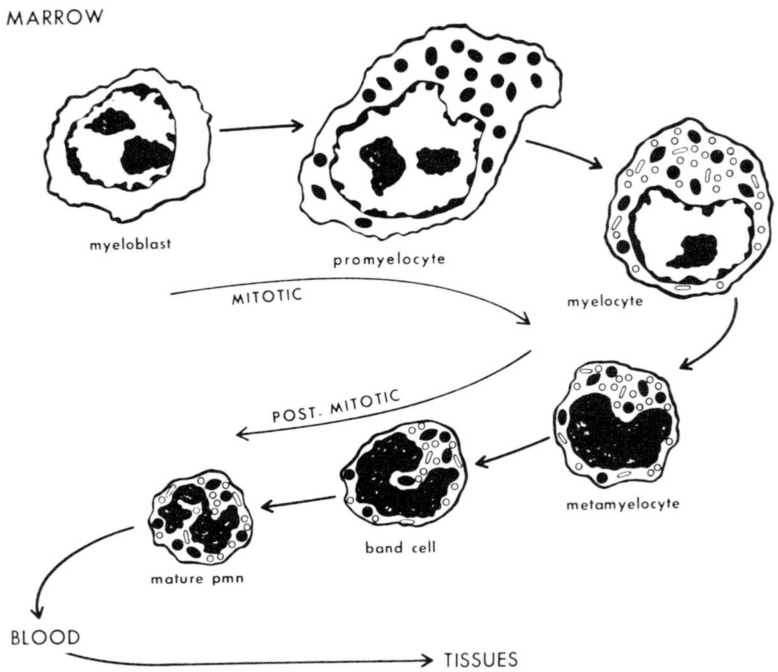

FIGURE 2. Diagramatic representation of neutrophil development. The myeloblast is an agranular undifferentiated cell with a large nucleus and prominent, multiple nucleoli. The first of two secretory phases, the promyelocyte stage, is characterized by the production of azurophil granules (dark granules). The second secretory phase, the myelocyte stage, is marked by the production of specific granules (light granules). The metamyelocyte and band stages are nonproliferating, nonsecretory phases characterized by nuclear chromatin clumping and changes in nuclear configuration. The segmented neutrophil contains both specific and azurophil granules in the approximate ratio of 2 to 1. (Modified from Bainton, D. F., Ullyot, J. L., and Farquhar, M. G., *J. Exp. Med.*, 134, 907, 1971. Reproduced with the permission of the author and the *Journal of Experimental Medicine.*)

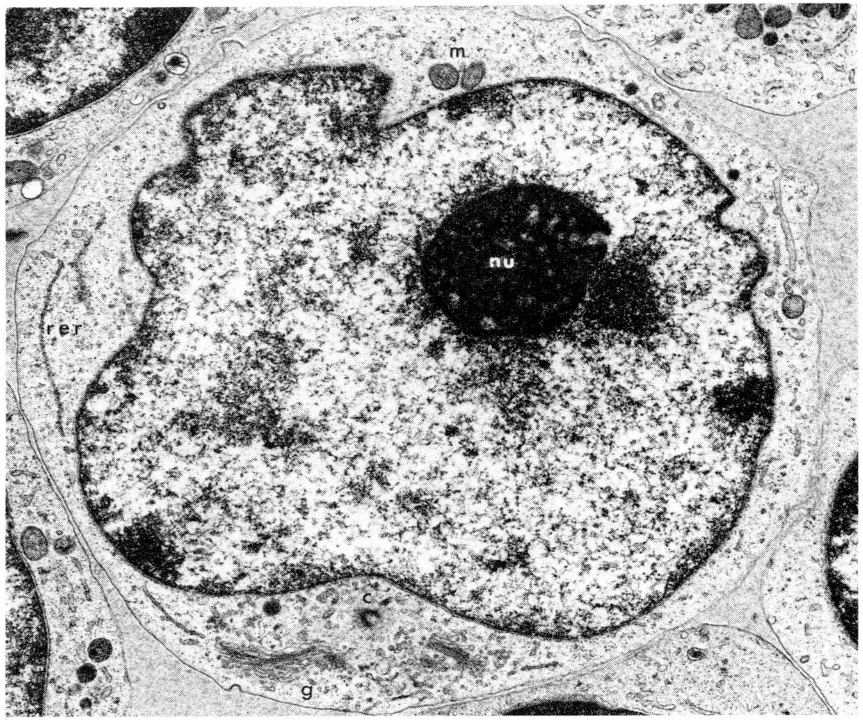

FIGURE 3. Myeloblast from the bone marrow of a patient with acute mylogenous leukemia. The nuclear chromatin is very finely dispersed with minimal condensation at the nuclear margin. A single prominent nucleolus (nu) is present. The cytoplasm contains a prominent Golgi (g), several mitochrondria (m), a few strands of rough endoplasmic reticulum (rer) and numerous mono- and polyribosomes. (Uranyl acetate-lead citrate; magnification × 13,400.)

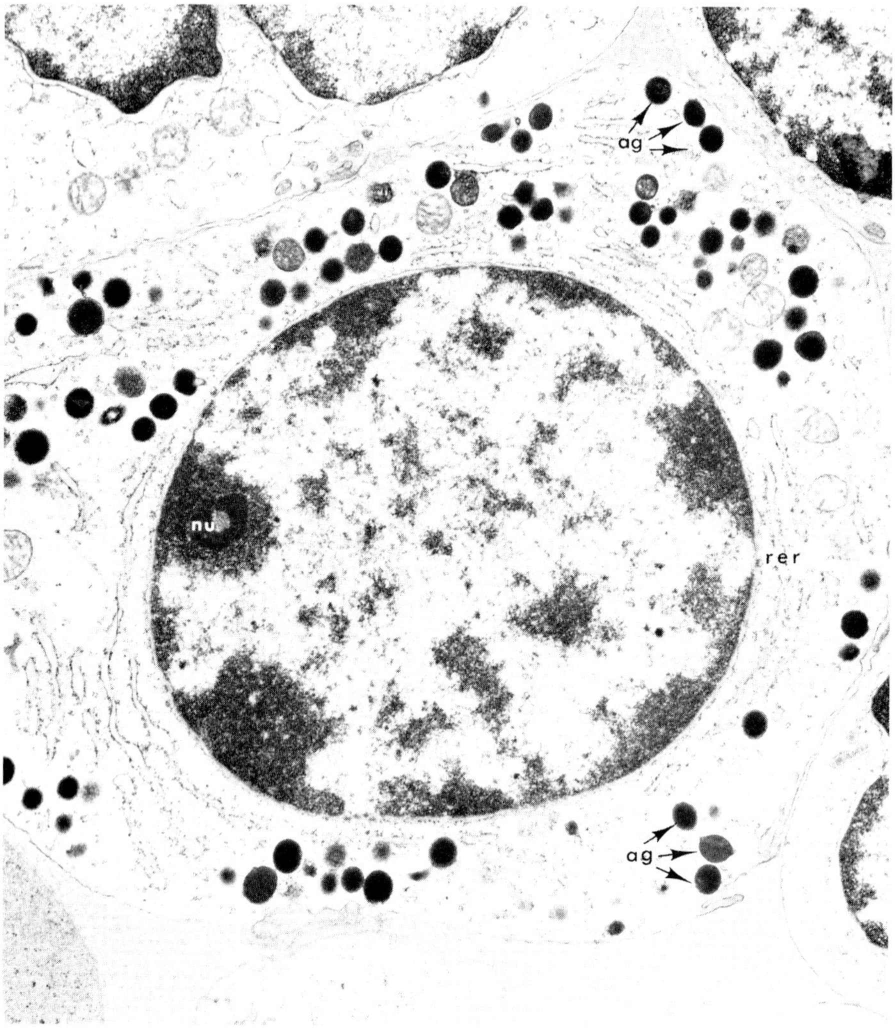

FIGURE 4. Neutrophil promyelocyte from the marrow of a patient with acute myelogenous leukemia. The nuclear chromatin is finely dispersed with clumping at the nuclear margin. One small nucleolus (nu) is present. The cytoplasm contains several strands of rough endoplasmic reticulum (rer). There are numerous dense granules (ag) scattered throughout the cytoplasm. These are peroxidase positive and correspond to the azurophilic granules of Romanowsky stained smears. The dense granules vary in size but are uniform in shape. An occasional granule contains a central crystalloid structure. (Uranyl acetate-lead citrate; magnification × 10,560.)

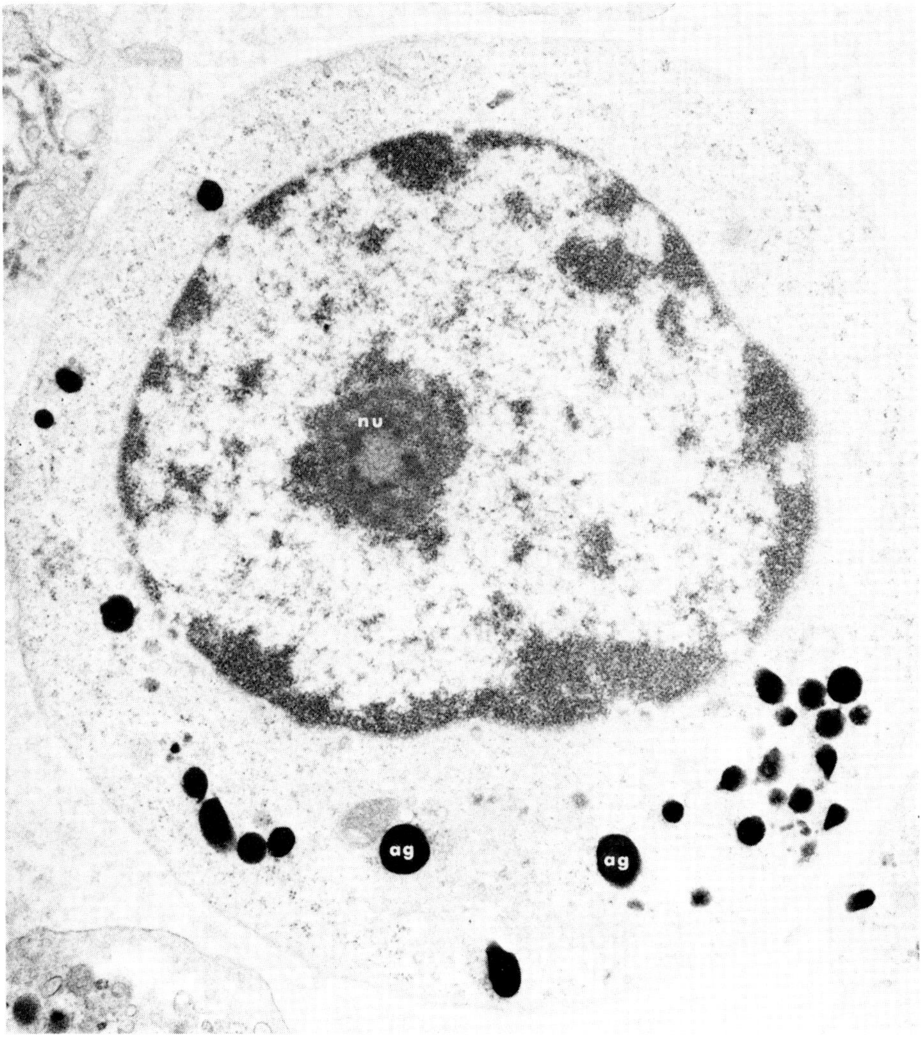

FIGURE 5. A neutrophil promyelocyte reacted for peroxidase. The granules arising at this stage of development (ag) react for peroxidase as evidenced by their electron density with this technique. These peroxidase-positive granules correspond to the azurophilic granules seen in Romanowsky stained smears. (Uranyl acetate; magnification × 16,750.)

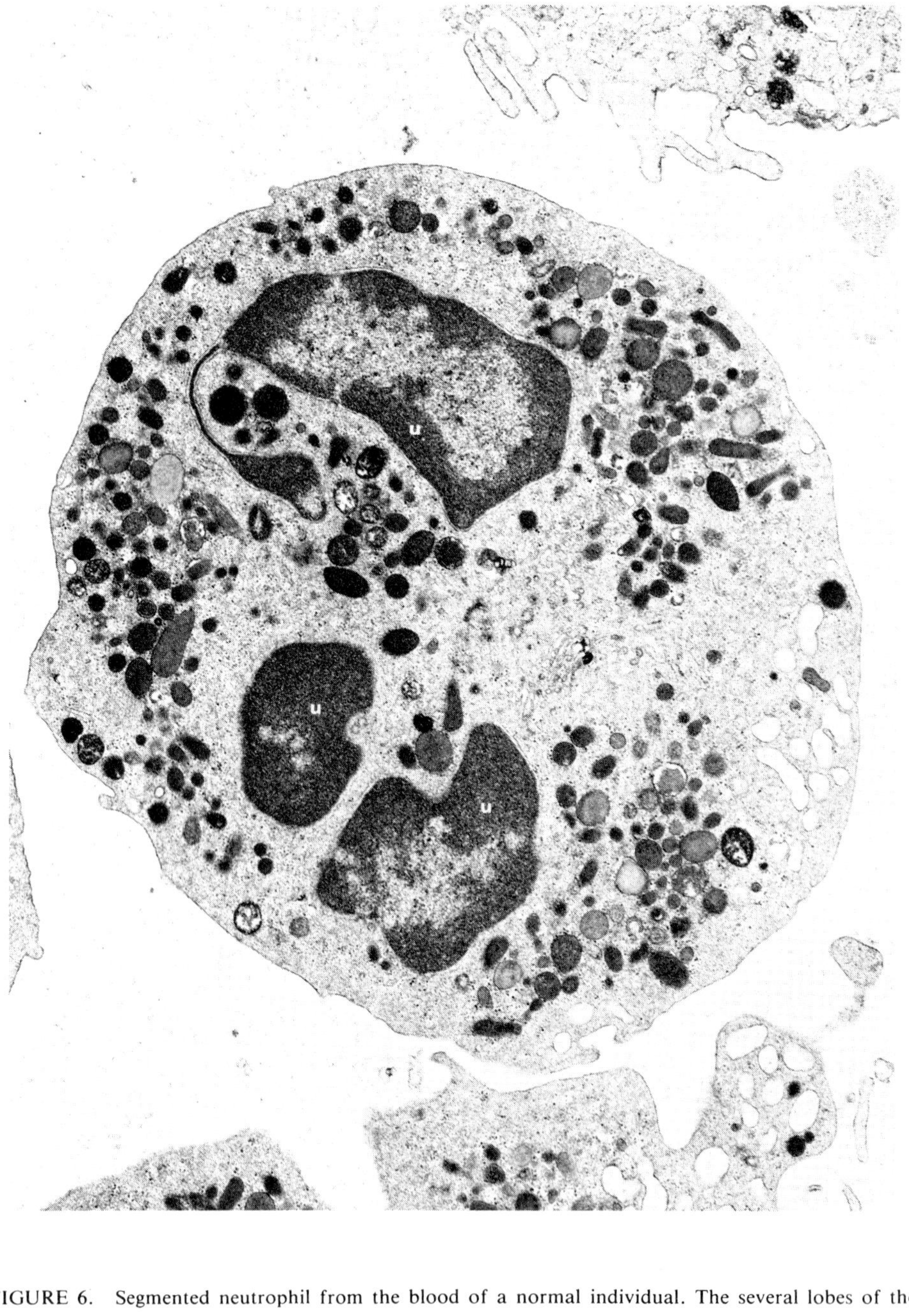

FIGURE 6. Segmented neutrophil from the blood of a normal individual. The several lobes of the nucleus (n) exhibit marked chromatin clumping. The cytoplasm contains numerous granules of varying density, size, and shape. Small particles of glycogen can be identified. The Golgi is small. (Uranyl acetate-lead citrate; magnification × 14,484.)

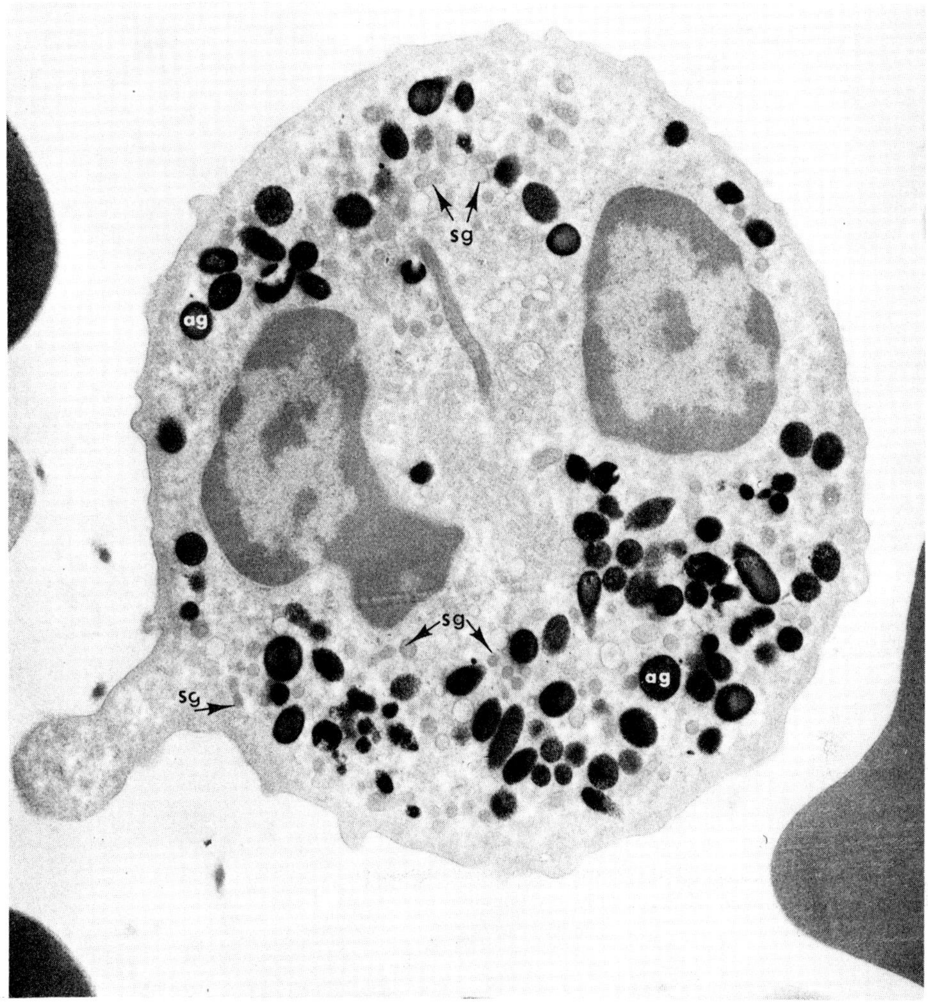

FIGURE 7. A segmented neutrophil reacted for peroxidase. The large peroxidase-positive dense granules (ag) correspond to the azurophilic granules of Romanowsky stained smears. The lighter, peroxidase nonreacting granules (sg) are the specific or neutrophil granules. The peroxidase negative granules are smaller and more irregular in shape than the peroxidase positive granules. (Unstained; magnification × 13,800.)

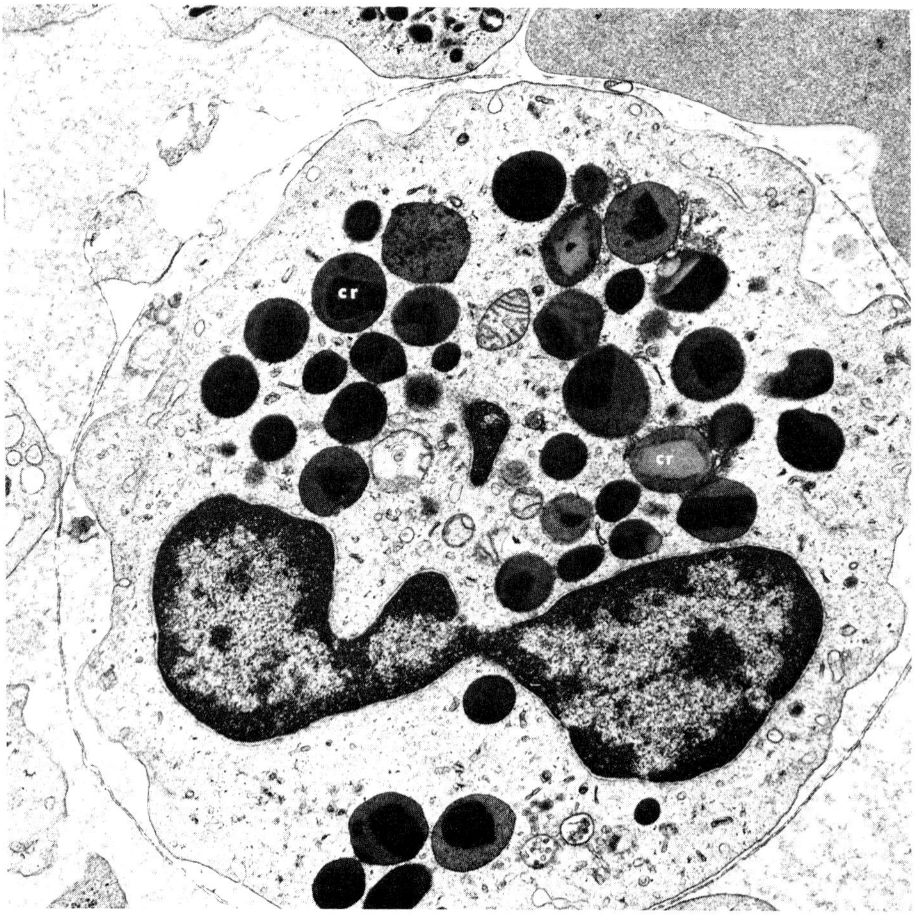

FIGURE 8. Mature eosinophil from the blood of a normal individual. The nucleus is lobulated and the chromatin shows marked clumping. The numerous granules vary somewhat in size but are generally large. The majority of the granules have a very dense crystalloid (cr) which is surrounded by a less dense matrix. (Uranyl acetate-lead citrate; magnification × 11,200.)

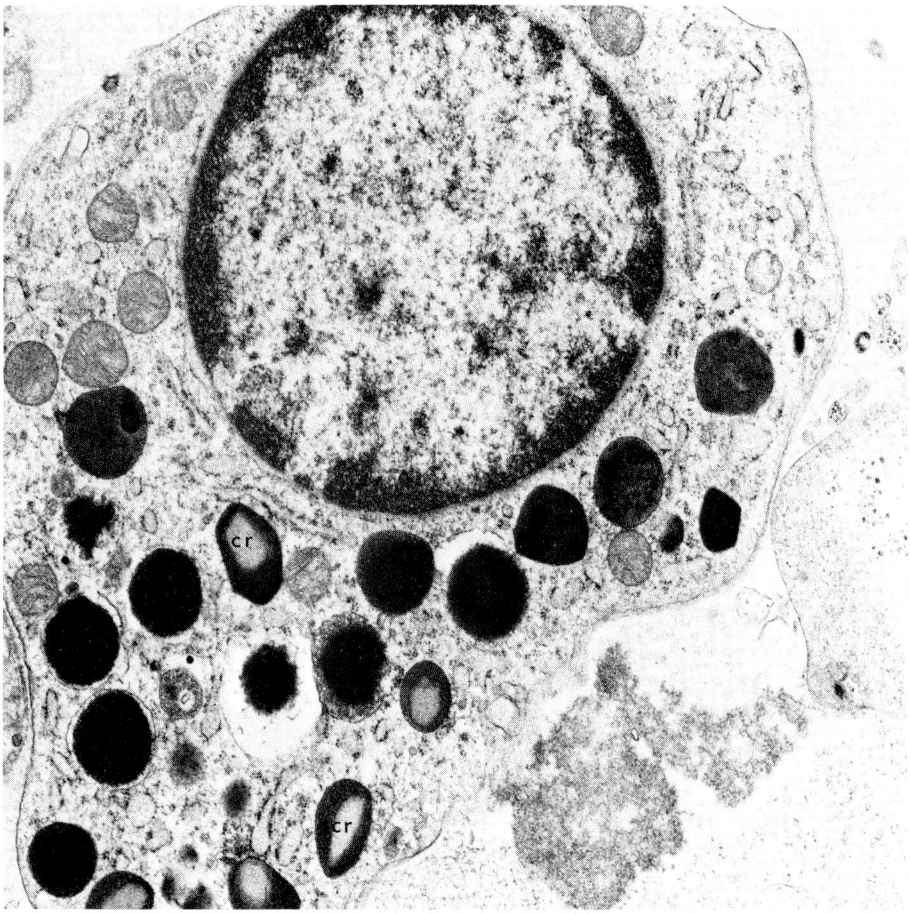

FIGURE 9. Eosinophil myelocyte from the bone marrow of a normal individual. The nucleus is round and the heterochromatin is fairly evenly dispersed; the cytoplasm contains mitochondria, strands of rough endoplasmic reticulum, and numerous large electron-dense granules. The granules are primarily spherical. The majority of the granules have a homogenous matrix; a small number have a central crystalloid structure (cr). (Uranyl acetate-lead citrate; magnification × 14,000.)

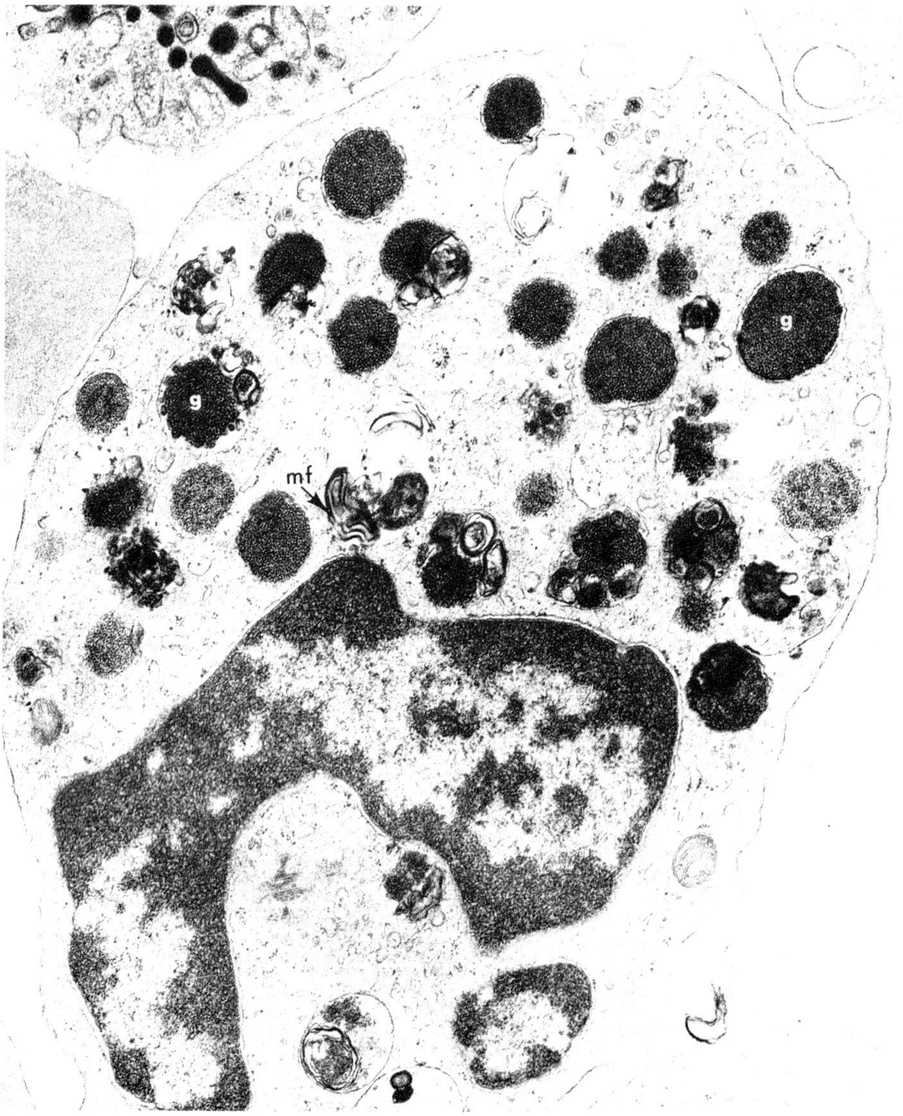

FIGURE 10. Basophil from the blood of a normal individual. The basophil granules (g) are large and consist of a membrane enclosing numerous smaller structures. Several of the granules contain myelin figures (mf). The nuclear chromatin shows marked clumping. (Uranyl acetate-lead citrate; magnification × 16,280.)

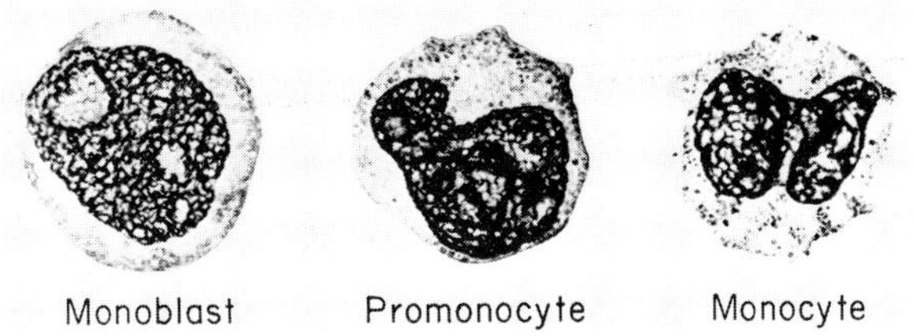

FIGURE 11. Monoblast, promonocyte, and monocyte as viewed in Romanowsky stained smear. (Reproduced from Diggs, L. W., Sturm, D., and Bell, A., *The Morphology of Human Blood Cells,* W. B. Saunders, Philadelphia, 1956. Reproduced with the permission of the authors and W. B. Saunders.)

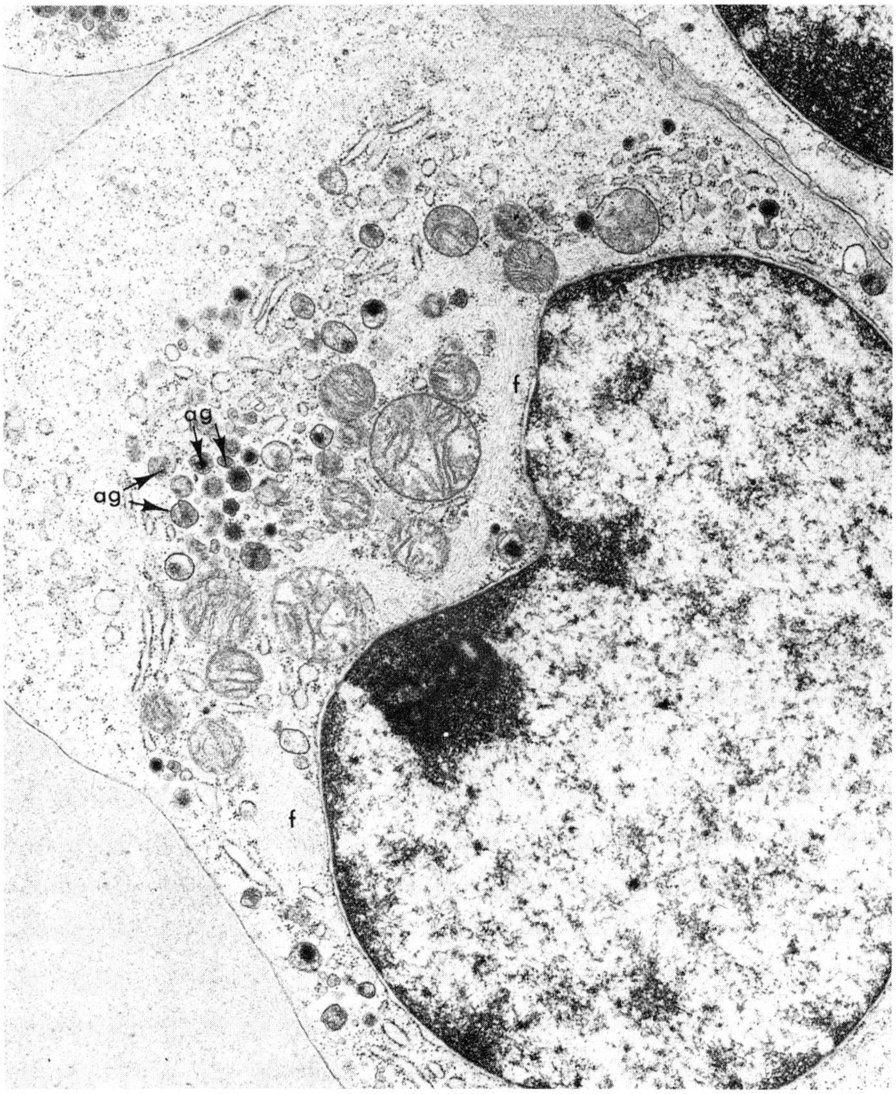

FIGURE 12. Monoblast from the bone marrow of a patient with acute monoblastic leukemia. The nuclear chromatin is very finely dispersed with slight condensation at the nuclear margin. A portion of a nucleolus is present at the nuclear margin. The cytoplasm contains numerous, some very large, mitochondria, several dense granules (ag), and strands of rough endoplasmic reticulum. Arrays of fibrillar structures (f) are located in a juxtanuclear location. (Uranyl acetate-lead citrate; magnification × 21,900.)

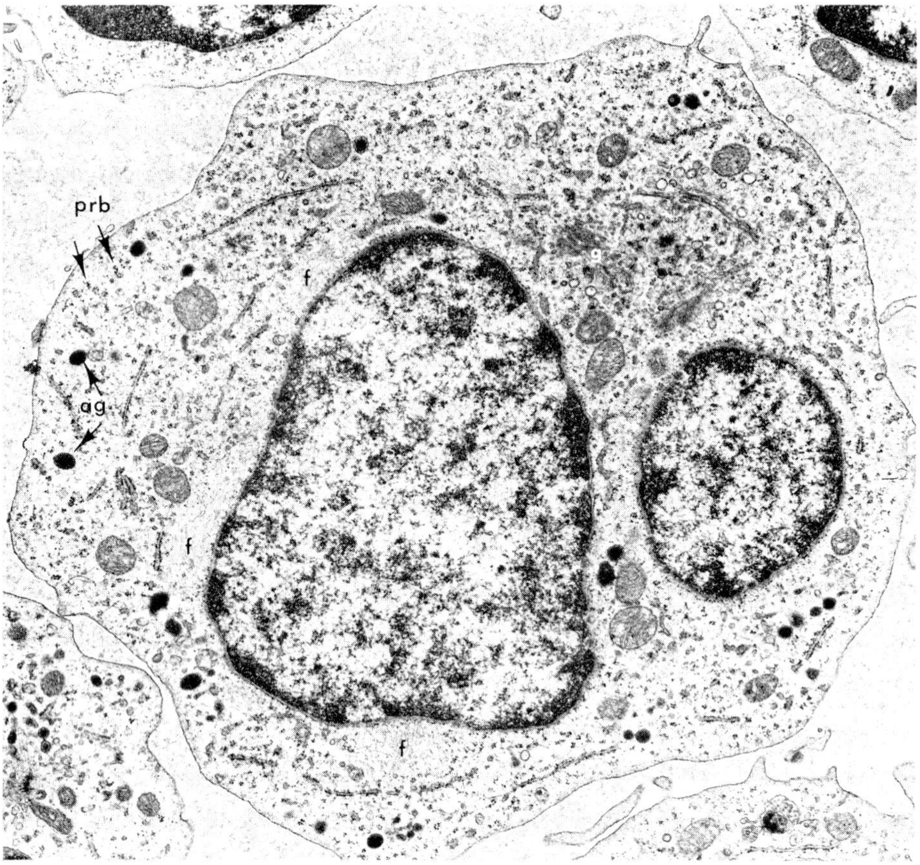

FIGURE 13. Immature monocyte from the marrow of a patient with acute monocytic leukemia. The nucleus, which is lobulated, has chromatin which is finely dispersed with slight condensation at the margin. The cytoplasm contains several mitochondria, short strands of rough endoplasmic reticulum, dense granules (ag), and numerous polyribosomes (prb). Arrays of fibrillar structures (f) can be identified in a paranuclear location. The plane of section is through the Golgi (g). (Uranyl acetate-lead citrate; magnification × 10,720.)

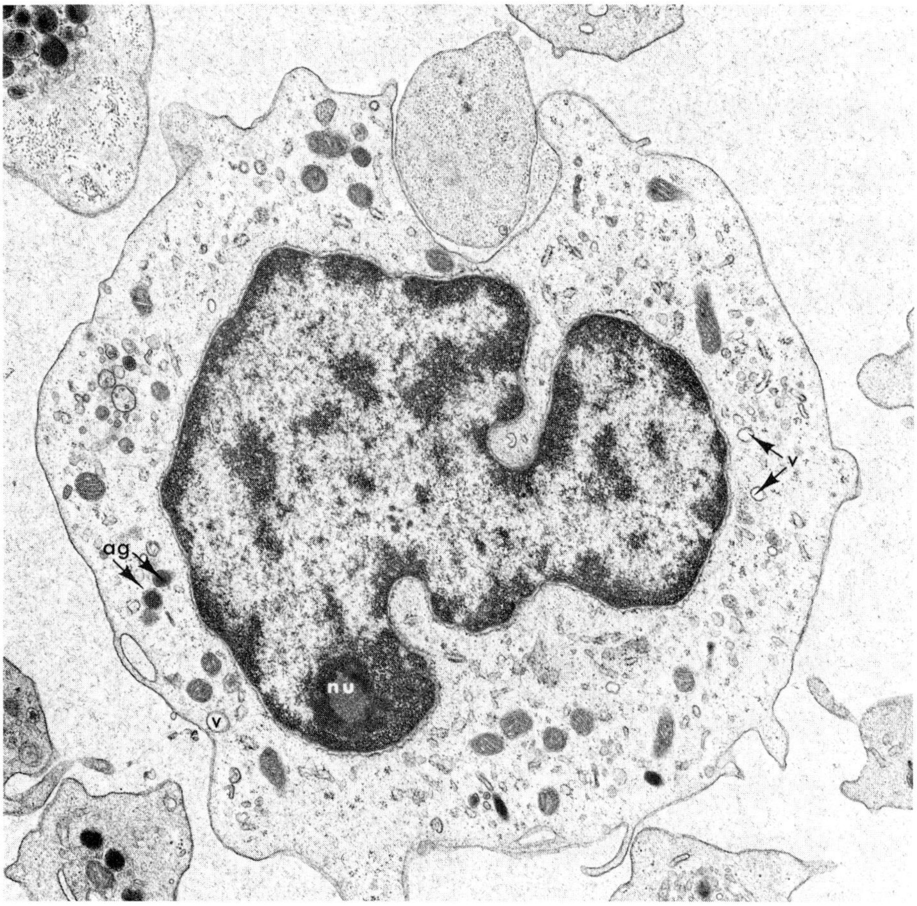

FIGURE 14. Monocyte from the blood of a normal individual. The lobulated nucleus contains moderately dispersed chromatin with somewhat uniform condensation at the nuclear margin. A distinct nucleolus (nu) can be identified. The cytoplasm contains several small mitochrondria, vesicles (v), short strands of rough endoplasmic reticulum, and a small number of dense granules (ag). The cell appears to be ingesting a fragment of a platelet. (Uranyl acetate-lead citrate; magnification × 11,360.)

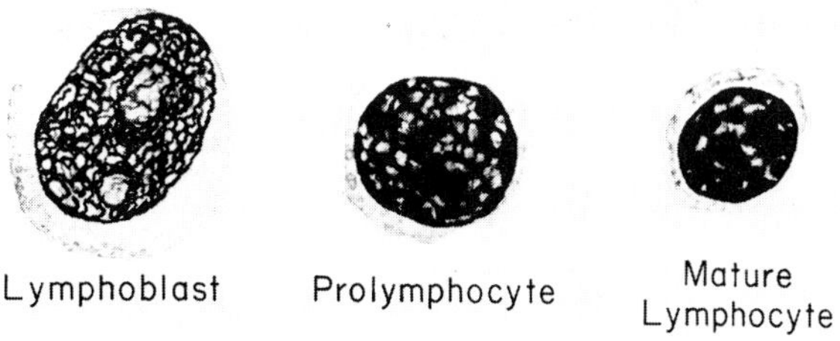

FIGURE 15. Lymphoblast, prolymphocyte, and mature lymphocyte as viewed in Romanowsky stained smear. (Reproduced from Diggs, L. W., Sturm, D., and Bell, A., *The Morphology of Human Blood Cells,* W. B. Saunders, Philadelphia, 1956. Reproduced with the permission of the authors and W. B. Saunders.)

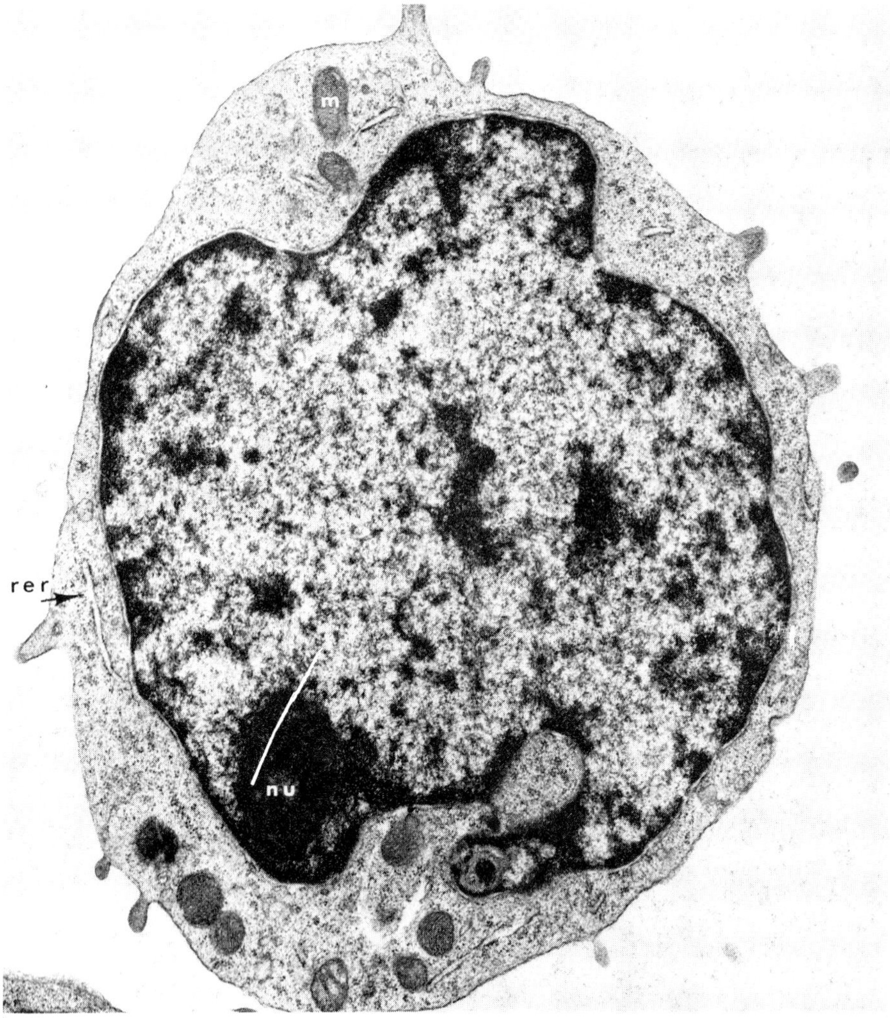

FIGURE 16. Lymphoblast from a patient with acute lymphocytic leukemia. The nucleus is indented and exhibits a small bleb formation. The nuclear chromatin is dispersed with some condensation at the nuclear margin. A single prominent nucleolus (nu) is present. The cytoplasm contains a few short strands of rough endoplasmic reticulum (rer) and several mitochondria (m). Numerous ribosomes are scattered throughout the cytoplasm. (Uranyl acetate-lead citrate; magnification × 14,800.)

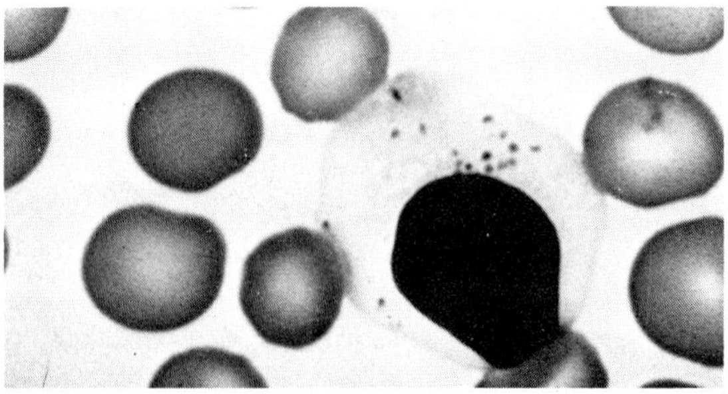

FIGURE 17. Large lymphocyte from the blood of a normal individual. The abundant, pale-staining cytoplasm contains several coarse, azurophilic granules. (Wright's Giemsa; magnification × 950.)

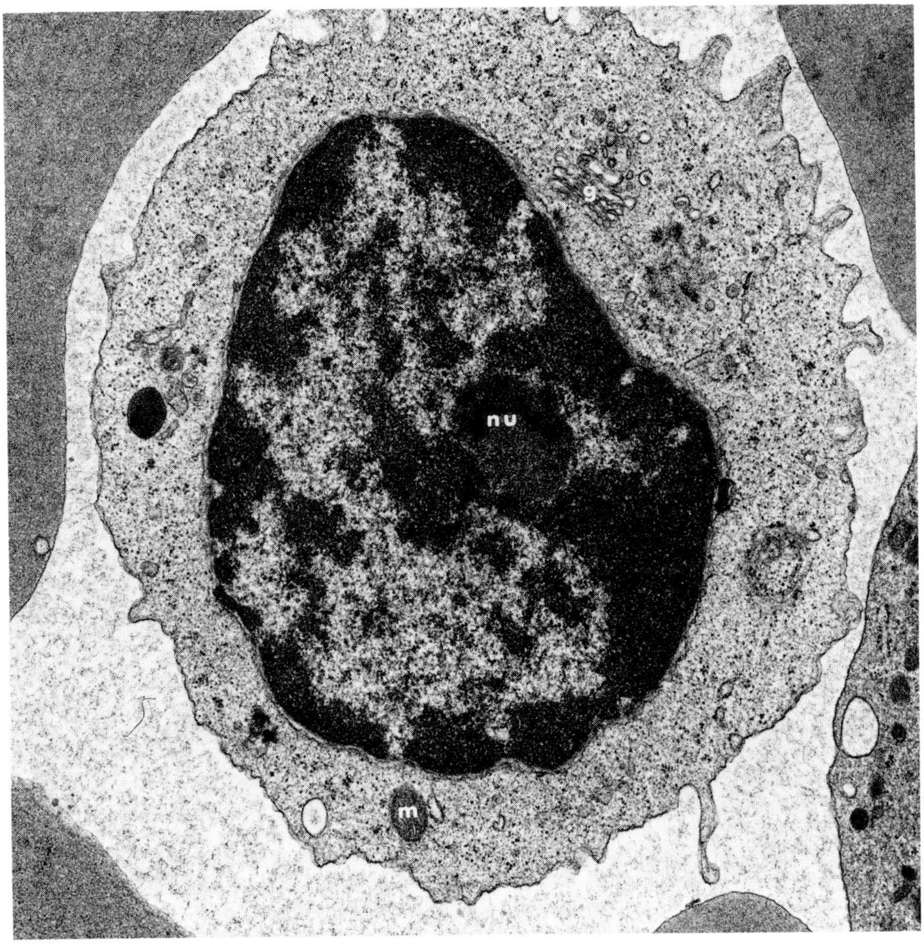

FIGURE 18. Small lymphocyte from the peripheral blood of a normal individual. The nuclear chromatin shows considerable clumping. A nucleolus (nu) is present and has a density similar to the chromatin. The moderate amount of cytoplasm contains scattered monoribosomes and a few polyribosomes, a small Golgi (g), and mitochondria (m). (Uranyl acetate-lead citrate; magnification × 15,800.)

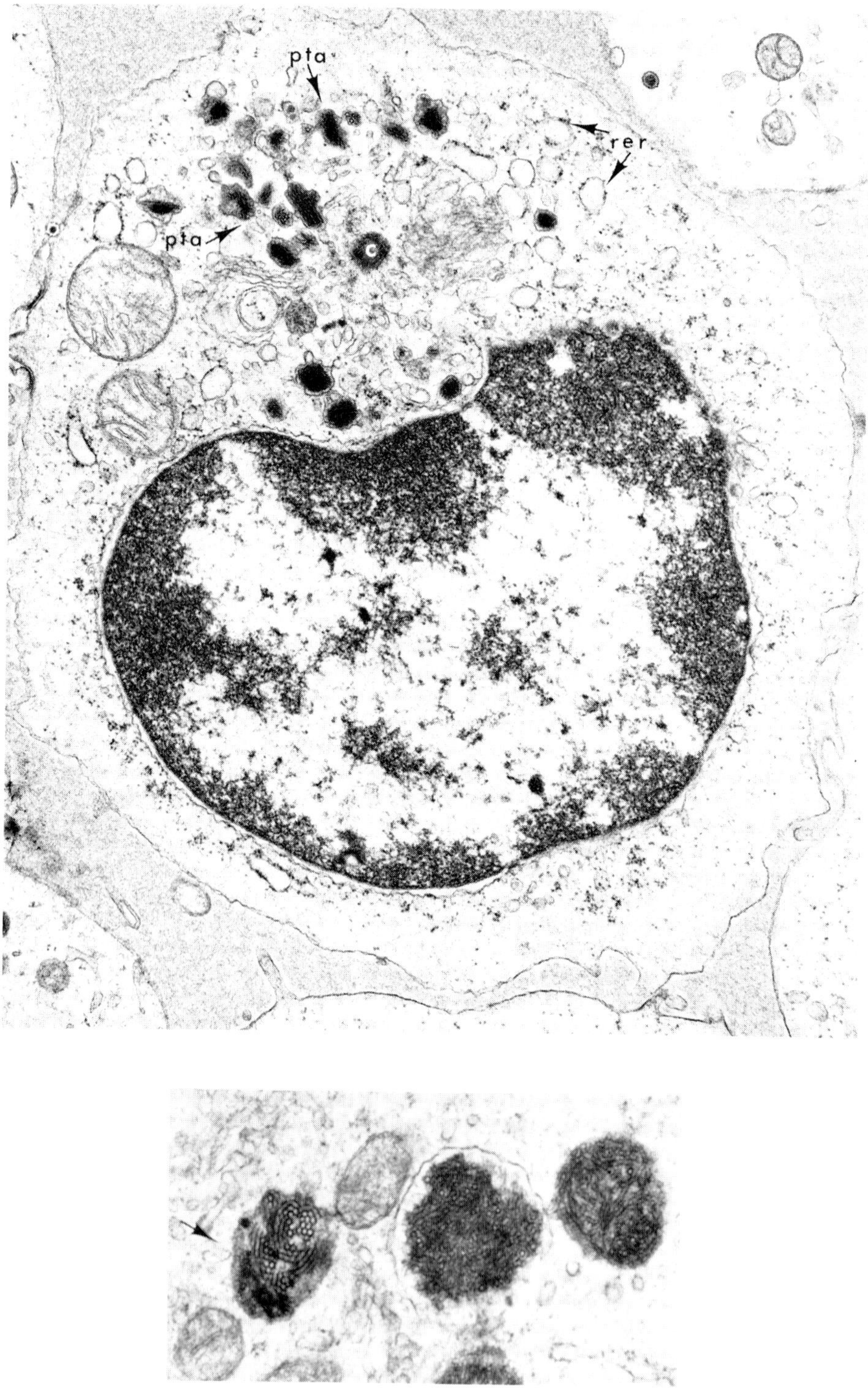

FIGURE 19. A large lymphocyte from the blood of a patient with infectious mononucleosis, which contains a prominent Golgi, and several dense granules, which have a substructure composed of parallel tubular arrays (pta). There are several dilated sacs of rough endoplasmic reticulum (rer) and a centriole (c). (Uranyl acetate-lead citrate × 18,000). Inset. High magnification of parallel tubular arrays. (Magnification × 29,750.)

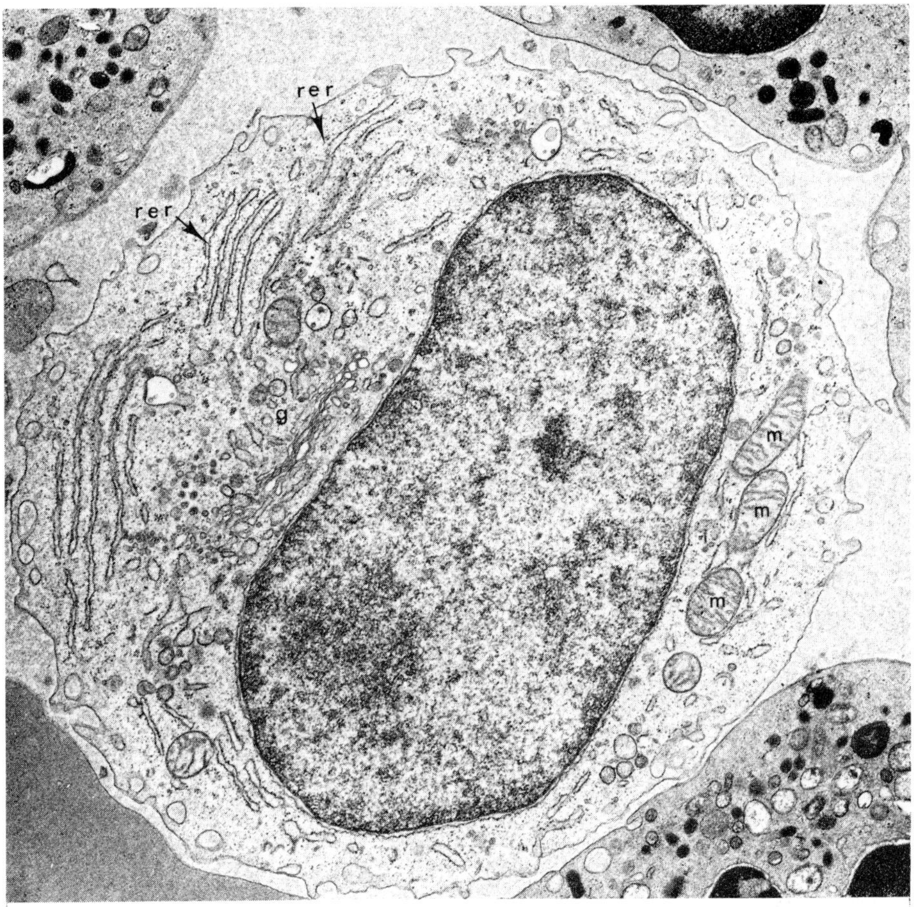

FIGURE 20. Large lymphoid cell from the blood of a normal individual. The nuclear chromatin is moderately dispersed with slight condensation at the nuclear margin. The cytoplasm contains numerous strands of rough endoplasmic reticulum (rer), a prominent Golgi (g), several mitochondria (m), and numerous ribosomes. Several small vesicles are present. (Uranyl acetate-lead citrate; magnification × 15,620.)

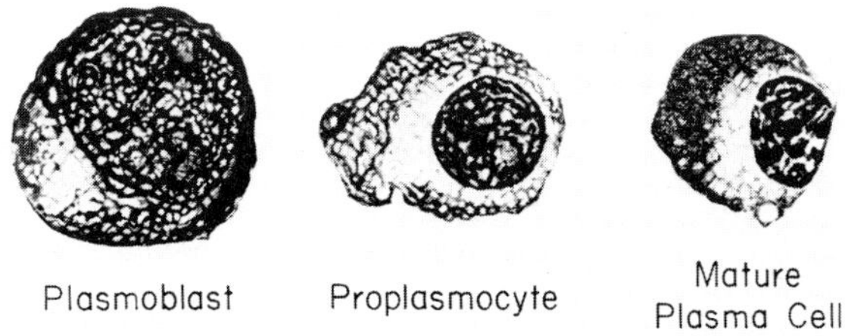

FIGURE 21. Plasmoblast, proplasmocyte, and mature plasma cell as viewed in Romanowsky stained smear. (Reproduced from Diggs, L. W., Sturm, D., and Bell, A., *The Morphology of Human Blood Cells,* W. B. Saunders, Philadelphia, 1956. Reproduced with permission of the authors and W. B. Saunders.)

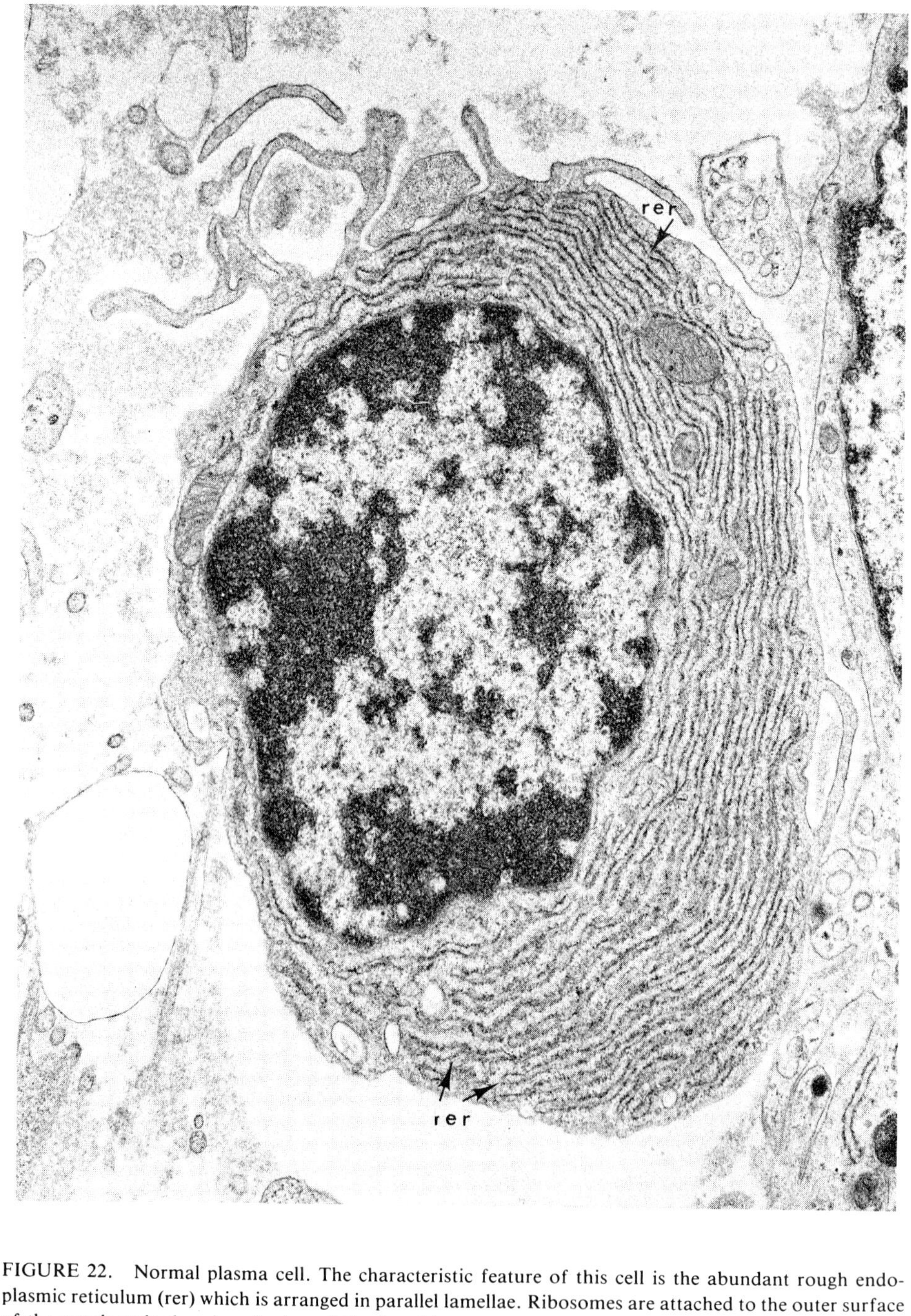

FIGURE 22. Normal plasma cell. The characteristic feature of this cell is the abundant rough endoplasmic reticulum (rer) which is arranged in parallel lamellae. Ribosomes are attached to the outer surface of the rough endoplasmic reticulum. Mitochondria are scattered throughout the cytoplasm. Clumping of the nuclear chromatin is present. (Uranyl acetate-lead citrate; magnification × 14,484.)

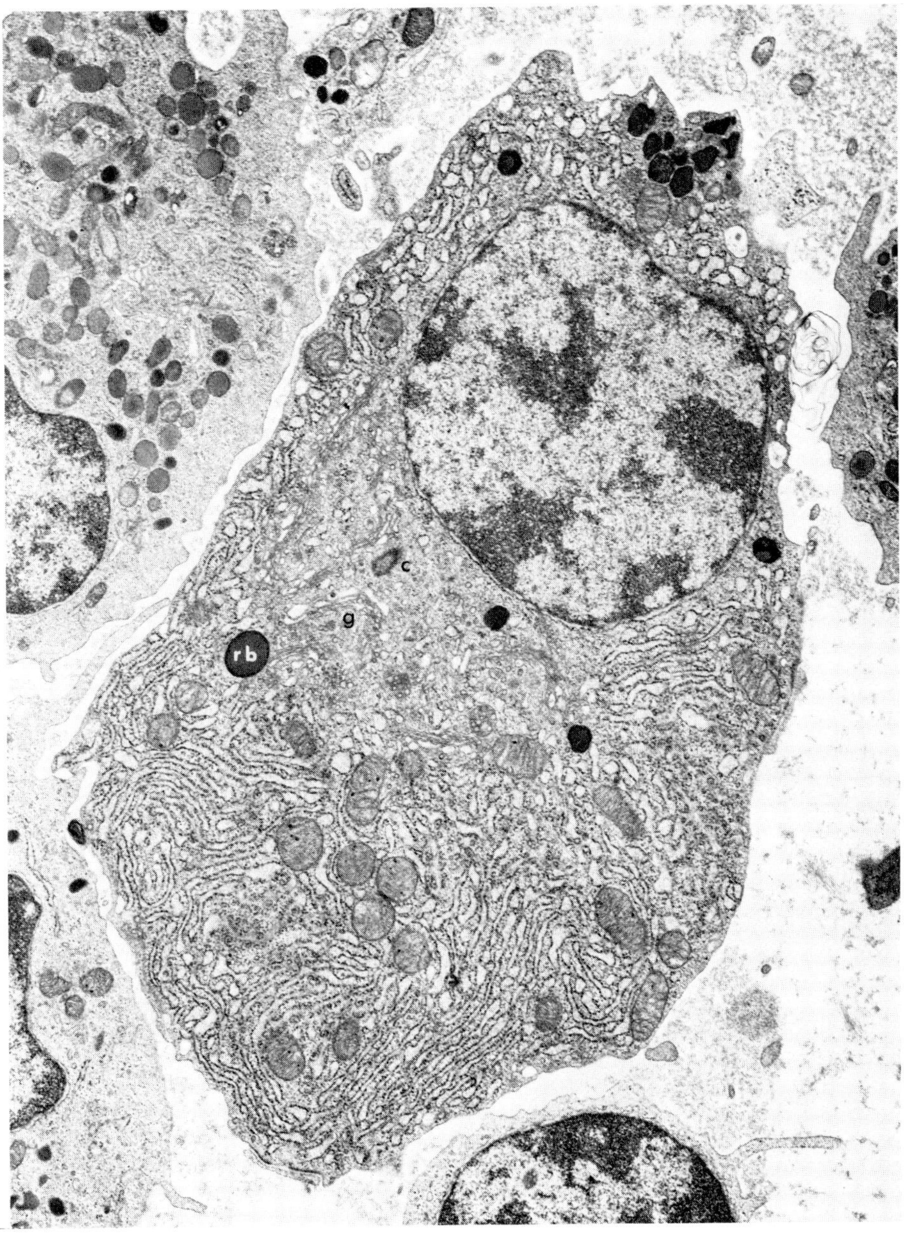

FIGURE 23. Plasma cell in which there is a prominent Golgi (g) adjacent to the nucleus. Several densely osmiophilic inclusions (rb) are present. The inclusions correspond to the Russell bodies of light microscopy. A centriole (c) and numerous mitochondria are present. (Uranyl acetate-lead citrate; magnification × 10,224.)

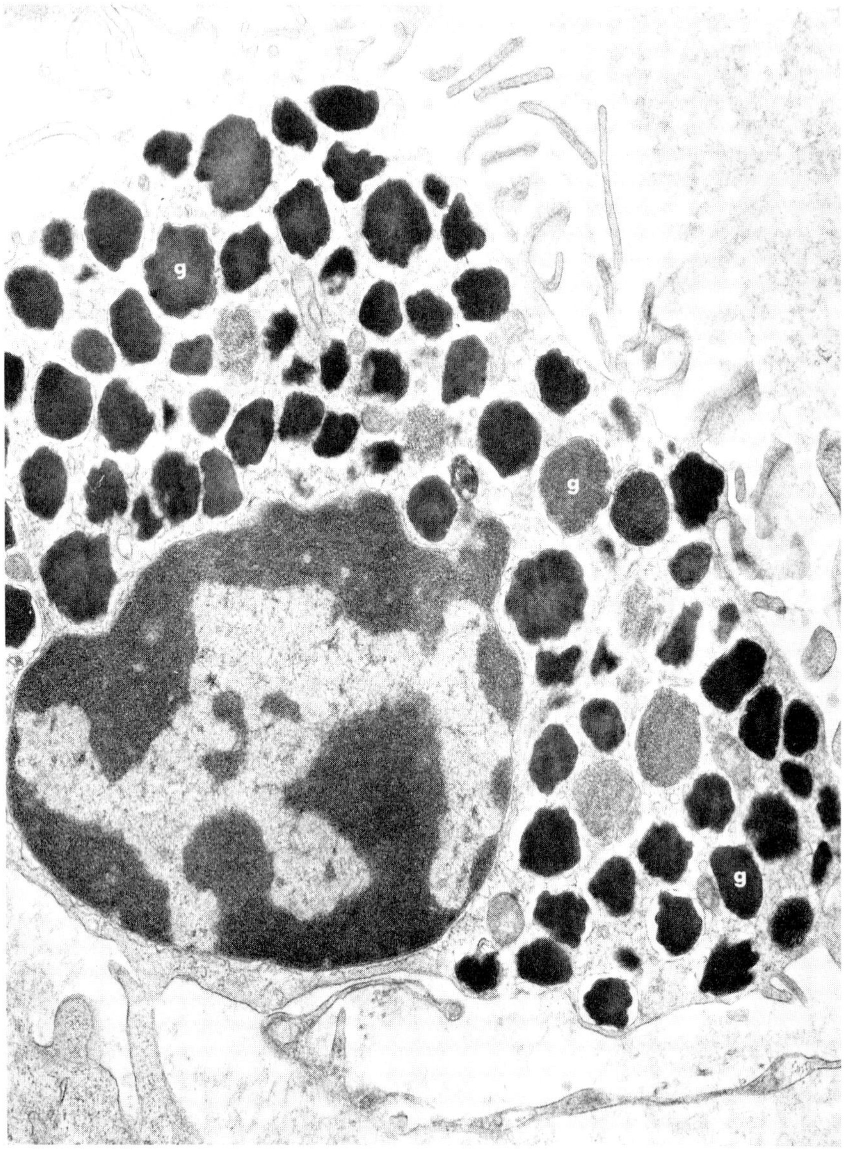

FIGURE 24. Mast cell. The cytoplasm contains numerous granules (g), the majority of which are markedly electron dense; a small number of the granules are more electron lucent. The nuclear chromatin shows marked clumping. Several delicate projections are arising from the cytoplasmic surface. (Uranyl acetate-lead citrate; magnification × 15,400.)

REFERENCES

1. **Metcalf, D.**, Regulation of granulocyte and monocyte-macrophage proliferation by colony stimulating factor (CSF). A review, *Exp. Hematol.*, 1, 185, 1973.
2. **Stanley, E. R., Hansen, G., Woodcock, J., and Metcalf, D.**, Colony stimulating factor and the regulation of granulopoiesis and macrophage production, *Fed. Proc.*, 34, 2272, 1975.
3. **Robinson, W. A. and Mangalik, A.**, The kinetics and regulation of granulopoiesis, *Semin. Hematol.*, 12, 7, 1975.
4. **Stossel, T. P.**, Phagocytosis: recognition and ingestion, *Semin. Hematol.*, 12, 83, 1975.
5. **Klebanoff, S. J.**, Antimicrobial mechanisms in neutrophilic polymorphonuclear leukocytes, *Semin. Hematol.*, 12, 117, 1975.
6. **Ebert, R. H. and Florey, H. W.**, The extravascular development of the monocyte observed in vitro, *Br. J. Exp. Pathol.*, 20, 342, 1939.
7. Editorial: What eosinophils do, *Lancet II*, 388, 1977.
8. **Wolf-Jurgensen, P.**, The basophilic leukocyte, *Ser. Hematol.*, 6, 4, 1968.
9. **Cooper, M. D., Perey, D. Y., Peterson, R. D. A., Gabrielson, A. E., and Good, R. A.**, The two-component concept of the lymphoid system, in *Immunologic Deficiency Diseases in Man*, Bergsma, D. and Good, R. A., Eds., National Foundation Press, New York, 1968.
10. **Whang, J., Frei, E., Tjio, J. H., Carbone, P. P., and Brecher, G.**, The distribution of the Philadelphia chromosome in patients with chronic myelogenous leukemia, *Blood*, 22, 664, 1963.
11. **Chervenick, P. A., Ellis, L., Pan, S., and Lawson, A. L.**, Human leukemic cells: in vitro growth of colonies containing the Philadelphia (Ph′.) chromosome, *Science*, 174, 1134, 1971.
12. **Golde, D. W., Burgaleta, C., Sparkes, R. S., and Cline, M. J.**, The Philadelphia chromosome in human macrophages, *Blood*, 49, 367, 1977.
13. **Boggs, D. R.**, Hematopoietic stem cell theory in relation to possible lymphoblastic conversion of chronic myeloid leukemia, *Blood*, 44, 449, 1974.
14. **Janossy, G., Roberts, M., and Greaves, M. F.**, Target cell in chronic myeloid leukemia and its relationship to acute lymphoid leukemia, *Lancet II*, 1058, 1976.
15. **Bloomfield, C. D., Peterson, L., Yunis, J., and Brunning, R.**, The Philadelphia chromosome (Ph) in adults presenting with acute leukemia: comparison of Ph+ and Ph− patients, *Br. J. Haematol.*, 36, 347, 1977.
16. **Hoffbrand, A. V., Ganeshaguru, K., Janossy, G., Greaves, M. F., Catovsky, D., and Woodruff, R. K.**, Terminal deoxynucleotidyl-transferase levels and membrane phenotypes in diagnosis of acute leukaemia, *Lancet II*, 520, 1977.
17. Committee for Clarification of the Nomenclature of Cells and Diseases of the Blood and Blood-Forming Organs. Report I, *Am. J. Clin. Pathol.*, 18, 443, 1948.
18. **Diggs, L. W., Sturm, D., and Bell, A.**, *The Morphology of Human Blood Cells*, W. B. Saunders, Philadelphia, 1956.
19. **Bainton, D. F., Ullyot, J. L., and Farquhar, M. G.**, The development of neutrophilic polymorphonuclear leukocytes in human bone marrow, *J. Exp. Med.*, 134, 907, 1971.
20. **Anderson, D. R.**, Ultrastructure of normal and leukemic leukocytes in human peripheral blood, *J. Ultrastruct. Res.*, 9 (Suppl.), 1, 1966.
21. **Watanabe, I., Donahue, S., and Hogatt, N.**, Method for electron microscopic studies of circulating human leukocytes and observations of their fine structure, *J. Ultrastruct. Res.*, 20, 366, 1967.
22. **Scott, R. E. and Horn, R. G.**, Ultrastructural aspects of neutrophil granulocytic development in humans, *Lab. Invest.*, 23, 202, 1970.
23. **Bainton, D. F.**, Annotation: neutrophil granules, *Br. J. Haematol.*, 29, 17, 1975.
24. **Yam, L. T., Li, C. Y., and Crosby, W. H.**, Cytochemical identification of monocytes and granulocytes, *Am. J. Clin. Pathol.*, 55, 283, 1971.
25. **Scott, R. E. and Horn, R. G.**, Fine structural features of eosinophilic granulocyte development in human bone marrow, *J. Ultrastruct. Res.*, 33, 16, 1970.
26. **Bainton, D. F. and Farquhar, M. G.**, Segregation and packaging of granule enzymes in eosinophilic leukocytes, *J. Cell Biol.*, 45, 54, 1970.
27. **Zucker-Franklin, D.**, Electron microscopic study of human basophils, *Blood*, 29, 878, 1967.
28. **Van Furth, R.**, Origin and kinetics of monocytes and macrophages, *Semin. Hematol.*, 7, 125, 1970.
29. **Cline, M. J. and Sumner, M. A.**, Bone marrow macrophage precursors. I. Some functional characteristics of the early cells of the mouse macrophage series, *Blood*, 40, 62, 1972.
30. **Schmazl, F. and Braunsteiner, H.**, The cytochemistry of monocytes and macrophages, *Ser. Hematol.*, 3, 93, 1970.
31. **Van Furth, R., Hirsch, J. G., and Fedorko, M. E.**, Morphology and peroxidase cytochemistry of mouse promonocytes, monocytes, and macrophages, *J. Exp. Med.*, 132, 794, 1970.

32. **Nichols, B. A. and Bainton, D. F.**, Differentiation of human monocytes in bone marrow and blood, *Lab. Invest.*, 29, 27, 1973.
33. **McKenna, R. W., Bloomfield, C. D., Dick, F., Nesbit, M. E., and Brunning, R. D.**, Acute monoblastic leukemia: diagnosis and treatment of ten cases, *Blood*, 46, 481, 1975.
34. **Li, C. Y., Lam, K. W., and Yam, L. T.**, Esterases in human leukocytes, *J. Histochem. Cytochem.*, 21, 1, 1973.
35. **Glick, A. D. and Horn, R. G.**, Identification of promonocytes and monocyte precursors in acute leukemia of adults. Ultrastructural and cytochemical observations, *Br. J. Haematol.*, 26, 395, 1974.
36. **Claman, H. N., Chaperon, E. A., and Triplett, R. F.**, Thymus-marrow cell combinations. Synergism in antibody production, *Proc. Soc. Exp. Biol. Med.*, 122, 1167, 1966.
37. **Feldman, M., Erb, P., and Kontiainen, S.**, Cell collaboration between T and B lymphocytes and macrophages in antibody production in vitro, *Lymphocytes and Their Interactions: Recent Observations*, Williams, R. C., Jr., Ed., Raven Press, New York, 1975, 1.
38. **Hansen, J. A. and Good, R. A.**, Malignant disease of the lymphoid system in immunological perspective, *Human Pathol.*, 5, 567, 1974.
39. **Raff, M. C.**, T and B lymphocytes and immune responses, *Nature (London)*, 242, 19, 1973.
40. **Kersey, J. H. and Gajl-Peczalska, K. J.**, T and B lymphocytes in humans. A review, *Am. J. Pathol.*, 81, 446, 1975.
41. **Aiuti, F., Cerotinni, J. C., Coombs, R. A. A., Cooper, M., Dickler, H. B., Froland, S. S., Fudenberg, H. H., Greaves, M. F., Grey, H. M., Kunkel, H. G., Natvig, J. B., Preud'homme, J. F., Rabellino, E., Ritts, R. B., Rowe, D. S., Seligman, M., Siegal, F. P., Stjernsward, J., Terry, W. D., and Wybran, J.**, Identification, enumeration and isolation of B and T lymphocytes from human peripheral blood, *Scand. J. Immunol.*, 3, 521, 1974.
42. **Greaves, M. F.**, Clinical applications of cell surface markers in *Progress in Hematology*, Vol. 9, Brown, E. B., Ed., Grune & Stratton, New York, 1975, 255.
43. **Bessis, M. C.**, *Living Blood Cells and Their Ultrastructure*, Springer-Verlag, New York, 1973, 418.
44. **Gowans, J. L. and McGregor, D. D.**, The immunological activities of lymphocytes, *Prog. Allergy*, 9, 1, 1965.
45. **Daniels, J. C., Ritzmann, S. E., and Levin, W. C.**, Lymphocytes: morphological, developmental and functional characteristics in health, disease, and experimental study. An analytical review, *Texas Rep. Biol. Med.*, 26, 5, 1968.
46. **Sundberg, R. D.**, Lymphocytes and plasma cells, *Ann. N.Y. Acad. Sci.*, 59, 671, 1955.
47. **Nathwani, B. N., Kim, H., and Rappaport H.**, Malignant lymphoma, lymphoblastic, *Cancer*, 38, 964, 1976.
48. **McKenna, R. W., Bloomfield, C. D., and Brunning, R. D.**, Nodular lymphoma: bone marrow and blood manifestation, *Cancer*, 36, 428, 1975.
49. **Zucker-Franklin, D.**, The ultrastructure of lymphocytes, *Semin. Hematol.*, 6, 4, 1969.
50. **Brunning, R. D. and Parkin, J.**, Ultrastructural studies of parallel tubular arrays in human lymphocytes, *Am. J. Pathol.*, 78, 59, 1975.
51. **McMillan, D. B. and Engelbert, V. E.**, The developmental history of the plasmacyte, *Am. J. Pathol.*, 42, 315, 1963.
52. **Birbeck, M. S. C. and Hall, J. G.**, Transformation in vivo, of basophilic lymph cells into plasma cells, *Nature (London)*, 214, 183, 1967.
53. **Kolouch, F., Good, R. A., and Campbell, B.**, The reticuloendothelial origin of the bone marrow plasma cells in hypersensitive states, *J. Lab. Clin. Med.*, 32, 749, 1947
54. **Leduc, E. H., Avrameas, S., and Bouteille, M.**, Ultrastructural localization of antibody in differentiating plasma cells, *J. Exp. Med.*, 127, 109, 1968.
55. **Leduc, E., Scott, G. B., and Avrameas, S.**, Ultrastructural localization of intracellular immunoglobulins in plasma cells and lymphoblasts by enzyme labelled antibodies, *J. Histochem. Cytochem.*, 17, 211, 1969.
56. **Brunning, R. D. and Parkin, J.**, Intranuclear inclusions in plasma cells and lymphocytes from patients with monoclonal gammopathies, *Am. J. Clin. Pathol.*, 66, 10, 1976.
57. **Cline, Martin J.**, *The White Cell*, Harvard University Press, Cambridge, Mass., 1975.
58. **Tanaka, Y. and Goodman, J. R.**, *Electron Microscopy of Human Blood Cells*, Harper & Row, New York, 1972.
59. **Cawley, J. C. and Hayhoe, F. G. J.**, *Ultrastructure of Haemic Cells*, W. B. Saunders, Philadelphia, 1973.
60. **Bessis, M. C.**, *Living Blood Cells and Their Ultrastructure*, Springer-Verlag, New York, 1973.

SEPARATION OF HUMAN LEUKOCYTES

Thomas F. Necheles

Table 1 describes the various techniques that can be used for the separation of human leukoyctes and lists the predominant cells that are recovered by each method.

Table 1
SEPARATION OF HUMAN LEUKOCYTES

Technique	Predominant cell recovered	Ref.
Sedimentation	—	14
Simple	All leukocytes	1, 2
Enhanced	—	—
Fibrinogen	All leukocytes	3—5
Dextran	All leukocytes	3, 6—8
Polyvinyl pyrrolidone	All leukocytes	9, 10
Gelatin	All leukocytes	11, 12
"Polybrene"	All leukocytes	13
Centrifugation, simple	All leukocytes	15
Special centrifuges	All leukocytes	16—18
Leukoadhesion	—	—
Cotton — wool	Lymphocytes	19
Glass — wool	Lymphocytes	20
Glass surface	Granulocytes and monocytes	21—24
Phagocytosis	Granulocytes or lymphocytes	25, 26
Differential centrifugation	—	—
Albumin	—	27, 28
Ficoll	—	29, 30
Ficoll—isopaque	Lympohcytes	31

REFERENCES

1. **Bessis, M. C.,** *Ann. N.Y. Acad. Sci.,* 59, 986, 1955.
2. **von Melen, J. and Unger, P.,** *Lancet,* 2, 313, 1967.
3. **Skogg, W. A. and Beck, W. S.,** *Blood,* 11, 436, 1956.
4. **Wells, W. and Wenzler, R. J.,** *Cancer Res.,* 19, 1086, 1959.
5. **Wenzler, R. J., Williams, A. D., and Best, W. R.,** *Cancer Res.,* 17, 108, 1957.
6. **Greenwald, T. J. and Polka, R.,** *Am. J. Clin. Pathol.,* 33, 358, 1960.
7. **Fleisher, G. A.,** *Methods Med. Res.,* 7, 150, 1958.
8. **Martin, S. P. and Green, R.,** *Methods Med. Res.,* 7, 136, 1958.
9. **Robineaux, R. and LeBrun-Pages, J.,** *Sang,* 21, 658, 1950.
10. **Gold, P. and Cole, M.,** *J. Lab. Clin. Med.,* 56, 319, 1960.
11. **Coulson, A. S. and Chalmers, D. G.,** *Lancet,* 1, 468, 1964.
12. **Sanderson, A. R.,** *Nature (London),* 215, 23, 1967.
13. **Lalezari, P.,** *Blood,* 19, 102, 1962.
14. **Tullis, J. L. and Bandanza, P.,** *Methods Med. Res.,* 7, 130, 1958.
15. **Dausset, J., Nenna, A., and Brecy, H.,** *Sang,* 24, 410, 1953.
16. **Perry, V. P., Kerby, C. C., and Gresham, R. B.,** *Ann. N.Y. Acad. Sci.,* 114, 651, 1964.
17. **Freireich, E. J., Judson, G., and Levine, R. H.,** *Cancer Res.,* 25, 1516, 1965.

18. **Buckner, D., Eisel, R., and Perry, S.,** *Blood,* 31, 653, 1968.
19. **Lamvick, J. O.,** *Acta Haematol.,* 35, 294, 1966.
20. **Johnson, T. M. and Garvin, J. E.,** *Proc. Soc. Exp. Biol. Med.,* 102, 333, 159.
21. **Wildy, P. and Ridley, M.,** *Nature (London),* 182, 1801, 1958.
22. **Rabenowitz, Y.,** *Blood,* 23, 811, 1964.
23. **Rabenowitz, Y.,** *Blood,* 26, 100, 1965.
24. **Rabenowitz, Y. and Dietz, A. A.,** *Blood,* 29, 182, 1967.
25. **Carstairs, K.,** *Lancet,* 1, 829, 1962.
26. **Cassen, B., Hitt, J., and Hays, E. F.,** *J. Lab. Clin. Med.,* 52, 778, 1958.
27. **Agranoff, B. W., Vallee, B. L., and Waugh, D. F.,** *Blood,* 9, 504, 1954.
28. **Spriggs, A. I. and Alexander, R. F.,** *Nature (London),* 188, 863, 1960.
29. **Nobel, P. B. and Cutts, J. H.,** *J. Lab. Clin. Med.,* 72, 533, 1968.
30. **Nobel, P. B., Cutts, J. H., and Carroll, K. K.,** *Blood,* 30, 465, 1967.
31. **Thorsky, E.,** *Vox Sang.,* 13, 194, 1967.

MORPHOLOGICAL AND BIOCHEMICAL FEATURES OF WHITE CELL ANOMALIES

William S. Beck

Table 1
MORPHOLOGICAL AND BIOCHEMICAL FEATURES OF WHITE CELL ANOMALIES

Anomalies	Morphology and staining characteristics	Genetics	Biochemical properties	Ref.
Alder-Reilly anomaly	Giant azurophilic granules (Alder-Reilly bodies) in neutrophils; stain dark lilac in Wright-Giemsa and metachromatically in toluidine blue; associated with other anomalies, e.g., Hurler's syndrome, Hunter's syndrome, and Maroteaux-Lamy syndrome; similar granules sometimes found in lymphocytes and monocytes (Gasser cells)	Autosomal recessive trait	Disorder of polysaccharide metabolism; deficiencies of specific catabolic enzymes lead to incomplete degradation of dermatan or heparan sulfates	1—7
Auer bodies (rods)	Rod-shaped cytoplasmic inclusions appearing in blasts of certain patients with acute myelocytic, myelomonocytic, or monocytic leukemia; may vary in size from round single granules to large diamond-shaped rods; surrounded by external limiting membranes; staining characteristics are those of normal azurophilic granules, though electron microscopy shows subtle differences of fine structure between Auer bodies and normal azurophilic granules	Acquired	Bodies contain acid phosphatase, peroxidase, and esterase	8—12
Chediak-Higashi anomaly	Giant lysosome-like granules appear in neutrophils and other leukocytes and in other granule-containing cells throughout the body; disorder associated with partial ocular and cutaneous albinism, leukopenia (perhaps due to increased destruction of granulocytes within the marrow), and increased susceptibility to infection; patients surviving repeated infections may die of hematologic malignancy; granules are abnormal azurophilic granules	Autosomal recessive trait	Granules peroxidase positive in neutrophils; large granules in Schwann cells, renal tubular cells, fibroblasts, and vascular endothelium contain glycolipid	13—23
Döhle bodies	Large, discrete, round or oval intracytoplasmic inclusions of granulocytes that stain pale blue with Romanowsky stains; usually located in the outer rim of the cytoplasm; appear following chemotherapy and in infection, pregnancy, trauma, burns, and other disorders	Acquired	Shown by electron microscopy to be lamellar aggregates of rough endoplasmic reticulum; rich in RNA	24—28

Table 1 (continued)
MORPHOLOGICAL AND BIOCHEMICAL FEATURES OF WHITE CELL ANOMALIES

Anomalies	Morphology and staining characteristics	Genetics	Biochemical properties	Ref.
Familial leukocyte vacuolization (Jordan's anomaly)	Vacuoles, 2—10 per cell (diameter 2—5 μm), appear in cytoplasm of granulocytes, monocytes, and some lymphocytes; should be distinguished from vacuoles occurring in infection and other diseases	Uncertain	Vacuoles contain lipid	29—30
Hereditary giant neutrophils	Large (diameter 17 μm) neutrophils occur rarely in normal individuals; in reported family 16% neutrophils per 100 were large; nuclei had 6—10 lobes with normal-appearing chromatin	Uncertain	Affected cells probably tetraploid; not due to vitamin B_{12} or folate deficiency	31—32
Hereditary nuclear hypersegmentation	Proportion of neutrophils containing 5 or more lobes exceeds 10% in heterozygotes and 14% in homozygotes; not associated with other clinical abnormalities; a similar condition involving eosinophils exists	Autosomal dominant trait	Not due to vitamin B_{12} or folate deficiency	32—35
May-Hegglin anomaly	Granulocytes contain 1—2 large (diameter 2—5 μm) intracytoplasmic pyroninophilic inclusions that resemble Döhle bodies; associated with leukopenia and large, bizarre platelets containing few granules; similar granulocytic inclusions of dense fibrils, diamater 50 Å, are seen in various acquired disorders	Autosomal dominant trait	Like Dohle bodies consist mainly of RNA derived from endoplasmic reticulum	36—46
Pelger-Huët anomaly	Nuclei of mature neutrophils display coarsely clumped chromatin and distinctive shape; heterozygotes have bilobed nuclei; homozygotes have round nuclei containing clumped chromatin; apparently due to failure of normal development of the nuclear lobes; common in the general population, occurring in 1 in 6,000 people; although abnormal morphologically, neutrophils have no functional impairment	Autosomal dominant trait	No biochemical abnormalities recognized	47—55
Pseudo-Pelger-Huët anomaly	Nuclei of neutrophils displaying morphologic changes resembling those in Pelger-Huët anomaly may appear in the course of several myeloproliferative diseases; single reports have associated this anomaly with severe myxedema, influenza, sulfisoxazole therapy, and other disorders	Acquired	No biochemical abnormalities recognized	56—63

Table 1 (continued)
MORPHOLOGICAL AND BIOCHEMICAL FEATURES OF WHITE CELL ANOMALIES

Anomalies	Morphology and staining characteristics	Genetics	Biochemical properties	Ref.
Toxic granulations	Coarse azurophilic granules in cytoplasm of neutrophils that are more darkly stained with Wright-Giemsa than granules of normal cells; seen in a variety of conditions, e.g., infections, burns, and acute inflammatory diseases; occasionally associated with vacuolization, especially in septicemia; in these cases vacuole may represent phagocytic vacuole in which an organism has been digested	Acquired	Increase in leukocyte alkaline phosphatase and acid phosphatase; latter is nongranule associated and hence, increase may be due to release from azuorophilic granules; granules are peroxidase positive	28, 64—68

REFERENCES

1. **Alder, A.**, Über konstitutionell bedingte Granulationsveranderungen der Leukocyten, *Dtsch. Arch. Klin. Med.*, 183, 372, 1939.
2. **Reilly, W. A.**, The granules in the leukocytes in gargoylism, *Am. J. Dis. Child.*, 62, 489, 1941.
3. **Reilly, W. A. and Lindsay, S.**, Gargoylism (lipochondrodystrophy): a review of clinical observations in eighteen cases, *Am. J. Dis. Child.*, 75, 595, 1948.
4. **Fricker-Alder, H.**, Die aldersche Granulationsanomalie, *Schweiz. Med. Wochenschr.*, 88, 989, 1958.
5. **Pearson, H. A. and Lorincz, A. E.**, A characteristic bone marrow finding in the Hurler Syndrome, *Pediatrics*, 34, 281, 1964.
6. **Groover, R. V., Burke, E. C., Gordon, H., and Berdon, W. E.**, The genetic mucopolysaccharidoses, *Semin. Hematol.*, 9, 371, 1972.
7. **Crocker, A. C.**, Histiocytoses and lipidoses, in *Hematology*, 2nd ed., Beck, W. S., Ed., MIT Press, Cambridge, 1977, 473.
8. **Harada, N.**, Histochemical studies on Auer body, *Nagoya J. Med. Sci.*, 14, 129, 1951.
9. **Goldberg, A. F.**, Acid phosphatase activity in Auer bodies, *Blood*, 24, 305, 1964.
10. **Fischer, R. et al.**, Der cytochemisch Nachweis von Naphthol-AS-D-Chloroacetat-Esterase in Auerstabchen, *Klin. Wochenschr*, 44, 1401, 1966.
11. **Freeman, J. A.**, Origin of Auer bodies, *Blood*, 27, 499, 1966.
12. **White, J. G.**, Fine structural demonstration of acid phosphatase activity in Auer bodies, *Blood*, 29, 667, 1967.
13. **Kritzler, R. A., Terner, J. Y., Lindenbaum, J. L., Magidson, J., Williams, R., Preisig, R., and Phillips, G. B.**, Chediak-Higashi syndrome. Cytologic and serum lipid observations in a case and family, *Am. J. Med.*, 36, 583, 1964.
14. **Windhorst, D. B., Zelickson, A. S., and Good, R. A.**, Chediak-Higashi syndrome: hereditary gigantism of cytoplasmic organelles, *Science*, 151, 81, 1966.
15. **Blume, R. S., Bennett, J. M., Yankee, R. A., and Wolff, S. M.**, Defective granulocyte regulation in the Chediak-Higashi syndrome, *N. Engl. J. Med.*, 279, 1009, 1968.
16. **White, J. G.**, The Chediak-Higashi syndrome: a possible lysosomal disease, *Blood*, 28, 143, 1966.
17. **Kanfer, J. N., Blume, R. S., Yankee, R. A., and Wolff, S. M.**, Alteration of sphingolipid metabolism in leukocytes from patients with the Chediak-Higashi syndrome, *N. Engl. J. Med.*, 279, 410, 1968.
18. **Efrati, P. and Danon, D.**, Electron-microscopical study of bone marrow cells in a case of Chediak-Higashi-Steinbrinck syndrome, *Br. J. Haematol.*, 15, 173, 1968.
19. **Douglas, S. D., Blume, R. S., and Wolff, S. M.**, Fine structural studies of leukocytes from patients and heterozygotes with the Chediak-Higashi syndrome, *Blood*, 33, 527, 1969.

20. **Blume, R. S. and Wolff, S. M.**, The Chediak-Higashi syndrome: studies in four patients and a review of the literature, *Medicine*, 51, 247, 1972.
21. **Davis, W. C. and Douglas, S. C.**, Defective granule formation and function in the Chediak-Higashi syndrome in man and animals, *Semin. Hematol.*, 9, 431, 1972.
22. **Kimball, H. R., Ford, G. H., and Wolff, S. M.**, Lysosomal enzymes in normal and Chediak-Higashi blood leukocytes, *J. Lab. Clin. Med.*, 86, 616, 1975.
23. **Oliver, J. M. and Zurier, R. B.**, Correction of characteristic abnormalities of microtubule function and granule morphology in Chediak-Higashi syndrome with cholinergic agonists. Studies in vitro in man and in vivo in the beige mouse, *J. Clin. Invest.*, 57, 1239, 1976.
24. **Döhle, H.**, Leukocyteneinschluse bei Scharlach, *Zentralbl. Bakteriol.*, 61, 63, 1911.
25. **Weiner, W. and Topley, E.**, Döhle bodies in the leukocytes of patients with burns, *J. Clin. Pathol.*, 8, 324, 1955.
26. **Itoga, T. and Laszlo, J.**, Döhle bodies and other granulocytic alterations during chemotherapy and cyclophosphamide, *Blood*, 20, 668, 1962.
27. **Abernathy, M. R.**, Döhle bodies associated with uncomplicated pregnancy, *Blood*, 27, 380, 1966.
28. **McCall, C. E., Katayama, I., Cotran, R. S., and Finland, M.**, Lysosomal and ultrastructural changes in human "toxic" neutrophils during bacterial infection, *J. Exp. Med.*, 129, 267, 1969.
29. **Jordans, G. H.**, The familial occurrence of fat containing vacuoles in the leukocytes, *Acta Med. Scand.*, 145, 419, 1953.
30. **Rozenszajn, L., Klajman, A., Yaffe, D., and Efrati, P.**, Jordans' anomaly in white blood cells, *Blood*, 28, 258, 1966.
31. **Davidson, W. M., Milner, R. D. G., and Lawler, S. D.**, Giant neutrophil leukocytes: an inherited anomaly, *Br. J. Haematol.*, 6, 339, 1960.
32. **Davidson, W. M.**, Inherited variations in leukocytes, *Semin. Hematol.*, 5, 255, 1968.
33. **Undritz, E.**, Les malformations héréditaires des éléments figurés du sang, *Le Sang*, 25, 296, 1954.
34. **Undritz, E.**, Eine neue Sippe mit erblichkonstitutioneller Hochsegmentierung der Neutrophilenkerne, *Schweiz. Med. Wochenschr.*, 88, 1000, 1958.
35. **Lüers, V. T.**, Das numerische Verhalten der geschlechtsspezifischen Kernanhange bei der erblich konstitutioneller Hochsegmentierung der neutrophilenkerne Undritz, *Schweiz. Med. Wochenschr.*, 90, 246, 1960.
36. **May, R.**, Leukocyteneinschlüsse, *Dtsch. Arch. Klin. Med.*, 96, 1, 1909.
37. **Hegglin, V. R.**, Gleichzeitige konstitutionelle Veränderungen an Neutrophilen und Thrombozyten, *Helv. Med. Acta*, 12, 439, 1945.
38. **Scholer, H., Imhof, H., and Schnös, M.**, Beobachtungen an einem weiterem Trager der May-Hegglinschen Anomalie der Leukocyten und Blutplättchen, *Schweiz. Med. Wochenschr.*, 90, 1269, 1960.
39. **Wassmuth, D. R., DeGroote, J. W., Hamilton, H. E., and Sheets, R. F.**, An anomaly of granulocytes and platelets: a newly established hereditary entity, *J. Lab. Clin. Med.*, 58, 969, 1961.
40. **Oski, F. A., Naiman, J. L., Allen, D. M., and Diamond, L. K.**, Leukocytic inclusions—Döhle bodies—associated with platelet abnormality (the May-Hegglin anomaly): report of a family and review of the literature, *Blood*, 20, 657, 1962.
41. **Buchanan, J. G., Pearce, L., and Wetherly-Mein, G.**, The May-Hegglin anomaly. A family report and chromosome study, *Br. J. Haematol.*, 10, 508, 1964.
42. **Jordan, S. W. and Larsen, W. E.**, Ultrastructural studies of the May-Hegglin anomaly, *Blood*, 25, 921, 1965.
43. **Lechner, K., Breddin, K., Moser, K., Stockinger, L., and Wenzel, E.**, May-Hegglinsche anomalie, *Acta Haematol.*, 42, 303, 1969.
44. **Gausis, N., Fortune, D. W., and Whiteside, M. G.**, The May-Hegglin anomaly. A case report and chromosome studies, *Br. J. Haematol.*, 16, 619, 1969.
45. **Jenis, E. H., Takeuchi, A., Dillon, D. E., Ruymann, F. B., and Rivkin, S.**, The May-Hegglin anomaly: ultrastructure of the granulocyte inclusion, *J. Clin. Pathol.*, 55, 187, 1971.
46. **Godwin, H. A. and Ginsburg, A. D.**, May-Hegglin anomaly: a defect in megakaryocyte fragmentation? *Br. J. Haematol.*, 26, 117, 1974.
47. **Pelger, K.**, Demonstratie van een paar zeldzaam voorkomende typen van bloedlichaampjes en bespreking der patienten, *Discuss. Med. Tijdschr. Geneesk.*, 72, 1178, 1928.
48. **Huët, G. J.**, Familial abnormality of leukocytes, *Ned. Tijdschr. Geneesk.*, 75, 5956, 1931.
49. **Huët, G. J.**, Uber eine bisher unbekannte familiare Anomalie der Leukocyten, *Klin. Wochenschr.*, 11, 1264, 1932.
50. **Begemann, N. H. and Campagne, A. van L.**, Homozygous form of Pelger-Huët's nuclear anomaly in man, *Acta Haematol.*, 7, 295, 1952.
51. **Harin, H.**, Beiträge zur Morphologie und Genetik der Pelger-Anomalie bei Mensch und Kaninchen, *Z. Menschl. Vereb.*, 30, 501, 1952.

52. **Klein, A., Hussar, A. E., and Bornstein, S.**, Pelger-Huët anomaly of the leukocytes, *N. Engl. J. Med.*, 253, 1057, 1955.
53. **Undritz, E. and de Sepibus, C.**, Das Resultat der Nachuntersuchung der vor 25 Jahren im Wallis gefundenen ersten schweizer Sippe mit Pelger-Huëtscher Kernanomalieder Blutköperchen und derzeitiger Stand der Erforschung der Anomalie, *Schweiz. Med. Wochenschr.*, 87, 1258, 1957.
54. **Skendzel, L. P. and Hoffman, G. C.**, The Pelger anomaly of leukocytes: forty one cases in seven families, *Am. J. Clin. Pathol.*, 37, 294, 1962.
55. **Schneiderman, L. J., Sampson, N. L., Schoene, W. C., and Haydon, G. B.**, Genetic studies of a family with two unusual autosomal dominant conditions: muscular dystrophy and Pelger-Huët anomaly, *Am. J. Med.*, 46, 380, 1969.
56. **Downey, H., Major, S. G., and Noble, J. F.**, Leukemoid blood pictures of the myeloid type, *Folia Haematol.*, 41, 493, 1930.
57. **Eliot, P. W. and Blackford, F.**, Nuclear alterations for the cells in peripheral blood associated with the virus of influenza A-1 Asian infection and inoculation, *J. Indiana State Med. Assoc.*, 51, 1651, 1958.
58. **Shanbrom, E., Collins, Z. and Miller, S.**, "Acquired Pelger-Huët cells in blood dyscrasias, *Am. J. Med. Sci.*, 240, 732, 1960.
59. **Dorr, A. D. and Moloney, W. C.**, Acquired pseudo-Pelger anomaly of granulocytic leukocytes, *N. Engl. J. Med.*, 261, 742, 1959.
60. **Shanbrom, E. and Tanaka, K. R.**, Acquired Pelger-Huët granulocytes in severe myxedema, *Acta Haematol.*, 27, 289, 1962.
61. **Stobbe, V. H. and Jorke, D.**, Befunde an homozygoten Pelger-Merkmalsträgern, *Schweiz. Med. Wochenschr.*, 95, 1524, 1965.
62. **Kaplan, J. M. and Barrett, O'N., Jr.**, Reversible pseudo-Pelger-Huët anomaly related to sulfisoxazole therapy, *N. Engl. J. Med.*, 277, 421, 1967.
63. **Kay, N. E., Nelson, D. A., and Gottlieb, A. J.**, Eosinophilic Pelger-Huët anomaly with myeloproliferative disorders, *Am. J. Clin. Pathol.*, 60, 663, 1973.
64. **Ponder, E. and Ponder, R.**, The cytology of the polymorphonuclear leukoycte in toxic conditions, *J. Lab. Clin. Med.*, 28, 316, 1942.
65. **Beck, W. S. and Valentine, W. N.**, Biochemical studies on leucocytes. II. Phosphatase activity in chronic lymphatic leucemia, acute leucemia, and miscellaneous hematologic conditions, *J. Lab. Clin. Med.*, 38, 245, 1951.
66. **Gordin, R.**, Toxic granulation in leukocytes, *Acta. Med. Scand. Suppl.*, 270, 1952.
67. **Malinin, T. I., Pekin, T. J., Jr., Bauer, H., and Zvaifler, N. J.**, Vacuoles in synovial fluid leukocytes *Am. J. Clin. Pathol.*, 45, 278, 1966.
68. **Zieve, P. D., Haghshenass, M., Blanks, M., and Krevans, J. R.**, Vacuolization of the neutrophil, *Arch. Intern. Med.*, 118, 356, 1966.

CHEMICAL CHARACTERISTICS OF THE LEUKOCYTES*

Lung T. Yam

Introduction

The human blood is an ideal tissue for chemical study. Blood cells can easily be obtained, homogenized, and analyzed. Since changes in blood may reflect many systemic diseases, the results of such analyses, compared in both healthy and diseased patients, may help to elucidate the biochemical behavior of the blood cells in various diseases. In addition, such studies can be repeated in the same patient, and changes can be sequentially observed. The use of "differential centrifugation" or "subcellular fractionation" techniques further permits observation of the enzymologic and metabolic changes in the subcellular components of blood cells. In this manner, quantitative biochemical studies of the blood cells have unveiled the pathophysiological mechanisms of many diseases. A notable example is the detection of enzyme deficiencies of the red cells in the congenital hemolytic anemias.

There are inherent shortcomings in the quantitative biochemical studies of the human blood cells. The quantitative approach can best be utilized to evaluate the chemical changes in a cell homogenate. In the erythrocytes, this approach may be sufficient, because a relatively homogeneous cell population can easily be obtained for analysis. Leukocytes, on the other hand, are heterogeneous and composed of various cell types: neutrophils, eosinophils, basophils, lymphocytes, and monocytes. Each type of cell has a considerably different chemical composition and metabolic behavior. A relative proportion of these cells may vary with time, in subjects, and in diseases — variables which may influence the results of analysis. This difficulty is further augmented when hemopoietic tissues such as marrow are studied due to the presence of many cells uncommonly seen in the blood, for example, plasma cells, megakaryocytes, macrophages, and mast cells. The chemical composition of many of these cells is still poorly understood. Furthermore, the leukocytes, especially the neutrophils and basophils, are very sensitive to technical manipulation. Analysis of the damaged cells is less than ideal, and the results should be interpreted with considerable reservation.

Many of the shortcomings related to leukocyte heterogeneity can be overcome by using a morphologic approach which permits direct observation of each individual cell. The inherent limitations of this approach are its relative insensitivity and poor quantitative ability. Although the sensitivity of the morphologic studies can be improved by the use of histochemistry, electron microscopy, and electron microscopic histochemistry, the majority of enzyme-catalyzed reactions still cannot be demonstrated histochemically by light or electron microscopy.

Much of our present knowledge concerning the chemical characteristics of the leukocytes is derived from biochemical quantitation. Efforts are needed to bridge the gap between biochemistry and morphology. More precise information can be obtained through the use of combined quantitative biochemical and qualitative morphologic approaches.

The main purpose of this chapter is to describe the cytochemical characteristics of the leukocytes and to show that a combined cytochemical, morphological, and biochemical study can lead to a better understanding of the structural and functional relationships of the leukocytes. First, the morphology of normal leukocytes is described, with emphasis on the close relationship between the subcellular components and the chemical composition of the cell. This is followed by a brief analytical survey

* Supported by the Medical Research Service of the Veterans Administration Fund No. 603-9850.

of the biochemical characteristics of the leukocytes in normal subjects and in patients with various diseases. Detailed morphology, composition, and metabolism of the leukocytes are not treated in great length, since this information is available elsewhere.[1-15] The chemical characteristics of the leukocytes are correlated with their subcellular structures. This discussion is followed by introductory remarks on the cytochemical characteristics of the leukocytes. The basic principles of cytochemistry are briefly discussed. Some of the useful cytochemical techniques which are not adequately discussed elsewhere are presented, and the indications and limitations of the clinical application of these techniques are examined.

Morphologic Characteristics of the Leukocytes

The morphologic charateristics of the leukocytes are listed in Table 1. Some pertinent features of the leukocytes are discussed below.

The Granulocytes[7-11,16]

The earliest granulocyte is the myeloblast. In air-dried smears stained by the Wright-Geimsa method, this cell has a small rim of blue cytoplasm without visible granules and a large nucleus with a fine chromatin network and prominent nucleolus. Ultrastructurally, this cell has no granules, but contains an abundance of free ribosomes and mitochondria. The Golgi system is poorly developed, and profiles of endoplasmic reticulum are either absent or few in number (Figure 1). As the cell matures into the promyelocyte, it becomes larger and its nucleus remains round with a fine nuclear chromatin network, but the nucleolus is less prominent. The Golgi system and the rough endoplasmic reticulum develop, giving rise to primary or azurophilic granules. Free ribosomes and mitochondria are abundant (Figure 2).

With further maturation, the cell becomes smaller, the nuclear cytoplasmic ratio decreases, the nucleus becomes irregular with new coarser chromatin network, and the nucleolus is inconspicuous or absent. Ribosomes and mitochondria diminish, and only a few are seen in mature neutrophils. The cytoplasmic ribonucleic acid (RNA) content is also reduced and in the Wright-Giemsa stained smear, the cytoplasm appears bluish to pink or reddish in color as the cell matures. The Golgi system becomes less conspicuous, and the endoplasmic reticulum decreases as the cell matures. Azurophilic granules are reduced as they cease to be formed, while the formation of specific granules proceeds with cell maturation. The cytoplasmic glycogen granules are visible in the myelocyte and plentiful in the neutophil. The eosinophils differ from the neutrophils in that they have the characteristic specific granules and more mitochondria.[6,17,18] The basophils are also distinct because of their specific basophilic granules. They have more mitochondria and less glycogen than neutrophils (Figure 3).[6,19-21]

The Lymphocytes[22-24]

These include small lymphocytes, atypical or large, active lymphocytes, and lymphoblasts. In air-dried smears stained with the Wright-Giemsa method, the small lymphocyte has a narrow rim of blue cytoplasm with a few ribosomes, mitochondria and lysosomes and a relatively large nucleus with clumped chromatin network. A small nucleolus may be visible. The Golgi system of the small lymphocytes is poorly developed, as is the endoplasmic reticulum. No specific granules are seen (Figure 4). In the activated lymphocyte, including the large or atypical lymphocyte and the lymphoblast, the cell is larger and has a round and relatively large nucleus which often contains a nucleolus. This cell is active metabolically, containing many free ribosomes, mitochondria, and endoplasmic reticulum. The Golgi system is also conspicuous and well-developed.

Table 1
MORPHOLOGIC CHARACTERISTICS OF THE LEUKOCYTES

Cell type	Nucleus	Chromati network	Nucleolus	Golgi system	Free ribosomes	Endoplasmi creticulum	Mitochondria	Glycogen	Azurophilic granules	Specific granules	Lysosome	Cytoplasmic vesicles
Myeloblast	Large, round	Fine	Large, prominent	Poorly developed	+ + + +[a]	+[a]	+ + + +	−[a]	−	−	—	−
Promyelocyte	Large, round	Fine	Small	Well-developed	+ + + +	+ + + +	+ + +[a]	−	+ + + +	−	—	−
Myelocytes	Small, often indented	Coarse	Inconspicuous or absent	Well-developed	+ + + +	+ + +	+ +	±[a]	+ + +	+	—	−
Metamyelocytes	Small, indented	Coarse	Absent	Small	+ +	+ +	+ +	+	+ +	+ +	—	−
Juvenile granulocytes	Small	Coarse	Absent	Small	+	+	+	+ + +	+	+ + +	—	−
Mature granulocytes	Small, lobulated	Coarse	Absent	Small	±	±	+	+ + + +	+	+ + +	—	−
Lymphoblast	Large, round	Fine	Large, prominent	Moderately developed	+ + +	+ + +	+ + +	±	±	−	±	±
Prolymphocyte	Round	Fine	Small, prominent	Small	+ + +	+	+ +	±	±	−	+	−
Lymphocyte	Round	Coarse	Often present, small	Small	+	+	+	±	±	−	+	−
Plasma cell	Round, eccentric	Coarse	Often present	Well-developed	±	+ + + +	+ +	±	±	−	—	±
Promonocyte	Oval	Fine	Prominent	Well-developed	+ + +	+	+ +	±	—	−	+ +	+
Monocyte	Kidney-shaped	Coarse	May be present	Well-developed	+	+	+ + +	±	—	−	+ + +	+
Macrophages	Oval or multiple	Coarse	Often present	Well-developed	+	+	+ + +	±	—	−	+ + +	+
Mast cell	—	—	—	—	—	—	—	—	−	+ + + +	—	−

[a] + + + + = Plentiful; + + + = many; + + = moderate; + = few; ± = scarce or sporadic; − = absent.

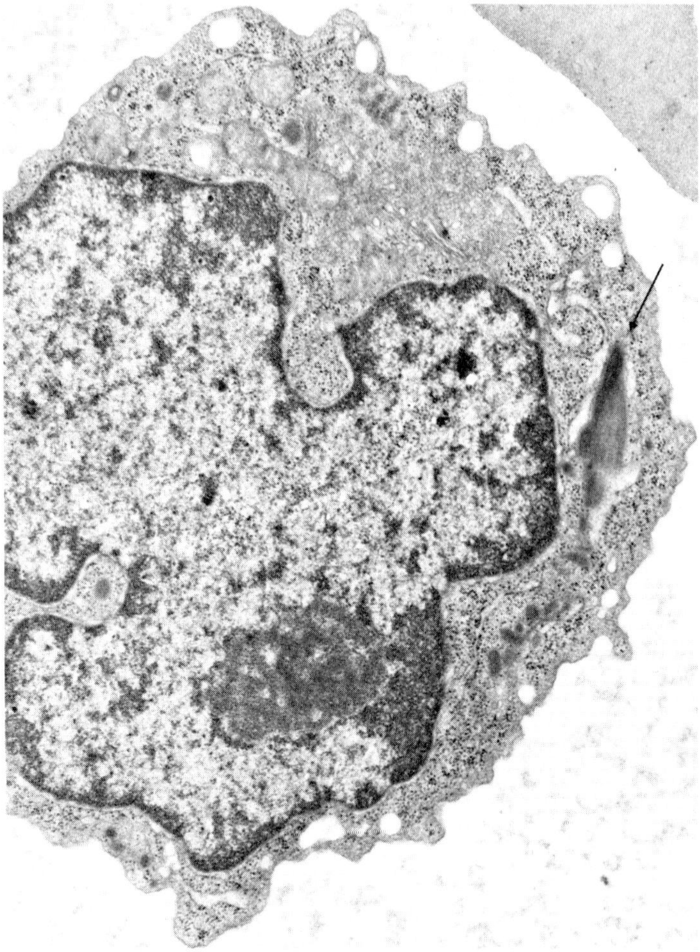

FIGURE 1. A myeloblast from a patient with acute granulocytic leukemia (AGL) showing the typical ultrastructural features and the presence of an Auer Rod (arrow). (Magnification × 14,000.) (Courtesy of Dr. M. Tavassoli.)

The Plasma Cells[2,25]

In air-dried smears stained by the Wright-Giemsa method, the plasma cell has an eccentric, round nucleus and abundant deep blue or purplish cytoplasm with a lightly stained perinuclear halo. Ultrastructurally, this cell has a highly developed Golgi system and abundant lamellar endoplasmic reticulum, suggesting that it is well equipped for protein synthesis.

The Monocytes and Macrophages[26-29]

Blood and marrow monocytes and tissue macrophages were considered to be different in origin. There is now ample evidence to indicate that they are of the same lineage, but have different degrees of maturation and differentiation.[30-33] The most primitive cell in the monocytic series is the marrow monoblast whose morphologic characteristics are similar to the myeloblast. In normal marrow, this cell has not been clearly identified, but its neoplastic equivalent is seen in acute monocytic leukemia, and it is characterized by having an abundance of lysosomal enzymes, including the nonspecific esterase in its cytoplasm.[27,34]

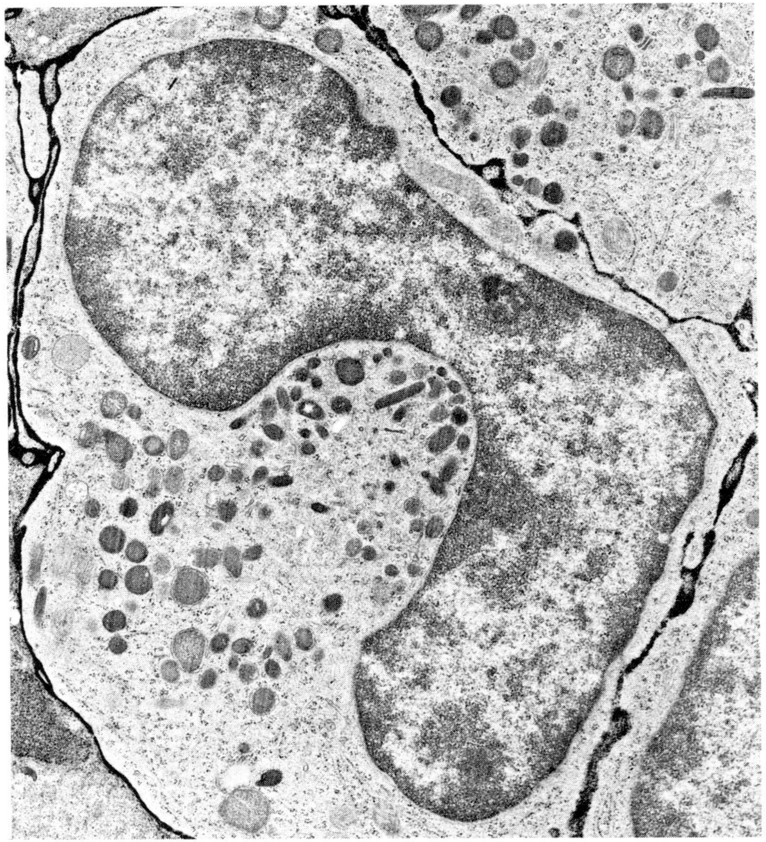

FIGURE 2. Neutrophilic metamyelocyte showing large, lucent, azurophilic granules at the periphery of the cell and small, electron-dense specific granules near the nucleus. The cell border was delineated by impregnation with colloidal lanthanum. (Magnification × 14,000.) (Courtesy of Dr. M. Tavassoli.)

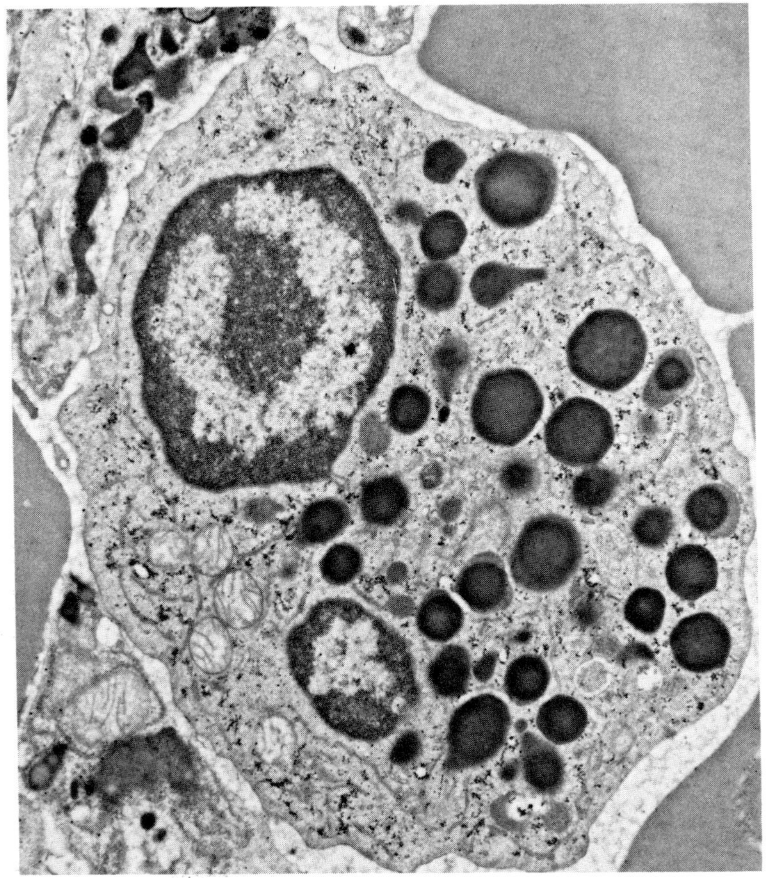

FIGURE 3. Mature basophil showing the presence of segmented nucleus and many specific granules and mitochondria. (Magnification × 14,000.) (Courtesy of Dr. M. Tavassoli.)

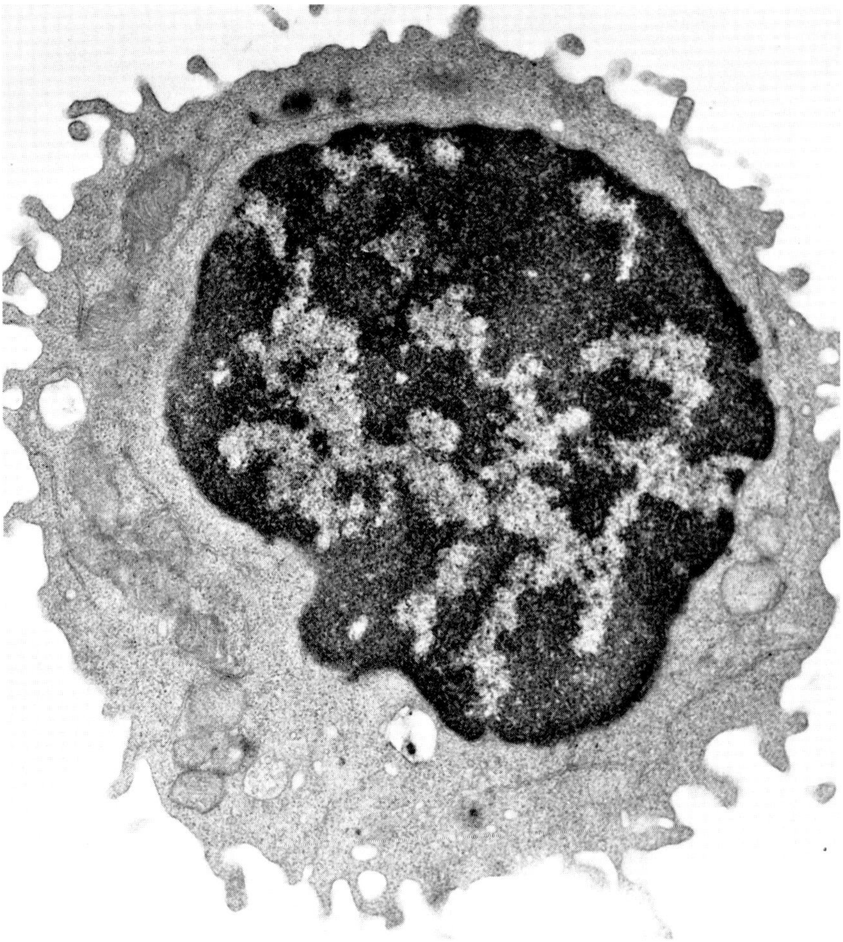

FIGURE 4. Lymphocyte. (Magnification × 14,000.) (Courtesy of Dr. M. Tavassoli.)

The promonocyte is relatively large with an indented nucleus and abundant cytoplasm. The chromatin structure is fine and frequently contains a conspicuous nucleolus. Its cytoplasm has an abundance of free ribosomes, primary and secondary lysosomes, many mitochondria, few profiles of endoplasmic reticulum, and a conspicuous Golgi system.

Maturation causes the nucleus to become more irregular with a coarser chromatin network. The monocyte has many mitochondria, a well-developed Golgi system, and many azurophilic granules or primary lysosomes and phagosomes. This cell also has a few free ribosomes and endoplasmic reticulum.

As the monocyte transforms into the tissue histiocyte or macrophage, the cell becomes larger with abundant cytoplasm and a relatively small nucleus (Figure 5). The chromatin network is usually very dense and the nucleolus is usually not seen. The Golgi system is well developed, and mitochondria and primary and secondary lysosomes are plentiful. There are a few free ribosomes and profiles of endoplasmic reticulum. Thus, as the monocyte matures, it loses its potential for deoxyribonucleic acid (DNA) synthesis, but maintains a limited degree of protein synthesis. Its phagocytic capacity is increased with maturation as evidenced by the numerous primary and secondary lysosomes in the macrophages. The abundance of mitochondria in the macro-

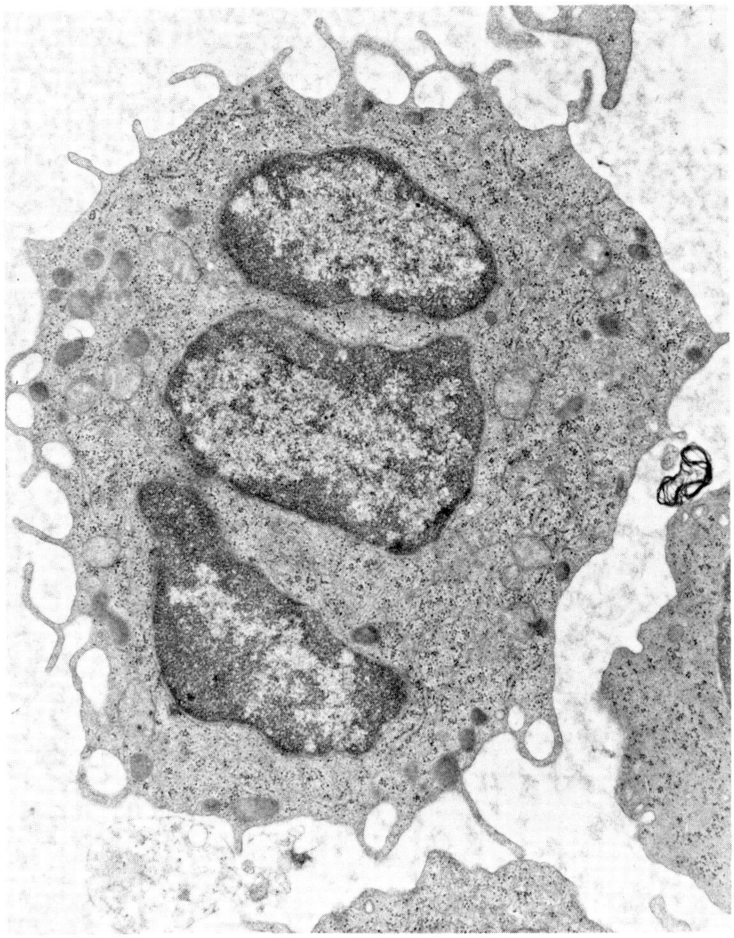

FIGURE 5. Monocyte showing many lysosomes and mitochondria. (Magnification × 14,000.) (Courtesy of Dr. M. Tavassoli.)

phages indicates that these cells are capable of providing adequate energy to support their highly specialized function.

The Mast Cells[1,2,20]

In air-dried smears stained with the Wright-Giemsa stain, the mast cell is round and has a relatively large, round, centrally located nucleus. Its cytoplasm has many coarse, purplish granules. Unlike the basophils, these cytoplasmic granules do not overlap or obscure the contour of the nucleus of the mast cells. Ultrastructurally, the mast cell has an oval nucleus with central euchromatin and peripheral heterochromatin. A nucleolus or several small ones may be present. The Golgi system is small, and mitochondria, free ribosomes, and endoplasmic reticulum are not abundant. Numerous specific granules are present in the cytoplasm. These granules vary greatly in size, shape, and content, probably reflecting the activity of the mast cell. The mast cell can be differentiated from the basophil by its round nucleus, fewer mitochondria, and more specific granules which vary greatly in morphology.[20] The origin of the mast cell is unclear. It has been proposed that this cell may be derived from the lymphocytes or the mesenchymal cells.

Biochemical Characteristics of the Leukocytes

The biochemical characteristics of the leukocytes are listed in Tables 2 to 5. The characteristics of each individual cell type are briefly discussed as follows.

The Neutrophilic Granulocytes[9,16,113,258]

The DNA content of normal mature or immature granulocytes is 0.7×10^{-12} g of DNA phosphorus per cell.[259] In acute leukemia, hyperdiploid leukemic cells have more DNA, but hypodiploid cells have less than the normal granulocytes.[259-262] The RNA content of the granulocytes varies with the type of cell and the degree of maturity of the cell.[196,263] In general, the RNA content of the cell diminishes with maturation. The neutrophilic granulocytes have been demonstrated to have many enzymes involved in nucleic acid metabolism (Table 4). Abnormalities of the nucleic acids and their related enzymes have been found in chronic granulocytic leukemia.[157,173,175,203,264] The granulocytes have a complete enzymatic machinery for pyrimidine metabolism.[560-562] They cannot carry out the early steps in purine biosynthesis, but they can metabolize purine intermediates from exogenous sources.[265-266]

Amino Acids and Proteins

The amino acid composition of neutrophils is similar to that of other tissues.[197-199,267] An exception is arginine, which is present in neutrophils in very small amounts, probably due to the presence of arginase in the leukocytes.[180,181] Immature neutrophils generally have a greater ability to incorporate amino acids than the mature granulocytes.[268,269] In several inborn errors of amino acid metabolism, examination of the leukocytes may be of diagnostic importance (Table 6).

Carbohydrates

Mature neutrophils have few mitochondria, but they can generate energy through glycolysis, the hexose monophosphate shunt, and, to some extent, the Krebs cycle. Many enzymes involving these metabolic pathways have been demonstrated in the neutrophils (Table 3). These cells use glucose, galactose, fructose, and glycogen as energy sources.[212,324,325] The neutrophils are rich in glycogen,[136,210] which is increased in infections and polycythemia vera,[136,326] but decreased in chronic granulocytic leukemia, and abnormally distributed in untreated cases of diabetes mellitus.[136,327,328] In several glycogen storage diseases, the activity of the affected enzymes may be decreased in the leukocytes with increased leukocyte glycogen.[252-257,329] Examination of the leukocytes may help to establish the diagnosis of several diseases with disturbance of carbohydrate metabolism (Table 6).

Lipids

Chemical analysis of neutrophil lipids indicates 30% neutral fat, 35% phospholipids, and 10% cholesterol.[216,330] Neutrophils are capable of lengthening fatty acid chains or degrading intracellular lipids, but are incapable of synthesizing fatty acids *de novo* due to the absence of acetyl CoA carboxylase.[331-333] Deficiency of enzymes related to lipid metabolism will cause systemic diseases (Table 6).

Enzymes in Granules

The neutrophils contain both azurophilic and specific granules (Table 2). These granules are very similar to the lysosomes in other types of cells, both in function and enzyme content. Many lysosomal storage diseases[252] with deficiency of activity of a specific lysosomal acid hydrolase in the leukocyte have been discovered (Table 6). In diseases such as Chediak-Higashi syndrome, activity of most of the hydrolytic enzymes may not be significantly altered, yet the distribution of these enzymes is abnormal.[334]

Table 2
HYDROLYTIC ENZYMES IN THE LEUKOCYTES

Enzymes	Neutrophils	Eosinophils	Basophils	Monocytes histiocytes	Lymphocytes	Plasma cells	Mast cells	Ref.
Ribonuclease	+[a]	+	—	+	—	—	—	35—39
Deoxyribonuclease	+	—	—	—	—	—	—	7, 36, 39, 40
Nucleotidase	+	—	—	—	±[a]	—	—	9, 41—45
Acid phosphatase	+	+	---	+	+	+	+	44, 46—50
Proteases	+	—	—	—	—	—	—	51—54
Peptidases	+	—	—	—	—	—	—	55, 56
Elastase	+	—	—	—	—	—	—	57—60
Chymotrypsin-like enzymes	+	—	---	—	—	—	+	61—64
Collagenase	+	—	—	—	—	—	+	65
"Chloroacetate esterase"	+	----	---	-	-	-	+	66—72
Cathepsins	+	—	—	+	—	—	—	36, 73—79
Naphthylamidase	+	+	±	+	±	—	+	44, 75, 80—83
Kinase	+	+	—	—	—	—	—	84, 85
Prolidase	+	—	—	—	—	—	—	75, 86
Lipase	+	—	—	+	—	—	—	67, 87, 88
Lecithinase A	+	—	—	—	—	—	—	88
Lysolecithinase	+	—	—	—	—	—	—	88
"Non-specific esterase"	-	---	---	+	±	±	±	44, 67, 69, 72, 89—92
Glucosidases	+	—	—	—	—	—	—	93, 94
Amylase	+	—	—	—	—	—	—	93, 95
Galactosidases	+	—	—	+	—	—	—	3, 93, 94, 96—98
Glucuronidase	+	+	---	+	+	+	+	7, 50, 93, 99
N-acetyl glucosaminidase	+	+	—	+	+	+	—	100—102

Table 2 (continued)
HYDROLYTIC ENZYMES IN THE LEUKOCYTES

Enzymes	Neutrophils	Eosinophils	Basophils	Monocytes histiocytes	Lymphocytes	Plasma cells	Mast cells	Ref.
Dextranase	+	—	—	—	—	—	—	93
Mannosidase	+	—	—	—	—	—	—	93, 103, 104
Fucosidase	+	—	—	—	—	—	—	105, 106
Lysozyme	+	---	—	+	−	—	—	112—116
Hyaluronidase	+	—	—	+	—	—	—	107
Adenosine triphosphatase	+	+	—	+	+	+	—	41—43, 108—111
Myeloperoxidase	+	+	±	+	−	−	−	72, 117—123
Catalase	+	+	—	—	—	—	—	125, 313
Arylsulfatases	+	+	+	+	+	+	—	9, 126—132
Thiamine pyrophosphatase	±	±	—	+	−	+	—	133
Alkaline phosphatase	+	−	---	−	−	−	+	44, 124, 134—136

[a] + = Positive or presence of enzyme; − = negative or absence of enzymes; ± = weak, sporadic or questionable presence of enzymes.

Table 3
DEHYDROGENASES AND RELATED GLYCOLYTIC ENZYMES IN THE LEUKOCYTES

	Neutrophils	Eosinophils	Basophils	Monocytes histiocytes	Lymphocytes	Plasma cells	Mast cells	Ref.
Hexokinase	+[a]	+	—	—	+	+	—	111
Phosphaglucomutase	—	+	—	—	—	+	—	111
Hexose phosphate isomerase	+	+	—	—	+	+	—	111
Fructose-6-phosphate kinase	+	+	—	—	+	+	—	111
Diphosphofructose aldolase	+	+	—	—	+	+	—	111
Triphosphate isomerase	+	+	—	—	+	+	—	111
Glycerine-1-phosphate dehydrogenase	+	+	+	+	+	0	—	44, 111, 137, 138
Glycerinaldehyde 3-phosphate dehydrogenase	+	+	—	—	+	+	—	44, 111, 138, 139
3-phosphoglycerate-1 kinase	+	+	—	—	+	+	—	111
Phosphoglyceromutase	+	+	—	—	+	+	—	111
Enolase	+	+	—	—	+	+	—	111
Pyruvate kinase	+	+	—	—	+	+	—	111
Lactate dehydrogenase	+	+	+	+	+	+	—	44, 111, 122, 140
Glucose 6-phosphate dehydrogenase	+	+	+	0—+	0—+	+	—	111, 122, 139, 140
6-phosphogluconate dehydrogenase	+	+	+	+	+	+	—	44, 111

Table 3 (continued)
DEHYDROGENASES AND RELATED GLYCOLYTIC ENZYMES IN THE LEUKOCYTES

	Neutrophils	Eosinophils	Basophils	Monocytes histiocytes	Lymphocytes	Plasma cells	Mast cells	Ref.
Glutathione reductase	+	+	—	—	+	+	—	111, 141
Aconitase	+	—	—	+	+	—	—	111, 142, 143
Isocitrate dehydrogenase	+	+	+	+	+	+	—	44, 108, 111
Succinate dehydrogenase	0— +	+	+	+	0— +	+	—	21, 44, 108, 111, 122, 137, 138
Fumerase	+	—	—	+	–	—	—	144
Malate dehydrogenase	+	+	+	+	+	+	—	21, 44, 108, 111, 145
Glutamate dehydrogenase	+	+	+	+	0— +	+	—	21, 44, 108, 111
Choline dehydrogenase	+	+	+	+	+	+	—	21, 111, 149, 150
Alcohol dehydrogenase	+	+	—	+	+	—	—	146
β-Hydroxybutyric acid	+	+	—	0— +	0— +	—	—	44, 108, 140, 146
Dihydrofolate reductase	+	+	+	+	+	—	—	147, 148
Dihydroorotic dehydrogenase	+	+	+	+	+	+	—	151
NAD cytochrome c diaphorase	+	+	+	+	+	—	—	21, 44, 138, 146, 153
NADP cytochrome c diaphorase	+	+	+	+	+	—	—	21, 44, 138, 46, 152

[a] + = Positive or presence of enzyme.

Table 4
MISCELLANEOUS ENZYMES IN THE LEUKOCYTES

Enzymes	Leukocytes	Neutrophils	Eosinophils	Basophils	Monocytes histiocytes	Lymphocytes	Plasma cells	Mast cells	Ref.
DNA polymerase	—	—	—	—	—	+[a]	—	—	139, 154—157
Reverse transcriptase	+	—	—	—	—	—	—	—	158—160
Nucleotidase	—	—	—	—	—	+	—	—	45, 161, 162
Terminal deoxynucleotidyl transferase	+	+ (Myeloblasts)	—	—	—	—	—	—	163—166
Adenylate kinase	—	+	+	—	—	+	+	—	111
Adenosine deaminase	—	+	—	—	—	+	—	—	167, 168
Xanthine oxidase	—	—	—	—	—	—	—	—	169
Uricase	—	—	—	—	—	—	—	—	169
Guanyl cyclase	+	—	—	—	—	0	—	—	170
Thymidine kinase	+	—	—	—	—	—	—	—	171—173
Thymine 7 hydroxylase	+	—	—	—	—	—	—	—	174
Thymidylate synthetase	+	—	—	—	—	—	—	—	175
Deoxycytidylate deaminase	+	—	—	—	—	—	—	—	175—177
Pyrimidine deoxyribosyl transferase	+	+	—	—	—	+	—	—	203—204
Deoxynucleoside phosphorylase	+	—	—	—	—	+	—	—	205
Ribonucleotide reductase	+	+	—	—	—	+	—	—	206, 207
Glyoxalase	+	+	+	+	+	+	—	—	178
Neuramidase	+	—	—	—	—	—	—	—	179
Arginase	+	—	—	—	—	—	—	—	180, 181, 292

Table 4 (continued)
MISCELLANEOUS ENZYMES IN THE LEUKOCYTES

Enzymes	Leukocytes	Neutrophils	Eosinophils	Basophils	Monocytes histiocytes	Lymphocytes	Plasma cells	Mast cells	Ref.
Histidine decarboxylase	—	—	—	+	—	—	—	+	182, 183
GOT[b]	—	+	—	—	—	+	+	—	111
GPT[c]	—	+	—	—	—	+	+	—	111
Superoxidase dimutase	—	+	—	—	—	—	—	—	184
Cytochrome oxidase	—	—	+	—	+	+	+	+	124, 185, 186
Monoamino oxidase	—	—	—	—	0	0	—	—	187
d-Amino oxidase	—	+	—	—	—	—	—	—	188
DOPA oxidase	—	—	+	+	—	—	—	—	186
Amylo-1,4,→1,6,trans-glucosidase	+	+	—	—	—	—	—	—	189
Phosphorylase	—	+	+	+	+	+	—	—	44, 190, 191, 192
Plasminogen	+	—	+	—	—	—	—	—	193, 194

[a] + = Positive or presence of enzyme.
[b] GOT = Glutamic oxaloacetic transaminase.
[c] GPT = Glutamic pyruvic transaminase.

Table 5
NONENZYMATIC CHEMICAL SUBSTANCES IN THE LEUKOCYTES

	"Leukocyte"	Neutrophils	Eosinophils	Basophils	Monocytes histiocytes	Lymphocytes	Plasma cells	Mast cells	Ref.
Ribonucleic acid	+[a]	+	+	+	+	+	+	+	195—196, 621
Deoxyribonucleic acid	+	+	+	+	+	+	+	+	195, 217
Free amino acids	+	—	—	—	—	—	—	—	197, 198, 199
Branched chain amino acids	+	—	—	—	—	—	—	—	200
Cationic protein	+	+	+	—	—	—	—	—	201
Cystine	+	—	—	—	—	—	—	—	202, 296, 297
Glycogen	+	+	+	+	+	+	0—+	—	124, 136, 208—211
Galactose-1-Phosphate	+[b]	—	—	—	—	—	—	—	212
Lipids	+	+	+	—	—	+	—[c]	—	124, 213—218
Lactoglyceramide	+[b]	—	—	—	—	—	—	—	219
Acid mucopolysaccharide	+	+	+	+	—	+[b]	—	+	220, 341
Histamine	—	+	+	+	—	—	—	+	221—226, 234
5-Hydroxytryptamine	—	—	—	—	—	—	—	+	227
Hyaluronic acid	—	—	—	—	—	—	—	+	228
Heparin	—	—	—	+	—	—	—	+	62, 223, 229, 230, 360
Sodium, potassium	+	+	+	—	—	+	—	—	231
Zinc, calcium, magnesium	—	+	+	+	—	+	—	+	231—236
Iron, copper	—	+	+	—	+	+	—	—	231, 344—347
Urate and pyrophosphate	—	+[b]	—	—	—	—	—	—	237

Table 5 (continued)
NONENZYMATIC CHEMICAL SUBSTANCES IN THE LEUKOCYTES

	"Leukocyte"	Neutrophils	Eosinophils	Basophils	Monocytes histiocytes	Lymphocytes	Plasma cells	Mast cells	Ref.
Heme	+	—	—	—	—	—	—	—	238
Sulfydryl group	+	+	+	+	+	+	—	—	239, 383, 392, 622
Cyclic adenosine monophosphate	+	—	—	—	—	—	—	—	240
Vitamin B_1	+	—	—	—	—	—	—	—	251
Vitamin B_2	+	—	—	—	—	—	—	—	241, 242
Vitamin B_6	+	—	—	—	—	—	—		243—246
Vitamin B_{12}	+	—	—	—	—	—	—	—	247
Vitamin C	+	—	—	—	—	—	—	—	248, 249
Folate	+	—	—	—	—	—	—	—	336, 337
Nicotinamide di-phosphonucleotide	+	—	—	—	—	—	—	—	250
Nicotinamide tri-phosphonucleotide	+	—	—	—	—	—	—	—	250

[a] + = Positive or presence of enzyme.
[b] In diseased states.
[c] − = Negative or absence of enzymes.

Table 6
DISEASES DIAGNOSED BY LEUKOCYTE ASSAYS

Disease	Enzyme or metabolite	Tissue examined	Ref.
	Nucleic acid metabolism		
Hereditary orotic aciduria	Orotidylic decarboxylase	Leukocyte	282
Gout (primary)	—	—	283
Lesch-Nyham Syndrome	Hypoxanthine guanine phosphoribosyl transferase	Lymphocyte	284
	Amino acid metabolism		
Maple syrup urine disease	Keto acid decarboxylase deficiency	Leukocyte	285
Isovaleric acidemia	Isovaleryl CoA dehydrogenase	Leukocyte	286
Hypervalinemia	Valine transaminase	Leukocyte	287
3-hydroxy-3-methyl glutaric aciduria	3-hydroxy-3-methyl glutaryl CoA lyase	Leukocyte	288
5-Oxprolinuria	Glutathione synthetase	Leukocyte	289
Homocystinuria	N-5,10, methylene tetrafolate reductase	Leukocyte	290
Glutaric aciduria	Glutaryl CoA dehydrogenase	Leukocyte	288, 291
Argininosuccinic aciduria	Argininosuccinase	Leukocyte	292
Methyl malonic aciduria	Methylmalonyl CoA racemase and isomerase	—	293
Ketotic hyperglycinemia	Propionyl CoA carboxylase	Leukocyte	294, 295
Cystinosis	Cystine	Leukocyte	202, 296, 297
	Carbohydrate metabolism		
Glycogen storage disease, II	α-Glucosidase	Leukocyte	252—254
Glycogen storage disease, III	Amylo-1-6-glucosidase	Leukocyte	252, 253
Glycogen storage disease, IV	Branching enzyme	Leukocyte	255
Glycogen storage disease, VI	Phosphorylase	Leukocyte	252—257, 259
Galactosemia	Galactose-1-P uridyl transferase	Leukocyte	270, 271
Fructose, 1,6, diphosphatase deficiency	Fructose 1-6 diphosphatase	Leukocyte	272—274
Glucose 6 phosphate dehydrogenase deficiency	Glucose 6 phosphate dehydrogenase	Leukocyte	275

Table 6 (continued)
DISEASES DIAGNOSED BY LEUKOCYTE ASSAYS

Disease	Enzyme or metabolite	Tissue examined	Ref.
	Carbohydrate Metabolism (continued)		
Triose phosphate isomerase deficiency	Triose phosphate isomerase	Leukocyte	276
Phosphohexose isomerase deficiency	Phosphohexose isomerase	Leukocyte	277
Phosphoglycerate kinase deficiency	Phosphoglycerate kinase	Leukocyte	278
Mannosidosis	α-Mannosidase	Leukocyte	104, 279, 280
Fucosidosis	Fucoidase	Leukocyte	105, 106, 281
	Lipids and Mucopolysaccharide Metabolism		
Gaucher's	β-Glucocerebrosidase	Leukocyte	298—300
Gaucher's	Lactosyl ceramide	Leukocyte	219
Niemann-Pick's	Sphinogmyelinase	Leukocyte	298—301
Wolman's	Acid esterase	Leukocyte	91
Cholesterol ester storage disease	Acid lipase	Leukocyte	87
Krabbe's	β-Galactocerebrosidase	Leukocyte	98, 300
Metachromatic leukodystrophy	Arylsulfatase A (sulfatidase)	Leukocyte	127, 128, 298, 302, 303
Mucopolysaccharidosis VI	Arylsulfatase B	Leukocyte	130
Mucopolysaccharidosis III A	Sulfamidase	Leukocyte	304
Tay-Sachs	N-acetyl hexasaminidase A	Leukocyte	305—308
Hurler-Hunter syndrome	α-L-Iduronidase	Leukocyte	309
Fabry's	α-Galactosidase	Leukocyte	96, 298
Familial Hypercholesterolemia	3-hydroxy 3 methylglutaryl CoA reductase	Leukocyte	310

Miscellaneous

Acid phosphatase deficiency	Acid phosphatase	Leukocyte	311
Hypophosphatasia	Alkaline phosphatase	Leukocyte	320, 321
Myeloperoxidase deficiency	Myeloperoxidase	Leukocyte	312
Primary agammaglobulinemia	5-Nucleotidase	Lymphocyte	162
Prolidase deficiency	Prolidase	Leukocyte	86
Acatalasia	Catalase	Leukocyte	125, 313
Chronic granulomatous disease	NAD oxidase	Leukocyte	314
	Glutathione peroxidase	Leukocyte	315, 316
	NADPH oxidase	Leukocyte	317
Leukemic reticuloendotheliosis	Tartrate resistant acid phosphatase	Hairy cells	318, 319
Cystic fibrosis of pancreas	Metachromasia	Leukocyte	323
Kuf's disease	Peroxidase	Leukocyte	322

Correction of impaired release of lysosomal enzymes such as β-glucuronidase has resulted in the enhancement of bactericidal capacity of the leukocytes in this disease.[335]

Vitamins and Coenzymes

Leukocyte folate content reflects the body folate storage (Table 5). Normal leukocytes contain 40 to 180 mμg of free and conjugated folate per milliliter of packed leukocytes.[336,337] This is decreased in megaloblastic disorders. Many folate-dependent enzymes and enzymes related to folate metabolism are present in the leukocytes.[147,148,338]

Normal leukocytes contain 400 pg of vitamin B12 per 10^8 leukocytes.[247] Proteins capable of binding vitamin B12 are present in mature neutrophils and, to a lesser extent, in immature granulocytes.[339]

Leukocytes also contain vitamin B1,[251] B2,[241,242] B6,[243-246] and vitamin C.[248,249] The intracellular concentration of these vitamins accurately reflects the body storage of some of these vitamins.[340] Nicotinamide adenine dinucleotide and nicotinamide adenine dinucleotide phosphate are also present in the leukocytes.[177]

Miscellaneous

The leukocytes contain histamine (Tables 4 and 5). Much of the histamine is found in basophils, but a considerable amount is also present in neutrophils.[222] In addition, neutrophils contain mucopolysaccharide, which does not show metachromasia readily.[220,341] The prominent granules in the neutrophils (Reilly bodies) in Alder-Reilly anomaly are due to accumulation of mucopolysaccharide in the cytoplasm of the netrophils.[342] These granules are different from the toxic granules of infection in that they have normal alkaline phosphatase activity.[343] Neutrophils also contain metals such as zinc, iron, copper, magnesium, and cobalt.[231,232,235,344-347,563] Disturbance of leukocyte zinc content has been observed in many hematologic diseases.[232,233,563] Iron is increased in neutrophils with heavy toxic granulation.[345]

The Eosinophils[18,348,349]

The eosinophil is an uncommon blood leukocyte. Quantitative chemical analysis of normal eosinophils is difficult due to the problem of obtaining a pure preparation of eosinophils in sufficient number. Most information concerning the chemical characteristics of eosinophils was obtained through experimental eosinophilia in animals or in patients with eosinophilia of diverse etiologies.[350-354] From these biochemical studies and the known morphologic characteristics of the eosinophils, it is generally assumed that the chemistry of the eosinophil is similar to that of the neutrophil. The eosinophil, however, has a well-developed Golgi system and many mitochondria; its capacity for protein synthesis is greater, and its ability to generate energy through the mitochondrial enzyme system is better than that of the neutrophil. It has been demonstrated[111] that activity of many of the mitochondrial enzymes in the eosinophil is much stronger than that in the neutrophil (Table 3). The eosinophil has a high content of arginine-rich basic proteins which enable the cell to attract more eosin than the neutrophil.[355] Its specific eosinophilic granules contain many enzymes and organic and inorganic substances (Tables 2-5). The eosinophil has a cyanide-resistant peroxidase in its specific granules which is different from the myeloperoxidase of the neutrophil and monocyte.[72,118,356] It has no activity of alkaline phosphatase[134] or chloroacetate esterase.[68,70,72]

The Basophils[21,357-359]

The basophil is a rare cell in the normal blood. Biochemical analysis of the basophil is incomplete; most information regarding the chemistry of this cell is derived from morphological and cytochemical studies (Tables 2-5). The basophil contains many water-soluble basophilic granules. It is rich in heparin,[224,360] histamine,[221,222,224-226] and mucopolysaccharides.[220,341] It also has histidine decarboxylase.[182] It does not contain periodic acid Schiff reaction (PAS) positive material in the granules, but it has a large number of cytoplasmic glycogen granules.[209,211] The basophil does not have alkaline phosphatase activity. It has many mitochondria and strong activity of many mitochondrial enzymes (Table 3). Increased serum histamine in patients with polycythemia vera and CGL with basophilia is believed to be responsible for itching and skin changes in these diseases. Symptoms attributed to hyperhistaminemia have been reported in patients wih basophilic leukemia.[361] Improved methods for purification of the normal basophils are now available.[224,362]

The Lymphocytes

The lymphocytes can be classified into small lymphocytes and large or activated lymphocytes according to their chemical characteristics (Tables 2 to 5).

The Small Lymphocytes

This cell is metabolically inactive. Chemical analysis of this cell tends to confirm this impression.

Nucleic acid — The lymphocyte has 8.0×10^{-12} g of DNA and 2.5×10^{-12} g of RNA per cell.[195,196,261] It synthesizes both DNA AND RNA, but the rate of DNA synthesis is very slow.[363-365] The mode of pyrimidine and purine synthesis is very simiar to that of neutrophil. Activity of terminal deoxynucleotidyl transferase is high in the thymus-derived (T) lymphocytes but low in the bone marrow-derived (B) lymphocytes and other types of granulocytes.[163-165] Elevated enzyme activity in the leukocytes has been demonstrated in acute lymphoblastic leukemia.[163-165] This enzyme is considered a marker for the T lymphocytes, although the blasts of acute granulocytic leukemia (AGL) and chronic granulocytic leukemia (CGL) in blastic crisis also have high enzyme activity.[166]

Amino acid and protein synthesis — Amino acid and protein synthesis in the lymphocyte is negligible. The ability of the cell to incorporate cystine and phenylalanine and the presence of glutamic acid dehydrogenase in the cell have been demonstrated.[44,366-367]

Carbohydrates — The small lymphocyte is capable of utilizing carbohydrates through the aerobic, anaerobic, and oxidative pathways, but at a rate less than the neutrophil.[111,368-370] Many of the mitochondrial enzymes and diaphorases are present in the lymphocyte (Table 3). Few normal lymphocytes contain glycogen. In types II, III, and IV glycogen storage diseases, the lymphocyte glycogen content is increased.[371]

Lipids — The small lymphocyte contains 11×10^{-12} g of lipid per cell. Normal cells have more lipids than cells in chronic lymphocytic leukemia (CLL) and acute lymphocytic leukemia (ALL).[215,216] Although lipid content of the lymphocytes is only half that of the neutrophils, it cannot be demonstrated cytochemically,[213,217,330,372-374] which suggests that the lymphocyte phospholipids are either too low or are different from those of the neutrophil. The ability of the lymphocyte to synthesize or utilize fatty acids is somewhat different from that of the neutrophil.[375] In Niemann-Pick's disease, lipid cytosomes have been observed in the lymphocytes.[301]

Hydrolytic enzymes — The lymphocyte lysosomes contain many hydrolytic enzymes (Table 2). In Wolman's disease, the esterase activity in the lymphocytes is characteristically absent.[91] Acid phosphatase, β-glucuronidase, and 5-nucleotidase activities are diminished in the lymphocytes of CLL.[45,376-380,599] Other studies suggest that these enzymes are decreased in B cell diseases, but normal or increased in T cell diseases.[45,379,381]

Miscellaneous — Lymphocytes also contain a variety of vitamins, coenzymes, and traces of zinc and iron (Tables 4 and 5). In patients with severe hemosiderosis or hemochromatosis, hemosiderin granules are demonstrable in the lymphocytes.[346,347]

Activated Lymphocytes

Typical of the activated lymphocyte is the phytohemagglutinin-stimulated (PHA) lymphocyte.[382] Other examples are atypical lymphocytes in infectious mononucleosis[383] and the "lymphoblasts" in reactive lymph nodes and in large cell lymphomas.[384-387] Metabolically, the PHA lymphocyte is a highly active cell. It incorporates amino acids and synthesizes DNA, RNA, lipids, and proteins.[154,364-366,389] Energy production is increased, and increased activity of many mitochondrial enzymes has been demonstrated.[24,44,122,140,369,370,390,391] The hexose monophosphate shunt, however, is not significantly altered. In the partially stimulated cells, the glycogen content is increased although little or no glycogen can be demonstrated cytochemically in the fully stimulated lymphocytes.[122,390,391] The activity of many hydrolytic enzymes other than β-glucuronidase and nonspecific esterase is increased.[44,389,390,391] Lymphocytes, small or activated, have no peptidase, peroxidase, alkaline phosphatase, or chloroacetate esterase.[55,68,70,72,134,392]

New Classification of the Lymphocytes

The lymphocytes can also be classified into long-lived or short-lived cells according to their life span in vivo.[393] No information is available concerning the differences in chemical and metabolic characteristics of these two classes. A more functional classification can be made according to sites of origin as either bone marrow derived (B) or thymus derived (T) cells (Table 7).[394] The B cells are involved in humoral immunity and have a rough cell surface which is often coated with immunoglobulin.[23,395-398,403] They have surface receptors for immunoglobulin,[396,399-402] complement,[410,411] and Fc fragment,[404,405] and may contain cytoplasmic immunoglobulins.[23,395-398] The T cells, on the other hand, are involved in cell-mediated immunity and have a smooth cell surface, surface receptors for measles virus,[406] and histamine[407] they are capable of forming rosettes with sheep red cells.[408,409] They have a high activity of acid phosphatase,[379] β-glucuronidase,[381] and terminal deoxynucleotidyl transferase.[163,164,165] On rare occasions, cells with markers for both T and B cells have been detected.[412,413] Lymphocytes without markers for either T or B cells are called Null cells.[384,414,415] Subtypes of T cells such as the helper cells and killer cells have been shown, although it is not certain whether they are new subtypes or are T cells at different stages of cell maturation.

Methods of preparing pure suspensions of lymphocytes[416-418] or T or B subtypes are now available.[419,420] Studies concerning the chemical characteristics of the T or B lymphocytes are, however, few and sporadic. The T cells can be activated by PHA and concanavalin A;[421,422] they have high activities of 5-nucleotidase[45] and have an isoenzyme pattern of lactic dehydrogenase different from that of the B cells.[423] The B cells, however, can be activated by PPD and other B cell activators[424] and have low activity of 5-nucleotidase.[45] Diseases of the lymphocytes or the immunoglobulins can be classified accordingly into T cell,[117,425-431] B cell,[404,426,427,432-438] or Null cell types.[384,414,415] Combined T and B cell leukemia has also been reported.[352,412,635]

The Plasma Cell

This cell constitutes 1% of all cells in the marrow. It is not present in normal blood, but is present in patients with plasma cell leukemia. Few biochemical analyses of the plasma cell are reported.[111,639] and most information regarding their chemical characteristics is derived from structural and cytochemical studies.[110,124,636-638] The plasma

Table 7
CHARACTERISTICS OF THE VARIOUS SUBTYPES OF LYMPHOCYTES

	T cell	B cell	Null cell	Monocytes	Ref.
Surface characteristics	Smooth	Rough, villous	—	Velvet	23, 397, 398, 403
Surface immunoglobulin	0[a]	P[b]	—	—	395, 396, 399—402
Surface receptors					
Immunoglobulins	0	P	0	P	398, 411
Theta[c]	P	0	0	0	642
Complement (C3)	0	P	0	P	404, 410, 411, 640
FC	0	P	0	P	405
Measles virus	P	0	—	—	406
Histamine	P	0	—	—	407
T Cell Antiserum	P	0	0	—	—
Sheep cell rosette	P	0	0	0	408, 409
Acid esterase	+ +[d]	±[e]	—	+ + + +[f]	641
Acid phosphatase	+ + +[g]	+[h]	—	+ + + +	379
β-Glucuronidase	+ + +	+	—	+ + + +	381
5-Nucleotidase	+ + +	+	—	—	45
Terminal deoxynucleotidyl transferase	+ + +	—	—	—	163—165
Phytohemagglutinin[i] activation	+ + +	—	—	0	421, 422
Activation by B cell[j] activators	—	+ + +	—	—	421, 422, 424

[a] 0 = Negative or absent.
[b] P = Positive or present.
[c] In mouse lymphocytes only.
[d] + + = Moderate.
[e] ± = Scarce or sporadic.
[f] + + + + = Plentiful.
[g] + + + = Many
[h] + = Few.
[i] T cell activators = Phytohemagglutinin, concanavalin A
[j] B cell activators = Purified protein derivatives, lipopolysaccharide endotoxins.

cell is capable of utilizing glucose through the Krebs cycle, glycolysis, and hexose monophosphate shunt.[111,639] Many mitochondrial enzymes have been demonstrated in the plasma cell (Table 3). In one patient with plasma cell leukemia, activities of mitochondrial enzymes in the plasma cells were shown to be much higher than in the lymphocytes.[111] The plasma cell has a well-devloped Golgi system and extensive endoplasmic reticulum. It incorporates amino acids and is highly active in protein synthesis. Many hydrolytic enzymes are present in the plasma cell (Table 2). The activity of these enzymes is usually higher than in the lymphocytes. The plasma cell also contains strong activity of α-naphthyl acetate esterase, but it has little or no activity of α-naphthyl butyrate esterase.[69,72] Adenosine triphosphatase has been demonstrated in the normal plasma cell. The activity of this enzyme is markedly reduced in the myeloma cell.[110]

The Monocytes and Macrophages[26,439,440]

It is technically difficult to obtain pure preparations of monocytes for biochemical analysis; therefore, most of the studies were made on macrophages from animal sources.[441,442] Methods of preparing monocyte-rich preparations are now available.[443,444]

Nucleic acids

Immature cells from marrow can synthesize DNA, but this synthesizing ability is lost in the blood monocytes.[28] Most cells in this system synthesize RNA.[39,445]

Amino Acids and Proteins

The macrophages have a prominent Golgi system and many profiles of endoplasmic reticulum and are capable of synthesizing proteins such as lysosomal enzymes, transferrin, and C3.[36,39,440]

Carbohydrates

These cells contain many enzymes necessary for a variety of energy-producing metabolic pathways (Table 3).[447-450] The monocytes and peritoneal macrophages obtain their energy largely through glycolysis, but the alveolar macrophages rely primarily on oxidation for energy supply.[368,451] During phagocytosis, hexose monophosphate shunt is activated to supply the necessary energy in the same way as in the neutrophils.[451-453] The alveolar macrophages are different from the peritoneal macrophages in that they have a very active aerobic oxidative pathway.[454,455] In heavy cigarette smokers, the activity of many mitochondrial enzymes in the alveolar macrophages is markedly reduced.[450]

Lipids

Monocytes contain lipids and are capable of utilizing fatty acids.[216,456,457] In patients with Gaucher's and Niemann-Pick's diseases, the abnormal lipid-containing macrophages accumulate in tissues as a result of specific enzyme deficiencies related to fatty acid metabolism.[298,299] In some patients with CGL, many Gaucher-like cells with normal or increased glucocerebrosidase activity accumulate in tissues due to a relative deficiency of the enzyme activity as a result of markedly increased lipid turnover in this disease.[298,299]

Hydrolytic Enzymes

Monocytes and histiocytes have many lysosomes and lysosomal enzymes (Table 2). Deficiency of these enzymes has been shown to cause a variety of disorders (Table 6).

The Mast Cells

This rare tissue cell is not present in blood except in mast cell leukemia (Tables 2 to 5). Information concerning its chemical characteristics is obtained through morphological and cytochemical studies. The mast cell and blood basophil are functionally similar but morphologically different. Both have many specific basophilic granules containing heparin, histamine, and serotonin.[223,227,230] The specific granules of the mast cell are less soluble in water than those of the basophil. The mast cell contains acid phosphatase,[50] alkaline phosphatase,[135] β-glucuronidase,[50] a chymotrypsin-like enzyme,[62,63] and a trypsin-like enzyme,[458] whereas the basophil has only a few of these enzymes but contains peroxidase which is absent in the mast cell.[123,135] Methods for obtaining and purifying the mast cells have been published.[459]

The "Hairy Cells"[460,461]

This mononuclear cell is present in the blood, marrow, and tissues from patients with leukemic reticuloendotheliosis (LRE) or "hairy cell leukemia".[319,462] It has a large, round nucleus, fine nuclear chromatin, and sometimes, a nucleolus. Its shaggy cytoplasm contains many mitochondria and vesicles.[319,463-465] A cytoplasmic inclusion, called the ribosome lamellar complex, is often present in the cell, although this structure is not unique to the hairy cells.[465-468] Cytochemically,[19,469-471] both succinate and lactate dehydrogenases are present in the hairy cell with activity that is stronger than that in the lymphocytes. The hairy cell does not have peroxidase, alkaline phosphatase, or chloroacetate esterase. It does not stain for Sudan Black B and stains weakly with PAS. It contains some nonspecific esterase and β-glucuronidase. This cell, however, has strong acid phosphatase activity;[47,469] most of it is resistant to tartaric acid inhibition.[48,18,319] The functional characteristics of the hairy cells have been examined.[472-474] At least some of the hairy cells are phagocytic.[466,475] Immunoglobulins have been demonstrated both on the surface and within the cell.[476-478] The origin of the cell is still debated.[318,469,475,479-482]

The "Histiocytes" or "Reticulum Cells"[385-387]

These are confusing terms that have been used interchangeably to denote cell types of diverse origin. The reticulum cell is sometimes considered a fixed tissue cell often found in germinal centers of lymph nodes or the malphigian follicle in the spleen.[483] However, the term "reticulum cell" has often been used to designate cells involved in hemopoietic neoplasms such as reticulum cell sarcoma, histiocytic medullary reticulosis, monocytic or histiocytic leukemias, or LRE. Occasionally, primitive granulocytes are also called reticulum cells. To some extent, the term "reticulum cell" becomes a vague, collective term used to indicate a poorly differentiated cell when proper identification by conventional methods has failed. Thus, this term may indicate cells that are heterogeneous in nature. The reticulum cells or histiocytes of the histiocytic lymphomas have weak activity of lysosomal enzymes, particularly the nonspecific esterases, but have no peroxidase or chloroacetate esterase.[384,387] The majority of these cells have been shown to be activated lymphocytes.[386,484,485] The leukemic monocytes or histiocytes in acute monocytic leukemia have strong activity of lysosomal enzymes; they may or may not have peroxidase or choloracetate esterase activity, but they do not have tartrate-resistant acid phosphatase (TAcP).[34,387] The primitive myeloblasts from acute myeloblastic leukemia do not have strong activity of lysosomal enzymes, but they often contain strong activity of peroxidase and chloroacetate esterase and may stain with Sudan Black B. The hairy cells of LRE have strong acid phosphatase and TAcP activity, although they have little or no activity of nonspecific esterase, chloroacetate esterase, or peroxidase.[47,48,469-471,474]

Cytochemical Characteristics of the Leukocytes

Introductory Remarks

Cytochemistry concerns the microscopic study of the chemical constituents in cells and tissues. In its narrowest sense, cytochemistry is limited to the study of individual cells, whereas histochemistry concerns the study of tissues. The earliest cytochemical studies were limited to inorganic substances; the results of some of these early studies, done more than 100 years ago, are still valid today.[486] Later, the scope of cytochemistry was extended to include enzymes and nonenzymic organic substances. The early enzyme cytochemistry was limited to the demonstration of the acid and alkaline phosphatases using Gomori's metal ion techniques and oxidases.[487-492] Due to the pioneering studies conducted by workers such as Gomori, Wachstein, and Burstone, the principles of cytochemistry were established, better and more sensitive substrates were synthesized, and more specific and sensitive methods were developed.[92,185,487,488,493-498] Many oxidases, dehydrogenases, hydrolases, peptidases, and many other enzymes can now be easily demonstrated. It is now possible to examine the cytochemical characteristics of individual cells in smears or tissue sections by light or electron microscopy, by visual examination, and by spectrophotometry.

Abundant information now exists on the cytochemistry of the hemopoietic system. This information comes from the study of individual cells in smears or cell suspensions,[217,499] the study of chemical or enzymic patterns of tissues in tissue sections by light microscopy,[41-43,356,500-502] and the study of the subcellu lar organelles by electron microscopy.[7,8,11,12,17,503] The basic principles involving cy tochemical studies of cell suspensions, tissue sections, or subcellular organelles are, however, very similar. In cytochemistry, cells are smeared on a glass slide, fixed, and reacted with the suitable substrates at optimal pH range for a specific period of time. The smear is then counterstained, dried, and examined. The type of fixative used depends on the desired cytochemical study. In general, a weak formalin solution at neutral pH buffered with phosphate is satisfactory.[72,504,585] Understandably, when the phosphatases are studied, it is necessary to replace the phosphate salts with citrate or acetate because of common-ion effect.[47,504]The dehydrogenases are very sensitive to formalin and alcohol; thus, cold, buffered acetone solution is a better fixative for these enzymes.[44,47,149,151,506] When studying the basophil and tissue mast cell, a specific fixative such as Mota's solution of cetyl pyridinium chloride may have to be used to preserve the metachromatic staining.[47,507] Occasionally, when one is studying enzymes that are very sensitive to fixatives, unfixed cells or fresh cells can be suspended in substrate solutions for enzymatic reaction and then smeared, fixed, and examined.[137,508,509] The morphology of the cells with postincubation fixation is usually less than optimal. In histochemical studies of tissue sections, the time of fixation of tissue is usually longer, and the tissue is sectioned with a cryostat and mounted to a glass slide before it is stained and examined.

In electron microscopic histochemistry, the tissue or cells may be briefly fixed with glutaraldehyde. They are then incubated for enzymatic reaction, after which the tissue or cells are further fixed, sectioned, stained, and examined. Gomori's metal-ion techniques are used for most of the cytochemical reactions.[8,10] Substrates and cytochemical methods that are useful in light microscopy may not necessarily be suitable for electron microscopy. At present, the scope of electron microscopic enzyme histochemistry is still limited and needs further improvement. By combining the cytochemical and biochemical techniques using pure cell suspensions, biochemical assays, and column chromatography to separate the isoenzymes for biochemical studies, it is now possible to understand the properties of many of the enzymes or isoenzymes and their subcellular localization.[47,48,69,113,318] It is also possible to determine a certain isoenzyme by its substrate or inhibitor specificity.[318,510] Several enzymes can be demonstrated in cells or tissues of the same slide by consecutive staining.[72,356,501,511]

Recent advances in immunology have extended cytochemistry even further. By reacting the intracellular substance with specific antibody which is conjugated with a chromogenic substance, it is now possible to demonstrate cell components with immunochemical techniques.[404,485,512-515] Any enzymes, isoenzymes, viral particles, and other cellular substances which are difficult to show by conventional cytochemical methods can now be successfully demonstrated.[112,512,516-521]

Cytochemical studies need not be limited to cells in smears or tissue sections; cells in agar medium or cell cultures can be examined.[522,523] Isoenzymes in cell lysate can also be examined in polyacrylamide gel columns and other media.[47,48,439,524-527] Specific antigen can be identified and studied in the agar plates after immunoelectrophoresis.[528,529]

The results of cytochemical studies can be evaluated under the microscope by comparison to suitable controls, but this method is neither objective nor sensitive. However, it is most suitable for the study of heterogeneous populations of cells such as the leukocytes. For example, when one is studying the lactate dehydrogenase activity in suspensions of leukocytes, one can readily appreciate that the enzyme activity in the monocytes is much higher than that in the lymphocytes, and that any leukocyte suspensions with higher percentages of monocytes will have more enzyme activity than the lymphocyte suspensions. Thus, the integration of morphology, biochemistry, and cytochemistry may help to clarify the behavior of the leukocytes much better than the use of any of these methods alone. By using marker enzymes such as succinate dehydrogenase for mitochondria, thiamine pyrophosphatase and acid phosphatase for the Golgi system, and β-glucuronidase and nonspecific esterase for the lysosomes, cytochemical studies can help to visualize the subcellular organelles in light microscopy. For instance, cells with numerous mitochondria have strong activity of succinate dehydrogenase, cells with a well-developed Golgi system have strong activity of thiamine pyrophosphatase and acid phosphatase near one pole of the nucleus,[110,133] and cells with many lysosomes invariably have strong activity of β-glucuronidase and other lysosomal enzymes.[36,108]

Cytochemical studies can also be extended to investigate the metabolism of the leukocytes. For example, in order to compare the mode of glucose metabolism through the glycolytic or oxidative pathways of the lymphocytes and monocytes, we can select and study key enzymes in these metabolic pathways and compare their activities in these two types of cells: glucose-6-phosphate dehydrogenase and 6-phosphoglucose mutase from the hexose monophosphate shunt, 3-glycerophosphate dehydrogenase and lactic acid dehydrogenase from the anaerobic glycolytic pathway, and succinate, maleate, or fumerate dehydrogenase from the Krebs cycle. The monocytes and macrophages have stronger activity of the Krebs cycle enzymes than the lymphocytes, indicating that they have more mitochondria and can utilize glucose more efficiently through the oxidative pathway than the lymphocytes. These cytochemical findings are in complete agreement with the ultrastructural and biochemical studies of these cells.[28,36,44,108,111,113]

Clinically, the cytochemical methods are the most useful for cell identification. They have been used to identify the various granulocytes instead of the conventional method of differential leukocyte counts.[530] They are also very useful in the differential diagnosis of acute leukemia by accurately identifying the primitive blast cells in these diseases.[72,499,531-533] Many histochemical studies have been made to investigate the cellular components of various hemopoietic tissues in neoplastic conditions. There are numerous cytochemical studies of the human blood and marrow cells. Some of the useful techniques will be discussed in detail later.

Leukocyte Alkaline Phosphatase (LAP)[134]

Human leukocytes contain alkaline phosphatase (Figure 6). Much of it is present in the mature neutrophils. Wachstein first noticed reduced activity of neutrophil alkaline phosphatase in CGL.[498] This finding was confirmed in subsequent studies.[134] The LAP is composed of several components with different electromobilities;[534-537] one of these components contains zinc and another contains magnesium.[536] Pure LAP has been prepared.[538,539] In humans, this enzyme is located in the specific granules of the neutrophilic granulocytes.[8-10] Normally, the enzyme activity is present in mature and juvenile neutrophils and, occasionally, in the metamyelocytes. It is almost undetectable in the myelocytes and is absent in younger cells. Thus, it may serve as an accurate measure of the granulocyte's age.[540,541] In myeloproliferative disorders with abnormal granule maturation, LAP activity may be present in myelocytes or younger cells.[542] Mast cells, osteoblasts, and vascular endothelial cells also contain alkaline phosphatase activity. The eosinophils, basophils, and monocytes do not have alkaline phosphatase activity.[134] The lymphocytes are generally considered to be devoid of alkaline phosphatase activity, although very weak enzyme activity has been demonstrated in the lymphocytes in blood and in the thymus.[543] Several cytochemical methods have been used to demonstrate LAP. The methods using naphtho-AS-phosphate-Fast Blue BBN[544] or naphthol-ASBI-phosphate-Fast Violet LB salt[545] are most promising. Rigid criteria for

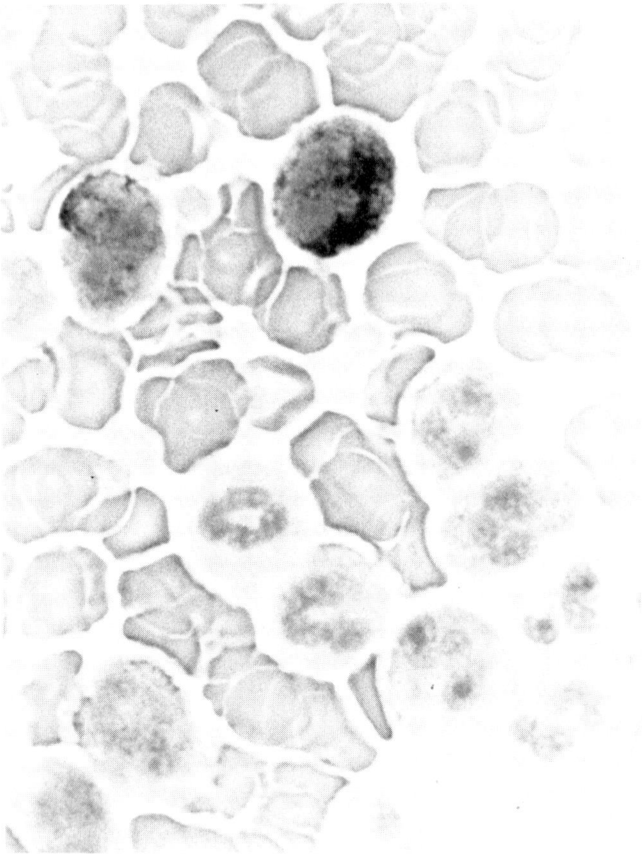

FIGURE 6. LAP. Leukocyte alkaline phosphatase showing neutrophils with various degrees of enzyme activity from the buffy coat smears of a normal subject. (Naphthol AS Phosphatase — Fast Blue BBN method.[544]) (Magnification ×1100.)

semiquantitating the leukocyte alkaline phosphatase activity have now been established.[545]

Cytochemical assessment of LAP activity is useful in diagnosing CGL.[134,546-548] It is also useful in differentiating CGL from granulocytic leukemoid reaction or polycythemia vera from benign erythrocytosis. Approximately 90% of the patients with CGL will have markedly decreased LAP activity.[134,546] As a rule, in juvenile CGL, chronic neutrophilic leukemia, or CGL with acute exacerbation, LAP activity is normal or increased.[134,547,549-552] Patients with negative pH′ often do not have reduced LAP activity.[541,546,553-555] The LAP activity may return to normal in about 50% of the patients with treated CGL in complete remission. Those with normal LAP usually have more sustained periods of remission than those with low LAP activity.[548] The return of LAP to normal can then be regarded as a favorable prognostic sign. In contrast to CGL, other types of leukemia usually have normal to elevated LAP activity.[134]

Low LAP may be seen in diseases other than CGL. These include paroxysmal nocturnal hemoglobinuria,[556] refractory sideroblastic anemia,[557] myelofibrosis with myeloid metaplasia,[558] familial hypophosphatasia[320,321] and, rarely, normal subjects.[371] It should be cautioned that one of the common causes of low LAP activity is technical failure resulting from improper staining or from assessing cells with little or no enzyme activity, such as the basophils and the eosinophils. Rigid quality control is therefore mandatory, and control smears with high enzyme activity should always be stained for comparison with the test smears.

High LAP is seen in polycythemia vera, thrombocythemia, myelofibrosis with myeloid metaplasia, bacterial infections, and in patients receiving corticosteroids. In Hodgkin's disease, LAP is markedly elevated during the active stage and normal during the inactive stage.[544,559] In reactive erythrocytosis and viral diseases, LAP is normal. The function of alkaline phosphotase in the neutrophils is not well understood, and the mechanism causing altered leukocyte enzyme activity remains unclear.

Peroxidase

This cytochemical test has been used with many technical modifications since 1902 to differentiate the lymphocytes from the monocytes and granulocytes.[490-492,564] Benzidine and its derivatives[120,565] have been used as the indicator for enzyme localization, but orthotoluidine,[566] α-naphthol-pyronin,[567] and 3-amino-9-ethylcarbazole[568] are also satisfactory. Many myeloblasts, promyeloblasts, and the more mature eosinophilic and neutrophilic granulocytes have peroxidase activity, while lymphocytes, plasma cells, and megakaryocytes do not. Monocytes contain moderate peroxidase activity, but the well-differentiated macrophages and histiocytes do not.[29,72,120,356] Enzyme activity in the basophils is weak or questionable.[117] Peroxidase isoenzymes in the granulocytes have been demonstrated.[121,569] Although monocytes generally have a weaker enzyme activity than granulocytes, chemical properties of the enzyme are similar in both cells.[72] Eosinophils have strong peroxidase activity. Part of the enzyme activity is resistant to cyanide treatment and is thus different from that in monocytes and neutrophils.[72,118]

Peroxidase stain is generally used for identifying monocytes and granulocytes and for the differential diagnosis of acute leukemias. For the latter, only the enzyme activity in the blasts is examined. This test is meaningful only when it is positive, indicating acute granulocytic or myelomonocytic leukemia. Cases with negative peroxidase stain may be acute lymphoblastic, monocytic (Schilling type), or acute granulocytic leukemia with very primitive myeloblasts. The peroxidase reaction does not differentiate granulocytes from monocytes. The myeloperoxidases are very sensitive to methanol.[570,571] Adding methanol to the staining solution abolishes the enzyme activity of the granulocytes but induces staining of the erythrocytes, which is due to a nonenzymatic reaction between the benzidine and the hemoglobin (Lephene's reaction).[571] This nonenzymatic staining can be used to identify hemoglobin in tissue sections.[356]

Myeloperoxidases are quite unstable and are sensitive to heat and organic solvents. When tissues are kept for several months at room temperature or embedded in paraffin, leukocyte enzyme activity is abolished. Deficiency of myeloperoxidase in the neutrophils and monocytes has been discovered.[312-316,322] Peroxidase from the horseradish plant can be demonstrated cytochemically by methods used for myeloperoxidase. This horseradish peroxidase is methanol insensitive and strongly antigenic and has been used successfully as an indicator to demonstrate specific antigens in a variety of tissues.[485,512,514,515,519,521]

Sudan Black B

Both Sudan Black B and Oil Red O have been used for the demonstration of lipids (Figure 7).[213,214,217,218,374,572,573] The substance demonstrable by Oil Red O is completely abolished by pretreatment with various lipid solvents, but the substance demonstrable by Sudan Black B is only slightly diminished. Oil Red O probably demonstrates neutral fats, whereas Sudan Black B demonstrates phospholipids. The cytochemical methods of Sudan Black B are more successful in smears than in sections. The method of Sheehan and Storey is the most widely used.[374] The Sudan Black B stain is useful for identification of granulocytes. Many myeloblasts, promyeloblasts, and the more mature

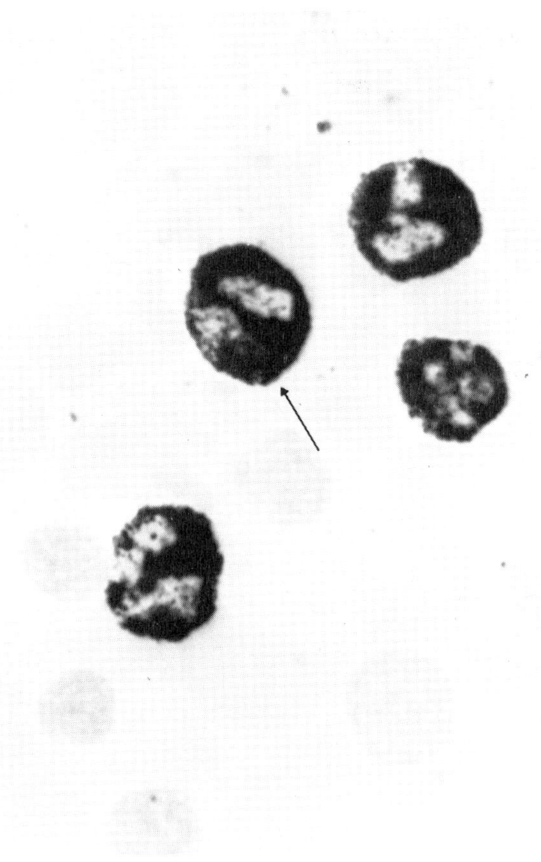

FIGURE 7. Sudan Black B stain showing three neutrophils and one eosinophil (arrow) with strong staining in contrast to the lymphocytes with round nucleus in the background showing no staining.[374] (Magnification × 1100.)

cells of the esoinophilic and neutrophilic granulocytes are stained. Monocytes and, rarely, basophils stain weakly. Lymphocytes and the plasma cells do not stain at all. Sudan Black B stain is as sensitive as the peroxidase stain and is more sensitive than chloroacetate esterase in identifying myeloblasts. It stains both the neutrophils and eosinophils and thus is less specific than chloroacetate esterase for identifying the neutrophilic granulocytes. Since it is a nonenzymatic reaction, it has an advantage over the peroxidase stain because it can be used in old smears with little or no peroxidase activity. For classifying acute leukemia in childhood, Sudan Black B stain is best used in combination with peroxidase and PAS reactions. Negative results with Sudan Black B and peroxidase and a positive PAS reaction in leukemic blasts suggest acute lymphoblastic leukemia.

Periodic Acid-Schiff (PAS) Reaction

The Schiff reagent reacts with the aldehyde group of a variety of complex carbohydrate compounds to give a pink color (Figure 8).[574] Carbohydrate-containing substances such as mucoproteins, glycoproteins, glycolipids, and polysaccharides can be stained by this method. Glycogen is also stained, but its reaction is sensitive to diastase digestion. Pretreatment of tissues by 1% diastase solution for 15 to 30 min results in complete hydrolysis of the glycogen, rendering the PAS reaction negative.

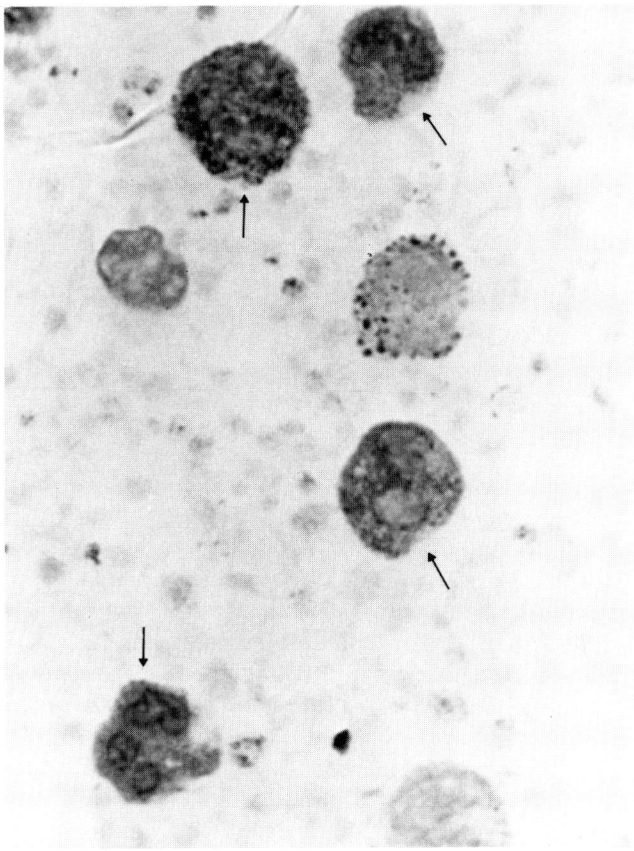

FIGURE 8. Periodic acid Schiff reaction showing one lymphocyte with granular cytoplasmic stain and several neutrophils (arrows) with diffuse stain. (Magnification × 1100.)

In human blood and marrow cells, PAS-positive substances are present in normal megakaryocytes, platelets, granulocytes, and a few erythroblasts, lymphoblasts, and monocytes.[496,575,577] Almost all the PAS-positive mateial in these cells is glycogen and thus is completely removable by diatase pretreatment. However, when formalin derivatives — formalin vapor in particular — are used as fixatives, removal of glycogen by diastase digestion may be incomplete. A positive PAS reaction in granulocytes exhibits a diffuse cytoplasmic pattern, while in lymphocytes and megakaryocytes, a granular pattern is seen. In CGL, neutrophil glycogen is subnormal. In untreated cases of diabetes mellitus, the neutrophil glycogen is not only decreased, but also located mainly in the periphery of the cell.[328] In polycythemia vera and reactive leukocytosis, neutrophil glycogen is increased.[136,326] However, quantitation of the neutrophilic glycogen content is difficult without the use of spectrophotometry.

In lymphosarcoma and in CLL, many of the neoplastic lymphocytes have increased glycogen content.[208,576] This finding however, is not unique to the neoplastic lymphocytes because the atypical lymphocytes of infectious mononucleosis and the activated normal lymphocytes also contain PAS-positive granules.[122,140,383,391] In AGL, the leukemic cells have little or no PAS-positive material, whereas the lymphoblasts of ALL have PAS-positive material.[214,499] In ALL, strong PAS positivity of cells is said to indicate a much better prognosis,[577,578] although this is disputed by others.[579,580] Few normal erythroblasts have PAS-positive granules. In patients with DiGuglielmo syndrome, sideroblastic anemias, thalessemia, hereditary spherocytosis, iron deficiency, and uremia, many erythroblasts may contain PAS-positive granules.[581,582] In iron deficiency and kidney diseases, positive PAS reaction in the erythroblasts disappears after appropriate therapy.[581] In patients with glycogen storage diseases (types II, III, and IV), glycogen content of leukocytes may be increased, and PAS-positive granules have been seen in lymphocytes.[371] The diagnostic significance of the PAS-positive material in the leukocytes in these groups of diseases has not been adequately investigated. It would appear that the PAS reaction may be of help in the differential diagnosis of some neoplastic hematologic diseases, but it should not be taken as a marker for neoplasia. Rather, a positive PAS reaction may simply indicate disturbance of glycogen metabolism in these cells, either due to increased production and storage or to decreased utilization.

Nonspecific Esterase

The esterases are a group of enzymes capable of hydrolyzing a variety of aliphatic or aromatic esters in acid or neutral pH. Those with a substrate preference for short chain esters such as acetate or butyrate are called nonspecific esterase. The exact nature of these enzymes and their physiologic role in the cell are not well understood. Many cytochemical methods have been designed to demonstrate the nonspecific esterases in the human blood cells.[69,72,89,90,92,583] Strong enzyme activity is seen in monocytes, and moderate to weak activity is seen in granulocytes and lymphocytes. Enzyme activity in monocytes is fluoride-sensitive, but in granulocytes and lymphocytes it is fluoride resistant.[583] Some studies suggest that the enzyme is demonstrable only in monocytes.[90] Using alpha-naphthyl acetate and hexazotized pararosanaline at pH 6.3, strong enzyme activity is demonstrable in monocytes, but there is only minimal activity in granulocytes.[72] By substituting alpha-naphthyl acetate with alpha-naphthyl butyrate, it becomes possible to eliminate or to keep the esterase activity minimal in the granulocytes and the megakaryocytes.[69]

The enzyme activity in blood or bone marrow monocytes is inhibited by sodium fluoride, whereas that in the tissue macrophages is not. At least nine different protein bands with esterase activity are demonstrable by polyacrylamide gel electrophoresis from the human leukocyte extracts. Several hydrolyze alpha naphthyl acetate or butyrate well.[69] Using purified suspensions of neutrophils, platelets, lymphocytes, and monocyte-rich preparations as enzyme sources, it appears that many of these leukocyte esterases are cell-specific.[60,69] The monocyte-specific esterases have an optimal pH at 6 to 6.3, are sensitive to fluoride inhibition, and can be best demonstrated by using alpha naphthyl butyrate as the substrate. The granulocyte-specific esterases have an optimal pH at 7.4 or greater, are resistant to fluoride inhibition, and can be best demonstrated by using naphthol AS-D chloroacetate as the substrate. By adjusting the pH of the incubation medium and by judicious selection of couplers for the cytochemical reaction, it is possible to stain the monocyte specifically with the nonspecific esterase reaction.

The enzyme activity in the monocytes varies from person to person and even from cell to cell (Figure 9).[511] The nonspecific esterase stain can be combined with other staining methods such as peroxidase and chloroacetate esterase for simultaneous demonstration of monocytes, granulocytes, and other cell types in smears and in tissue sections.[69,72,356,501,502] Methods for ultrastructural histochemistry are also available.[503]

The nonspecific esterase stain is most useful for the identification of monocytes and histiocytes.[41-43,69,72,356,511,584] The clinical features of the pure monocytic leukemia have been recognized, and the leukemic cells have been characterized.[27,34,584] The leukemic cells in this disease stain strongly for nonspecific esterase, but negatively for peroxidase

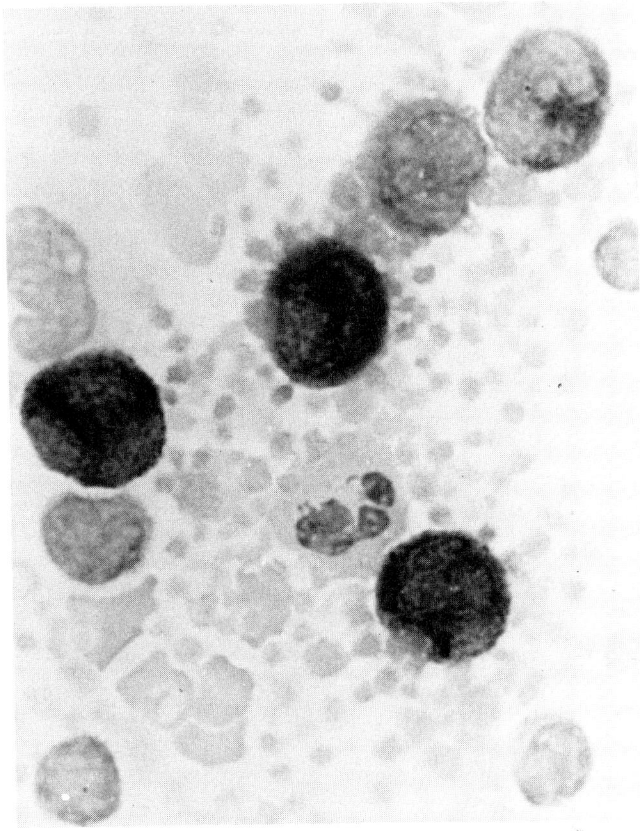

FIGURE 9. Nonspecific esterase stain showing various degrees of staining in the monocytes and no staining in a neutrophil. (α-Naphthyl Butyrate-Hexazotized Pararosaniline method.[69]) (Magnification × 1100.)

and Sudan Black B. In Wolman's disease, the nonspecific esterase activity in the lymphocytes is characteristically absent.[91]

Chloroacetate Esterase

In 1951, Gomori demonstrated esterase activity in the human leukocytes by using naphthol AS-D chloroacetate as the substrate.[66] Subsequent studies showed that leukocyte chloroacetate esterase is present almost exclusively in neutrophils.[68,70,72,585] Although Benditt et al. have reported its presence in mast cells in rats and concluded that its chemical properties are very similar to those of the chymotrypsins,[62] others have shown that this esterase has properties of chymotrypsin, elastase, and protease.[52-54,58-60,64,71] The exact nature of this enzyme(s), however, remains unclear. Polyacrylamide gel electrophoresis of the human granulocyte extracts demonstrates several protein bands with chloroacetate esterase activity[60,69] some resembling either elastase or chymotrypsin.[54,60,64,69,71] Several cytochemical methods are now available for the demonstration of the chloroacetate esterase in human leukocytes.[68-72] The methods using either naphthol-AS-D chloroacetate-hexazotized pararosanaline at pH 6.3[68] or naphthol AS-D chloroacetate-hexazotized new fuchsin at pH 7.4[72] are most satisfactory (Figure 10).

In human blood cells, activity of chloroacetate esterase is predominantly present in neutrophilic granulocytes and mast cells. The promyelocytes and some myeloblasts

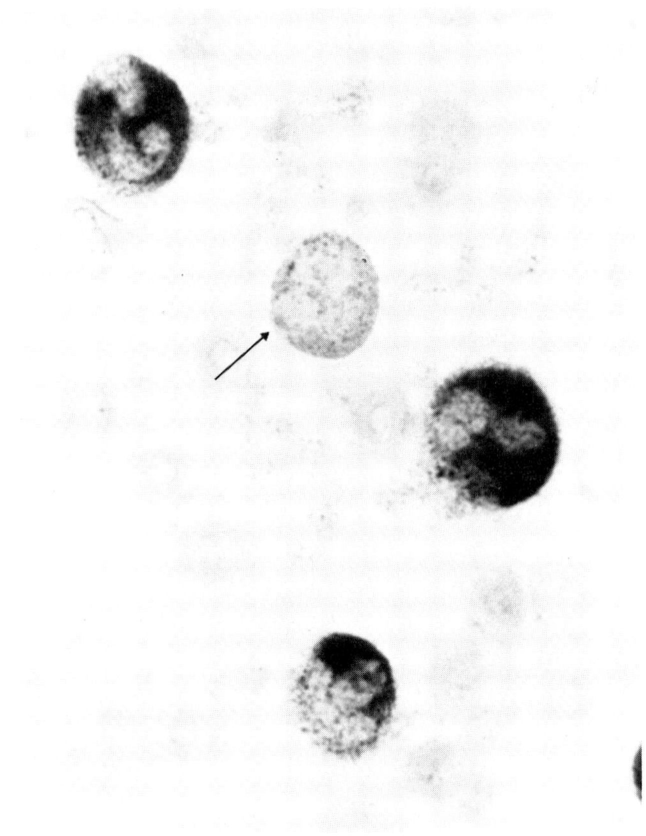

FIGURE 10. Chloroacetate esterase showing strong enzyme activity in three neutrophils and weak activity in one (arrow) neutrophil. (Naphthol AS-D-Chloroacetate — Fast Blue BBN method.[72]) (Magnification × 1100.)

also have enzyme activity. The blood monocytes and the tissue histiocytes have minimal or no enzyme activity. Positive reaction in these cells may indicate ingestion of neutrophils. An exception is the alveolar macrophage, which normally contains significant chloroacetate esterase activity. Lymphocytes, plasma cells, basophils, eosinophils, and erythroblasts have little or no enzyme activity. However, in a rare case of eosinophilic leukemia, the leukemic eosinophils may have strong chloroacetate activity.[586] It should be remembered that in granulocytic leukemia with severe disturbance in granule formations and maturation, neutrophils may have granules simulating those of the true eosinophils. Chloroacetate esterase activity has been demonstrated in such abnormal neutrophils or ''pseudoeosinophils''.[587]

Chloroacetate esterase is a useful marker for the neutrophils. It is not as sensitive as the peroxidase stain or Sudan Black B in identifying myeloblasts, but it may be present in myeloblasts which do not have peroxidase activity. Thus, combined demonstration of the chloroacetate esterase with the peroxidase stain increases the sensitivity for identification of myeloblasts in acute leukemia.[72] Since eosinophils and monocytes do not have chloroacetate esterase activity, this enzyme has specificity for identification of neutrophilic granulocytes while peroxidase and Sudan Black B do not. Chloroacetate esterase is very stable and is well-preserved in blood smears and in paraffin-embedded tissues kept for long periods of time. For this reason, chloroacetate esterase stain is particularly useful in demonstrating myeloid cells in paraffin-embedded tissue sections.[588]

Acid Phosphatase

The acid phosphatases are a group of enzymes capable of hydrolyzing phosphate ester at an acid pH. In human leukocytes, they are located in the lysosomes, but are also present in the Golgi system and the endoplasmic reticulum. Biochemical studies show that leukocyte acid phosphatase activity is increased in CGL and acute monocytic leukemia, and decreased in CLL.[380,589] Acid phosphatase activity can be demonstrated both by light microscopy in smears and in tissue sections, and by electron microscopy,[46-49,356,590,591] Enzyme activity is strong in monocytes and moderate to weak in eosinophils, neutrophils, lymphocytes, basophils, and platelets (Figure 11). In CLL, the total leukocyte acid phosphatase activity is markedly decreased.[380,589] This is attributed to the increase in enzyme-poor leukemic lymphocytes concomitant with the decrease of enzyme-rich monocytes and neutrophils in this disease.[47,48] Enzyme activity is increased in CGL and monocytic leukemia. These findings are, however, quantitative and not qualitative. Strong activity of acid phosphatase is present in PHA-stimulated lymphocytes and the T lymphocytes.[24,44,122,379,391]

The leukocyte acid phosphatase can be separated by disc gel electrophoresis into several isoenzymes.[47,48,439,592] Some are cell-specific; for example, isoenzymes 2 and 4 in neutrophils, isoenzyme 4 in monocytes, isoenzyme 3 in lymphocytes and platelets, isoenzyme 3B in primitive blast cells, and isoenzyme 5 in the reticulum cells of leukemic reticuloendotheliosis (LRE).[48] The total serum acid phosphatase may not reflect the otherwise altered isoenzyme patterns observed in Hodgkin's disease, CGL, AGL, infectious mononucleosis, and LRE.[47] A genetically determined deficiency of acid phosphatase has been reported.[311]

Tartrate-Resistant Acid Phosphatase (TAcP)[47,48,318]

The human leukocytes contain seven different fractions of acid phosphatase. All isoenzymes in lymphocytes, monocytes, granulocytes, and platelets (isoenzymes 1, 2, 3, 3B, and 4) are sensitive to tartaric acid inhibition. Isoenzyme 5 is resistant to tartaric acid inhibition and is derived almost exclusively from the leukocyte extract in patients with LRE. It originates from the characteristic hairy cells and not from the lymphocytes, monocytes, or neutrophils from patients with this disease (Figure 12).[48,318] It can be demonstrated in the hairy cells on smears, in tissue sections, and in tissue extracts.[48,318,319,356,593]

Cytochemical demonstration of the TAcP has become an essential diagnostic criterion for LRE.[470,594] The method using naphthol AS-BI phosphate-Fast Garnet GBC is most satisfactory for this purpose.[48,594,595] In normal blood, enzyme activity is absent in the erythrocytes, platelets, neutrophils, most lymphocytes and monocytes, and only weakly positive in some lymphocytes, monocytes, and most eosinophils. In normal marrow, enzyme activity is absent in the megakaryocytes, erythroblasts, plasma cells, and young neutrophilic granulocytes, and only weakly positive in some immature eosinophils, but strongly positive in a few histiocyte-like cells. Enzyme activity is strongly positive in the Gaucher-like cells in CGL, in Gaucher's disease, and in the epithelioid cells in granuloma of Hodgkin's disease and sarcoidosis. Enzyme activity is weak or moderate in the atypical lymphocytes of infectious mononucleosis. In 22 patients with LRE, cells containing strong TAcP activity are demonstrated in every patient, although the number of cells with strong enzyme activity varied. The presence of cells in blood, even as few as one or two with strong enzyme activity, should be considered presumptive evidence for the diagnosis of LRE.[594] The TAcP isoenzyme of LRE has been purified and partially characterized.[596,597] It is an acid pyrophosphatase with some unusual biochemical characteristics. Most of the enzyme activity is present in the lysosomal

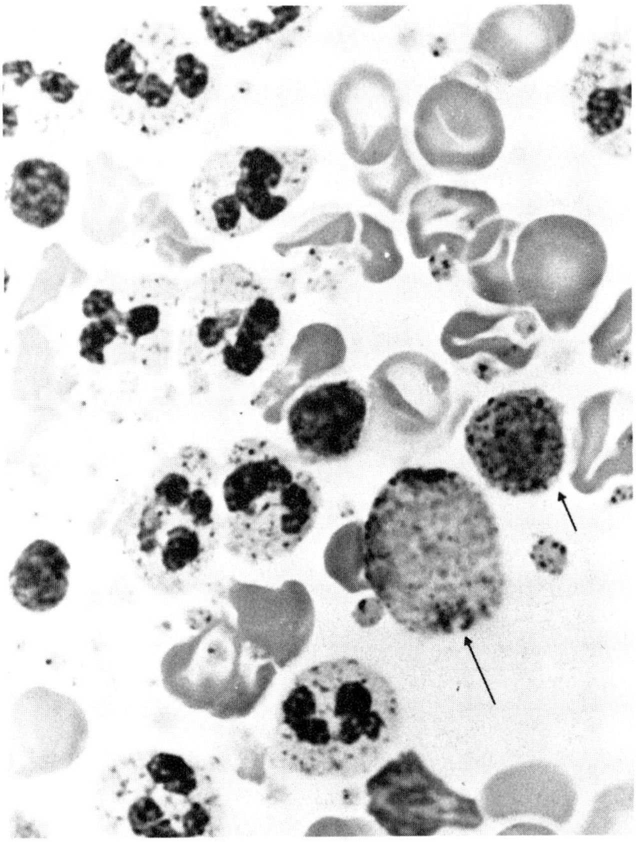

FIGURE 11. Acid phosphatase stain of a buffy coat smear from a normal subject showing strong and moderate activity in two monocytes (arrows) and moderate-to-weak enzyme activity in the neutrophils and lymphocytes. (Naphthol ASBI Phosphoric Acid — Fast Garnet GBC method.[47]) (Magnification × 1100.)

fraction, although a small portion of the isoenzyme is also observed in the microsomal fraction. Ultrastructural observation showed that most of the TAcP activity is located in the cytoplasmic vesicles and the Golgi saccules of the cell.[510]

Beta-Glucuronidase

Beta-glucuronidase is a lysosomal enzyme capable of hydrolyzing the glucuronide group from glucuronide-containing compounds at an acid pH. It is present in the human blood cells, with most of its activity in the leukocytes.[99,376-378,598,599] Blood leukocyte β-glucuronidase activity in CLL is significantly less than in normal subjects.[99,376-378,598,599] This finding is also true for cells in spleen tissue.[589] A dependable cytochemical method was developed in which naphthol AS-BI β-glucuronidase was used as substrate and hexazotized pararosanaline as the coupling agent.[99,600] Beta-glucuronidase is present in most blood and marrow cells. Enzyme activity is very strong in macrophages, monocytes, plasma cells, and some lymphocytes. It is moderate in the granulocytes and platelets and weak in the erythroblasts. In human lymphocytes, a positive reaction has a granular pattern, whereas in monocytes and granulocytes it is diffuse. Semiquantitative estimation indicates a heterogeneous distribution of enzyme activity in lymphocytes.[378,599] In normal lymphocytes, enzyme activity is strong in approximately one

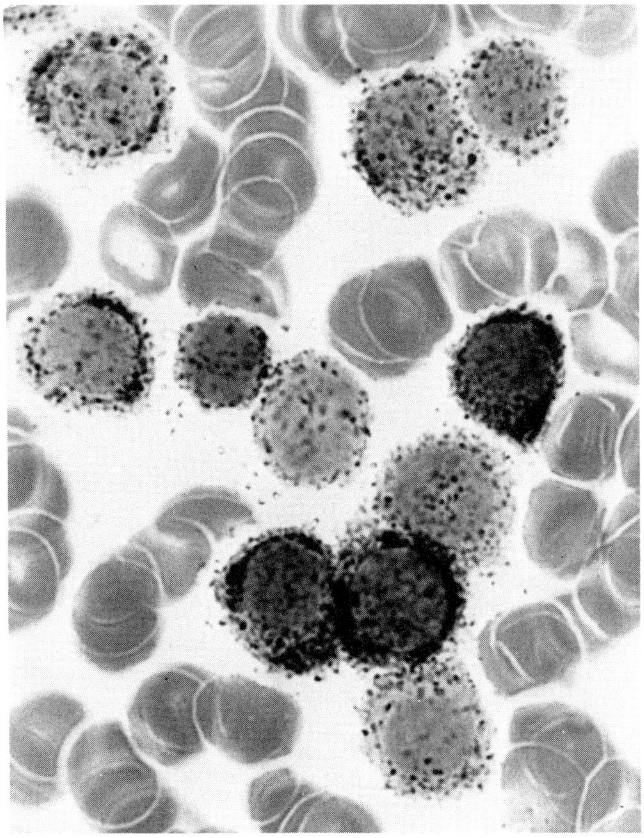

FIGURE 12. Tartrate-resistant acid phosphatase showing strong enzyme activity in most of the hairy cells from one patient with leukemic reticuloendotheliosis. (Naphthol ASBI Phosphoric Acid — Fast Garnet GBC in the presence of 0.05 M L(+) tartrate.[595]) (Magnification × 1100.)

third of the cells and weak in the other two thirds. In patients with CLL, lymphosarcoma, and in some with reticulum cell sarcoma, the enzyme activity is low due to an increase in the proportion of cells with low enzyme activity.[377,378,599] The low β-glucuronidase activity of lymphocytes is usually associated with decreased ability of these cells to undergo blast transformation upon phytohemagglutinin stimulation.[378] Low lymphocyte β-glucuronidase activity is said to be characteristic of the B cells, while high enzyme activity may be indicative of T cells.[381]

Muramidase (Lysozyme)

This lysosomal enzyme is present in many mammalian tissues such as lungs, kidneys, and blood. In human blood cells, much of the enzyme activity is in the leukocytes. Cytochemical and immunochemical studies have shown that enzyme activity is strong in the monocytes and the mature granulocytes, weak in the myeloblasts, and not detectable in the lymphocytes.[112,115] A rapid turnover of cells rich in muramidase will result in leakage of the enzymes into the serum.[601] Muramidase is a cationic protein with a molecular weight of 17,000 and is easily excreted by the kidneys. Rapid destruction of a large number of cells with strong muramidase activity may result in increased enzyme activity, both in the serum and in the urine. Excessive renal excretion of muramidase may cause kidney damage with impairment of renal excretory functions. High serum muramidase activity is characteristic of acute monocytic leukemia.[116] In AGL, CGL, Hodgkin's disease, sarcoidosis, tuberculosis, and several renal diseases, the serum muramidase activity is increased. In ALL and in some cases of AGL, however, the serum enzyme activity may be normal or low. Assessment of serum muramidase activity may be of prognostic significance in adult patients with AGL.

Dehydrogenases

Many dehydrogenases in blood cells have been studied biochemically or cytochemically (Table 3). They are present in different quantities in almost all blood cells. The lactate dehydrogenases are the most extensively studied. Markedly increased enzyme activity is seen in the granulocytes and in megaloblasts, as well as in serum of megaloblastic anemia. Markedly increased serum lactate dehydrogenase activity in megaloblastic anemia is probably due to ineffective hemopoiesis and premature cell death with the release of enzymes from the cells into the blood.[602,603] Isoenzymes of the lactate dehydrogenase have been studied and five isoenzymes have been identified in the human leukocytes.[145,423,604-608]

In several hemolytic anemias due to enzyme deficiencies in the erythrocytes, similar enzyme deficiencies can be demonstrated in the leukocytes.[275-278] Many cytochemical studies have been made on the human blood cells.[137,138,146-152,449,450,509,609] The clinical significance of changes of the dehydrogenases is rather limited. An interesting observation has been made on dihydroortic acid dehydrogenase.[151] Increased enzyme activity is noted in the leukemic blasts of the corresponding acute leukemias, in the myeloblasts and erythroblasts of erythroleukemia, and in the myeloblasts, erythroblasts, and megakaryocytes in aplastic anemia. The reason for this alternation is unknown.

Miscellaneous Enzymes

These include aminopeptidase,[80,83,494,637] cytochrome oxidase,[185] monoamino oxidase,[187] adenosine triphosphatase,[109,110] thiamine phyrophosphatase,[133] aminocaproate esterase,[458] 5-nucleotidase,[9,45,610,611] cathepsin,[75-79] glucosaminidase,[100-102] phosphorylase,[44,190,192] amylo-14-16 transglucosidase,[189] cholinesterase,[612] galactosidase,[9] arylsulfatase,[9,126,127,129] and α-glutamyl transpeptidase.[55] The clinical significance of these enzymes has not been fully evaluated.

Iron Stain

This test is used to evaluate marrow iron stores and is equally useful for demonstrating iron in urine, tissues, and blood siderocytes. The Prussian Blue (Perls' stain) method is widely used for this purpose.[613] It stains iron in the form of hemosiderin and ferritin. Hemoglobin-bound iron is not stained. The stainable iron is seen in the marrow, both extracellularly in stroma and intracellularly in macrophages and erythroblasts. Decreased or absent stainable iron in the marrow invariably denotes iron deficiency. Increased marrow iron content may result from increased supply or from decreased utilization. It is often seen in aplastic anemia with frequent blood transfusion, chronic inflammatory diseases, and malignant diseases. In familial hemochromatosis, marrow iron is normal or slightly increased, although the liver and other tissues are overloaded with iron. In blood buffy coat smears from patients with hemochromatosis, stainable iron granules are often detectable in circulating monocytes.

The iron granules in blood and marrow monocytes and macrophages in hemochromatosis are relatively small, whereas iron granules in hemosiderosis are large.[344,347] This difference may indicate an alteration in iron metabolism related to the fundamental defect in hemochromatosis. In erythremic myelosis and erythroleukemia, marrow iron is often increased in stroma, macrophages, and erythroblasts. In erythroblasts, iron is deposited in mitochondria appearing as a ring surrounding the nuclei (ringed sideroblasts). Other diseases such as thalassemia, lead poisoning, pyridoxine responsive anemia, chloramphenicol toxicity, and severe alcoholic intoxication with megaloblastosis may also have increased iron deposition in the marrow and many ringed sideroblasts.[614,615] Thus, ringed sideroblasts per se simply indicate a disturbance of iron utilization and are not diagnostic of neoplasia of the erythroblasts. In patients suspected of having Di Guglielmo syndrome, the absence of ringed sideroblasts together with a negative PAS stain of the erythroblasts strongly argues against (and tends to rule out) this diagnosis.

Toluidine Blue Stain

Toluidine Blue O is a substance which can bind with the acid mucopolysaccharides to give a metachromatic staining. Although human eosinophils, neutrophils, and basophils all contain mucopolysaccharides,[220] only the basophils react with toluidine Blue O in an acid pH to give metachromasia. Mast cells are also strongly metachromatic. The toluidine blue stain is useful in identifying basophils and their precursors and tissue mast cells.[72] A specially modified method is now available specifically for the mast cells.[616] In Hurler-Hunter disease, the lymphocytes characteristically contain large metachromatic granules.[388,617-619] In several mucopolysaccharidoses, demonstration of metachromatic granules in the Reilly bodies in the granulocytes is of diagnostic significance.[342] Demonstration of metachromatic granules in fibroblasts and in other cell cultures helps to establish the diagnosis of many inherited diseases.[323,620]

Miscellaneous Nonenzymatic Stains

These include oil red O,[214,218] methyl green pyronin for DNA and RNA,[621] Feulgen's reaction for DNA,[217] dihydroxy, dinaphthyl disulphide reaction for sulfhydryl groups,[383,392,622] ubiquinone,[623] and Amido Black 10B.[624] Clinical applications of these stains are rather limited.

Lymphocyte Immunochemistry

Morphologic study suggests that the small lymphocyte does not have high metabolic activity, although it contains most of the subcellular organelles commonly present in monocytes and granulocytes. Extensive biochemical and cytochemical studies of the lymphocyte reveal quantitative, but not major qualitative, chemical differences between the lymphocytes, granulocytes, and monocytes. No specific cytochemical markers for the lymphocytes have been detected.

Recent advances in immunology have created a new impetus for the study of the lymphocyte.[394] Lymphocytes are now divided into B and T subtypes (Table 7). The immunofluorescent techniques for immunoglobulins require fresh cell preparations and immediate examination after the cells have been labelled with fluorescein-conjugated antibodies to the immunoglobulins. In addition, these preparations cannot be kept permanently for future reference because of fading of fluorescence. These problems can be avoided by the use of immunoperoxidase techniques in which horseradish peroxidase is used as an indicator. It is possible to demonstrate the immunoglobulins in the lymphocytes on smears, fresh tissue sections, or paraffin-embedded sections.[512,514,515] Methods of demonstrating surface receptors by red cell rosette techniques which identify T or B cells are also available.[404,405] These immunochemical techniques vary somewhat in sensitivity and specificity, and care must be taken to interpret the results. Surface immunoglobulins may be due to nonspecific adsorption of immunoglobulins to cells other than the lymphocytes. Blood monocytes normally have surface receptors to complement.[640] Thus, surface immunoglobulins or receptors are not unique to the lymphocytes, since they may be seen in granulocytes and monocytes as well.[625,626,640]

Combined immunological and cytochemical techniques are now available which should enhance the accuracy of identification of the lymphocytes, granulocytes, and monocytes.[484,627-631] These techniques may be clinically useful for both prediction of prognosis and therapeutic decision-making. In acute childhood leukemia, for example, those with mediastinal tumor (T cell disease) are relatively resistant to treatment and have a worse prognosis than those with the B cell type.[425,632-634]

Concluding Remarks

From the discussion in this review, and from data presented in Tables 2-5, it is evident that much information has been gained in the past several decades from either biochemical or morphologic studies of the leukocytes. On the other hand, this brief review also demonstrates that the data on the chemical characteristics of many of the leukocytes are still incomplete. Even in an extensively studied cell such as the neutrophil and its cytoplasmic granules, our understanding of its chemical characteristics is still insufficient. This void is indicated in the recent studies on inborn errors of metabolism (Table 6) showing that these cells have many lysosomal enzymes whose chemical characteristics are still poorly understood. Some studies on the leukocytes are in need of reexamination, because they were carried out many years ago using relatively crude techniques. Other studies were made on mixed leukocyte preparations, which made it extremely difficult to understand the chemical characteristics of each individual type of leukocyte. The improvement in methodology of cell separation should make it possible to obtain various types of pure leukocyte preparations for precise chemical studies.

Leukocytes are now used for the diagnosis of a variety of lysosome storage diseases and other disorders (Table 6). In some instances, the diagnosis can be reached without resorting to the examination of the leukocytes; nevertheless, it is reassuring to know that this can be done. Sensitive automated enzyme assay methods have been developed for the purpose of screening the inborn errors of metabolism.[643] In the future, examination of the leukocytes may replace other tedious and time-consuming techniques such as tissue culture and surgical biopsies of the affected organs for the diagnosis of many of the inborn errors of metabolism.[644]

Many studies of the enzymatic make-up of the leukocytes are now being directed towards the isoenzymes. Since isoenzymes may be located in different subcellular organelles — and also because some are organelle-specific — a combined morphologic and biochemical study of the isoenzymes may be most rewarding. At present, morphologic studies have not been truly integrated into biochemistry and often lag behind biochemistry in obtaining crucial information. This is probably because the potential of many morphologic investigative techniques has not been developed to the fullest extent; there is also insufficient communication between the biochemists and the morphologists. Few biochemists know the properties and the clinical implications of the "chloroacetate esterase" in the leukocytes although they may be familiar with chymotrypsin and elastase in these cells. On the other hand, the clinician or the histochemist seldom makes extensive biochemical studies on chloroacetate esterase. If the chemical characteristics of this enzyme(s) can be examined adequately by an integral morphologic and biochemical approach, its function and subcellular localization can be better delineated, and more precise histochemical methods may be devised for its localization in leukocytes and tissues.

The potential for further investigation of the leukocytes by morphologic techniques has not been exhausted. It is entirely possible that more information can be gained from transmission electron microscopy, surface scanning electron microscopy, freeze fracture microscopy, and histochemistry. The present limitations of histochemistry are mainly technical in nature and may be resolved by an integral biochemical-morphologic approach. For example, it is difficult to demonstrate enzymes involved in nucleic acid metabolism cytochemically because of a lack of suitable substrates. This problem may be solved, at least partially, by immunohistochemistry if specific, pure enzymes or antigens are available for the preparation of the corresponding antibodies. Further immunohistochemical studies on the leukocyte should be extremely helpful in the understanding of chemical characteristics of the human leukocyte.

ACKNOWLEDGMENT

To Mrs. Julia Yam and Patricia Streips for their patience and assistance, and to Dr. Mehdi Tavassoli for his electron micrographs and critique of this manuscript.

REFERENCES

1. **Huhn, D. and Stich, W.,** *Fine Structure of Blood and Bone Marrow,* Hefner Publishing, New York, 1969.
2. **Tanaka, Y. and Goodman, J. R.,** *Electron Microscopy of Human Blood Cells,* Harper and Row, New York, 1972.
3. **Cline, M. J.,** *The White Cell,* Harvard University Press, 1975.
4. **Beck, W. S.,** Morphological and biochemical features of white cell anomalies, in *CRC Handbook Series in Clinical Laboratory Science, Section 1: Hematology,* Vol. 2, in press.
5. **Anderson, D. R.,** Ultrastructure of normal and leukemic leukocytes in human peripheral blood, *J. Ultrastruct. Res.,* 27, 205, 1969.
6. **Wetzel, B. K., Horn, R. G., and Spicer, S. S.,** Fine stuctural studies on the development of heterophil, eosinophil and basophil granulocytes in rabbit, *Lab Invest.,* 16, 349, 1967.
7. **Bainton, D. F. and Farquhar, M. G.,** Differences in enzyme content of azurophil and specific granules of polymorphonuclear leukocytes. I. Histochemical staining of bone marrow smears, *J. Cell. Biol.,* 39, 286, 1968.
8. **Bainton, D. F. and Farquhar, M. G.,** Differences in enzyme content of azurophil and specific granules of polymorphonuclear leukocytes. II. Cytochemistry and electron microscopy of bone marrow cells, *J. Cell Biol.,* 39, 299, 1968.
9. **Bainton, D. F., Ullyot, J. L., and Farquhar, M. G.,** The development of neutrophilic polymorphonuclear leukocytes in human bone marrow, *J. Exp. Med.,* 134, 907, 1971.
10. **Spicer, S. S. and Hardin, J. H.,** Ultrastructure, cytochemistry, and function of neutrophil leukocyte granules, *Lab. Invest.,* 20, 488, 1969.
11. **Scott, R. E. and Horn, R. G.,** Ultrastructural aspects of neutrophil granulocyte development in humans, *Lab. Invest.,* 23, 202, 1970.
12. **Beck, W. S.,** Leukocyte metabolism, *Ser. Haematol.,* 1, 69, 1968.
13. **Cline, M. J.,** Metabolism of the circulating leukocytes, *Physiol. Rev.,* 45, 674, 1965.
14. **Weissmann, G.,** Lysosomal mechanisms of tissue injury in arthritis, *N. Engl. J. Med.,* 286, 141, 1972.
15. **Sbarra, A. J.,** White cell metabolism, in *CRC Handbook Series in Clinical Laboratory Science. Section 1: Hematology,* Vol. 2, in press.
16. **Zucker-Franklin, D.,** Electron microscopic studies of human granulocytes: structural variations related to function, *Semin. Hematol.,* 5, 109, 1968.
17. **Bainton, D. F., and Farquhar, M. G.,** Segregation and packing of granule enzymes in eosinophilic leukocytes, *J. Cell Biol.,* 45, 54, 1970.
18. **Zucker-Franklin, D.,** Eosinophil function and disorders, *Adv. Intern. Med.,* 19, 1, 1974.
19. **Zucker-Franklin, D.,** Electron microscopic study of human basophils, *Blood,* 29, 878, 1967.
20. **Parmley, R. T., Spicer, S. S., and Wright, N. J.,** The ultrastructural identification of tissue basophils and mast cells in Hodgkin's disease, *Lab. Invest.,* 32, 469, 1975.
21. **Parwaresch, M. R.,** The Human Basophils, Springer-Verlag, Berlin, 1976.
22. **Zucker-Franklin, D.,** The ultrastructure of lymphocytes, *Semin. Hematol.,* 6, 4, 1969.
23. **Polliack, A., Lampen, N., Clarkson, B. D., and De Harven, E.,** Identification of human B and T lymphocytes by scanning electron microscopy, *J. Exp. Med.,* 138, 607, 1973.

24. **Parker, J. W., Wakasa, H., and Lukes, R. J.**, The morphologic and cytochemical demonstration of lysosomes in lymphocytes incubated with phytohemagglutinin by electron microscopy, *Lab. Invest.*, 14, 1736, 1965.
25. **Feldman, J. D.**, Morphology of plasma cells, in *Hematology*, Williams, W. J., Beutler, E., Erslev, A. J., and Rundles, R. W., Eds., McGraw-Hill, 1972, 771.
26. **Albrecht, R. M. and Hong, R.**, Basic and clinical considerations of the monocyte-macrophage systems in man, *J. Pediatr.*, 88, 751, 1976.
27. **Glick, A. D. and Horn, R. G.**, Identification of promonocytes and monocytoid precursors in acute leukaemia of adults: ultrastructural and cytochemical observations, *Br. J. Haematol.*, 26, 395, 1974.
28. **Van Furth, R.**, The origin and turnover of promonocytes, monocytes and macrophages in normal mice, in *Mononuclear Phagocytes*, Van Furth, R., Ed., F. A. Davis, Philadelphia, 1970, 151.
29. **Van Furth, R., Hirsch, J. G., and Fedorko, M. E.**, Morphology and peroxidase cytochemistry of mouse promonocytes, monocytes and macrophages, *J. Exp. Med.*, 132, 794, 1970.
30. **Hetherington, D. C. and Pierce, E. J.**, The transformation of monocytes into macrophages and epithelioid cells in tissue cultures of buffy coat (demonstrated by trypan blue), *Arch. Exp. Zellforsch.*, 12, 1, 1931.
31. **Leder, L. D.**, The origin of blood monocytes and macrophages, *Blut*, 16, 86, 1967.
32. **Nichols, B. A., Bainton, D. F., and Farquhar, M. G.**, Differentiation of monocytes. Origin, nature, and fate of their azurophil granules, *J. Cell Biol.*, 50, 498, 1971.
33. **Weiss, L. P. and Fawcett, D. W.**, Cytochemical observations on chicken monocytes, macrophages and giant cells in tissue culture, *J. Histochem. Cytochem.*, 1, 47, 1953.
34. **McKenna, R. W., Bloomfield, C. D., Dick, F., Nesbit, M. E., and Brunning, R. D.**, Acute monoblastic leukemia: diagnosis and treatment of ten cases, *Blood*, 46, 481, 1975.
35. **Archer, G. T. and Hirsch, J. G.**, Isolation of granules from eosinophil leucocytes and study of their enzyme content, *J. Exp. Med.*, 118, 277, 1963.
36. **Cohn, Z. A. and Benson, B.**, The differentiation of mononuclear phagocytes. Morphology, cytochemistry and biochemistry, *J. Exp. Med.*, 121, 153, 1965d.
37. **Drake, W. P.**, A white blood cell RNAse assay for the possible monitoring of malignancy, *J. Natl. Cancer Inst.*, 54, 1475, 1975.
38. **Reddi, K. K.**, Human granulocyte ribonuclease, *Biochem. Biophys. Res. Comm.*, 68, 1119, 1976.
39. **Cohn, Z. A.**, The structure and function of monocytes and macrophages, *Adv. Immunol.*, 9, 163, 1968.
40. **Bornstein, D. L., Weinberg, A. N., and Swartz, M. N.**, A deoxyribonuclease from rabbit leukocytes, *Proc. Soc. Exp. Biol. Med.*, 121, 677, 1966.
41. **Braunstein, H., Freiman, D. G., and Gall, E. A.**, Histochemical studies of enzymatic activity of lymph nodes. II. Further investigation of normal and hyperplastic lymph nodes, *Cancer*, 15, 130, 1962.
42. **Braunstein, H., Freiman, D. G., and Gall, E. A.**, A histochemical study of the enzymatic activity of lymph nodes. I. The hyperplastic lymph node, *Cancer*, 11, 829, 1958.
43. **Braunstein, H., Freiman, D. G., Thomas, W. J., Jr., and Gall, E. A.**, A histochemical study of the enzymatic activity of lymph nodes. III. Granulomatous and primary neoplastic conditions of lymphoid tissue, *Cancer*, 15, 139, 1962.
44. **Gough, J. and Elves, M. W.**, Studies of lymphocytes and their derivative cells in vitro. II. Enzyme cytochemistry, *Acta Haematol.*, 37, 42, 1967.
45. **Kramers, M. T., Catovsky, D., Foa, R., Cherchi, M., and Jalton, D. A. G.**, 5′ Nucleotidase activity in leukemic lymphocytes, *Biomedicine*, 25, 363, 1976.
46. **Goldberg, A. F. and Barka, T.**, Acid phosphatase activity in human blood cells, *Nature (London)*, 195, 297, 1962.
47. **Li, C. Y., Yam, L. T., and Lam, K. W.**, Acid phosphatase isoenzyme in human leukocytes in normal and pathologic conditions, *J. Histochem. Cytochem.*, 18, 473, 1970.
48. **Li, C. Y., Yam, L. T., and Lam, K. W.**, Studies of acid phosphatase isoenzymes in human leukocytes demonstration of isoenzyme cell specificity, *J. Histochem. Cytochem.*, 18, 901, 1970.
49. **Rozenszajn, L., Marshak, G., and Efrati, P.**, Acid phosphatase activity in normal human blood and bone marrow cells as demonstrated by the azo dye method, *Acta Haematol.*, 30, 310, 1963.
50. **Schauer, A.**, *Die Mast Zelle*, Gustav Fischer Verlag, Stuttgart, 1964.
51. **Folds, J. D., Welsh, I. R. H., and Spitznagel, J. K.**, Neutral proteases confined to one class of lysosomes of human polymorphonuclear leukocytes, *Proc. Soc. Exp. Biol. Med.*, 139, 461, 1972.
52. **Mounter, L. A. and Atiyeh, W.**, Proteases of human leukocytes, *Blood*, 15, 52, 1960.
53. **Pryce-Jones, R. H. and Wood, G. C.**, Purification of granulocyte neutral protease from human blood and rheumatoid synovial fluid, *Biochim. Biophys. Acta*, 397, 449, 1975.
54. **Rindler-Ludwig, R., Schmalzl, F., and Braunsteiner, H.**, Esterases in human neutrophil granulocytes: evidence for their protease nature, *Br. J. Haematol.*, 27, 57, 1974.

55. **Bona, C.**, Histochemical demonstration of γ-glutamyltranspeptidase in leukocytes of guinea pig peritoneal exudate, *J. Histochem. Cytochem.*, 13, 298, 1965.
56. **Shrader, R. E. and Hurley, L. S.**, Enzyme histochemistry of peripheral blood and bone marrow in zinc-deficient rats, *Lab. Invest.*, 26, 566, 1972.
57. **Baugh, R. J. and Travis, J.**, Human leukocyte elastase: rapid isolation and characterization, *Biochemistry*, 15, 836, 1976.
58. **Feinstein, G. and Janoff, A.**, A rapid method of purification of human granulocyte cationic neutral proteases: purification and further characterization of human granulocyte elastase, *Biochim. Biophys. Acta*, 403, 493, 1975.
59. **Kruze, D., Menninger, H., Fehr, K., and Böni, A.**, Purification and some properties of a neutral protein from human leukocyte granules and its comparison with pancreatic elastase, *Biochim. Biophys. Acta*, 438, 503, 1976.
60. **Sweetman, F. and Ornstein, L.**, Electrophoresis of elastase-like esterases from human neutrophils, *J. Histochem. Cytochem.*, 22, 327, 1974.
61. **Feinstein, G. and Janoff, A.**, A rapid method for purification of human granulocyte cationic neutral proteases: purification and characterization of human granulocyte chymotrypsin-like enzyme, *Biochim. Biophys. Acta*, 403, 477, 1975.
62. **Benditt, E. P. and Arase, M.**, An enzyme in mast cells with properties like chymotrypsin, *J. Exp. Med.*, 110, 451, 1959.
63. **Lagunoff, D. and Benditt, E. P.**, Histochemical examination of chymotrypsin-like esterases, *Nature, (London)*, 192, 1198, 1961.
64. **Rindler-Ludwig, R. and Braunsteiner, H.**, Cationic proteins from human neutrophil granulocytes. Evidence for their chymotrypsin-like properties, *Biochim. Biophys. Acta*, 379, 606, 1975.
65. **Lazarus, G. S., Brown, R. S., Daniels, J. R., and Fullmer, H. M.**, Human granulocyte collagenase, *Science*, 159, 1483, 1968.
66. **Gomori, G.**, Chloroacyl esters as histochemical substrates, *J. Histochem. Cytochem.*, 1, 469, 1953.
67. **Gomori, G.**, Histochemistry of human esterases, *J. Histochem. Cytochem.*, 3, 479, 1955.
68. **Leder, L. D. and Nicolas, R.**, Fermentcytochemische untersuchungen zur genese fer macrophagen un haufenster präparaten, *Frankf. Z. Pathol.*, 73, 228, 1963.
69. **Li, C. Y., Lam, K. W., and Yam, L. T.**, Esterases in human leukocytes, *J. Histochem. Cytochem.*, 21, 1, 1973.
70. **Moloney, W. C., McPherson, K., and Fliegelman, L.**, Esterase activity in leukocytes demonstrated by the use of naphthol AS-D chloroacetate substrate, *J. Histochem. Cytochem.*, 8, 200, 1960.
71. **Rindler, R., Schmalzl, F., Hortnagl, H., and Braunsteiner, H.**, Naphthol AS-D chloroacetate esterases in granule extracts from human neutrophil leukocytes, *Blut*, 23, 223, 1971.
72. **Yam, L. T., Li, C. Y., and Crosby, W. H.**, Cytochemical identification of monocytes and granulocytes, *Am. J. Clin. Pathol.*, 55, 283, 1971.
73. **Fraenkel-Conrat, J. and Chew, W. B.**, Catheptic activity of leukocytes in normal and leukemic subjects, *Blood*, 16, 1447, 1960.
74. **Fraenkel-Conrat, J., Chew, W. B., Pitlick, F., and Barber, S.**, Certain properties of leukocytic cathepsins in health and disease, *Cancer*, 19, 1393, 1966.
75. **Haschen, R. J. and Krug, K.**, Distribution patterns of proteolytic enzymes of normal and leukemic human leukocytes, *Nature, (London)*, 209, 511, 1966.
76. **Ishikawa, I. and Cimasoni, G.**, Isolation of cathepsin D from human leukocytes, *Biochim. Biophys. Acta*, 480, 228, 1977.
77. **Stiles, M. A. and Fraenkel-Conrat, J.**, Subcellular distribution of human leukocytic cathepsins, *Blood*, 32, 119, 1968.
78. **Sylven, B. and Spellman, O.**, Studies on the histochemical 'leucine aminopeptidase' reaction. V. Cathepsin B as potential effector of LNA hydrolysis, *Histochemie*, 12, 240, 1968.
79. **Vanha-Perttula, T., Hopsu, V. K., Sonninen, V., and Glenner, G. G.**, Cathepsin C. Activity as related to some histochemical substrates, *Histochemie*, 5, 170, 1965.
80. **Ackerman, G. A.**, Histochemical demonstration of aminopeptidase activity in the cells of the blood and bone marrow from various hematological disorders, *Nature, (London)*, 197, 189, 1963.
81. **Braun-Falco, O. and Salfeld, K.**, Leucine aminopeptidase activity in mast cells, *Nature, (London)*, 183, 51, 1959.
82. **Brok-Simoni, F., Ashkenazi, Y. E., Holtzman, F., and Ramot, B.**, Blood leukocyte enzymes. II. Activities at 8-9 A.M. in cells of normal subjects, chronic lymphatic, leukemic, and chronic myeloid leukemia patients, *Br. J. Haematol.*, 29, 293, 1975.
83. **Rutenberg, A. M. and Rosales, C. L.**, A histochemical method for the demonstration of leucocyte naphthylamidase using two substrates: alanyl- and methionyl-4-methoxy-2-naphthylamide, *Br. J. Haematol.*, 12, 595, 1966.
84. **Melmon, K. L. and Cline, M. J.**, Interaction of plasma kinins and granulocytes, *Nature, (London)*, 213, 90, 1967.

85. **Melmon, K. L. and Cline, M. J.**, The interaction of leukocytes and the kinin system, *Biochem. Pharmacol.*, (Suppl.), 271, 1968.
86. **Powell, G. F., Kurosky, A., and Maniscalco, R. M.**, Prolidase deficiency: report of a second case with quantitation of the excessively excreted amino acids, *J. Pediatr.*, 91, 242, 1977.
87. **Beaudet, A. L, Ferry, G. D., Nichols, B. L., Jr., and Rosenberg, H. S.**, Cholesterol ester storage disease: clinical, biochemical and pathological studies, *J. Pediatr.*, 90, 910, 1977.
88. **Elsbach, P. and Rizack, M. A.**, Acid lipase and phospholipase activity in homogenates of rabbit polymorphonuclear leukocytes, *Am. J. Physiol.*, 205, 1154, 1963.
89. **Ackerman, G. A.**, Histochemical demonstration of indoxyl acetate esterase in normal human blood and bone marrow, *Lab. Invest.*, 9, 298, 1960.
90. **Braunstein, H.**, Esterase in leukocytes, *J. Histochem. Cytochem.*, 7, 202, 1959.
91. **Lake, B. D.**, Histochemical detection of the enzyme deficiency in blood films in Wolman's disease, *J. Clin. Pathol.*, 24, 617, 1971.
92. **Wachstein, M. and Wolf, G.**, The histochemical demonstration of esterase activity in human blood and bone marrow smears, *J. Histochem. Cytochem.*, 6, 457, 1958.
93. **Clarke, A. E.**, Hydrolytic enzymes of human pol).norphonuclear leukocytes and rat monocytes, *Aust. J. Exp. Biol. Med. Sci.*, 43, 201, 1965.
94. **Hsia, D. Y. Y., Monteleone, J., and Farquhar, J.**, The nature of disaccharidoses in human leukocytes, *J. Lab. Clin. Med.*, 73, 111, 1969.
95. **Barnes, J. M.**, The enzymes of lymphocytes and polymorphonuclear leukocytes, *Br. J. Exp. Pathol.*, 21, 264, 1940.
96. **Kint, J. A.**, Fabry's disease: alpha-galactosidase deficiency, *Science*, 167, 1268, 1970.
97. **Singern H. S. and Shaffer, I. A.** White cell β-galactosidase activity, *N. Engl.J. Med.*, 282, 571, 1970.
98. **Suzuki, Y., Fukuoka, K., Wey, J. J., and Hauda, S.**, β-Galactosidase in mucopolysaccharidoses and mucolipidoses. Deficiency of GMI β-galactosidase in liver and leukocytes, *Clin. Chim. Acta*, 75, 91, 1977.
99. **Lorbacher, P., Yam, L. T., and Mitus, W. J.**, Cytochemical demonstration of β-glucuronidase activity in blood and bone marrow cells, *J. Histochem. Cytochem.*, 15, 680, 1967.
100. **Hayashi, M.**, Histochemical demonstration of N-acetyl-β-gluco-saminidase employing napthol AS-BI N-acetyl-β-glucosaminidine as substrate, *J. Histochem. Cytochem.*, 13, 355, 1965.
101. **Platt, D., Platt, M., and Loffler, H.**,Cytochemischer Nachweis der beta-acetyl-Glucosaminidase in menschlichen Blut- und Knochenmarkszellen, *Klin. Wochenshr.*, 46, 617, 1961.
102. **Reed, C. E. and Bennett, J. M.**, N-acetyl-β-glucosaminidase activity in normal and malignant leukocytes, *J. Histochem. Cytochem.*, 23, 752, 1975.
103. **Avila, J. L. and Convit, J.**, Characterization and Properties of α-D-mannosidase of human polymorphonuclear leucocytes, *Clin. Chim. Acta*, 47, 335, 1973.
104. **Hultberg, B., Autio, S., Berg, B., and Öckerman, P. A.**, White blood cell acid hydrolases in leukemias, mucopolysaccharidoses and mannosidosis, *Scand. J. Haematol.*, 10, 265, 1973.
105. **Beratis, N. G., Turner, B. M., and Hirschhorn, K.**, Fucosidosis: detection of the carrier state in peripheral blood leukocytes, *J. Pediatr.*, 87, 1193, 1975.
106. **Troost, J., van der Heijden, M. C. M., and Staal, G. E. J.**, Characterization of α-L-Fucosidase from two different families with fucosidosis, *Clin. Chim. Acta*, 73, 329, 1976.
107. **Goggins, J. F., Lazarus, G. S., and Fullmer, H. M.**, Hyaluronidase activity of alveolar macrophages, *J. Histochem. Cytochem.*, 16, 688, 1968.
108. **Braunstein, H. and Schmalzl, F.**, Cytochemistry of monocytes and macrophages , in *Mononuclear Phagocytes*, Van Furth, R., Ed., F. A. Davis, Philadelphia, 1970, 62.
109. **Freiman, D. G. and Kaplan, N.**, Studies on histochemical differentiation of enzymes hydrolyzing adenosine triphosphate, *J. Histochem. Cytochem.*, 8, 159, 1960.
110. **Von Schubert, J. C. F. and Schubert, H.**, Die Zytologische Diagnose des Plasmozytoms am Knochenmarkausstrich mit Hilfe der Adenosintriphosphatase-Reaktion, *Blut*, 19, 78, 1969.
111. **Seitz, J. F.**, *The Biochemistry of the Cells of Blood and Marrow*, Charles C Thomas, Springfield, 1969, 132.
112. **Asamer, H., Schmalzl, F., and Braunsteiner, H.**, Der Immunozytologische Lysozymnachweis in menschlichen Blutzellen, *Acta Haematol.*, 41, 49, 1969.
113. **Baggiolini, M.**, The enzymes of the granules of polymorphonuclear leukocytes and their functions, *Enzyme*, 13, 132, 1972.
114. **Briggs, R. S., Perillie, P. E., and Finch, S. C.**, Lysozyme in bone marrow and peripheral blood cells, *J. Histochem. Cytochem.*, 14, 167, 1966.
115. **Mason, D. Y.**, Intracellular lysozyme and lactoferrin in myeloproliferative disorders, *J. Clin. Pathol.*, 30, 541, 1977.
116. **Osserman, E. F. and Lawlor, D. P.**, Serum and urinary lysozyme (muramidase) in monocytic and monomyelocytic leukemia, *J. Exp. Med.*, 124, 921, 1966.

117. **Ackerman, G. A. and Clark, M. A.**, Ultrastructural localization of peroxidase activity in human basophil leukocytes, *Acta Haematol.*, 45, 280, 1971.
118. **Archer, R. K. and Broome, J.**, Studies on the peroxidase reaction of living eosinophils and other leucocytes, *Acta Haematol.*, 29, 147, 1963.
119. **Dunn, W. B., Hardin, J. H., and Spicer, S. S.**, Ultrastructural localization of myeloperoxidase in human neutrophil and rabbit heterophil and eosinophil leukocytes, *Blood*, 32, 935, 1968.
120. **Kaplow, L. S.**, Simplified myeloperoxidase stain using benzidine dihydrochloride, *Blood*, 26, 215, 1965.
121. **Malmquist, J.**, Serum myeloperoxidase in leukaemia and polycythemia vera, *Scand. J. Haematol.*, 9, 311, 1972.
122. **Quaglino, D., Hayhoe, F. G. J., and Flemans, R. J.**, Cytochemical observations on the effect of phytohemagglutinin in short-term tissue cultures, *Nature, (London)*, 196, 338, 1962.
123. **Tokue, K.**, The blood mast cell and its oxidase and peroxidase reaction, *J. Exp. Med.*, 12, 459, 1929.
124. **Quaglino, D., Torelli, U., Sauli, S., and Mauri, C.**, Cytochemical and autoradiographic investigations on normal and myelomatous plasma cells, *Acta Haematol.*, 38, 79, 1967.
125. **Nishimura, E. T., Whest, G. M., and Yang, H-Y.**, Ultrastructural localization of peroxidatic catalase in human peripheral blood leukocytes, *Lab. Invest.*, 34, 60, 1976.
126. **Austin, J. H. and Bischel, M.**, A histochemical method for sulfatase activity in hemic cells and organ imprints, *Blood*, 17, 216, 1961.
127. **Austin, J., McAffe, D., Armstrong, D., O'Rourke, M., Shearer, L., and Bachawat, B.**, Abnormal sulphatase activities in two human diseases. (Metachromatic leucodystrophy and gargoylism), *Biochem. J.*, 93, 15c , 1964.
128. **Dubois, G., Harzer, K., and Baumann, N.**, Very low aryl sulfatase A acid cerebroside sulfatase activities in leukocytes of healthy members of metachromatic leukocystrophy family, *Am. J. Hum. Genet.*, 29, 191, 1977.
129. **Ekert, H. and Denett, X.**, An evaluation of nuclear aryl sulfatase activity as an aid to the cytological diagnosis of acute leukemia, *Aust. Ann. Med.*, 15, 152, 1966.
130. **Humbel, R.**, Rapid method for measuring arylsulfatase A and B in leukocytes as a diagnosis for sulfatidosis, mucosulfatidosis and mucopolysaccharidosis VI, *Clin. Chim. Acta*, 68, 339, 1976.
131. **Tanaka, K. R., Valentine, W. N., and Fredericks, R. E.**, Human leucocyte arylsulphatase activity, *Br. J. Haematol.*, 8, 86, 1962.
132. **Tanaka, K. R., Valentine, W. N., and Fredericks, R. E.**, Arylsulfatase activity of human leukocytes: distinctive pattern in eosinophils, *J. Clin. Invest.*, 39, 1034, 1960.
133. **Fischer, R. and Hennekeuser, H. H.**, Uber den Nachweis der Thiaminpyrophosphatase (<<Golgiphosphatase>>) in Blut- und Knochenmarkszellen, *Acta Haematol.*, 40, 177, 1968.
134. **Kaplow, L. S.**, Leukocyte alkaline phosphatase cytochemistry: applications and methods, *Ann. N.Y. Acad. Sci.*, 155, 911, 1968.
135. **Noback, C. R. and Montagna, W.**, Some histochemical aspects of the mast cells with special reference to alkaline phosphatase and cytochrome oxidase, *Anat. Rec.*, 96, 279, 1946.
136. **Valentine, W. N., Follette, J. H., and Lawrence, J. S.**, The glycogen content of human leukocytes and various disease states, *J. Clin. Invest.*, 32, 251, 1953.
137. **Balogh, K. and Cohen, R. B.**, Histochemical demonstration of diaphorases and dehydrogenases in normal human leukocytes and platelets, *Blood*, 17, 491, 1961.
138. **Wulff, H. R.**, Histochemical studies of leukocytes from an inflammatory exudate. II. Succinic dehydrogenase, mitochondrial α-glycerophosphate dehydrogenase and di- and triphosphopyridine nucleotide diaphorases, *Acta Haematol.*, 29, 208, 1963.
139. **Rabinowitz, Y.**, DNA polymerase and carbohydrate metabolizing enzyme content of normal and leukemic glass column separated leukocytes, *Blood*, 27, 470, 1966.
140. **Barker, B. E. and Farnes, P.**, Histochemistry of blood cells treated with pokeweed mitogen, *Nature, (London)*, 214, 787, 1967.
141. **Shapiro, B. L., Smith, Q. T., and Martinez, A.**, White cell glutathione reductase in cystic fibrosis, *Lancet*, 2, 1020, 1974.
142. **Beutler, E. and Yeh, M. K. Y.**, Aconitase in human blood, *J. Lab. Clin. Med.*, 54, 456, 1959.
143. **Tanaka, K. R. and Valentine, W. N.**, Aconitase activity of human leukocytes, *Acta Haematol.*, 26, 12, 1961.
144. **Tanaka, K. R. and Valentine, W. N.**, Fumarase activity of human leukocytes and erythrocytes, *Blood*, 17, 328, 1961.
145. **Rabinowitz, Y. and Dietz, A. A.**, Malic and lactic dehydrogenase isoenzymes of normal and leukemic leukocytes separated on glass bead columns, *Blood*, 29, 182, 1966.
146. **Rozenszajn, L. and Shoham, D.**, The demonstration of dehydrogenases and diaphorases in cells of peripheral blood and bone marrow, *Blood*, 29, 737, 1967.

147. **Tzortzatou, F. and Hayhoe, F. G. J.**, Cytochemical demonstration of dihydrofolate reductase activity, *Br. J. Haematol.*, 28, 199, 1974.
148. **Tzortzatou, F. and Hayhoe, F. G. J.**, The effect of folate antagonists on dihydrofolate reductase activity demonstrated cytochemically, *Br. J. Haematol.*, 28, 209, 1974.
149. **Castoldi, G. L. and Merker, H.**, Nachweis und bedeutung Histochemisch Darstellbarer cholin-dehydrogenase in Menschlichen Blut- und Knochenmarkszellen, *Klin. Wochenschr.*, 43, 368, 1965.
150. **Merker, V. H., Castoldi, G. L., and Linde, A. H.**, Cholindehydrogenase in den Phagocyten des Blutes und des Entzundlichen exsudats, *Schweiz. Med. Wochenschr.*, 95, 1446, 1965.
151. **Castoldi, G. L., Yam, L. T., and Mitus, W. J.**, Cytochemical demonstration of dihidroorotic dehydrogenase in blood and bone marrow cells, *Acta Haematol.*, 39, 203, 1968.
152. **Nachlas, M. M., Walker, D. G., and Seligman, A. M.**, The histochemical localization of triphosphopyridine nucleotide diaphorase, *J. Biophys. Biochem. Cytol.*, 4, 467, 1958.
153. **Nachlas, M. M., Walker, D. G., and Seligman, A. M.**, A histochemical method for the demonstration of diphosphopyridine nucleotide diaphorase, *J. Biophys. Biochem. Cytol.*, 4, 29, 1958.
154. **Agarwal, S. S., Blumberg, B. S., Gerstley, B. J. S., London, W. T., Sutnick, A. I., and Loeb, L. A.**, DNA polymerase activity as an index of lymphocyte stimulation: studies in Down's syndrome, *J. Clin. Invest.*, 49, 161, 1970.
155. **Chuang, R. Y., Laszlo, J., and Keller, P.**, Effect of nitrosoureas on human DNA polymerase activities from acute and chronic granulocytic leukemia cells, *Biochim. Biophys. Acta*, 425, 463, 1976.
156. **Wantzin, G. L., Karle, H., and Killmann, S-A.**, Nuclear DNA-polymerase estimation in human leukaemic myeloblasts, *Br. J. Haematol.*, 33, 329, 1976.
157. **Ove, P., Kremer, W. B., and Laszlo, J.**, Increased DNA polymerase activity in human leukemic cells, *Nature, (London)*, 220, 713, 1968.
158. **Gallo, R. C., Yang, S. S., and Ting, R. C.**, RNA dependent DNA polymerase of human acute leukaemic cells, *Nature, (London)*, 288, 927, 1970.
159. **Guyton, J. R.**, Role of reverse transcriptase, *New Engl. J. Med.*, 294, 902, 1976.
160. **Viola, M. V., Frazier, M., Wiernik, P. H., McCredie, K. B., and Spiegelman, S.**, Reverse transcriptase in leukocytes of leukemic patients in remission, *N. Engl. J. Med.*, 294, 75, 1976.
161. **Swendseid, M. E., Wright, P. D., and Bethell, F. H.**, Variations in nucleotidase activity of leukocytes. Studies with leukemic patients, *J. Lab. Clin. Med.*, 40, 515, 1952.
162. **Johnson, S. M., Asherson, G. G. L., Watts, R. W. E., North, M. E., Allsop, J., and Webster, A. D. B.**, Lymphocyte purine 5′-nucleotidase deficiency in primary hypogammaglobulinemia, *Lancet*, 1, 168, 1977.
163. **Gallo, R. C.**, Terminal transferase and leukemia, *N. Engl. J. Med.*, 292, 804, 1975.
164. **Marcus, S. L.**, Terminal deoxyribonucleotidyl transferase activity in acute undifferentiated leukemia, *Biochem. Biophys. Res. Comm.*, 70, 37, 1976.
165. **McCaffrey, R., Smoler, D. F., and Baltimore, D.**, Terminal deoxynucleotidyl transferase in a case of childhood acute lymphoblastic leukemia, *Proc. Natl. Acad. Sci. U.S.A.*, 70, 521, 1973.
166. **Srivastava, B. I. and Henderson, E. S.**, High terminal deoxynucleotidyl transferase activity in acute myelogenous leukemia, *Cancer Res.*, 36, 3847, 1976.
167. **Meier, J., Colman, M. S., and Hutton, J. J.**, Adenosine deaminase activity in peripheral blood cells of patients with hematological malignancies, *Br. J. Cancer*, 33, 312, 1976.
168. **Zimmer, J., Khalifa, A. S., and Lightbody, J. J.**, Decreased lymphocyte adenosine deaminase activity in acute lymphocytic leukemia, children and their parents, *Cancer Res.*, 35, 68, 1975.
169. **Ultmann, J. E. and Feigelson, P.**, Cellular xanthine oxidase and uricase levels in leukemic and normal mouse leukocytes, *Blood*, 15, 418, 1960.
170. **DeViller, P.**, Guanyl cyclase activity of human blood leukocytes, *Enzyme*, 19, 300, 1975.
171. **Bianchi, P. A.**, Thymidine phosphorylation and deoxyribonucleic acid synthesis in human leukemic cells, *Biochim. Biophys. Acta*, 55, 547, 1962.
172. **Bresnick, E. and Kariala, R. J.**, End-product inhibition of thymidine kinase activity in normal and leukemic human leukocytes, *Cancer Res.*, 24, 841, 1964.
173. **Wilmanns, W.**, Die Thymidin-kinase in Normalen und Leukamischen myeloischen Zellen, *Klin. Wochenschr.*, 45, 505, 1967.
174. **Schandl, E. K.**, Thymine 7-hydroxylase activity in normal and leukemic leukocytes, *Biochem. Biophys. Res. Comm.*, 52, 524, 1973.
175. **Silber, R., Gabrio, B. W., and Huennekens, F. M.**, Studies on normal and leukemic leukocytes. VI. Thymidylate synthetase and deoxycytidylate deaminase , *J. Clin. Invest.*, 42, 1913, 1963.
176. **Bernengo, M. G. and Pegoraro, L.**, Deoxycytidylate deaminase activity and its template stability in human acute lymphoblastic and myeloblastic leukaemic cells, *Eur. J. Cancer*, 12, 611, 1976.
177. **Silber, R.**, Regulatory mechanisms in the human leukocyte. I. The feedback control of deoxycytidylate deaminase, *Blood*, 29, 896, 1967.
178. **McKinney, G. R.**, Glyoxalase activity in human leukocytes, *Arch. Biochem. Biophys.*, 46, 246, 1953.

179. **Gielen, W. and Schaper, R.**, Neuramidase, Acrylneuraminat-dytidylytransferase und Neuraminyltransferase in den Leukozyten des Menschen, *Hoppe Seylers Z. Physiol. Chem.*, 355, 660, 1974.
180. **Reynolds, J., Follette, J. H., and Valentine, W. H.**, The arginase activity of erythrocytes and leukocytes with particular reference to pernicious anemia and thalassemia major, *J. Lab. Clin. Med.*, 50, 78, 1957.
181. **Tanaka, K. R. and Valentine, W. N.**, The arginase activity of human leukocytes, *J. Lab. Clin. Med.*, 56, 754, 1960.
182. **Hartman, W. J., Clark, W. G., and Cyr, S. S.**, Histidine decarboxylase activity of basophils from chronic myelogenous leukemia patients: origin of blood histamine, *Proc. Soc. Exp. Biol. Med.*, 107, 123, 1961.
183. **Schayer, R. W.**, Histidine decarboxylase in mast cells, *Ann. N.Y. Acad. Sci.*, 103, 164, 1963.
184. **Salin, M. L. and McCord, J. M.**, Superoxide dismutases in polymorphonuclear leukocytes, *J. Clin. Invest.*, 54, 1005, 1974.
185. **Burstone, M. S.**, Histochemical demonstration of cytochrome oxidase with new amine reagents, *J. Histochem. Cytochem.*, 8, 63, 1960.
186. **Vercauteren, R. A.**, A cytochemical approach to the problem of the significance of blood and tissue eosinophilia, *Enzymologia*, 14, 340, 1951.
187. **Glenner, G. G., Burtner, H. J., and Brown, G. W., Jr.**, Histochemical demonstration of monoamine oxidase activity by tetrazolium salt, *J. Histochem.*, 5, 591, 1957.
188. **Cline, M. J. and Lehrer, R. I.**, D-amino acid oxidase in leukocytes. *Proc. Natl. Acad. Sci. U.S.A.*, 62, 756, 1969.
189. **Takeuchi, T.**, Histochemical demonstration of branching enzyme (Amylo-1,4-1,6-transglucosidase) in animal tissues, *J. Histochem. Cytochem.*, 6, 208, 1958.
190. **Quaglino, D. and Hayhoe, F. G. J.**, Phosphorylase activity in hemic cells, *Nature, (London)*, 194, 929, 1962.
191. **Williams, H. E., Kendig, E. M., and Field, J. B.**, Leukocyte debranching enzyme in glycogen storage disease, *J. Clin. Invest.*, 42, 656, 1963.
192. **Wulff, H. R. and Sorensen, M.**, A new technique for the histochemical demonstration of phosphorylase in blood films, *Acta Haematol.*, 35, 304, 1966.
193. **Barnhart, M. I. and Riddle, J. M.**, Cellular localization of profibrinolysin (plasminogen), *Blood*, 21, 306, 1963.
194. **Wohl, R. C., Arzadon, L., Summaria, L., and Robbins, K. C.**, Comparison of the esterase and human plasminogen activator activities of various activated forms of human plasminogen and their equimolar streptokinase complexes, *J. Biol. Chem.*, 252, 1141, 1977.
195. **Glen, A. C. A.**, Measurement of DNA and RNA in human peripheral blood lymphocytes, *Clin. Chem.*, 13, 299, 1967.
196. **Kiss, K., Astaldi, G., and Airo, R.**, The RNA nucleotide composition in human leukocytes from normal and leukemic cases, *Blood*, 30, 707, 1967.
197. **Iyer, G. Y. N.**, Free amino acids in leukocytes from normal and leukemic leukocytes, *J. Lab . Clin. Med.*, 54, 229, 1959.
198. **McMenamy, R. H., Lund, C. C., Neville, G. J., and Wallach, D. F. H.**, Studies of unbound amino acid distribution in plasma, erythrocytes, leukocytes, and urine of normal human subjects, *J. Clin. Invest.*, 39, 1675, 1960.
199. **McMenamy, R. H., Lund, C. C., and Wallach, D. F. H.**, Unbound amino acid concentrations in plasma, erythrocytes, leukocytes and urine of patients with leukemia, *J. Clin. Invest.*, 39, 1688, 1960.
200. **Dancis, J., Hutzler, J., and Rokkones, T.**, Intermittent branched chain ketonuria, *N. Engl. J. Med.*, 276, 84, 1967.
201. **Zeya, H. I. and Spitznagel, J. K.**, Characterization of cationic protein-bearing granules of polymorphonuclear leukocytes, *Lab. Invest.*, 24, 229, 1971.
202. **Mateles, R. I., Baruah, J. N., and Tannenbaum, S. R.**, Increased cystine in leukocytes from individuals homozygous and heterozygous for cystinosis, *Science*, 157, 1321, 1967.
203. **Gallo, R. C. and Perry, S.**, Enzyme abnormality in human leukaemia, *Nature, (London)*, 218, 465, 1968.
204. **Marsh, J. C. and Perry, S.**, Thymidine catabolism by normal and leukemic leukocytes, *J. Clin. Invest.*, 43, 267, 1964.
205. **Gallo, R. C. and Perry, S.**, The enzymatic mechanisms for deoxythymidine synthesis in human leucocytes. IV. Comparisons between normal and leukemic leukocytes, *J. Clin. Invest.*, 48, 105, 1969.
206. **Fujioka, S. and Silber, R.**, Leukocyte ribonucleotide reductase: studies in normal subjects and a subject with leukemia by pernicious anemia, *J. Lab. Clin. Med.*, 77, 59, 1971.
207. **Fujioka, S. and Silber, R.**, Ribonucleotide reductase in human bone marrow: lack of stimulation by 5′-deoxyadenosyl B_{12}, *Biochem. Biophys. Res. Comm.*, 35, 759, 1969.
208. **Astaldi, G. and Verga, L.**, The glycogen content of the cells of lymphatic leukaemia, *Acta Haematol.*, 17, 129, 1957.

209. **Kaung, D. T.**, Periodic acid-schiff reaction in human basophilic leucocytes, *Acta Haematol.*, 42, 269, 1969.
210. **Scott, R. B.**, Glycogen in human peripheral blood leukocytes. I. Characteristics of the synthesis and turnover of glycogen in vitro, *J. Clin. Invest.*, 47, 344, 1968.
211. **Smith, C.**, Glycogen in basophilic leucocytes in human blood smears, *Proc. Soc. Exp. Biol. Med.*, 72, 209, 1949.
212. **Weinberg, A. N. and Segal, S.**, Effect of galactose-1-phosphate on glucose oxidation by normal and galactosemic leukocytes, *Science*, 132, 1015, 1960.
213. **Ballif, R. N. and Kimbrough, C.**, Studies on leukocyte granules after staining with Sudan Black B and May-Grunwald Giemsa, *J. Lab. Clin. Med.*, 32, 155, 1947.
214. **Bennett, J. M. and Dutcher, T. F.**, The cytochemistry of acute leukemia: observations on glycogen and neutral fat in bone marrow aspirates, *Blood*, 33, 341, 1969.
215. **Blomstrand, R.**, Fatty acid synthesis in human lymphocytes, *Acta Chem. Scand.*, 20, 1122, 1966.
216. **Gottfried, E. L.**, Lipid patterns of leukocytes in health and disease, *Semin. Hematol.*, 9, 241, 1972.
217. **Rheingold, J. J. and Wislocki, G. B.** Histochemical methods applied to hematology, *Blood*, 3, 641, 1948.
218. **Wright, D. H.**, Cytology and histochemistry of the Burkitt lymphoma, *Br. J. Cancer*, 17, 50, 1963.
219. **Klibansky, C., Ossimi, Z., Matoth, Y., Pinkhas, J., and De Vries, A.**, Accumulation of lactosyl ceramide in leukocytes of patients with adult Gaucher's disease, *Clin. Chim. Acta*, 72, 141, 1976.
220. **Dunn, W. B. and Spicer, S. S.**, Histochemical demonstration of sulfated mucosubstances and cationic proteins in human granulocytes and platelets, *J. Histochem. Cytochem.*, 17, 668, 1969.
221. **Code, C. F. and Mitchell, R. G.**, Histamine, eosinophils and basophils in the blood, *J. Physiol.*, 136, 449, 1957.
222. **Graham, H. T., Lowry, O. H., Wheelwright, F., Lenz, M. A., and Parish, H. H., Jr.**, Distribution of histamine among leukocytes and platelets, *Blood*, 10, 467, 1955.
223. **Riley, J. F.**, Functional significance of histamine and heparin in tissue mast cells, *Ann. N.Y. Acad. Sci.*, 103, 151, 1963.
224. **Sampson, D. and Archer, G. T.**, Release of histamine from human basophils, *Blood*, 29, 722, 1967.
225. **Valentine, W. N., Pearce, M. L., and Lawrence, J. S.**, Studies on the histamine content of blood with special reference to leukemia, leukemoid reactions and leukocytosis, *Blood*, 5, 623, 1950.
226. **Valentine, W. N., Lawrence, J. S., Pearce, M. L., and Beck, W. S.**, The relationship of the basophil to blood histamine in man, *Blood*, 10, 154, 1955.
227. **Benditt, E. P., Wong, R. L., Arase, M., and Roeper, E.**, 5-Hydroxy-tryptamine in mast cells, *Proc. Soc. Exp. Biol. Med.*, 90, 303, 1955.
228. **Laves, W. and Thoma, K.**, Histoenzymatische Untersuchungen un der Mastzellen des Blutes, *Klin. Wochenschr.*, 28, 95, 1950.
229. **Parekh, A. C. and Glick, D.**, Heparin and hexosamine in isolated mast cells: determination, intracellular distribution and effects of biological state, *J. Biol. Chem.*, 237, 280, 1962.
230. **Tas, J. and Geenen, L. H. M.**, Microspectrophotometric detection of heparin in mast cells and basophilic granulocytes stained metachromatically with toluidine blue O, *Histochem J.*, 7, 231, 1975.
231. **Broome, J., Archer, R. K., Burnett, S., and LeRiche, H. H.**, On some metallic constituents of leukocytes, *J. Histochem. Cytochem.*, 11, 446, 1963.
232. **Fredericks, R. E., Tanaka, R. K., and Valentine, W. N.**, Variations of human blood cell zinc in disease, *J. Clin. Invest.*, 43, 304, 1964.
233. **Dennes, E., Tupper, R., and Wormall, A.**, The zinc content of erythrocytes and leukocytes of blood from normal and leukemic subjects, *Biochem. J.*, 78, 578, 1961.
234. **Kerp, L.**, Bedeutung von Zink für die Histaminspeicherung in Mastzellen, *Int. Arch. Allergy*, 22, 112 , 1963.
235. **McNary, W. F.**, Dithizone staining of myeloid granules, *Blood*, 12, 644, 1957.
236. **Pihl, E., Gustafson, G. T., Josefsson, B., and Paul, K. G.**, Heavy metals in the granules of eosinophilic granulocytes, *Scand. J. Haematol.*, 4, 371, 1967.
237. **Schumacher, H. R., Fishbein, P., Phelps, P., Tse, R., and Krauser, R.**, Comparison of sodium urate and calcium pyrophosphate crystal phagocytosis by polymorphonuclear leukocytes, *Arth. Rheum.*, 18, (Suppl.), 783, 1975.
238. **Walters, T. R., Welland, F. H., Gribble, T. J., and Schwartz, H. C.**, Biosynthesis of heme in leukemic leukocytes, *Cancer*, 20, 1117, 1967.
239. **Hardin, E. B., Valentine, W. N., Follette, J. H., and Lawrence, J. S.**, Studies on the sulfhydryl content of human leukocytes and erythrocytes, *Am. J. Med. Sci.*, 228, 73, 1954.
240. **Bourne, H. R., Lehrer, R. I., Cline, M. H., and Melmon, K. L.**, Cyclic 3′,5′-adenosine monophosphate in the human leukocytes; synthesis degradation, and effects on neutrophil candidacidal activity, *J. Clin. Invest.*, 50, 920, 1971.

241. **Burch, H. B., Bessey, O. A., and Lowry, O. H.**, Fluorometric measurements of riboflavin and its natural derivatives in small quantities of blood serum and cells, *J. Biol. Chem.*, 175, 457, 1948.
242. **Prager, M. D., Malicky, M., Goemer, M., and Hill, H. M.**, Riboflavin activity in normal and leukemic human leukocytes and nuclei, *J. Lab. Clin. Med.*, 53, 926, 1959.
243. **Chabner, B. A., DeVita, V. T., Livingston, D. M., and Oliverio, V. T.**, Tryptophan metabolism and plasma pyridoxal phosphate in Hodgkin's disease, *N. Engl. J. Med.*, 282, 838, 1970.
244. **Donald, E. A. and Ferguson, R. F.**, A micromethod for determination of pyridoxal phosphate in leukocytes and liver, *Ann. Biochem.*, 7, 335, 1964.
245. **Wachstein, M., Kellner, J. D., and Ortiz, J. M.**, Pyridoxal phosphate in plasma and leukocytes of normal and pregnant subjects following B_6 load tests, *Proc. Soc. Exp. Biol. Med.*, 103, 350, 1960.
246. **Wachstein, M., Kellner, J. D., and Ortiz, J. M.**, Pyridoxal phosphate in patients with leukemia and other diseases, *Proc. Soc. Exp. Biol. Med.*, 105, 563, 1960.
247. **Kidd, H. M. and Thomas, J. W.**, The level of vitamin B_{12} in circulating leukemic leukocytes, *Br. J. Haematol.*, 8, 64, 1962.
248. **Butler, A. M. and Cushman, M.**, Distribution of ascorbic acid in the blood and its nutritional significance, *J. Clin. Invest.*, 19, 459, 1941.
249. **Crandon, J. H., Lennikan, R., Jr., Mikal, S., and Reif, A. E.**, Ascorbic acid economy in surgical patients, *Ann. N.Y. Acad. Sci.*, 92, 246, 1961.
250. **Silber, R., Gabrio, B. W., and Huennekens, F. M.**, Studies on normal and leukemic leukocytes. III. Pyridine nucleosides, *J. Clin. Invest.*, 41, 230, 1962.
251. **Gorham, A. T., Abels, J. C., Robins, A. L., and Rhoads, C. P.**, The measurement and metabolism of thiamin and of a pyrimidine stimulating yeast fermentation found in the blood cells and urine of normal individuals, *J. Clin. Invest.*, 21, 161, 1942.
252. **Hers, H. G. and Van Hoof, E.**, *Lysosomes and Storage Diseases*, Academic Press, New York, 1973.
253. **Steinitz, K.**, Laboratory diagnosis of glycogen storage diseases, *Adv. Clin. Chem.*, 9, 227, 1967.
254. **Hulsman, W. C., Oei, T. L., and van Creveld, S.**, Phosphorylase activity in leukocytes from patients with glycogen storage disease, *Lancet*, 2, 581, 1961.
255. **Brown, B. I. and Brown, D. H.**, Lack of α-1,4 glucan: α^1 4 glucan 6 glycosyl transferase in a case of Type IV glycogenosis, *Proc. Natl. Acad. Sci. U.S.A.*, 56, 725, 1966.
256. **Williams, H. E. and Field, J. B.**, Low leukocyte phosphorylase in hepatic phosphorylase-deficient glycogen storage disease, *J. Clin. Invest.*, 40, 1841, 1961.
257. **Williams, H. E. and Field, J. B.**, Further studies on leukocyte phosphorylase in glycogen storage disease, *Metabolism*, 12, 464, 1963.
258. **Estes, F. L., Austin, N. S., and Gast, J. H.**, Metabolic characterization of polymorphonuclear leukocytes, *Clin. Chem.*, 6, 501, 1960.
259. **Davidson, J. N., Leslie, J., and White, J. C.**, Quantitative studies on the content of nucleic acids in normal and leukemic cells from blood and bone marrow, *J. Pathol. Bacteriol.*, 63, 471, 1951.
260. **Hale, A. J. and Wilson, S. J.**, The desoxyribonucleic acid content of the nuclei of leukemic leukocytes, *Lancet*, 1, 577, 1960.
261. **Petrakis, N. L.**, Microspectrophotometric estimation of the desoxyribonucleic acid content of individual normal and leukemic human lymphocytes, *Blood*, 8, 905, 1953.
262. **Reisman, L. E., Mitani, M., and Zueler, W. W.**, Chromosome studies in leukemia. I. Evidence for the origin of leukemic stem lines from aneuploid mutants, *N. Engl. J. Med.*, 270, 591, 1964.
263. **Rigas, D., Duerst, M. L., Jump, M. E., and Osgood, E. E.**, The nucleic acids and other phosphorus compounds of human leukemic leukocytes: relationship to cell maturity, *J. Lab. Clin. Med.*, 48, 356, 1956.
264. **Polli, E. E., Rosoff, M., DeMayorca, G., and Cavalieri, L. F.**, Physiochemical characterization of deoxyribonucleic acids from human leukemic leukocytes, *Cancer Res.*, 19, 159, 1959.
265. **Scott, J. L.**, Human leukocyte metabolism in vitro. I. Incorporation of adenine-8-C^{14} and formate-C^{14} into the nucleic acids of leukemic leukocytes, *J. Clin. Invest.*, 41, 67, 1962.
266. **Williams, W. J. and Buchanan, J. M.**, Biosynthesis of the purines. V. The conversion of hypoxanthine to inosinic acid by liver enzyme, *J. Biol. Chem.*, 203, 583, 1953.
267. **Nour-Eldin, F. and Wilkinson, J. F.**, Amino acid content of white blood cells in human leukemias, *Br. J. Haematol.*, 1, 358, 1955.
268. **Weisberger, A. S. and Levine, B.**, Incorporation of radioactive L-cystine by normal and leukemic leukocytes in vivo, *Blood*, 9, 1082, 1954.
269. **Weisberger, A. S., Suhrland, L. G., and Griggs, R. C.**, Incorporation of radioactive L-cystine and L-methione by leukemic leukocytes in vivo, *Blood*, 9, 1095, 1954.
270. **Inouye, T., Nadler, H. L., and Hsia, Y. Y.**, Galactose-1-phosphate uridyltransferase in red and white blood cells, *Clin. Chim. Acta*, 19, 169, 1968.
271. **Mellman, W. J. and Tedesco, T. A.**, An improved assay of erythrocyte and leukocyte galactose-1-phosphate uridyl transferase: stabilization of the enzyme by a thiol protective reagent, *J. Lab. Clin. Med.*, 66, 980, 1965.

272. **Melancon, S. B., Khachadurian, A. K., Nadler, H. L., and Brown, B. I.**, Metabolic and biochemical studies in fructose 1,6-diphosphatase deficiency, *J. Pediatr.*, 82, 650, 1973.
273. **Schrijver, J. and Hommes, F. A.**, Activity of fructose 1-6-diphosphatase in human leukocytes, *N. Engl. J. Med.*, 292, 1298, 1975.
274. **Cahill, J. and Kirtley, M. E.**, FDPase activity in human leukocytes, *N. Engl. J. Med.*, 292, 212, 1975.
275. **Monteleone, P. L., Nadler, H. L., Justice, P., and Hsia, D. Y.**, Glucose 6 phosphate dehydrogenase. Electrophoretic mobility of glucose 6 phosphate dehydrogenase in lymphocytes and granulocytes, *Clin. Chim. Acta*, 18, 275, 1967.
276. **Schneider, A. S., Valentine, W. N., Hattori, M., and Heins, H. L.**, Triose phosphate isomerase. 'Hereditary hemolytic anemia with triophosphate isomerase deficiency, *N. Engl. J. Med.*, 272, 229, 1965.
277. **Baughan, M. A., Valentine, W. N., Paglia, D. E., Ways, P. O., Simon, E. R., and DeMarsh, Q. B.**, Phosphohexose isomerase. Hereditary hemolytic anemia associated with glucose phosphate isomerase deficiency. A new enzyme defect of the erythrocytes, *Blood*, 30, 850, 1967.
278. **Valentine, W. N., Hsieh, H. S., Paglia, D. E., Anderson, H. M., Baughan, M. A., Jaffee, E. R., and Garson, A. M.**, Phosphoglycerate kinase. Hereditary hemolytic anemia associated with phosphoglycerate kinase deficiency in erythrocytes and leukocytes, *N. Engl. J. Med.*, 280, 528, 1969.
279. **Masson, P. K. and Lundblad, A.**, Mannosidosis: detection of the disease and of heterozygotes using serum and leucocytes, *Biochem. Biophys. Res. Comm.*, 56, 296, 1974.
280. **Vidgoff, J., Lovrien, E. W., Beals, R. K., and Buist, N. R. M.**, Mannosidosis in three brothers — a review of the literature, *Medicine*, 56, 335, 1977.
281. **Matsuda, I., Arashima, S., Anakura, M., and Oka, Y.**, α-L-Fucosidase and α-D mannosidase activity in the white blood cells in the disease and carrier state of fucosidosis, *Clin. Chim. Acta*, 48, 9, 1973.
282. **Fallon, H. J., Lotz, M., and Smith, L. H., Jr.**, Congenital orotic aciduria: demonstration of an enzyme defect in leukocytes and comparison with drug-induced orotic aciduria, *Blood*, 20, 700, 1962.
283. **Kelley, W. N., Rosenbloom, F. M., Henderson, J. F., and Seegmiller, J. E.**, A specific enzyme defect in gout associated with overproduction of uric acid, *Proc. Natl. Acad. Sci. U.S.A.*, 57, 1735, 1967.
284. **Choi, K. W. and Bloom, A. D.**, Biochemically marked lymphocytoid lines: establishment of Lesch-Nyhan cells, *Science*, 170, 89, 1970.
285. **Dancis, J., Hutzler, J., and Levitz, M.**, The diagnosis of Maple-Syrup Urine disease by the *in vitro* study of peripheral leukocytes, *Pediatrics*, 32, 234, 1963.
286. **Budd, M. A., Tanaka, K., Holmes, L. B., Efron, M. L., Crawford, J. D., and Isselbacher, K. J.**, Isovaleric aciduria. Clinical features of a new genetic defect of leucine metabolism, *N. Engl. J. Med.*, 277, 321, 1967.
287. **Dancis, J., Hutzler, J., Tada, K., Wada, Y., Morikawa, T., and Arakawa, T.**, Hypervalinemia. A defect in valine transamination, *Pediatrics*, 39, 813, 1967.
288. **Wysocki, S. J. and Hahnel, R.**, 3-Hydroxy-3-methylglutaric aciduria. 3-Hydroxy-3-methylglutaryl-coenzyme A lyase levels in leukocytes, *Clin. Chim. Acta*, 73, 373, 1976.
289. **Spielberg, S. P., Kramer, L. I., Goodman, S. I., Butler, J., Tietze, F., Quinn, P., and Shulman, J. D.**, 5-Oxoprolinuria: biochemical observations and case report, *J. Pediatr.*, 91, 237, 1977.
290. **Narisawa, K., Wada, Y., Saito, T., Suzuki, H., Kudo, M., Arakawa, T., Katsushima, N., and Tsuboi, R.**, Infantile type of homocystinuria with N.5,10-methylene tetrahydrofolate reductase defect, *Tohoku J. Exp. Med.*, 121, 185, 1977.
291. **Gregersen, N., Brandt, N. J., Christensen, E., Grøn, I., Rasmusen, K., and Brandt, S.**, Glutaric aciduria: clinical and laboratory findings in two brothers, *J. Pediatr.*, 90, 740, 1977.
292. **Tomlinson, S. and Westall, R. G.**, Argininosuccinic aciduria. Argininosuccinase and arginase in human blood cells, *Clin. Sci.*, 26, 261, 1964.
293. **Rosenberg, L. E., Lilljeqvist, A. C., and Hsia, Y. E.**, Methylmalonic aciduria, *N. Engl. J. Med.*, 278, 1319, 1968.
294. **Oberholzer, V. G., Levin, B., Burgess, E. A., and Young, W. F.**, Methylmalonic aciduria. An inborn error of metabolism leading to chronic metabolic acidosis, *Arch. Dis. Child.*, 42, 492, 1967.
295. **Morrow, G. and Barness, L. A.**, Studies in a patient with methylmalonic acidemia, *J. Pediatr.*, 74, 691, 1969.
296. **Schulman, J. D., Wong, V. G., Kuwabara, T., Bradley, K. H., and Seegmiller, J. E.**, Intracellular cystine content of leukocyte populations in cystinosis, *Arch. Intern. Med.*, 125, 660, 1970.
297. **Schneider, J. A., Bradley, K., and Seegmiller, J. E.**, Increased cystine in leukocytes from individuals homozygous and heterozygous for cystinosis, *Science*, 157, 1321, 1967.
298. **Brady, R. O.**, Genetics and the sphingolipidoses, *Med. Clin. North Am.*, 53, 827, 1969.
299. **Kampine, J. P., Brady, R. O., Kanfer, J. N., Feld, M., and Shapiro, D.**, Diagnosis of Gaucher's disease and Niemann-Pick disease with small samples of venous blood, *Science*, 155, 86, 1967.

300. **Poulos, A. and Pollard, A. C.**, A rapid method for the estimation of β-galactocerebrosidase, β-glucocerebrosidase and sphingomyelinase activities in leukocytes, *Clin. Chim. Acta*, 72, 327, 1976.
301. **Lazarus, S. S., Vehtamany, F. B., Schneck, L., and Volk, B. W.**, Fine structure and histochemistry of peripheral blood cells in Niemann-Pick disease, *Lab. Invest.*, 17, 155, 1967.
302. **Lott, I. T., Dulaney, J. T., Milunsky, A., Hoefnagel, D., and Moser, H. W.**, Apparent biochemical homozygosity in two obligatory heterozygotes for metachromatic leukodystrophy, *J. Pediatr.*, 89, 438, 1976.
303. **Percy, A. K. and Brady, R. O.**, Metachromatic leukodystrophy: diagnosis with samples of venous blood, *Science*, 161, 594, 1968.
304. **Kresse, H.**, Mucopolysaccharidosis IIIA (San Filippo A Disease): deficiency of heparin sulfamidase in skin fibroblasts and leucocytes, *Biochem. Biophys. Res. Comm.*, 54, 1111, 1973.
305. **Friedland, J., Schneck, L., Saifer, A., Pourfar, M., and Volk, B. W.**, Identification of Tay-Sachs' disease carriers by acrylamide gel electrophoresis, *Clin. Chim. Acta*, 28, 397, 1970.
306. **Okada, S. and O'Brien, J. S.**, Tay-Sachs' disease: generalized absence of a Beta-D-N-Acetylhexosaminidase component, *Science*, 165, 698, 1969.
307. **Okada, S. and O'Brien, J. S.**, Generalized gangliosidosis: beta-galactosidase deficiency, *Science*, 160, 1002, 1968.
308. **Tallman, J. F., Brady, R. O., Navon, R., and Padeh, B.**, Ganglioside catabolism in hexosaminidase A-deficient adults, *Nature (London)*, 252, 254, 1974.
309. **Dulaney, J. T., Milunsky, A., and Moser, H. W.**, Detection of the carrier state of Hurler's syndrome by assay of α-L-Iduronidase in leukocytes, *Clin. Chim. Acta*, 69, 305, 1976.
310. **Fogelman, A. M.**, Abnormal induction of 3-hydroxy-3-methyl glutaryl coenzyme A reductase in leukocytes from subjects with heterozygous familial hypercholesterolemia, *J. Biol. Chem.*, 250, 2045, 1975.
311. **Nadler, H. L. and Egan, T. J.**, Deficiency of lysosomal acid phosphatase, *N. Engl. J. Med.*, 282, 302, 1970.
312. **Salmon, S. E., Cline, M. J., Schultz, J., and Lehrer, R. I.**, Myeloperoxidase deficiency: immunologic study of a genetic leukocyte defect, *N. Engl. J. Med.*, 282, 250, 1970.
313. **Aebi, H., Jeunet, F., Richterich, R., Suter, H., Butler, R., Frie, J., and Marti, H. R.**, Observations in two Swiss families with acatalasia, *Enzymol. Biol. Clin.*, 2, 1, 1962.
314. **Baehner, R. L. and Karnovsky, M. L.**, Deficiency of reduced nicotinamide-adenine dinucleotide oxidase in chronic granulomatous disease, *Science*, 162, 1277, 1968.
315. **Holmes, B., Park, B. H., Malawista, S. E., Quie, P. G., Nelson, D. L., and Good, R. A.**, Chronic granulomatous disease in females. A deficiency of leukocyte glutathione peroxidase, *N. Engl. J. Med.*, 283, 217, 1970.
316. **Matsuda, I., Oka, Y., Taniguchi, N., Furuyama, M., Kodama, S., Aroshima, S., and Mitsuyama, T.**, Leukocyte glutathione peroxidase deficiency in a male patient with chronic granulomatous disease, *J. Pediatr.*, 88, 581, 1976.
317. **McPhail, L. C., DeChatelet, R., Shirley, P. S., Wilfert, C., Johnston, R. B., Jr., and McCall, C. E.**, Deficiency of NADPH oxidase activity in chronic granulomatous disease, *J. Pediatr.*, 90, 213, 1977.
318. **Yam, L. T., Li, C. Y., and Lam, K. W.**,Tartrate-resistant acid phosphatase isoenzyme in the reticulum cells of leukemic reticuloendotheliosis, *N. Engl. J. Med.*, 284, 357, 1971.
319. **Yam, L. T., Li, C. Y., and Finkel, H. E.**, Leukemic reticuloendotheliosis. The role of tartrate-resistant acid phosphatase in diagnosis and splenectomy in treatment, *Arch. Intern. Med.*, 130, 248, 1972.
320. **Kretchmer, N., Stone, M., and Bauer, C.**, Hereditary enzymatic effects as illustrated by hypophosphatasia, *Ann. N. Y. Acad. Sci.*, 75, 279, 1958.
321. **Beisel, W. R., Benjamin, N., and Austen, K. R.**, Absence of leukocyte alkaline phosphatase activity in hypophosphatasia, *Blood*, 14, 975, 1959.
322. **Armstrong, D., Dimmitt, S., Boehme, D. H., Leonberg, S. C., Jr., and Vogel, W.**, Leukocyte peroxidase deficiency in a family with a dominant form of Kuf's disease, *Science*, 186, 155, 1974.
323. **Danes, B. S., Foley, K. M., Dillon, S. D., and Bearn, A. G.**, Genetic study of cystic fibrosis of the pancreas using white blood cell cultures, *Nature, (London)*, 222, 685, 1969.
324. **Kalant, H. and Schucher, R.**, Concentration of galactose by leukocytes, *Can. J. Biochem. Physiol.*, 41, 849, 1963.
325. **Stjernholm, R. L. and Noble, E. P.**, Carbohydrate metabolism in leukocytes. IV. The metabolism of glucose and galactose in polymorphonuclear leukocytes from rabbits, *J. Biol. Chem.*, 236, 3093, 1961.
326. **Wulff, H. R.**, Histochemical studies of leukocytes from an inflammatory exudate. Glycogen and phosphorylase, *Acta Haematol.*, 28, 86, 1962.
327. **Esmann, V.**, The diabetic leukocyte, *Enzyme*, 13, 32, 1972.

328. **Gartner, I. and Norden, A.**, Studies on Periodic Acid-Schiff reactive material in white blood cells from the peripheral blood of patients with diabetes, polycythemia and chronic lymphocytic leukaemia, *Acta Med. Scand.*, 169, 289, 1961.
329. **Wagner, R.**, Glycogen content of isolated white blood cells in glycogen storage disease, *Am. J. Dis. Chld.*, 73, 559, 1947.
330. **Bloom, M. L. and Wislocki, G. B.**, The localization of lipids in human blood and bone marrow cells, *Blood*, 5, 79, 1950.
331. **Buchanan, A. A.**, Lipid synthesis by human leucocytes *in vitro*, *Biochem. J.*, 75, 315, 1960.
332. **Majerus, P. W. and Lastra, R.**, Fatty acid biosynthesis in human leukocytes, *J. Clin. Invest.*, 46, 1596, 1967.
333. **Marks, P. A, Gelhorn, A., and Kidson, C.**, Lipid synthesis in human leukocytes, platelets, and erythrocytes, *J. Biol. Chem.*, 235, 2579, 1960.
334. **Kimball, H. R., Ford, G. H., and Wolff, S. M.**, Lysosomal enzymes in normal and Chediak-Higashi blood leukocytes, *J. Lab. Clin. Med.*, 86, 616, 1975.
335. **Boxer, L. A., Rister, M., Allen, J. M., and Baehner, R. L.**, Improvement of Chediak-Higashi leukocyte function by cyclic guanosine monophosphate, *Blood*, 49, 9, 1977.
336. **Hoffbrand, A. V. and Newcomb, B. F. A.**, Leukocyte folate in vitamin B_{12} and folate deficiency in leukemia, *Br. J. Haematol.*, 13, 954, 1967.
337. **Swenseid, M. E., Bethell, F. H., and Bird, O. D.**, The concentration of folic acid in leukocytes: observations in normal subjects and persons with leukemia, *Cancer Res.*, 11, 864, 1951.
338. **Bertino, J. R., Silber, R., Freedman, M., Alenty, A., Albrecht, M., Gabrio, B. W., and Huennekens, F. M.**, Studies on normal and leukemic leukocytes. IV. Tetrahydrofolate-dependent enzyme systems and dihydrofolic reductase, *J. Clin. Invest.*, 42, 1899, 1963.
339. **Hall, C. A.**, Annotation: transport of vitamin B12 in man, *Br. J. Haematol.*, 16, 429, 1969.
340. **Lowry, O. H., Bessey, O. A., Brock, M. J., and Lopez, J. A.**, The interrelationship of dietary, serum, white blood cell and total body ascorbic acid, *J. Biol. Chem.*, 166, 111, 1946.
341. **Horn, R. G. and Spicer, S. S.**, Sulfonated mucopolysaccharide and basic protein in certain granules of rabbit leukocytes, *Lab. Invest.*, 13, 1, 1964.
342. **Groover, R. V., Burke, E. C., Gordon, H., and Berdon, W. E.**, The genetic mucopolysaccharidoses, *Semin. Hematol.*, 9, 371, 1972.
343. **Donahue, S., Watanabe, I., and Zeman, W.**, Morphology of leukocytic hypergranulation in Batten's disease, *Ann. N. Y. Acad. Sci.*, 155, 847, 1968.
344. **Cooperberg, A. A., Rosenberg, A., and Schwartz, J. P.**, Diagnostic value of bone marrow iron deposits in idiopathic hemochromatosis, *Arch. Intern. Med.*, 137, 748, 1977.
345. **Koszewski, B. J., Vahabzedeh, H., and Willrodt, B. S.**, Hemosiderin content of leukocytes in animals and man and its significance in the physiology of granulocytes, *Am. J. Clin. Pathol.*, 48, 474, 1967.
346. **Koszewski, B. J.**, Blood changes resulting from intravenous iron therapy: storage of hemosiderin in lymphocytes and monocytes, *Acta Haematol.*, 13, 217, 1955.
347. **Yam, L. T., Finkel, H. E., Weintraub, L. R., and Crosby, W. H.**, Circulating iron containing macrophages in hemochromatosis, *N. Engl. J. Med.*, 279, 514, 1968.
348. **Archer, R. K.**, The eosinophil leukocytes, *Ser. Haematol.*, 1, 3, 1968.
349. **Kay, A. B.**, Functions of the esoinophil leucocyte, *Br. J. Haematol.*, 33, 313, 1976.
350. **Mickenberg, I. D., Root, R. K., and Wolff, S. M.**, Bactericidal and metabolic properties of human eosinophils, *Blood*, 39, 67, 1972.
351. **Baehner, R. L. and Johnston, R. B., Jr.**, Metabolic and bactericidal activities of human eosinophils, *Br. J. Haematol.*, 20, 277, 1971.
352. **Bass, D. A.**, Behavior of eosinophil leukocytes in acute inflammation. I. Lack of dependence on adrenal function, *J. Clin. Invest.*, 55, 1229, 1975.
353. **Cline, M. J., Hanifin, J., and Lehrer, R. I.**, Phagocytosis by human eosinophils, *Blood*, 32, 922, 1968.
354. **Herion, J. C., Glasser, R. M., Walker, R. I., and Palmer, J. G.**, Eosinophil kinetics in two patients with eosinophilia, *Blood*, 36, 361, 1970.
355. **Seligman, A. M., Wasserkrug, H. L., Deb, C., and Hanker, J. S.**, Osmium containing compounds with multiple basic or acidic groups as stains for ultrastructure, *J. Histochem. Cytochem.*, 16, 87, 1968.
356. **Li, C. Y., Yam, L. T., and Crosby, W. H.**, Histochemical characterization of cellular and structural elements of the human spleen, *J. Histochem. Cytochem.*, 20, 1049, 1972.
357. **Ackerman, G. A.**, Cytochemical properties of the blood basophilic granulocytes, *Ann. N.Y. Acad. Sci.*, 103, 376, 1963.
358. **Wolf-Jurgensen, P.**, The basophilic leukocyte, *Ser. Haematol.*, 1, 4, 1968.
359. **Thonnard, N. E.**, Studies of basophils: variations with age and sex, *Acta Haematol.*, 30, 221, 1963.

360. **Behrens, M. and Taubert, M.**, Der Nachweiss von Heparin in den basophilen Leukocyten, *Klin. Wochenschr.*, 30, 76, 1952.
361. **Olinger, E. J., McCarthy, D. M., Younger, R. C., and Gardner, J. D.**, Hyperhistaminemia and hyperchlorhydria in basophilic granulocytic leukemia, *Gastroenterology*, 71, 667, 1976.
362. **Dvorak, H. F., Selvaggio, S. S., Dvorak, A. M., Colvin, R. B., Lean, D. B., and Rypysc, J.**, Purification of basophilic leukocytes from guinea pig blood and bone marrow, *J. Immunol.*, 113, 1694, 1974.
363. **Bond, V. P., Fliedner, T. M., Cronkite, E. P., Rubini, J. R., Bretcher, G., and Schork, P. K.**, Proliferation potentials of bone marrow and blood cells studied by *in vitro* uptake of ^{3}H thymidine, *Acta Haematol.*, 21, 1, 1959.
364. **McIntyre, O. R. and Ebaugh, F. G., Jr.**, The effect of phytohemagglutinin on leukocyte cultures as measured by ^{32}P incorporation in the DNA, RNA and acid soluble fractions, *Blood*, 19, 443, 1962.
365. **Torelli, U. L., Henry, P. H., and Weissman, S. M.**, Characteristics of the RNA synthesized *in vitro* by the normal human small lymphocyte and the changes induced by phytohemagglutinin stimulation, *J. Clin. Invest.*, 47, 1083, 1968.
366. **Weisberger, A. S. and Levine, B.**, Incorporation of radioactive L cystine by normal and leukemic leukocytes *in vitro*, *Blood*, 9, 1082, 1954.
367. **Bach, F. and Hirschhorn, K.**, γ-Globulin production by human lymphocytes *in vitro*, *Exp. Cell Res.*, 32, 592, 1963.
368. **Frei, J., Borel, C., Horvath, G., Cullity, B., and Vannotti, A.**, Enzymatic studies on the different types of normal and leukemic human white cells. *Blood*, 18: 317, 1961.
369. **Hedeskov, C. J. and Essman, V.**, Respiration and glycolysis of normal human lymphocytes, *Blood*, 28, 163, 1966.
370. **Packman, L. M.**, The carbohydrate metabolism and respiration of isolated small lymphocytes: *in vitro* studies of normal and PHA stimulated cells, *Blood*, 30, 691, 1967.
371. **Yam, L. T.**, unpublished observation.
372. **Hayhoe, F. G. J.**, The cytochemical demonstration of lipids in blood and bone marrow cells, *J. Pathol. Bacteriol.*, 65, 413, 1953.
373. **Sehrt, E.**, Die histologische Darstellung der lipoiden der weissen Blutzellen (Neutro u Eosinophile Leukocyten, Mastzellen, uberganszellen u Mononukleäre) ud Beziehungdiese lipoide zur Oxydase Reaktion, *Münch Med. Woschenschr.*, 74, 139, 1927.
374. **Sheehan, H. L. and Storey, G. W.**, An improved method of staining leukocyte granules with Sudan Black B, *J. Pathol. Bacteriol.*, 59, 336, 1947.
375. **Burns, C. P., Welshman, I. R., and Spector, A. A.**, Differences in free fatty acid and glucose metabolism of human blood neutrophils and lymphocytes, *Blood*, 47, 431, 1976.
376. **Anlyan, A. J., Gamble, J., and Hoster, H. A.**, Beta-glucuronidase activity of the leukocytes in human leukemias and Hodgkin's disease, *Cancer*, 3, 116, 1950.
377. **Woessner, S., Milla, F., and Rozman, C.** A study of lymphocytic β-glucuronidase in various benign and malignant lymphatic processes, *Acta Haematol.*, 51, 84, 1974.
378. **Yam, L. T. and Mitus, W. J.**, The lymphocyte β-glucuronidase activity in lymphoproliferative disorders, *Blood*, 31, 480, 1968.
379. **Catovsky, D.**, T cell origin of acid phosphatase — positive lymphoblasts, *Lancet*, 2, 327, 1975.
380. **Valentine, W. N. and Beck, W. S.**, Biochemical studies on leukocytes. I. Phosphatase activity in health, leukocytosis and myelocytic leukemia, *J. Lab. Clin. Med.*, 38, 39, 1951.
381. **Flandrin, G. and Daniel, M. T.**, β-Glucuronidase activity in Sezary cells, *Scand. J. Haematol.*, 12, 23, 1974.
382. **Nowell, P. C.**, Phytohemagglutinin: an imitator of mitosis in cultures of normal human leukocytes, *Cancer Res.*, 20, 462, 1960.
383. **Galbraith, P., Mitus, W. J., Gollerkeri, M., and Dameshek, W.**, The "infectious mononucleosis cell". A cytochemical study, *Blood*, 22, 630, 1963.
384. **Davey, F. R. and Gottlieb, A. J.**, Lymphocyte surface markers in acute lymphocytic leukemia, *Am. J. Clin. Pathol.*, 62, 818, 1974.
385. **Glick, A. D. Leech, J. H., Waldron, J. A., Flexner, J. M., Horn, R. G., and Collins, R. D.**, Malignant lymphomas of follicular center cell origin in man. II. Ultrastructural and cytochemical studies, *J. Natl. Cancer Inst.*, 54, 23, 1975.
386. **Lukes, R. J. and Collins, R. D.**, Immunologic characterization of human malignant lymphomas, *Cancer*, 34, 1488, 1974.
387. **Yam, L. T., Tavassoli, M., and Jacobs, P.**, Differential characterization of the reticulum in lymphoreticular neoplasms, *Am. J. Clin. Pathol.*, 64, 171, 1975.
388. **Belcher, R. W.**, Ultrastructure and cytochemistry of lymphocytes in the genetic mucopolysaccharidoses, *Arch. Pathol.*, 93, 1, 1972.

389. **Nadler, H. L., Dowben, R. M., and Hsia, D. Y. Y.**, Enzyme changes and polyribosome profiles in phytohemagglutinin stimulated lymphocytes, *Blood*, 34, 52, 1969.
390. **Fischer, R. and Gropp, A.**, Cytochemie des lymphocyten in vitro, *Klin. Wochenschr.*, 13, 733, 1966.
391. **Rozenszajn, L. A. and Fischer, D.**, Enzymatic and chemical changes in human lymphocyte cultures, *Acta Haematol.*, 42, 138, 1969.
392. **Ackerman, G. A.**, Histochemistry of normal and leukemic lymphocytes, *J. Histochem. Cytochem.*, 7 (Abstr.), 318, 1959.
393. **Christensen, B. and Ottesen, J.**, The age of leukocytes in the bloodstream of patients with chronic lymphocytic leukemia, *Acta Haematol.*, 13, 289, 1955.
394. Editorial, Membrane markers in lymphoproliferative disorders, *Lancet*, 1, 670, 1975.
395. **Pernis, B., Forni, L., and Amante, L.**, Immunoglobulin spots on the surface of rabbit lymphocytes, *J. Exp. Med.*, 132, 1001, 1970.
396. **Raff, M. C., Sternberg, M., and Taylor, R. B.**, Immunoglobulin determinants on the surface of mouse lymphoid cells, *Nature, (London)*, 225, 553, 1970.
397. **Sciorra, L. and Eckert, C.**, Distinguishing T and B lymphocytes by light microscopy and Normarski optics, *Lancet*, 2, 1526, 1974.
398. **Vila, J. M. and Taub, R. N.**, Normarski optics and T and B markers, *Lancet*, 1, 977, 1975.
399. **Basten, A., Miller, J. F. A. P., Sprent, M. J., and Pye, J.**, A receptor for antibody on B lymphocytes. I. Method of detection and functional significance, *J. Exp. Med.*, 135, 610, 1972.
400. **Papamichail, M., Brown, J. C., and Holborow, E. J.**, Immunoglobulins on the surface of human lymphocytes, *Lancet*, 2, 850, 1971.
401. **Raff, M. C.**, Two distinct populations of peripheral lymphocytes in mice distinguishable by immunofluorescence, *Immunology*, 19, 637, 1970.
402. **Unanue, E. R., Grey, H. M., Rabellino, E., Campbell, P., and Schmidtke, J.**, Immunoglobulins on the surface of lymphocytes. II. The bone marrow as the main source of lymphocytes with detectable surfacebound immunoglobulin, *J. Exp. Med.*, 133, 1188, 1971.
403. **Warfel, A. H. and Elberg, S. S.**, Macrophage membranes viewed through a scanning electron microscope, *Science*, 170, 446, 1970.
404. **Jaffe, E. S., Shevach, E. M., Frank, M. M., Berard, C. W., and Green, I.**, Nodular lymphoma — evidence for origin from follicular B lymphocytes, *N. Engl. J. Med.*, 290, 813, 1974.
405. **Itoh, G., Miura, S., and Suzuki, I.**, Immunohistochemical detection of Fc receptor. I. Light microscopic demonstration of Fc receptor by using soluble immune complexes of peroxidase-antiperoxidase immunoglobulin G, *J. Histochem. Cytochem.*, 25, 252, 1977.
406. **Valdimarsson, H., Agnarsdottir, G., and Lachmann, P. J.**, Measles virus receptor on human T lymphocytes, *Nature, (London)*, 255, 554, 1975.
407. **Plaut, M., Lichtenstein, L. M., and Henney, C. S.**, Properties of a subpopulation of T cells bearing histamine receptors, *J. Clin. Invest.*, 55, 856, 1975.
408. **Jondal, M., Holm, G., and Wigzell, H.**, Surface markers on human T and B lymphocytes. I. A large population of lymphocytes forming nonimmune rosettes with sheep red blood cells, *J. Exp. Med.*, 136, 207, 1972.
409. **Wybran, J., Carr, M. C., and Fudenberg, H. H.**, The human rosette-forming cell as a marker of a population of thymus-derived cells, *J. Clin. Invest.*, 51, 2537, 1972.
410. **Bianco, C., Patrick, R., and Nussenzweig, V.**, A population of lymphocytes bearing a membrane receptor for antigen-antibody-complement complexes. I. Separation and characterization, *J. Exp. Med.*, 132, 702, 1970.
411. **Shevach, E. M., Herberman, R., Frank, M. M., and Green, I.**, Receptor for complement and immunoglobulin on human leukemic cells and human lymphoblastoid cell lines, *J. Clin. Invest.*, 51, 1933, 1972.
412. **Haegert, D. G., Cawley, J. C., Karpas, A., and Goldstone, A. H.**, Combined T and B cell acute lymphoblastic leukaemia, *Br. Med. J.*, 4, 79, 1974.
413. **Stein, H. and Müller-Hermelink, H. K.**, Simultaneous presence of receptors for complement and sheep red blood cells on human fetal thymocytes, *Br. J. Haematol.*, 36, 225, 1977.
414. **Collins, R. D., Smith, J. L., Clein, G. P., and Barker, C. R.**, Absence of B and T cell markers on acute lymphoblastic leukaemic cells and persistence of the T cell marker on mitogen transformed T lymphocytes, *Br. J. Haematol.*, 26, 615, 1974.
415. **Kaplan, J., Ravindranath, Y., and Peterson, W. D., Jr.**, T and B lymphocyte antigen positive Null cell leukemias, *Blood*, 49, 371, 1977.
416. **Böyum, A.**, Isolation of mononuclear cells and granulocytes from human blood, *Scand. J. Clin. Invest.*, 21 (Suppl. 97), 77, 1968.
417. **Chanarat, P. and Chiewsilp, P.**, A simple method for the elimination of platelets from the lymphocyte platelet mixture by sucrose, *Am. J. Clin. Pathol.*, 63, 237, 1975.

418. **Zucker-Franklin, D.**, The percentage of monocytes among "mononuclear" cell fractions obtained from normal human blood, *J. Immunol.*, 112, 234, 1974.
419. **Greaves, M. F. and Brown, G.**, Purification of human T and B lymphocytes , *J. Immunol.*, 112, 420, 1974.
420. **Wybran, J., Chantler, S., and Fudenberg, H. H.**, Isolation of normal T cells in chronic lymphatic leukaemia, *Lancet*, 1, 126, 1973.
421. **Oppenheim, J. J. and Schecter, B.**, Lymphocyte transformation, in *Manual of Clinical Immunology*, Rose, N. R. and Friedman, H., Eds., American Society for Microbiology, Washington, D.C., 1976, 81.
422. **Greaves, M., Janossy, G., and Doenhoff, M.**, Selective triggering of human T and B lymphocytes *in vitro* by polyclonal mitogens, *J. Exp. Med.*, 140, 1, 1974.
423. **Ringoir, S. and Plum, J.**, LDH isozymes of human T and B lymphocytes, *Clin. Chim. Acta*, 60, 379, 1975.
424. **Moller, G.**, Effect of B cell mitogens on lymphocyte subpopulations possessing C'3 and Fc receptors, *J. Exp. Med.*, 139, 969, 1974.
425. **Catovsky, D., Goldman, J. M., Okos, A., Frisch, B., and Galton, D. A. G.**, T Lymphoblastic leukaemia: a distinct variant of acute leukaemia, *Brit. Med. J.*, 2, 643, 1974.
426. **Gajl-Peczalska, K. J., Park, B. H., Biggar, W. D., and Good, R. A.**, B and T lymphocytes in primary immunodeficiency disease in man, *J. Clin. Invest.*, 52, 919, 1973.
427. **Gajl-Peczalska, K. J., Bloomfield, C. D., Coccia, P. F., Sosin, H., Brunning, R. D., and Kersey, J. H.**, B and T cell lymphomas. Analysis of blood and lymph nodes in 87 patients, *Am. J. Med.*, 59, 674, 1975.
428. **Kaplan, J., Mastrangelo, R., and Peterson, W. D., Jr.**, Childhood lymphoblastic lymphoma, a cancer of thymus-derived lymphocytes, *Cancer Res.*, 34, 521, 1974.
429. **Kersey, J. H., Sabad, A., Gajl-Peczalska, K., Hallgren, H. M., Yunis, E. J., and Nesbit, M. E.**, Acute lymphoblastic leukemic cells with T (thymus-derived) lymphocyte markers, *Science*, 182, 1355, 1973.
430. **Wybran, J. and Fudenberg, H. H.**, T cells in chronic lymphatic leukemia, *Lancet*, 2, 265, 1973.
431. **Wybran, J. and Fudenberg, H. H.**, Thymus-derived rosette-forming cells in various human disease states: cancer, lymphoma, bacterial and viral infections, and other diseases, *J. Clin. Invest.*, 52, 1026, 1973.
432. **Flandrin, G., Brouet, J. C., Daniel, M. T., and Preud'homme, J. L.**, Acute leukemia with Burkitt's tumor cells: a study of six cases with special reference to lymphocyte surface markers, *Blood*, 43, 183, 1975.
433. **Gajl-Peczalska, K. J., Bloomfield, C. D., Nesbit, M. E., and Kersey, J. H.**, B cell markers on lymphoblasts in acute lymphoblastic leukemia, *Clin. Exp. Immunol.*, 17, 561, 1974.
434. **Grey, H. M., Rabellino, E., and Pirofsky, B.**, Immunoglobulins on the surface of lymphocytes. IV. Distribution in hypogammaglobulinemia, cellular immune deficiency and chronic lymphatic leukemia, *J. Clin. Invest.*, 50, 2368, 1971.
435. **Pincus, S., Bianco, C., and Nussenzweig, V.**, Increased proportion of complement-receptor lymphocytes in the peripheral blood of patients with chronic lymphocytic leukemia, *Blood*, 40, 303, 1972.
436. **Preud'homme, J. L. and Seligmann, M.**, Surface bound immunoglobulins as a cell marker in human lymphoproliferative diseases, *Blood*, 40, 777, 1972.
437. **Stein, H., Lennert, K., and Parwaresch, M. R.**, Malignant lymphomas of B cell type, *Lancet*, 2, 855, 1972.
438. **Wilson, J. D. and Hurdle, D. F.**, Surface immunoglobulins on lymphocytes in chronic lymphocytic leukemia and lymphosarcoma, *Br. J. Haematol.*, 24, 563, 1973.
439. **Axline, S. G.**, Functional biochemistry of the macrophage, *Semin. Hematol.*, 7, 142, 1970.
440. Editorial, Proliferating and phagocytic histiocytes, *Lancet*, 2, 937, 1974.
441. **Myrvik, Q. N., Leake, E. S., and Fariss, B.**, Pulmonary alveolar macrophages from the normal rabbit: a technique to procure them in a high state of purity, *J. Immunol.*, 86, 128, 1961.
442. **Myrvik, Q. N., Leake, E. S., and Oshima, S.**, A study of macrophages and epithelioid-like cells from granulomatous lungs of rabbits, *J. Immunol.*, 89, 745, 1962.
443. **Bennett, W. E. and Cohn, Z. A.**, The isolation and selected properties of blood monocytes, *J. Exp. Med.*, 123, 145, 1964.
444. **Loos, H., Blok-Schut, B., Van Doorn, R., Hoksbergen, R., de la RiViere, A. B., and Meerhof, L.**, A method for recognition and separation of human blood monocytes and density gradient, *Blood*, 48, 731, 1976.
445. **Askonas, B. A. and Rhodes, J. M.**, Immunogenicity of antigen containing ribonucleic acid preparations from macrophages, *Nature, (London)*, 205, 470, 1965.

446. **Stecher, V. J.,** Synthesis of proteins by mononuclear phagocytes, in *Mononuclear Phagocytes,* Van Furth, V., Ed., F. A. Davis, Philadelphia, 1970, 133.
447. **Dannenberg, A. M., Burstone, M. S., Walter, P. C., and Kinsley, J. W.,** A histochemical study of phagocytic and enzymatic functions of rabbit mononuclear and polymorphonuclear exudate cells and alveolar macrophages, *J. Cell. Biol.,* 17, 465, 1963.
448. **Dannenberg, A. M., Jr. and Bennett, W. E.,** Hydrolytic enzymes of rabbit mononuclear exudate cells, *J. Cell Biol.,* 21, 1, 1964.
449. **Jansa, P. and Kratky, J.,** Enzyme pattern of macrophages in the course of inflammation, *Blut,* 18, 218, 1969.
450. **Roque, A. L. and Pickren, J. W.,** Enzymatic changes in fluorescent alveolar macrophages of the lungs of cigarette smokers, *Acta Cytol.,* 12, 420, 1968.
451. **Cline, M. J. and Lehrer, R. I.,** Phagocytosis by human monocytes, *Blood,* 32, 423, 1968.
452. **Karnovsky, M. L.,** Metabolic basis of phagocytic activity, *Physiol. Rev.,* 42, 143, 1962.
453. **Iyer, G. Y. N., Islam, M. E., and Quastel, J. H.,** Biochemical aspects of phagocytosis, *Nature, (London),* 192, 535, 1961.
454. **Oren, R., Farnham, A. E., Saito, K., Milosky, E., and Karnovsky, M. L.,** Metabolic patterns in three types of phagocytizing cells, *J. Cell Biol.,* 17, 487, 1963.
455. **Ouchi, E., Selvaraj, R. J., and Sbarra, A. J.,** The biochemical activities of rabbit alveolar macrophages during phagocytosis, *Exp. Cell. Res.,* 40, 456, 1965.
456. **Byers, S. O.,** Lipids and the reticuloendothelial system, *Ann. N. Y. Acad. Sci.,* 88, 240, 1960.
457. **Day, A. J.,** Lipid metabolism by macrophages and its relation to atherosclerosis, *Adv. Lipid Res.,* 5, 185, 1967.
458. **Hopsu, V. K. and Glenner, G. G.,** Further observations on histochemical esterase and amidase activities with similarities to trypsin, *J. Histochem. Cytochem.,* 11, 520, 1963.
459. **Uvnas, B. and Thon, I.,** Isolation of "biologically intact" mast cells, *Exp. Cell Res.,* 18, 512, 1959.
460. **Schrek, R. and Donnelly, W. J.,** "Hairy" cells in blood and in lymphoreticular neoplastic disease and "flagellated" cells of normal lymph nodes, *Blood,* 27, 199, 1966.
461. **Mitus, W. J.,** Hairy cells and isoenzymes, *N. Engl. J. Med.,* 284, 389, 1971.
462. **Bouroncle, B. A., Wiseman, B. K., and Doan, C. A.,** Leukemic reticuloendotheliosis, *Blood,* 13, 609, 1958.
463. **Burns, C. P. and Hoak, J. C.,** Freeze-etching, scanning and thin-section electron microscopic studies of the "hairy" leukocytes in leukemic reticuloendotheliosis, *J. Natl. Cancer Inst.,* 51, 743, 1973.
464. **Golomb, H. M., Braylan, R., and Polliack, A.,** "Hairy" cell leukaemia (leukaemic reticuloendotheliosis): a scanning electron microscopic study of eight cases, *Br. J. Haematol.,* 29, 455, 1975.
465. **Katayama, I., Li, C. Y., and Yam, L. T.,** Ultrastructural characteristics of the hairy cells of leukemic reticuloendotheliosis, *Am. J. Pathol.,* 67, 361, 1972.
466. **Daniel, M. T. and Flandrin, G.,** Fine structure of abnormal cells in hairy cell (tricholeukocytic) leukemia , with special reference to their *in vitro* phagocytic capacity, *Lab. Invest.,* 30, 1, 1974.
467. **Brunning, R. D. and Parkin, J.,** Ribosome lamella complexes in neoplastic hemopoietic cells, *Am. J. Pathol.,* 79, 565, 1975.
468. **Stefani, S., Chandra, S., Schrek, R., Tonaki, H., and Knospe, W. H.,** Endoplasmic reticulum-associated structures in lymphocytes from patients with chronic lymphocytic leukemia, *Blood,* 50, 125, 1977.
469. **Mitus, W. J., Mednicoff, I. B., Wittels, B., and Dameshek, W.,** Neoplastic lymphoid reticulum cells in the peripheral blood: a histochemical study, *Blood,* 17, 206, 1961.
470. **Schmalzl, F., Huhn, D., Asamer, H., and Braunsteiner, H.,** Hairy cell leukemia ("leukemic reticuloendotheliosis"), reticulosarcoma and monocytic leukemia. Cytochemical and ultrastructural investigations, *Acta Haematol.,* 53, 257, 1975.
471. **Trubowitz, S., Masek, B., and Frasca, J. M.,** Leukemic reticuloendotheliosis, *Blood,* 38, 288, 1971.
472. **Burns, C. P., Maca, R. D., and Hoak, J. C.,** Biochemical, morphological and immunological observations of leukemic reticuloendotheliosis, *Cancer Res.,* 33, 1615, 1973.
473. **Debusscher, L., Bernheim, J. L., Collard-Ronge, E., Covaerts, A., Hooghe, R., Lejeune, F. J., Zeicher, M., and Stryckmans, P. A.,** Hairy cell leukemia: functional, immunologic, kinetic and ultrastructural characterization, *Blood,* 46, 495, 1975.
474. **Yam, L. T., Castoldi, G. L., Garvey, M. B., and Mitus, W. J.,** Functional, cytogenetic and cytochemical study of the leukemic reticulum cells, *Blood,* 32, 90, 1968.
475. **Utsinger, P. D., Yount, W. J., Fuller, C. R., Logue, M. J., and Orringer, E. P.,** Hairy cell leukemia: B-lymphocyte and phagocytic properties, *Blood,* 49, 19, 1977.
476. **Aisenberg, A. C. and Bloch, K. J.,** Immunoglobulins on the surface of neoplastic lymphocytes, *N. Engl. J. Med.,* 287, 272, 1972.
477. **Golde, D. W., Stevens, R. H., Quan, S. G., and Saxon, A.,** Immunoglobulin synthesis in hairy cell leukemia, *Br. J. Haematol.,* 35, 359, 1977.

478. **Haak, H. L., De Man, J. D. H., Hijmans, W., Knapp, W., and Speck, B.,** Further evidence for the lymphocytic nature of leukaemic reticuloendotheliosis (hairy cell leukemia), *Br. J. Haematol.*, 27, 31, 1974.
479. **Catovsky, D., Pettit, J. E., Galetto, J., Okos, A., and Galton, D. A. G.,** The B-lymphocyte nature of the hairy cell of leukaemic reticuloendotheliosis, *Br. J. Haematol.*, 26, 29, 1974.
480. **Jaffe, E. S., Shevach, E. M., Frank, M. M., and Green, I.,** Leukemic reticuloendotheliosis: presence of a receptor for cytophilic antibody, *Am. J. Med.*, 57, 108, 1974.
481. **Scheinberg, M., Brenner, A. I., Sullivan, A. L., Cathcart, E. S., and Katayama, I.,** The heterogeneity of leukemic reticuloendotheliosis, "hairy cell leukemia". Evidence for its monocytic origin, *Cancer*, 37, 1302, 1976.
482. **Seshadri, R. S., Brown, E. J., and Zipursky, A.,** Leukemic reticuloendotheliosis. A failure of monocyte production, *N. Engl. J. Med.*, 295, 181, 1976.
483. **Streefkerk, J. G. and Veerman, A. J. P.,** Histochemistry and electron microscopy of follicle lining reticular cells in the rat spleen, *Z. Zellforsch.*, 115, 524, 1971.
484. **Morris, M. W. and Davey, F. R.,** Immunologic and cytochemical properties of histiocytic and mixed histiocytic-lymphocytic lymphomas, *Am. J. Clin. Pathol.*, 63, 403, 1975.
485. **Taylor, C. R.,** The nature of Reed-Sternberg cells and other malignant "reticulum" cells, *Lancet*, 2, 802, 1974.
486. **Perls, M.,** Nachweis von Eisenoxyd in gewissen Pigmenten, *Virchows Arch. Pathol. Anat. Physiol.*, 39, 42, 1867.
487. **Gomori, G.,** Microtechnical demonstration of phosphatase in tissue sections, *Proc. Soc. Exp. Biol. Med.*, 42, 23, 1939.
488. **Gomori, G.,** Histochemical staining methods, in *Methods in Medical Research*, Vol. 4, Visscher, M. B., Ed., The Year Book Publishers, Chicago, 1951, 14.
489. **Rabinovitch, M. and Andreucci, D.,** A histochemical study of acid and alkaline phosphatase distribution in normal human bone marrow smears, *Blood*, 4, 580, 1949.
490. **Richter, M. N.,** Leukemia, the relative values of cell morphology and the peroxidase reaction as diagnostic aids, *Arch. Intern. Med.*, 36, 13, 1925.
491. **Sato, A. and Sekiya, S.,** A simple method for differentiation of myeloid and lymphatic leukocytes, *Tohoku J. Exp. Med.*, 7, 111, 1926.
492. **Washburn, A. H.,** A combined peroxidase and Wright's stain for routine blood smears, *J. Lab. Clin. Med.*, 14, 246, 1928.
493. **Burstone, M. S.,** *Enzyme Histochemistry and Its Application in the Study of Neoplasms*, Academic Press, New York, 1962.
494. **Burstone, M. S. and Folk, J. E.,** Histochemical demonstration of aminopeptidase, *J. Histochem.*, 4, 217, 1956.
495. **Burstone, M. S.,** New histochemical techniques for demonstration of tissue oxidase (cytochrome oxidase), *J. Histochem. Cytochem.*, 7, 112, 1959.
496. **Wachstein, M.,** The distribution of histochemically demonstrable glycogen in human blood and bone marrow cells, *Blood*, 4, 54, 1949.
497. **Wachstein, M. and Meisel, E.,** Histochemistry of hepatic phosphatases of physiological pH: with special reference to demonstration of bile canaliculi, *Am. J. Clin. Pathol.*, 27, 13, 1957.
498. **Wachstein, M.,** Alkaline phosphatase activity in normal and abnormal human blood and bone marrow cells, *J. Lab. Clin. Med.*, 31, 1, 1946.
499. **Hayhoe, F. G. J.,** Quaglino, D., and Doll, R., *The Cytology and Cytochemistry of Acute Leukemias*, Her Majesty's Stationery Office, London, 1964, 25.
500. **Dorfman, R. F.,** Enzyme Histochemistry of Normal, Hyperplastic, and Neoplastic Lymphoreticular Tissues, Symp. Lymph Tumours in Africa, 1963, 304.
501. **Stutte, H. J. and Gluck, W.,** Uber Gitterfaserdarstellung an Fermenthistochemischen Praparaten, *Histochemie*, 5, 130, 1965.
502. **Stutte, H. J.,** Nature of human spleen red pulp cells with special reference to sinus lining cells, *Z. Zellforschung*, 91, 300, 1968.
503. **Deimling, O. V. and Böcking, A.,** Esterases in histochemistry and ultrahistochemistry, *Histochem. J.*, 8, 215, 1976.
504. **Kaplow, L. S. and Burstone, M. S.,** Acid buffered acetone as a fixative for enzyme cytochemistry, *Nature, (London)*, 200, 690, 1963.
505. **Burstone, M. S.,** The relationship between fixation and techniques for the histochemical localization of hydrolytic enzymes, *J. Histochem. Cytochem.*, 6, 322, 1958.
506. **Gough, J. and Elves, M. W.,** Studies of lymphocytes and their derivative cells *in vitro*. I. Biochemical constituents, *Acta Haematol.*, 36, 344, 1966.
507. **Pease, A. G. E.,** Cetyl pyridinium salt for fixative of metachromasia, in *Histochemistry*, Vol. 1, 3rd ed., Little, Brown, Boston, 1968, 604.

508. **Kaplow, L. S. and Burstone, M. S.**, Cytochemical demonstration of acid phosphatase in hemopoietic cells in health and in various hematological disorders using azo dye techniques, *J. Histochem. Cytochem.*, 12, 805, 1964.
509. **Stuart, J. and Simpson, J. S.**, Dehydrogenase enzyme cytochemistry of unfixed leucocytes, *J. Clin. Pathol.*, 23, 517, 1970.
510. **Katayama, I., Li, C. Y., and Yam, L. T.**, Ultrastructural cytochemical demonstration of tartrate resistant acid phosphatase isoenzyme activity in hairy cells of leukemic reticuloendotheliosis, *Am. J. Pathol.*, 69, 471, 1972.
511. **Kaplow, L. S.**, Cytochemical heterogeneity of human circulating monocytes, *Acta Cytol.*, 19, 358, 1975.
512. **Avrameas, S.**, Coupling of enzymes to proteins with glutaraldehyde. Use of the conjugates for the detection of antigens and antibodies, *Immunochemistry*, 6, 43, 1969.
513. **Nakane, P. K. and Kawaoi, A.**, Peroxidase-labeled antibody. A new method of conjugation, *J. Histochem. Cytochem.*, 22, 1084, 1974.
514. **Sternberger, L. A., Hardy, P. H., Cuculis, J. J., and Meyer, H. G.**, The unlabeled antibody enzyme method of immunohistochemistry, *J. Histochem. Cytochem.*, 18, 315, 1970.
515. **Taylor, C. R. and Burns, J.**, The demonstration of plasma cells and other immunoglobulin-containing cells in formalin fixed paraffin-embedded tissues using peroxidase-labelled antibody, *J. Clin. Pathol.*, 27, 14, 1974.
516. **Baba, N., Hurtubise, P., and Myser, T.**, Immunofluorescence and immunoperoxidase observations of anti-lactic dehydrogenase-1 antibody, *J. Histochem. Cytochem.*, 24, 572, 1976.
517. **Erlandsen, S. L., Parsons, J. A., Burke, J. P., Redick, J. A., Van Orden, D. E., and Van Orden, L. S.**, A modification of the unlabeled antibody enzyme method using heterologous antisera for the light microscopic and ultrastructural localization of insulin, glucagon and growth hormone, *J. Histochem. Cytochem.*, 23, 666, 1975.
518. **Lin, C. T., Chang, J. P., and Chen, J. P.**, Ultrastructural localization of γ-chain and immunoglobulin G in human lymphocytes using enzyme labeled Fab fragment, *J. Histochem. Cytochem.*, 23, 624, 1975.
519. **Miller, M. H., Karnovsky, M. J., and Diamandopoulos, G. T.**, An improved immunoperoxidase technique for identifying SV40V and T antigens by light microscopy, *Proc. Soc. Exp. Biol. Med.*, 146, 432, 1974.
520. **Pickel, V. M., Joh, T. H., Field, P. M., Becker, C. G., and Reis, D. J.**, Cellular localization of tyrosine hydroxylase by immunohistochemistry, *J. Histochem. Cytochem.*, 23, 1, 1975.
521. **Wendelschafer-Crabb, G., Erlandsen, S. L., and Walker, D. H., Jr.**, Ultrastructural localization of viral antigens using the unlabeled antibody-enzyme method, *J. Histochem. Cytochem.*, 24, 517, 1976.
522. **Wilcox, M. B., Golde, D. W., and Cline, M. J.**, Cytochemical reactions of hemopoietic cells in liquid culture, *J. Histochem. Cytochem.*, 2, 979, 1976.
523. **Zucker-Franklin, D. and Grusky, G.**, The identification of eosinophil colonies in soft agar cultures by differential staining for peroxidase, *J. Histochem. Cytochem.*, 24, 1270, 1976.
524. **Allen, J. M. and Hunter, R. L.**, A histochemical study of enzymes in the epididymis of normal, castrated, and hormone replaced castrated mice separated by zonal electrophoresis in starch gel, *J. Histochem. Cytochem.*, 8, 50, 1960.
525. **Allen, R. C., Popp, R. A., and Moore, D. J.**, Separation and relative quantitation of mouse plasma esterases with disc electrophoresis, *J. Histochem. Cytochem*, 13, 249, 1965.
526. **Hunter, R. L. and Burstone, M. S.** The zymogram as a tool for the characterization of enzyme substrate specificity, *J. Histochem. Cytochem.*, 8, 58, 1960.
527. **Markert, C. L. and Hunter, R. L.**, The distribution of esterases in mouse tissue, *J. Histochem. Cytochem.*, 7, 42, 1959.
528. **Milisauskas, V. and Rose, N. R.**, Immunochemical quantitation of prostatic phosphatase, *Clin. Chem.*, 18, 1529, 1972.
529. **Lanzerotti, R. H. and Gulliano, P. M.**, Immunochemical quantitation of enzymes using multispecific antisera, *Anal. Biochem.*, 50, 344, 1972.
530. **Tycko, D. H., Anbalagan, S., Liu, H. C., and Ornstein, L.**, Automatic leukocyte classification using cytochemically stained smears, *J. Histochem. Cytochem.*, 24, 178, 1976.
531. **Grusovin, G. D. and Castoldi, G. L.**, Characterization of blast cells in acute non-lymphoid leukemias by consecutive cytochemical methods, *Acta Haematol.*, 55, 338, 1976.
532. **James, V. and Price, P. W.**, Esterase and acid phosphatases in the identification of cell types in leukemia, *J. Clin. Pathol.*, 27, 928, 1974.
533. **Yam, L. T., Li, C. Y., Wolfe, H. J., and Moy, P. W.**, Histochemical study of acute leukemia, *Arch. Pathol.*, 97, 129, 1974.
534. **Bottomley, R. H., Lovig, C. A., Holt, R., and Griffin, M. J.**, Comparison of alkaline phosphatase from human normal and leukemic leukocytes, *Cancer Res.*, 29, 1866, 1969.

535. **Lyons, R. B., Weaver, D. D., and Beck, J. H.**, Isoenzymes of human leukocyte alkaline phosphatase, *Ann. N. Y. Acad. Sci.*, 155, 948, 1968.
536. **Rosner, F. and Lee, S. L.**, Zinc and magnesium content of leukocyte alkaline phosphatase isoenzymes, *J. Lab. Clin. Med.*, 79, 228, 1972.
537. **Weaver, D. D. and Lyons, R. B.**, Leukocyte alkaline phosphatase isoenzymes, *Lancet*, 1, 1196, 1968.
538. **Rosenblum, D. and Petzold, S. J.**, Neutrophil alkaline phosphatase: comparison of enzymes from normal subjects and patients with polycythemia vera and chronic myelogenous leukemia, *Blood*, 45, 335, 1975.
539. **Trubowitz, S., Feldman, D., Morgenstern, S. W., and Hunt, V. M.**, The isolation, purification and properties of the alkaline phosphatase of human leukocytes, *Biochem. J.*, 80, 369, 1961.
540. **Spiers, A. S. D., Liew, A., and Baikie, A. G.**, Neutrophil alkaline phosphatase score in chronic granulocytic leukemia: effects of splenectomy and antileukemic drugs, *J. Clin. Pathol.*, 28, 517, 1975.
541. **Williams, D. M.**, Leucocyte alkaline phosphatase as a marker of cell maturity: a quantitative cytochemical and autoradiographic study, *Br. J. Haematol.*, 31, 371, 1975.
542. **Malaskova, V. and Fuksova, J.**, Alkaline phosphatase activity in immature granulocytes, *Br. J. Haematol.*, 15, 119, 1968.
543. **Kaplow, L. S.**, Alkaline phosphatase activity in peripheral blood lymphocytes, *Arch. Pathol.*, 88, 69, 1969.
544. **Bennett, J. M., Nathanson, L., and Rutenburg, A. M.**, Significance of leukocyte alkaline phosphatase in Hodgkin's disease, *Arch. Intern. Med.*, 121, 338, 1968.
545. **Kaplow, L. S.**, Cytochemistry of leukocyte alkaline phosphatase. Use of complex naphthol AS phosphates in azo dye-coupling technics, *Am. J. Clin. Pathol.*, 39, 439, 1963.
546. **Mitus, W. J. and Kiossoglou, K. A.**, Leukocyte alkaline phosphatase in myeloproliferative syndrome, *Ann. N. Y. Acad. Sci.*, 155, 976, 1968.
547. **Rosner, F., Schreiber, Z. R., and Parise, F.**, Leukocyte alkaline phosphatase, *Arch. Intern. Med.*, 130, 892, 1972.
548. **Xefteris, E., Mitus, W. J., Mednicoff, I. B., and Dameshek, W.**, Leukocytic alkaline phosphatase in busulfan induced remissions of chronic granulocytic leukemia, *Blood*, 18, 202, 1961.
549. **Hammouda, F., Quaglino, D., and Hayhoe, F. G. J.**, Blastic crisis in chronic granulocytic leukemia. Cytochemical, cytogenetic, and autoradiographic studies in four cases, *Br. Med. J.*, 1, 1275, 1964.
550. **Jackson, I. M. D. and Clark, B. M.**, A case of neutrophilic leukemia, *Am. J. Med. Sci.*, 249, 172, 1965.
551. **Rosen, R. B. and Nishiyama, H.**, Leukocyte alkaline phosphatase in chronic granulocytic leukemia of childhood, *Ann. N. Y. Acad. Sci.*, 155, 992, 1968.
552. **Rubin, H.**, Chronic neutrophilic leukemia, *Ann. Intern. Med.*, 65, 93, 1966.
553. **Ezdinli, E. Z., Sokal, J. E., Crosswhite, L., and Sandberg, A. A.**, Philadelphia chromosome positive and negative chronic myelocytic leukemia, *Ann. Intern. Med.*, 72, 175, 1970.
554. **Krauss, S.**, The Philadelphia chromosome and leukocyte alkaline phosphatase in chronic myelocytic leukemia and related disorders, *Ann. N. Y. Acad. Sci.*, 155, 983, 1968.
555. **Krauss, S., Sokal, J. E., and Sandberg, A. A.**, Comparison of Philadelphia chromosome positive and negative patients with myelocytic leukemia, *Ann. Intern. Med.*, 61, 625, 1964.
556. **Lewis, S. M. and Dacie, J. V.**, Neutrophil (leucocyte) alkaline phosphatase in paroxysmal nocturnal haemoglobinuria, *Br. J. Haematol.*, 11, 549, 1965.
557. **Dacie, J. V., Smith, M. D., White, J. C., and Mollin, D. L.**, Refractory normoblastic anemia: a clinical and hematological study of seven cases, *Br. J. Haematol.*, 5, 56, 1959.
558. **Mitus, W. J., Bergna, L. J., Mednicoff, I. B., and Dameshek, W.**, Alkaline phosphatase of mature neutrophils in chronic forms of the myeloproliferative syndrome, *Am. J. Clin. Pathol.*, 30, 285, 1958.
559. **Lacher, M. J. and Ley, A. B.**, The value of leukocyte alkaline phosphatase determinations in the malignant lymphomas, *Cancer*, 17, 402, 1964.
560. **Cooper, H. L., Perry, S., and Breitman, T. R.**, Pyridimine metabolism in human leukocytes. II. Metabolism of the thymine nucleotide pools in normal and leukemic leukocytes, *Cancer Res.*, 26, 2276, 1966.
561. **Smith, L. H., Jr., Baker, F. A., and Sullivan, M.**, Pyrimidine metabolism in man. I. The biosynthesis of orotic acid, *J. Clin. Invest.*, 38, 798, 1959.
562. **Smith, L. H., Jr., Baker, F. A., and Sullivan, M.**, Pyrimidine metabolism in man. II. Studies of leukemic cells, *Blood*, 15, 360, 1960.
563. **Vallee, B. L. and Gibson, J. G.**, The zinc content of whole blood, plasma, leukocytes and erythrocytes in the anemias, *Blood*, 4, 445, 1949.
564. **Goodpasture, E. W.**, A peroxidase reaction with sodium nitroprusside and benzidine in blood smears and tissues, *J. Clin. Lab. Med.*, 4, 442, 1919.

565. **Graham, R. C. and Karnovsky, M. J.**, The early stages of absorption of injected horseradish peroxidase in the proximal tubules of mouse kidney: ultrastructural cytochemistry by a new technique, *J. Histochem. Cytochem.*, 14, 291, 1966.
566. **Quaglino, D. and Flemans, R.**, Peroxidase staining in leukocytes, *Lancet*, 2, 1020, 1958.
567. **Lillie, R. D.**, *Histopathological Technic and Practical Histochemistry*, 3rd ed., McGraw-Hill, London, 1965, 371.
568. **Graham, R. C., Jr., Lundholm, U., and Karnovsky, M.**, Cytochemical demonstration of peroxidase activity with 3-amino-9-ethylcarbazole, *J. Histochem. Cytochem.*, 13, 150, 1965.
569. **Himmelhoch, S. R., Evans, W. H., Mage, M. G., and Peterson, E. A.**, Purification of myeloperoxidases from the bone marrow of the guinea pig, *Biochemistry*, 8, 914, 1969.
570. **Streefkerk, J. G. and Van der Ploeg, M.**, The effect of methanol on granulocyte and horseradish peroxidase quantitatively studied in a film model system, *Histochemistry*, 40, 105, 1974.
571. **Undritz, E.**, Peroxidase reaction of lepehne for erythroblasts, in *Sandoz Atlas of Haematology*, Sandoz, Basel, Switzerland, 1952, 28.
572. **Lillie, R. D. and Burtner, H. J.**, Stable sudanophilia of human neutrophil leucocytes in relation to peroxidase and oxidase, *J. Histochem. Cytochem.*, 1, 8, 1953.
573. **Storti, E. and Perugini, S.**, Cytochemical researches on the lipids of the hematic cells with particular attention to those of acute leukosis, *Acta Haematol.*, 5, 321, 1951.
574. **Pearse, A. G. E.**, *Histochemistry*, Vol. 1, 3rd Ed., Little, Brown, Boston, 1968, 307.
575. **Wislocki, G. B., Rheingold, J. J., and Dempsey, E. W.**, The occurrence of the periodic acid schiff reaction in various normal cells of blood and connective tissues, *Blood*, 4, 562, 1949.
576. **Mitus, W. ., Bergna, L. J., Mednicoff, I. B., and Dameshek, W.**, Cytochemical studies of glycogen content of lymphocytes in lymphocyte proliferations, *Blood*, 13, 748, 1958.
577. **Feldges, A. J., Aur, R. J. A., Verzosa, M. S., and Daniels, S.**, Periodic acid-schiff reaction, a useful index of duration of complete remission in acute childhood lymphocytic leukemia, *Acta Haematol.*, 52, 8, 1974.
578. **Vowels, M. R. and Willoughby, M. L. N.**, Cyclic chemotherapy in acute lymphoblastic leukaemia of childhood. Five year survivals, *Arch. Dis. Child.*, 48, 436, 1973.
579. **Bennett, J. M. and Henderson, E. S.**, Lymphoblastic leukaemia, *Br. Med. J.*, 2, 513, 1969.
580. **Humphrey, G. B., Nesbit, M. E., and Brunning, R. D.**, Prognostic value of the periodic acid-schiff (PAS) reaction in acute lymphoblastic leukemia, *Am. J. Clin. Pathol.*, 61, 393, 1974.
581. **Klein, H. O. and Heller, A.**, PAS-positive erythroblasts in kidney diseases, *Acta Haematol.*, 37, 225, 1967.
582. **Quaglino, D. and Hayhoe, F. G. J.**, Periodic acid-schiff positivity in erythroblasts with special reference to Di Guglielmo's disease, *Br. J. Haematol.*, 6, 26, 1960.
583. **Fischer, R. and Schmalzl, F.**, Über die hemmbarkeit der esterase-aktivität in blutmonocyten durch natriumfluorid, *Klin. Wochenschr.*, 44, 751, 1964.
584. **Schmazl, F. and Braunsteiner, H.**, Zur Diagnose Monozytarer Leukamien mit Zytochemischen Methoden , *Acta Haematol.*, 40, 121, 1968.
585. **Rozenszajn, L., Leibovich,M., Shoham, D., and Epstein, J.**, The esterase activity in megaloblasts, leukaemic and normal hemopoietic cells, *Br. J. Haematol.*, 14, 605, 1968.
586. **Löffler, H., Luck, R., and Syed, A. S.**, Eosinophilenleukamie mit Chloracetat-Esterase-Positiven Granula bei Einem Kinde, *Dtsch. Med. Wochenschr.*, 100, 2092, 1975.
587. **Yam, L. T., Li, C. Y., Necheles, T. F., and Katayama, I.**, Pseudoeosinophilia, eosinophilic endocarditis and eosinophilic leukemia, *Am. J. Med.*, 53, 193, 1972.
588. **Leder, L. D.**, Uber die Sclcktive Fermentcytochemische Darstellung von Neutrophilen Myeloischen Zennen und Gewebsmastzellen un Paraffinschnitt, *Klin. Wochenschr.*, 42, 553, 1964.
589. **Salvidio, E. and Bladini, M.**, Quantitative determinations of phosphatase and β-glucuronidase activities in spleens from patients with myelofibrosis and myeloid metaplasia and other haematological disorders, in *Current Research in Leukemia*, Hayhoe, F. G. J., Ed., Cambridge University Press, London, 1965, 241.
590. **Barka, T. and Anderson, P. J.**, Histochemical methods for acid phosphatase using hexazonium pararosanalin as coupler, *J. Histochem. Cytochem.*, 10, 741, 1962.
591. **White, J. G.**, Fine structural demonstration of acid phosphatase activity in Auer bodies, *Blood*, 29, 667, 1967.
592. **Barka, T.**, Studies of acid phosphatase. I. Electrophoretic separation of acid phosphatases of rat liver on polyacrylamide gels, *J. Histochem. Cytochem.*, 9, 542, 1961.
593. **Katayama, I., Li, C. Y., and Yam, L. T.**, Histochemical study of acid phosphatase isoenzyme in leukemic reticuloendotheliosis, *Cancer*, 29, 157, 1972.
594. **Mover, S., Li, C. Y., and Yam, L. T.**, Semiquantitative evaluation of tartrate-resistant acid phosphatase activity in human blood cells, *J. Lab. Clin. Med.*, 80, 711, 1972.

595. **Janckila, A. J., Lam, K. W., Li, C. Y., and Yam, L. T.**, The cyochemistry of tartrate-resistant acid phosphatase. I. Technical considerations, *Am. J. Clin. Pathol.*, in press.
596. **Lam, K. W. and Yam, L. T.**, Biochemical characterization of the tartrate-resistant acid phosphatase of human spleen with leukemic reticuloendotheliosis as a pyrophosphatase, *Clin. Chem.*, 23, 89, 1977.
597. **Lam, K. W., Lai, L. C., Burkart, P. T., and Yam, L. T.**, Kinetic properties of tartrate-resistant acid phosphatase isolated from human spleen with leukemic reticuloendotheliosis, *J. Biol. Chem.*, 252, 3371, 1977.
598. **Follette, J. H., Valentine, W. N., and Lawrence, J. S.**, The beta-glucuronidase content of human leukocytes in health and in disease, *J. Lab. Clin. Med.*, 40, 825, 1952.
599. **Lorbacher, P., Yam, L. T., and Quaynor, E.**, Cytochemischer Nachweis von β-Glucuronidase in Normalen und Leukamische Blutlymphocyten, *Klin. Wochenschr.*, 46, 1046, 1968.
600. **Hayashi, M.**, Distribution of β-glucuronidase activity in rat tissues employing the naphthol ASBI glucuronide hexazonium pararosanalin method, *J. Histochem. Cytochem.*, 12, 659, 1964.
601. **Crowder, J. G. and White, A. C.**, Selective changes in white cell lysosomal enzymes in man, *Am. J. Med. Sci.*, 255, 327, 1968.
602. **Goldfarb, T. G. and Papp, B. J.**, Excessively high levels of lactic acid dehydrogenase activity in pernicious anemia, *Am. J. Med.*, 34, 578, 1963.
603. **Libnoch, J. A., Yakulis, V. J., and Heller, P.**, Lactate dehydrogenase in megaloblastic bone marrow, *Am. J. Clin. Pathol.*, 45, 302, 1966.
604. **Bottomley, R. H., Locke, S. J., and Ingram, H. C.**, Lactic dehydrogenase of human chronic lymphocytic leukemic leukocytes, *Blood*, 27, 85, 1966.
605. **Dioguardi, N., Agostoni, A., and Fiorelli, G.**, Characterization of lactic dehydrogenase in cells of myeloid leukemia, *Enzymol. Biol. Clin.*, 2, 116, 1962—1963.
606. **Hellung-Larsen, R. and Andersen, P.**, Kinetics of oxygen-induced changes in lactate dehydrogenase isoenzymes of human lymphocytes in culture, *Exp. Cell. Res.*, 54, 201, 1969.
607. **Kerppola, W.**, Oxidative and glycolytic phosphorylation and lactic dehydrogenase isoenzymes in neoplastic tissue, *Ann. Med. Exp. Biol. Fenn.*, 44, 567, 1966.
608. **Starkweather, W. H., Spencer, H. H., and Schoch, H. K.** The lactate dehydrogenase of hemopoietic cells, *Blood*, 28, 860, 1966.
609. **Ackerman, G. A.**, Histochemical demonstration of dehydrogenase activity in the cells of normal blood and bone marrow, *J. Biophys. Biochem. Cytol.*, 8, 61, 1960.
610. **Hardonk, M. J.**, 5′ Nucleotidase, *Histochemie*, 12, 1, 1968.
611. **Hardonk, M. J. and Koudstaal, J.**, 5′ Nucleotidase *Histochemie*, 12, 18, 1968.
612. **Lehrer, G. M. and Ornstein, L.**, A diazo coupling method for the electron microscopic localization of cholinesterase, *J. Biochem. Biophys. Cytol.*, 6, 399, 1959.
613. **Beutler, E.**, Peripheral blood, bone marrow and urine iron stains, in *Hematology*, Williams, W. J., Beutler, E., Erslev, A. J., and Rundles, R. S., Eds., McGraw-Hill, New York, 1972, 1360.
614. **Mollin, D. L.**, Sideroblasts and sideroblastic anemia, *Br. J. Haematol.*, 11, 41, 1965.
615. **Bowman, W. D.**, Abnormal (ringed) sideroblasts in various hematologic and non-hematologic disorders, *Blood*, 18, 662, 1961.
616. **Blumenkrantz, N. and Asboe Hansen, G.**, A selective stain for mast cells, *Histochem. J.*, 7, 277, 1975.
617. **Mittwoch, U.**, Abnormal lymphocytes in gargoylism, *Br. J. Haematol.*, 5, 365, 1959.
618. **Mittwoch, U.**, The demonstration of mucopolysaccharide inclusions in the lymphocytes of patients with gargoylism, *Acta Haematol.*, 29, 202, 1963.
619. **Zelson, J. and Dekaban, A. S.**, Biological behavior of lymphocytes in Hunter-Hurler's disease, *Arch. Neurol.*, 20, 358, 1969.
620. **Nitowsky, H. M.**, Use of cell culture techniques in diagnosis and studies of inherited disease, *Semin. Hematol.*, 9, 403, 1972.
621. **Perry, S. and Reynolds, J.**, Methyl green pyronin as a differential nucleic acid stain for peripheral blood smears, *Blood*, 11, 1132, 1956.
622. **Ackerman, G. A. and Sveringer, S. C.**, Histochemical localization of sulfhydryl groups in the cells of normal human blood and bone marrow, *Lab. Invest.*, 9, 356, 1960.
623. **Hernadez, F. and Morentin, J. M.**, Cytochemical localization of ubiquinone in human peripheral blood cells, *Stain Technol.*, 42, 241, 1967.
624. **Mundkur, B. and Greenwood, H.**, Amido black 10B as a nucleolar stain for lymph nodes in Hodgkin's disease, *Acta Cytol.*, 12, 218, 1968.
625. **Gupta, S., Ross, G. C., Good, R. A., and Siegal, F. P.**, Surface markers of human eosinophils, *Blood*, 48, 755, 1976.
626. **Messner, R. P. and Jelinek, J.**, Receptors for human γG globulin on human neutrophils, *J. Clin. Invest.*, 49, 2165, 1970.

627. **Davey, F. R., Huntington, S. J., Maccallum, J., and MacMath, J. M.,** Cytochemical reactions of normal and neoplastic lymphocytes, *J. Clin. Pathol.*, 30, 653, 1977.
628. **Mendes, N. F., Miki, S. S., and Peixinho, Z. F.,** Combined detection of human T and B lymphocytes by rosette formation with sheep erythrocytes and zymosan-C3 complexes, *Immunology*, 113, 531, 1974.
629. **Papamichail, M., Holborrow, E. J., Keith, H. I., and Currey, H. L. F.,** Subpopulations of human peripheral blood lymphocytes distinguished by combined rosette formation and membrane immunofluorescence, *Lancet*, 2, 64, 1972.
630. **Preud'Homme, J. L., and Flandrin, G.,** Identification by peroxidase staining of monocytes in surface immunofluorescence tests, *J. Immunol.*, 113, 1650, 1974.
631. **Ross, G. D., Rabellino, E. M., Polley, M. J., and Grey, H. M.,** Combined studies of complement receptor and surface immunoglobulin-bearing cells and sheep erythrocyte rosette-forming cells in normal and leukemic human lymphocytes, *J. Clin. Invest.*, 52, 377, 1973.
632. **Catovsky, D., Goldman, J. M., Okos, A., Frisch, B., and Galton, D. A. G.,** T-lymphoblastic leukaemia: a distinct variant of acute leukaemia, *Br. Med. J.*, 2, 643, 1974.
633. **Murphy, S. B., Borella, L., Sen, L., and Mauer, A.,** Lack of correlation of lymphoblast cell size with presence of T-Cell markers or with outcome in childhood acute lymphoblastic leukaemia, *Br. J. Haematol.*, 31, 95, 1975.
634. **Sen, L. and Borella, L.,** Clinical importance of lymphoblasts with T markers in childhood acute leukemia, *N. Engl. J. Med.*, 292, 828, 1975.
635. **Barrett, S. G., Schwade, J. G., Ranken, R., and Kadin, M. E.,** Lymphoblasts with both T and B markers in childhood leukemia and lymphoma, *Blood*, 50, 71, 1977.
636. **Loeffler, H. and Schubert, J. C. F.,** Cytochemische Unterschiede Swischen Plasmazellen und Myelomzellen, *Klin. Wochenschr.*, 41, 484, 1963.
637. **Schubert, J. C. F. and Katzenmier, F.,** Der Zytochemische Nachweis der Leucinaminopeptidase in Menschlichen Blut- und Knochenmarkausstrichen, in *Zyto- und Histochemie in der Hamatologie 9 Freiburger Symp.*, Springer, Berlin/Gottingen, Heidelberg, 1963.
638. **Shaw, M. T., Twele, T. W., and Nordquist, R. E.,** Plasma cell leukemia: detailed studies and response to therapy, *Cancer*, 33, 619, 1974.
639. **Stjernholm, R. L.,** Carbohydrate metabolism in leukocytes. VII. Metabolism of glucose, acetate, and propionate by human plasma cells, *J. Bacteriol.*, 93, 1657, 1967.
640. **Huber, H., Polley, M. J., Linscott, W. D., Fudenberg, H. H., and Muller-Eberhard, H. J.,** Human monocytes: distinct receptor sites for the third component of complement and for immunoglobulin G, *Science*, 162, 1281, 1968.
641. **Kulenkampff, J., Janossy, G., and Greaves, M. F.,** Acid esterase in human lymphoid cells and leukaemic blasts: a marker for T lymphocytes, *Br. J. Haematol.*, 36, 231, 1977.
642. **Bianco, C. and Nussenzweig, V.,** Theta-bearing and complement-receptor lymphocytes are distinct populations of cells, *Science*, 173, 154, 1971.
643. **Kolodny, E. H. and Mumford, R. A.,** Human leukocyte acid hydrolases: characterization of eleven lysosomal enzymes and study of reaction conditions for their automated analysis, *Clin. Chim. Acta*, 70, 247, 1976.
644. **Ryman, B. E.,** Leukocyte enzyme assay as a means of diagnosis, *J. Clin. Pathol.*, 28, 758, 1975.

TESTS OF LEUKOCYTE FUNCTION

James P. Crowley, James D. Simon, and Maurice M. Albala

Introduction

Peripheral blood leukocytes are a heterogeneous group of nucleated cells that collectively perform a number of functions essential for the health and survival of the larger organism. On the basis of nuclear morphology, these cells may be classified into polymorphonuclear leukocytes (PMN), lymphocytes, monocytes, eosinophils, and basophils. Since these cells differ from each other in their physical and biological characteristics, methods for the pure isolation of each leukocyte type are feasible. Density gradient centrifugation allows the clean separation of the lighter lymphocytes and monocytes from the more dense PMN and eosinophils. Monocytes can be separated from lymphocytes by allowing the sticky monocytes to adhere to a suitable surface, leaving the lymphocytes in pure form. Standardized isolation techniques are important for reducing the variability of many tests of leukocyte function. Some tests, notably chemotaxis, are affected by the technique used to purify the leukocytes. Depending on the circumstances, it may be advisable to work with a less purified population in order to ensure against a loss of activity.

Polymorphonuclear Leukocyte Function Tests

The great increase in knowledge of intermediary metabolism that occurred in the 1930s and 1940s stimulated a wide variety of biochemical studies of human leukocytes. Initially, little effort was made to separate observed effects due to PMN from those due to lymphocytes. Basic concepts of leukocyte function remained little changed from the ideas of Metchnikoff, who worked at the turn of the present century.

In the late 1950s, several laboratories began reporting the results of experiments in which the newer knowledge of intermediary metabolism was specifically related to phagocytosis and other leukocyte functions. The subsequent description of hereditary chronic granulomatous disease (CGD) and Chediak-Higashi syndrome, in which the major defect leading to frequent infection was suspected of residing in the PMN, stimulated these efforts enormously. Many new methods for assessing leukocyte function were developed. Table 1 shows specific assays of PMN function representative of those currently in use. Tables 2 to 5 show the principal diseases or conditions in which abnormalities in PMN function have been described.

Defects in phagocytosis have been demonstrated in a very large number of diseases, and only the principal categories could be listed in Table 4. In terms of clinical frequency, most defects in phagocytosis are probably due to impaired opsonization rather than cellular defects in the PMN. Occasionally, more than one factor that depresses phagocytosis is present. An extreme example of this is the patient with systemic lupus erythematosus in whom low complement levels, defective alternate pathway activation, circulating immune complexes, neutrophil autoantibodies, and acute infection all may be present simultaneously. It is not surprising that these patients are notably prone to septicemia and infection.

While many specific assay systems for assessing isolated functions exist, these methods are merely convenient ways of categorizing and quantitating parts of the continuum of interactions that exist among bacteria, serum factors, cell membranes, lysosomes, microtubules, microfilaments, and cellular metabolism. Sharp distinctions in functional defects are sometimes difficult to make, and a fundamental alteration of any one component may lead to multiple defects in function at the cellular level.

Table 1
POLYMORPHONUCLEAR LEUKOCYTE FUNCTION TESTS

	Method	Results	Comment	Ref.
I. Tests of inflammatory function				
A. Adhesion	Nylon fiber column	28—70%PMNS adhere	Amount of nylon critical	1
B. Mobilization	Blood count	WBC doubles	Epinephrine may raise blood pressure	2, 3
1. Marginal pool	1. 30-min post i.v. epinephrine			
2. Marrow reserve	2. 6-hr post i.v. steroid			
C. Migration	Superficial abrasion skin	72×10^6 WBC/cm²/day	Test may leave unsightly scars	4, 5
D. Random movement	Capillary tube	10—15 mm in 4 hr	—	6, 7
E. Chemotaxis	Migration thru millipore filter	Fivefold increase in PMN movement when stimulated	51Cr method technically simpler but less sensitive	8, 9
II. Tests of phagocytosis and killing				
A. Mechanical ingestion	Spectrophotometric measurement of red paraffin oil	0.14 mg oil/10^7 WBC/min	—	10
B. Bactericidal activity	Bacterial colony count post phagocytosis	Less than 15% alive at 60 min	Ratio bacteria to cells critical	11
C. Candidacidal activity	Intracellular organisms take up dye	—	—	12
D. Opsonic function	Modification of above + antibody or complement	Base-line activity enhanced 50—100%	—	13—16
III. Tests of metabolic activation during phagocytosis				
A. Oxygen consumption	Polarographic electrode	These studies generally show a two- to tenfold increase over resting state	True absolute values cannot be stated with certainty and, for reproducible results, specific conditions must be kept rigidly constant	17
B. Peroxide formation	Scopoletin fluorescence			18
C. Superoxide formation	Reduction of cytochrome C			19
D. Iodination	TCA precipitable fixed 131,			20
E. Hexose monophosphate shunt	Alkali trapping of CO_2 post (1-14C) glucose oxidation			21
F. NBT reduction	Colormetric measure of purple formazan dye			14, 22

Table 2
ALTERATIONS IN GRANULOCYTE ADHESIVENESS

	Ref.
Drugs that Diminish Adhesion of Granulocytes	
Iodoacetamide	23
Ethanol	24
Prednisone	24
Aspirin	24
cAMP	25
Diseases with Diminished Adhesion of Granulocytes	
Chronic Myelogenous L[illegible]	[illegible]
Multiple M[illegible]	[illegible]

Table 3
DISORDERS OF CHEMOTAXIS

	Ref.
Associated with Plasma or Serum Defects in the Generation or Inactivation of Chemotactic Factors	
Complement deficiency states	33, 34
Excess chemotactic factor inactivator	
Idiopathic	35
Hodgkin's disease	36
Sarcoidosis	37
Alcoholic liver disease	38
[illegible]irrhosis	39
[illegible]ular Defects Leading to Impaired Chemotaxis	
[illegible]norphologic alterations	
[illegible]liak-Higashi syndrome	40
[illegible]leukocyte syndrome	6
[illegible] morphologic alteration	
[illegible]phil actin dysfunction syndrome	41
[illegible]ciation with thermal injury	42
[illegible]rsus host disease	43
[illegible]atoid arthritis	44
Hypophosphatemia	45
Viral hepatitis	46
Diabetes mellitus	47
In Association with Hyperimmunoglobulin E and Dermatitis	
Recurrent mucocandidiasis and eczema	48—50
Congenital ichthyosis	51
Variant icthyosis	52
Incontinentia pigmenti	53

BUY BOOKS • DO GOOD • BUY BOOKS • DO GOOD
Help keep knowledge free.
The Internet Archive preserves millions of books, web pages, and recordings—free, forever.
LEARN MORE

Table 4
DISORDERS OF PHAGOCYTOSIS

	Ref.
Impaired Opsonization	
Deficient antibody formation	54, 55
Complement component deficiency	54, 56
Defective alternate pathway activation	16, 57
Cellular Defects	
Circulating immune complexes	58
Hyperosmolar states	59, 60
Acute infection	61
Neutrophil autoantibodies	62

Table 5
ALTERATIONS IN GRANULOCYTE BACTERICIDAL ACTIVITY

	Ref.
Hereditary or Congenital	
Chronic granulomatous disease (sex-linked)	63, 64
CGD variants (not sex-linked)	65, 66
Lipochrome histiocytosis	67
Selective staphylococcal bactericidal defect	68, 69
Chediak-Higashi syndrome	70
Neutrophil actin dysfunction	41
Glucose-6 phosphate dehydrogenase deficiency	71
Acquired	
During craniospinal irradiation	72
In association with mixed cryoglobulinemia	73
With refractory dysmyelopoeitic anemia	74
In neonates	75
Felty's syndrome	76
Severe neutropenia	11
Acute infection	77
Severe iron deficiency	78

Monocyte Function

The monocyte is the largest peripheral blood leukocyte and may be thought of as the precursor cell of the relatively long-lived tissue macrophage. It shares with the PMN the capacity for both random and directed movement, as well as phagocytosis and bacterial killing. It is relatively sluggish in these functions, however (Table 6). Most in vivo tests of phagocytosis and chemotaxis are basically modifications of existing methods developed in the study of PMN.

In addition, monocytes and macrophages are particularly abundant at the sites of delayed hypersensitivity reactions, implying important interactions with lymphocytes. While the precise relation of the monocyte to lymphocyte in vivo remains controversial, a number of specific in vitro interactions of monocytes with lymphocyte-derived factors have been described, most notably the interaction of monocytes with the migratory inhibitory factor (MIF). The monocyte-macrophage may also be involved with

Table 6
MONOCYTE FUNCTION

	Ref.
Monocyte macrophage transformation	79
Interaction with lymphocytes	
Interaction with migration inhibitory factor	80
Stimulation of lymphoid blastogenesis	81
Interaction with lymphokines	82
Immune recognition	
Spreading reaction	83
Fc receptor and IgG binding	84—86
C_3 receptor	86
Tumor recognition	87, 88
Antibody-dependent cytotoxicity	89
Phagocytic function	
Pinocytosis	90
Mechanical engulfment	91
Bactericidal activity	91
Fungicidal activity	92
Chemotaxis	93
Myelopoeitic function	94

lymphocytes in immune surveillance and the destruction of preneoplastic cells. They also play a role in normal hematopoeisis.

Eosinophils and Basophils

Knowledge about the function of eosinophils and basophils remains scanty, despite a recent revival of interest in their study. A major difficulty associated with attempts to study human eosinophils and basophils is the usual paucity of these cells in the peripheral blood. Most workers have been forced to rely on the occasional occurrence of marked eosinophilia in certain types of patients. Recent studies have emphasized factors affecting or mediating eosinophil chemotaxis, since these cells are not believed to play a significant role in bacterial clearance. Nevertheless, eosinophils share with monocytes and PMN the property of phagocytosis. These and other eosinophil functions, for which specific tests have been described, are listed in Table 7.

Basophils represent the least studied of the peripheral leukocytes. Most published reports have dealt either with the interaction of these cells with IgE[113] or their role in histamine release in allergic reactions.[112] It is not established whether normal basophils have the capacity for in vitro phagocytosis, chemotaxis, or related functions.

Secretory (Lysosomal) Function of the Leukocyte

A prominent feature of PMN is their abundant granules seen on light microscopic examination. Granules are also present in monocytes. The granules, or lysosomes, contain various constituents (Table 8) that can be released or secreted when the cell is stimulated in certain ways, particularly by phagocytosis. These secretory products may serve diverse functions, but they are thought to be released primarily to promote bacterial killing. Alterations in lysosomal function have been noted in only a few disease states, most notably the Chediak-Higashi syndrome.[70] However, a large number of substances have been described that will alter the secretory function of the normal PMN (Table 9).

Tests of Lymphocyte Function

While blood lymphocytes appear to be morphologically similar, they are in fact a

Table 7
EOSINOPHIL FUNCTION

	Ref.
Chemotaxis and Chemotactic Factors[95]	
Histamine	96
Complement	97
Noncomplement serum factors	98
Tumor factor	99
Polymorphonuclear leukocyte derived	100
Lymphocyte derived	101, 102
Phagocytosis	
Bacteria	103
Candida	104, 105
Immune complexes	106, 107
Miscellaneous	
Fibrinolysis	108
Histamine neutralization	109
Prostaglandin release	110
Antibody mediated cytotoxicity	111

diverse group of cells in which distinct functions are mediated by specific subpopulations. Most lymphocytes are classified as either B (bursal-derived) or T (thymic-derived) lymphocytes. T lymphocytes are those that have been processed by the thymus and that mediate delayed hypersensitivity and associated immune function. Immunological activation of T cells results in the production and secretion of nonimmunoglobulin factors (lymphokines) that modulate and mediate cytotoxicity. Lymphokines also affect the interaction of T lymphocytes with other lymphocytes, monocytes, and eosinophils. B lymphocytes originate in extrathymic sites (bone marrow, fetal liver) and presumably are not processed by the thymus. B lymphocytes and plasma cells synthesize and secrete immunoglobulins that serve as specific antibodies. These cells mediate humoral immunity. Much of their activity is regulated by suppressor and helper lymphocytes that are of thymic origin. A small percentage of lymphocytes ($< 2\%$) lack either B or T cell markers and are therefore referred to as "null" cells. Table 10 summarizes the in vitro methods used for the detection of lymphocyte surface markers. In addition to surface markers, a variety of other assays of lymphocyte function have been developed (Table 11). Most of these functions are associated with T lymphocytes. In Table 12 are listed some relatively common, acquired clinical conditions in which cell surface markers and assays of lymphocyte function have been found to be abnormal. Hereditary immunological disorders have been the subject of a recent review.[237]

Table 8
MAJOR CONSTITUENTS OF HUMAN LEUKOCYTE[a] GRANULES

Constituent	Granule: Primary (azurophilic)	Granule: Secondary (specific)	Granule: Tertiary	Granule: Basophil	Modal density in sucrose gradient	Function	Ref.
Myeloperoxidase	+	—	—	—	1.20—1.23	Antibacterial, virucidal, fungicidal	115—122
Acid hydrolases	+	—	+	—	1.20—1.23	Carbohydrate, protein, lipid, and nucleic acid degradation	115—122
Neutral proteases	+	—	—	—	1.23	Protein degradation	115,120,122
NADPH and NADH oxidases	+	—	—	—	1.22	Involved in microbicidal mechanisms	118
Cationic antibacterial proteins	+	—	—	—	—	Antibacterial	119—122
Lysozyme	+	+	—	—	1.18—1.23	Degrades bacterial cell wall	115—112
Lactoferrin	—	+	—	—	—	Iron and copper chelator	120,123
Collagenase	—	+	—	—	—	Hydrolyzes nondenatured collagen fibrils	120,122, 124
Unsaturated Vitamin B_{12} binding proteins	—	+	—	—	1.19	Serves role in vitamin B_{12} metabolism	115
Alkaline phosphatase[b]?	—	+	—	—	1.145	May hydrolyze certain phosphoesters	115,116,125
α-Glucosidase	—	+	—	—	1.20	May hydrolyze polysaccharide α (1 → 6) linkages	115,118,122
Histamine	—	—	—	+	—	Vasodilates vessels, contracts smooth muscle, stimulates gastric secretion, and modulates function of variety of cells	126—129
Heparin	—	—	—	+	—	Prevents coagulation of blood	129,130

[a] Leukocytes: neutrophils, eosinophils, and basophils.

[b] Cytochemistry suggests alkaline phosphatase in granules; subfractionation experiments localize this enzyme in agranular fraction.

Table 9
MODULATION OF RELEASE OF SUBSTANCES FROM HUMAN LEUKOCYTE[a] GRANULES

Agents that increase release	**Ref.**
Compounds that promote accumulation of intracellular cyclic GMP	131—136
cGMP	
Phorbol myristate acetate	
Carbamylcholine chloride	
Cholinergic agonists	
Compounds that promote assembly of cytoplasmic microtubules	135
Deuterium oxide	
Compounds that may disrupt lysosomal membranes	134,137
Monosodium urate crystals	
Polyene antibiotics	
Endotoxin	
Substances that promote an increase in intracellular calcium	138—144
Ca^{++}	
Ionophore A23187	
Substances that are phagocytosed	136, 145—148
Serum-coated zymosan	
Immune complexes	
Bacteria	
Substances that interact with the cytoplasmic membrane	149—151
Phagocytic stimulus + cytochalasin B	
Complement components	
Immune reactants on nonphagocytosable surfaces	
Agents that decrease release	**Ref.**
Compounds that iromote accumulation of cAMP	132,134,136,152
cAMP	
Theophylline	
Prostaglandin E_1	
Cholera enterotoxin	
Histamine	
Adrenergic agonists	
Compounds that promote disassembly of cytoplasmic microtubules	132,134,135,137
Colchicine	
Vinblastine	
Compounds that may stabilize lysosomal membranes	132,153,154
Adrenal corticosteroids	

[a] Leukocytes: neutrophils, eosinophils, and basophils.

Table 10
METHODS OF DETECTION OF T and B CELLS BY SURFACE MARKERS

Marker	Principle of test	Interpretation	Comments	Ref.
EAC rosettes	Sheep erythrocytes (E) coated with antibody (A) and complement (C) yield EAC that form rosettes with complement receptor lymphocytes (CRL)	Three or more sensitized RBC bound to lymphocytes; normal range: 6—18%;	Contamination of preparation with monocytes, PMNs and human RBC falsely increases the proportion of EAC rosettes	155
EA rosettes	Human erythrocytes (E) are coated with human IgG (A); receptors are specific only for IgG	Five or more erythrocytes bound to lymphocytes; normal range: 4—39%;	Monocytes and granulocytes also form EA rosettes. "K" cells and certain "T" cells may also be detected	156
Surface immunoglobulins (SIg)	Immunoglobulin fraction of rabbit antihuman globulin sera conjugated with fluorescein isothiocyanate (F.I.T.C.) is incubated with a predetermined volume of lymphocytes	200—500 cells are counted with fluorescent illumination. Membrane fluorescence is detected; normal range: IgG 7.2—12.8%, IgD 5.2—13.3%, IgM 4.5—12.4%, and IgA < 1%	Caution must be exercised when using commercial antisera. The use of monospecific antisera is critical for accurate analysis. Lymphocytes must be thoroughly washed since exogenous Ig may bind to cell surface	157
Surface immunoglobulins (SIg) with aggregated Ig	Fluorescein-conjugated heat aggregated human Ig mixed with a predetermined volume of lymphocytes is incubated at 23° for 30 min	200—500 cells are counted with fluorescent illumination; normal range 11—38%	Binding of aggregated human Ig to lymphocytes is dependent on an intact Fc portion of the IgG molecules. It is not dependent on complement. Uptake of aggregated Ig is inhibited by Ag-Ab complexes. Aggregates of IgG tend to precipitate in storage	158
E rosettes	Incubation of peripheral blood lymphocytes with sheep erythrocytes (E) causes sheep erythrocytes to bind to individual lymphocytes	At least three SRBC must bind to each lymphocyte; normal range: 88 ± 6%	Rosetting can be modified by pretreatment of RBC or lymphocytes with neuraminidase, sulfhydral reagents (AET), etc.	159
Anti T cell sera (anti HULTA)	Rabbit antisera against monkey thymocytes is obtained. The antiserum is extensively absorbed with cultured human B lymphoid cells, CLL cells, etc.	Antisera reacts with 95—100% of normal human thymocytes, with T cells in peripheral blood and spleen	Not tested extensively as yet. Relationship between E-rosette markers and anti-T cell marker is unknown	160

Table 11
TESTS THAT DETECT FUNCTIONAL POPULATIONS OF LYMPHOCYTES

Test	Principle	Results	Comment	Ref.
Lymphocyte transformation	In vitro lymphocyte response to specific or nonspecific mitogens	Stimulated lymphocytes proliferate and undergo blastic transformation	Pokeweed mitogen (PWM) stimulates proliferation of "T" and "B" lymphocytes. PHA stimulates "T" lymphocytes. Measures undefined mechanisms of lymphocyte functions. Most probably relates to interaction of stimulatory agents at the membrane surface	161—164
One way MLC	Mitomycin-C treated or X-irradiated lymphocytes (stimulating cells) can stimulate proliferation of normal allogeneic lymphocytes (responding cells)	Measures antigeneic disparity at the HLA locus determinants between two or more allogeneic cell lines	There is usually good to excellent correlation between antigeneic disparity and lymphocyte stimulation in one-way MLC test	165—167
Macrophage Migration Inhibition (M.I.F.)	Migration of macrophages of individuals sensitized to specific antigens is inhibited in the presence of the specific sensitizing antigens. The area of migration out of a capillary tube after 24 hr of incubation is projected onto paper through a projecting prism mounted on a microscope and measured.	Considered as an in vitro correlate of delayed hypersensitivity	This technique can detect delayed hypersensitivity tumor specific antigens to soluble antigens	168—171

Table 11 (continued)
TESTS THAT DETECT FUNCTIONAL POPULATIONS OF LYMPHOCYTES

Test	Principle	Results	Comment	Ref.
	Percent migration is calculated from the ratio of sensitized cells to normal controls			
^{51}Cr release assay for quantitative measurement of cell mediated cytolysis in vitro	Appropriate target cells in suspension cultures or purified blood leukocytes, incubated with ^{51}Cr are mixed with appropriate dilutions of effector cells. Shaking of tubes is necessary to assure adequate cell-to-cell contact	Maximum release (%) of ^{51}Cr in supernatant at 3 hr is determined. Percent ^{51}Cr release is directly related to cytolytic activity of effector cells	Detects cytolytic activity of sensitized T cells, K cells, and activated macrophages	172, 173
Antibody-dependent cellular cytotoxicity (ADCC)	Lymphocytes (effector cells) incubated with labeled target cells sensitized against target cell antigens (antibody coated) induce cytotoxicity of normal lymphocytes. Maximum ^{51}Cr release of target cells is obtained 4—5 hr	Test demonstrates K cell activity of normal lymphocytes	"Null" cell subset of peripheral blood lymphocytes have "K" cell activity	174—176
Assay to demonstrate immunoglobulin secretion by lymphocytes	A predetermined concentration of washed lymphocytes is incubated with and without pokeweed mitogen for 7 days. IgG, IgM, and IgA secreted into the culture medium is determined by	Normal range (nanograms): IgG 672—5702, IgA 1002—2877, IgM 834—16500	This technique measures immunoglobulin secretion by B lymphocytes	177

Table 11 (continued)
TESTS THAT DETECT FUNCTIONAL POPULATIONS OF LYMPHOCYTES

Test	Principle	Results	Comment	Ref.
	double radioimmunoassay			
Assay to demonstrate suppression of immunoglobulin secretion by normal lymphocytes	Lymphocytes from affected patients are incubated with lymphocytes from normal individuals for 7 days. Immunoglobulin secreted into culture medium is then determined by a double radioimmunoassay	Secretion of immunoglobulins by normal lymphocytes is markedly inhibited	Results indicate an active suppression of B cell maturation and antibody secretion by lymphocytes from affected patients	178

Table 12
LYMPHOCYTE ABNORMALITIES ASSOCIATED WITH ACQUIRED DISORDERS AND DRUGS

Clinical disease	Defect	Comment	Ref.
Hodgkin's Disease	E-rosette formation by peripheral blood lymphocytes is decreased. Decreased lymphocyte response to PHA stimulation. Macrophage migration inhibitory activity is detected in serum of affected individuals	Patients with constitutional symptoms (B symptoms) have lower mean percentage of E rosettes. Defect is more pronounced in patients with more extensive disease (Stages III and IV)	179—181
Non-Hodgkin's lymphoma	Variable: increase in B cell markers in some patients (SIg-EAC rosettes) SIg may be polyclonal. Macrophage migration inhibitory activity detected in serum of affected individuals	B cell lymphomas appear to survive longer. T cell lymphomas are more prone to development of leukemia. Mediastinal masses are usually present	182—186
Chronic lymphocytic leukemia (CLL)	Increase in lymphocytes with B cell markers (SIg and EAC rosettes). No EA receptors are present. Lymphosarcoma cells contain greater concentrations of immunoglobulin on its surface when compared to CLL. Occasional patients show only E-rosette formation. Patients' lymphocytes show delayed and subnormal reactivity to PHA stimulation	Marker is usually SIg M. Either K or λ light chain determinants. Lymphocyte hyporeactivity becomes more pronounced with progressive lymphocytosis	187—193
Sjögren's Syndrome	Increase in SIg markers in lymphocytes. Lymphocyte transformation is significantly impaired	Some of the lymphocytes appear to have more than one heavy chain class on their surface	194, 195
Acute lymphoblastic leukemia (ALL)	In most patients with untreated acute lymphoblastic leukemia, blasts show neither T nor B cell markers (Null cells)	E-rosette formation may be increased, especially in remission	196—199
Sèzary Syndrome	E-rosette formation in peripheral blood lymphocytes is normal or increased. SIg markers usually not present in peripheral blood lymphocytes. Coculture of normal B lymphocytes and Sezary cells results in marked increase in Ig	Helper T cell activity appears to be exaggerated	200, 201
Multiple myeloma	SIg markers are decreased in peripheral blood lymphocytes. Marked decrease of immunoglobulin secretion by lymphocytes from affected individuals. Circulating mononuclear cells from patients with multiple myeloma cocultured with normal lymphocytes suppress immunoglobulin synthesis by normal lymphocytes	The nature of the suppressive effect of normal lymphocytes by patient's lymphocytes is unknown	178, 202

Table 12 (continued)
LYMPHOCYTE ABNORMALITIES ASSOCIATED WITH ACQUIRED DISORDERS AND DRUGS

Clinical disease	Defect	Comment	Ref.
Solid tumors	Variable: low number of E-rosettes. Low number of EAC rosette forming lymphocytes. Decreased number of lymphocytes with SIg markers. Macrophage migration inhibitory activity demonstrated in the presence of tumor antigens	Depression of E-rosettes tends to correlate with worsening of clinical status. Number of E-rosette forming cells may improve following X-ray irradiation or surgical excision of malignant tumor	181, 203—209
Common variable hypogammaglobulinemia	Lymphocytes from affected individuals show marked decreased immunoglobulin secretion. Coculture of normal allogeneic lymphocytes with lymphocytes from affected individuals results in marked reduction of Ig synthesis by normal lymphocytes. Patient's lymphocytes fail to transform with PHA. A small group of patients shows no lymphocyte markers	B cell maturation and antibody production by normal lymphocytes may be suppressed by an abnormality of regulatory T cell activity	210—212
Systemic Lupus erythematosus (SLE) and rheumatoid arthritis (RA)	Variable number of T cells. They may be quantitatively depressed in some patients. Lymphocyte transformation to PHA may be reduced	In RA, low number of T cells appears to correlate with severity of clinical disease. In SLE there is no correlation with disease activity. T cell suppressor cells may be depleted in SLE	213, 214
Hashimoto's thyroiditis and Graves' disease	Increase in E-rosettes	These results need confirmation	215
Sarcoidosis	E-rosettes are decreased in peripheral blood lymphocytes	Cause of T cell deficiency is unknown	216
Glomerulonephritis	Macrophage migration inhibitory activity detected in the presence of glomerular basement membrane antigen	Results indicate cellular hypersensitivity in some patients with glomerulonephritis	217, 218
Chronic renal failure	Patient's plasma decreases lymphocyte transformation by PHA	This defect is improved by dialysis	219, 220
Crohn's disease and chronic ulcerative colitis	Peripheral blood T lymphocytes are decreased and cells with SIg markers are increased in Crohn's disease. In chronic ulcerative colitis, there are normal proportions of T lymphocytes	T cell depression in Crohn's disease does not correlate with disease activity	221
Multiple sclerosis	Autologous and normal allogeneic peripheral blood lymphocyte transformation is decreased in the presence of serum from patients with multiple sclerosis	Nature of serum inhibitory factor in patients with multiple sclerosis is unknown	222
Guillain—Barre Syndrome	Lymphocytes of affected individuals incubated with peripheral nerve antigen show increased blastogenesis	Lymphocyte mediated hypersensitivity may play a role in the etiology of this disorder	223

Table 12 (continued)
LYMPHOCYTE ABNORMALITIES ASSOCIATED WITH ACQUIRED DISORDERS AND DRUGS

Clinical disease	Defect	Comment	Ref.
Lepromatous leprosy	Lymphocytes with SIg markers are increased in peripheral blood	Probable deficiency of T cell population is suggested	224
Chronic mucocutaneous candidiasis	Peripheral blood E-rosettes are decreased. Lymphocyte transformation with PHA is depressed	E-rosettes do not improve after therapy with transfer factor	225, 226
Primary and secondary syphilis	Autologous and allogeneic lymphocytes incubated with patients' plasma show significant reduction of PHA lymphocyte transformation	Nature of the defect is unknown	227
Infectious mononucleosis	Increase in T cell markers. Transient increase in SIg M marker in lymphocytes	Findings are suggestive of depression in cell-mediated immunity	228, 229
Therapy with chloramphenicol (CPL)	Decreased lymphocyte transformation with PHA and PWM. Lymphocytes incubated with PHA and various concentrations of CPL show marked inhibition of lymphocyte blastogenesis	Nature of the defect is unknown	230
Aspirin ingestion	Lymphocyte blastogenesis with PHA and PWM stimulation is significantly decreased after aspirin ingestion	Blastogenesis response returns to normal values 36 hr after discontinuation of aspirin	231
Therapy with L-asparaginase	Autologous and allogeneic lymphocytes incubated with plasma of patients treated with L-asparaginase and PHA show marked inhibition of lymphocyte blastogenesis	Nature of the defect is unknown	232
Cytoxan therapy	Lymphocytes with SIg markers and E-rosette formation are decreased	Therapeutic effect may depend mainly on reduction of B cells	233
Chronic marijuana smokers	E-rosettes are decreased in 37% of marijuana smokers	No correlation was found between decreased E-rosette formation and other parameters of cell-mediated immunity	234
Halothane exposure	Lymphocytes incubated with plasma of individuals exposed to halothane show increased transformation	Stimulation of lymphocytes in the presence of halothane is helpful in the differential diagnosis of halothane and viral hepatitis	235
Surgical postop period	PHA lymphocyte response is depressed	Operative trauma is thought to be responsible for this change in lymphocyte reactivity	236

REFERENCES

1. **MacGregor, R. R., Spagnuolo, P. J., and Lentnek, A. L.,** Inhibition of granulocyte adherence by ethanol, prednisone and aspirin, measured with an assay system, *N. Engl. J. Med.,* 291, 642, 1974.
2. **Godwin, H. A., Zimmerman, T. S., Kimball, H. R., Wolff, S. M., and Perry, S.,** The effect of etiocholanolone on the entry of granulocytes into the peripheral blood, *Blood,* 31, 461, 1968.
3. **Athens, J. W., Haab, O. P., Raab, S. O., Mauer, A., Ashenbrucker, H., Cartwright, G. E., and Wintrobe, M. M.,** Leukokinetic studies. IV. The total blood circulating and marginal pools and granulocyte turnover rate in normal subjects, *J. Clin. Invest.,* 40, 989, 1961.
4. **Brayton, R. G., Stokes, P. E., Schwartz, M. S., and Louria, D. B.,** Effect of alcohol and various diseases on leukocyte mobilization, phagocytosis and intracellular bacterial killing, *N. Engl. J. Med.,* 282, 123, 1970.
5. **Holland, J. F., Hansjoerg, S., and Banerjee, T.,** Quantitative studies of localized leukocyte mobilization in acute leukemia, *Blood,* 37, 499, 1971.
6. **Miller, M. E., Oski, F. A., and Harris, M. B.,** Lazy leukocyte syndrome. A new disorder of neutrophil function, *Lancet,* 1, 665, 1971.
7. **Ketchel, M. M., Favour, C. B., and Sturgis, S. H.,** The in vitro action of hydrocortisone on leukocyte migration, *J. Exp. Med.,* 107, 211, 1958.
8. **Gallin, J. I., Clark, R. A., and Kimball, H. R.,** Granulocyte chemotaxis: an improved in vitro assay employing chromium 51 labeled granulocytes, *J. Immunol.,* 110, 233, 1973.
9. **Hill, H. R., Hogan, N., Mitchell, T. G., and Quie, P. G.,** Evaluation of a cytocentrifuge method for measuring neutrophil granulocyte chemotaxis, *J. Lab. Clin. Med.,* 86, 703, 1975.
10. **Stossel, T. P.,** Evaluation of opsonic and leukocyte function with a spectrophotometric test in patients with infection and with phagocytic disorders, *Blood,* 42, 121, 1973.
11. **Clawson, C. C., Repine, J. E., and Kunce, J.,** Quantitation of maximal bactericidal capability in human neutrophils, *J. Lab. Clin. Med.,* 88, 316, 1976.
12. **Lehrer, R. I. and Cline, M. J.,** Interaction of Candida albicans with human leukocytes and serum, *J. Bacteriol.,* 98, 996, 1969.
13. **Weinstein, R. J. and Young, L. S.,** Neutrophil function in gram-negative rod bacteremia: the interaction between phagocytic cells, infectious organisms, and humoral factors, *J. Clin. Invest.,* 58, 190, 1976.
14. **Johnston, R. B., Klemperer, M. R., Alper, C. A., and Rosen, F. S.,** The enhancement of bacterial phagocytosis by serum, *J. Exp. Med.,* 129, 1275, 1969.
15. **Messner, R. P., Laxdal, T., Quie, P. G., and Williams, R. C.,** Serum opsonin, bacteria and polymorphonuclear leukocyte interactions in subacute bacterial endocarditis: anti-globulin factors and their interaction with specific opsonins, *J. Clin. Invest.,* 47, 1109, 1968.
16. **Stossel, T. P., Alper, C. A., and Rosen, F. S.,** Opsonic activity in the newborn: the role of properdin, *Pediatrics,* 52, 134, 1973.
17. **Crowley, J. P., Skrabut, E. M., and Valeri, C. R.,** The determination of leukocyte phagocytic oxidase activity by measurement of the initial rate of stimulated oxygen consumption, *J. Lab. Clin. Med.,* 86, 586, 1975.
18. **Root, R. K., Metcalf, J., Oshino, N., and Chance, B.,** H_2O_2 release from human granulocytes during phagocytosis, *J. Clin. Invest.,* 55, 945, 1975.
19. **Babior, B. M., Kipnes, R. S., and Curnutte, J. T.,** The production by leukocytes of superoxide, a potential bactericidal agent, *J. Clin. Invest.,* 52, 741, 1973.
20. **Pincus, S. H. and Klebanoff, S. J.,** Quantitative leukocyte iodination, *N. Engl. J. Med.,* 284, 743, 1971.
21. **Skeel, R. T., Yankee, R. A., and Spivak, W. A.,** Leukocyte preservation. I. Phagocytic stimulation of the hexose monophosphate shunt as a measure of cell viability, *J. Lab. Clin. Med.,* 73, 327, 1969.
22. **Steigbigel, R. T., Johnson, P. K., and Remington, J. S.,** The nitroblue tetrazolium reduction test versus conventional hematology in the diagnosis of bacterial infection, *N. Engl. J. Med.,* 290, 235, 1974.
23. **Garvin, J. E.,** Factors affecting the adhesiveness of human leukocytes and platelets in vitro, *J. Exp. Med.,* 114, 51, 1961.
24. **McGregor, R. R., Spagnuolo, P. J., and Lentnek, A. L.,** Inhibition of granulocyte adherence by ethanol, prednisone, and aspirin, measured with an assay system, *N. Engl. J. Med.,* 291, 642, 1974.
25. **Bryant, R. E. and Sutcliffe, M. C.,** The effect of 3′, 5′-adenosine monophosphate on granulocyte adhesion, *J. Clin. Invest.,* 54, 1241, 1974.
26. **Brandt, L.,** Adhesiveness to glass and phagocytic activity of neutrophilic leukocytes in myeloproliferative diseases, *Scand. J. Haematol.,* 2, 126, 1965.
27. **Penny, R. and Galton, D. A. G.,** Studies on neutrophil function. II. Pathological aspects, *Br. J. Haematol.,* 12, 633, 1966.

28. **Provisor, D., Boxer, L., Strawbridge, R., Allen, J., Watanabe, A., Besch, H., and Baehner, R.,** Granulocyte adherence in the Chediak-Higashi Syndrome, *Clin. Res.*, 25 (Abstr.), 382, 1977.
29. **Buckley, R. M. and MacGregor, R. R.,** Propanolol prolongs the survival of infected intoxicated animals, *Clin. Res.*, 25 (Abstr.), 373, 1977.
30. **Craddock, P., Fehr, J., Brigham, K., and Jacob, H.,** Pulmonary capillary leukostasis: a complement (C') mediated complication of hemodialysis, *Clin. Res.*, 23 (Abstr.), 402, 1975.
31. **Lentnek, A. L., Schreiber, A. D., and MacGregor, R. R.,** The induction of augmented granulocyte adherence by inflammation: mediation by a plasma factor, *J. Clin. Invest.*, 40, 159, 1976.
32. **MacGregor, R. R.,** The effect of anti-inflammatory agents and inflammation on granulocyte adherence: evidence for regulation by plasma factors, *Am. J. Med.*, 61, 597, 1976.
33. **Miller, M. E.,** Leukocyte movement — in vitro and in vivo correlates, *J. Pediatr.*, 83, 1104, 1973.
34. **Alper, C. A., Abramson, N., Johnston, R. B., Jandl, J. H., and Rosen, F. S.,** Increased susceptibility to infection associated with abnormalities of complement-mediated functions and of the third component of complement (C3), *N. Engl. J. Med.*, 282, 349, 1970.
35. **Ward, P. A.,** Natural and synthetic inhibitors of leukotaxis, *Inflammation: Mechanisms and Control,* Lepow, I. H. and Ward, P. A., Eds., Academic Press, New York, 1972, 301.
36. **Ward, P. A. and Berenberg, J. L.,** Defective regulation of inflammatory mediators in Hodgkin's Disease, *N. Engl. J. Med.*, 290, 76, 1974.
37. **Maderazo, E., Ward, P. A., Woronick, C. L., Kubik, J., and DeGraff, A. C.,** Leukotactic dysfunction in sarcoidosis, *Ann. Intern. Med.*, 84, 414, 1976.
38. **Van Epps, D. E., Strickland, R. G., and Williams, R. C.,** Inhibitors of leukocyte chemotaxis in alcoholic liver disease, *Am. J. Med.*, 59, 200, 1975.
39. **DeMeo, A. N. and Anderson, B. R.,** Defective chemotaxis associated with a serum inhibitor in cirrhotic patients, *N. Engl. J. Med.*, 286, 735, 1972.
40. **Wolff, S. M., Dale, D. C., Clark, R. A., Root, R. K., and Kimball, H. R.,** The Chediak-Higashi syndrome: studies of host defenses, *Ann. Intern. Med.*, 76, 293, 1972.
41. **Boxer, L. A., Hedley-White, E. T., and Stossel, T. P.,** Neutrophil actin dysfunction and abnormal neutrophil behavior, *N. Engl. J. Med.*, 291, 1093, 1974.
42. **Warden, G. D., Mason, A. D., and Pruitt, B. A.,** Evaluation of leukocyte chemotaxis in vitro in thermally injured patients, *J. Clin. Invest.*, 54, 1001, 1974.
43. **Clark, R. A., Johnson, F. L., Klebanoff, S. J., and Thomas, E. D.,** Defective neutrophil chemotaxis in bone marrow transplant patients, *J. Clin. Invest.*, 58, 22, 1976.
44. **Mowat, A. G. and Baum, J.,** Chemotaxis of polymorphonuclear leukocytes from patients with rheumatoid arthritis, *J. Clin. Invest.*, 50, 2541, 1971.
45. **Craddock, P. R., Yawatta, Y., Silvis, S., and Van Santen, L.,** Acquired phagocyte dysfunction. A complication of the hypophosphatemia of parenteral hyperalimentation, *N. Engl. J. Med.*, 290, 1403, 1974.
46. **Magliuo, E. and Benzi-Cipelli, R.,** Impaired leukotaxis in viral hepatitis B, *N. Engl. J. Med.*, 293, 303, 1975.
47. **Mowat, A. G. and Baum, J.,** Chemotaxis of polymorphonuclear leukocytes from patients with diabetes mellitus, *N. Engl. J. Med.*, 284, 621, 1971.
48. **Hill, H. R., Ochs, H. D., Quie, P. G., Clark, R. A., Pabst, H. F., Klebanoff, S. J., and Wedgwood, R. J.,** Defect in neutrophil granulocyte chemotaxis in Job's syndrome of recurrent "cold" staphylococcal abscesses, *Lancet II*, 617, 1974.
49. **Hill, H. R. and Quie, P. G.,** Raised serum IgE levels and defective neutrophil chemotaxis, *Lancet*, 1, 183, 1974.
50. **Buckley, R. H., Wray, B. B., and Belmaker, E. Z.,** Extreme hyperimmunglobulinemia E and undue susceptibility to infection, *Pediatrics*, 49, 59, 1972.
51. **Miller, M. E., Normal, M. E., Koblenzer, P. J., and Schonauer, S.,** A new familial defect of neutrophil movement, *J. Lab. Clin. Med.*, 82, 1, 1973.
52. **Pincus, S. H., Thomas, I. T., Clark, R. A., and Ochs, H. D.,** Defective neutrophil chemotaxis with variant ichthyosis, hyperimmunoglobulinemia E and recurrent infections, *J. Pediatr.*, 87, 908, 1975.
53. **Dahl, M. V., Matula, G., Leonards, R., and Tuffanelli, D. L.,** Incontinentia pigmenti and neutrophil chemotaxis, *Arch. Dermatol.*, 111, 1603, 1975.
54. **Rosen, F. S., Alper, C. A., and Janeway, C. A.,** The primary immunodeficiencies and the serum complement defects, *Hematology of Infancy and Childhood,* Nathan, D. G. and Oski, F. A., Eds., W. B. Saunders, Philadelphia, 1975, 529.
55. **McCracken, G. H., Jr. and Eichenwald, H. F.,** Leukocyte function and the development of opsonic and complement activity in the neonate, *Am. J. Dis. Child.*, 121, 120, 1971.
56. **Forman, M. L. and Stiehm, E. R.,** Impaired opsonic activity but normal phagocytosis in low-birth-weight infants, *N. Engl. J. Med.*, 281, 926, 1969.

57. **Johnston, R. B., Jr., Newman, S. L., and Struth, A. G.,** An abnormality of the alternate pathway of complement activation in sickle-cell disease, *N. Engl. J. Med.*, 288, 803, 1973.
58. **Turner, R. A., Schumacher, H. R., and Myers, A. R.,** Phagocytic function of polymorphonuclear leukocytes in rheumatic diseases, *J. Clin. Invest.*, 52, 1632, 1973.
59. **Drachman, R. H., Root, R. K., and Wood, W. B., Jr.,** Studies on the effect of experimental nonketotic diabetes mellitus on antibacterial defense. I. Demonstration of a defect in phagocytosis, *J. Exp. Med.*, 124, 227, 1966.
60. **Chernew, I. and Braude, A. I.,** Depression of phagocytosis by solutes found in the kidney and urine, *J. Clin. Invest.*, 41, 1945, 1962.
61. **McCall, C. E., Caves, J., Cooper, R., and DeChatelet, L.,** Functional characteristics of human toxic neutrophils, *J. Infect. Dis.*, 124, 68, 1971.
62. **Boxer, L. A., Greenberg, M. S., Boxer, G. J., and Stossel, T. P.,** Autoimmune neutropenia, *N. Engl. J. Med.*, 293, 748, 1975.
63. **Good, R. A., Quie, P. G., Windhorst, D. G., Page, A. R., Rodey, G. E., White, J., Wolfson, J. J., and Holmes, B. H.,** Fatal (chronic) granulomatous disease of childhood: a hereditary defect of leukocyte function, *Semin. Hematol.*, 5, 215, 1968.
64. **Klebanoff, S. J. and White, L. R.,** Iodination defect in leukocytes of a patient with chronic granulomatous disease of childhood, *N. Engl. J. Med.*, 280, 460, 1969.
65. **Douglas, S. D., Davis, W. C., and Fudenberg, H. H.,** Granulocytopathies: pleomorphism of neutrophil dysfunction, *Am. J. Med.*, 46, 901, 1969.
66. **van Der Meer, J. W. M., van Zwet, T. L., and van Furth, R.,** New familial defect in microbicidal function of polymorphonuclear leukocytes, *Lancet*, 2, 630, 1975.
67. **Rodey, G. E., Holmes, B., Park, B. H., Ford, D., and Good, R. A.,** Leukocyte function in lipochrome histiocytosis (abstr.), *Clin. Res.*, 17, 375, 1969.
68. **Davis, W. C., Douglas, S. D., and Fudenberg, H. H.,** A selective neutrophil dysfunction syndrome: impaired killing of staphylococci, *Ann. Intern. Med.*, 69, 1237, 1968.
69. **Mandell, G. L.,** Staphylococcal infection and leukocyte bactericidal defect in a 22-year old woman, *Arch. Int. Med.*, 130, 754, 1972.
70. **Root, R. K., Rosenthal, A. S., and Balestra, D. J.,** Abnormal bactericidal, metabolic, and lysosomal functions of Chediak-Higashi syndrome leukocytes, *J. Clin. Invest.*, 51, 649, 1972.
71. **Baehner, R. L., Johnston, R. B., and Nathan, G. D. G.,** Comparative study of the metabolic and bactericidal characteristics of severely glucose-6-phosphate dehydrogenase deficient polymorphonuclear leukocytes and leukocytes from children with chronic granulomatous disease, *J. Reticuloendothelial Soc.*, 12, 150, 1972.
72. **Baehner, R. L., Neiburger, R. G., Johnson, D. E., and Murrman, S. M.,** Transient bactericidal defect of peripheral blood phagocytes from children with acute lymphoblastic leukemia receiving craniospinal irradiation, *N. Engl. J. Med.*, 289, 1209, 1973.
73. **Douglas, S. D., Lahav, M., and Fudenberg, H. H.,** A reversible neutrophil bactericidal defect associated with a mixed cryoglobulin, *Am. J. Med.*, 49, 274, 1970.
74. **Lehrer, R. I., Goldberg, L. S., Apple, M. A., and Rosenthal, N. P.,** Refractory megaloblastic anemia with myeloperoxidase deficient neutrophils, *Ann. Intern. Med.*, 76, 447, 1972.
75. **Coen, R., Grush, O., and Kauder, E.,** Studies of bactericidal activity and metabolism of the leukocyte in full-term neonates, *J. Pediatr.*, 75, 400, 1969.
76. **Gupta, R. C., Laforce, F. M., and Mills, D. M.,** Polymorphonuclear leukocyte inclusions and impaired bacterial killing in patients with Felty's syndrome, *J. Lab. Clin. Med.*, 88, 183, 1976.
77. **Solberg, C. O. and Hellum, C. O.,** Neutrophil granulocyte function in bacterial infections, *Lancet*, 2, 727, 1972.
78. **Chandra, R. K.,** Reduced bactericidal capacity of polymorphs in iron deficiency, *Arch. Dis. Child.*, 48, 864, 1973.
79. **Cohn, Z. A. and Benson, B.,** The differentiation of mononuclear phagocytes: morphology, cytochemistry and biochemistry, *J. Exp. Med.*, 121, 153, 1965.
80. **David, J. R.,** Macrophage activation by lymphocyte mediators, *Fed. Proc.*, 34, 1730, 1975.
81. **Unanue, E. R. and Calderon, J.,** Evaluation of the role of macrophages in immune induction, *Fed. Proc.*, 34, 1737, 1975.
82. **Altman, L. C., Syndermann, R., and Blaese, R. M.,** Abnormalities of chemotactic lymphokine synthesis and mononuclear leukocyte chemotaxis in Wiskott-Aldrich syndrome, *J. Clin. Invest.*, 54, 486, 1974.
83. **Dekaris, D., Silobucic, V., Mazuran, R., Kadrnka, R., and Lovrenic, M.,** Inhibition of monocyte spreading: a direct in vitro test for assaying delayed type hypersensitivity in man, *Clin. Exp. Immunol.*, 16, 311, 1974.
84. **LoBuglio, A. F., Cotran, R. S., and Jandl, J. H.,** Red cells coated with immunoglobulin G., binding and sphering by mononuclear cells in man, *Science*, 158, 282, 1967.

85. **Abramson, N., LoBuglio, A. F., Jandl, J. H., and Cotran, R. S.**, The interaction between monocytes and red cell binding characteristics, *J. Exp. Med.*, 132, 1191, 1970.
86. **Huber, H., Polley, M. I., Linscott, N. D., Fudenberg, H. H., and Muller-Eberhard, H. J.**, Human monocytes: distinct receptor sites for the third component of complement and for immunoglobulin G, *Science*, 162, 282, 1967.
87. **Hibbs, J. B., Lambert, C. H., and Remington, J. S.**, Control of carcinogenesis: a possible role for the activated macrophage, *Science*, 177, 998, 1972.
88. **Evans R. and Alexander, P.**, Mechanism of immunlogically specific killing of tumor cells by macrophages, *Nature (London)*, 236, 168, 1972.
89. **Poplack, D. G., Bonnard, G. D., Holiman, B. J., and Blaese, R. M.**, Monocyte mediated antibody dependent cellular cytotoxicity: a clinical test of monocyte function, *Blood*, 48, 809, 1976.
90. **Edelson, P. J., Swiebel, R., and Cohn, Z. A.**, The pinocytic rate of activated macrophages, *J. Exp. Med.*, 142, 1150, 1975.
91. **Steigbigel, R. T., Lambert, L. H., and Remington, J. S.**, Phagocytic and bactericidal properties of normal human monocytes, *J. Clin. Invest.*, 53, 131, 1974.
92. **Lehrer, R. I.**, Fungicidal mechanisms of human monocytes, *J. Clin. Invest.*, 55, 338, 1975.
93. **Snyderman, R. L., Altman, C., Hausman, M. S., and Mergenhagen, S. E.**, Human mononuclear leukocyte chemotaxis: a quantitive assay for humoral and cellular chemotactic factors, *J. Immunol.*, 108, 857, 1972.
94. **Golde, D. W. and Cline, M. J.**, Identification of the colony-stimulating cells in human peripheral blood, *J. Clin. Invest.*, 51, 2981, 1972.
95. **Ward, P. A.**, Chemotaxis of human eosinophils, *Am. J. Pathol.*, 54, 121, 1969.
96. **Clark, R. A., Gallin, J. I., and Kaplin, A. P.**, The selective eosinophil chemotactic activity of histamine, *J. Exp. Med.*, 142, 1462, 1975.
97. **Kay, A. B.**, Studies on eosinophil leukocyte migration. II. Factors specifically chemotactic for eosinophils and neutrophils generated from guinea pig serum by antigen antibody complexes, *Clin. Exp. Immunol.*, 7, 723, 1970.
98. **Robinson, I. O. and Miller, M. E.**, SECA, a new mediator of the human eosinophil response, *J. Allergy Clin. Immunol.*, 56, 317, 1975.
99. **Wasserman, S., Goetzl, E. J., Ellman, L., and Austen, K. F.**, Tumour associated eosinophilotactic factor, *N. Engl. J. Med.*, 290, 420, 1974.
100. **Czarnetski, B. M., Konig, W., and Lichtenstein, L. M.**, Release of eosinophil chemotactic factor from human polymorphonuclear neutrophils by calcium ionophore A23187 and phagocytosis, *Nature (London)*, 258, 725, 1976.
101. **Cohen, S. and Ward, P. A.**, In vitro and in vivo activity of a lymphocyte and immune complex-dependent chemotactic factor for eosinophils, *J. Exp. Med.*, 133, 133, 1971.
102. **Basten, A. and Beeson, P. B.**, Mechanism of eosinophilia. II. Role of the lymphocyte, *J. Exp. Med.*, 131, 1288, 1970.
103. **Cohen, S. G. and Sapp, T. M.**, Phagocytosis of bacteria by eosinophils in infectious related asthma, *J. Allergy*, 44, 113, 1969.
104. **Lehrer, R. I.**, Measurement of candidacidal activity of specific leukocyte types in mixed cell populations. II. Normal and chronic granulomatous disease eosinophils, *Infect. Immun.*, 3, 800, 1971.
105. **Ishizaka, T., Dalton, A. C., and Arbesman, C. E.**, Phagocytosis of C. albicans by eosinophil leukocytes, *J. Allergy Clin. Immunol.*, 49, 311, 1972.
106. **Litt, M.**, Studies in experimental eosinophilia. VI. Uptake of immune complexes by eosinophils, *J. Cell Biol.*, 23, 355, 1964.
107. **Saresin, S. M.**, A function of the eosinophil. Phagocytosis of antigen antibody complexes, *Proc. Soc. Exp. Biol. Med.*, 112, 667, 1963.
108. **Riddle, J. M. and Barnhart, M. I.**, The eosinophil as a source for profibrinolysin in acute inflammation, *Blood*, 25, 776, 1965.
109. **Archer, R. K.**, *The eosinophil leukocytes*, F. A. Davis, Philadelphia, 1963.
110. **Hubscher, T.**, Role of the eosinophil in allergic reactions. II. Release of prostaglandin from human eosinophilic leukocytes, *J. Immunol.*, 114, 1389, 1975.
111. **Butterworth, A. E., Sturroch, R. F., and Houba, V.**, Eosinophils as mediators of antibody dependent damage to schistosomula, *Nature (London)*, 256, 727, 1975.
112. **Sampson, D. and Archer, G. T.**, Release of histamine from human basophils, *Blood*, 29, 722, 1967.
113. **Ishizaka, T.**, Degranulation of human basophil leukocytes by anti-IgE antibody, *J. Immunol.*, 106, 705, 1971.
114. **Ishizaka, T., DeBernaro, R., Tomioka, H., Lichtenstein, L., and Ishizaka, K.**, Identification of basophil granulocytes as a site of allergic histamine release, *J. Immunol.*, 108, 1000, 1972.
115. **Kane, S. P. and Peters, T. J.**, Analytical subcellular fractionation of human granulocytes with reference to the localization of Vitamin B_{12} binding proteins, *Clin. Sci. Mol. Med.*, 49, 171, 1975.

116. **West, B. C., Rosenthal, A. S., Gelb, N. A., and Kimball, H. R.,** Separation and characterization of human neutrophil granules, *Am. J. Pathol.*, 77, 41, 1974.
117. **Rausch, P. G. and Moore, T. G.,** Granule enzymes of polymorphonuclear neutrophils: a phylogenetic comparison, *Blood*, 46, 913, 1975.
118. **Segal, A. W. and Peters, T. J.,** Analytical subcellular fractionation of human granulocytes with special reference to the localization of enzymes involved in microbicidal mechanisms, *Clin. Sci. Mol. Med.*, 52, 429, 1977.
119. **Welsh, I. R. H. and Spitznagel, J. K.,** Distribution of lysosomal enzymes, cationic proteins, and bactericidal substances in subcellular fractions of human polymorphonuclear leukocytes, *Infect. Immun.*, 4, 97, 1971.
120. **Bainton, D. F., Nichols, B. A., and Farquhar, M. G.,** Primary lysosomes of blood leukocytes, in *Lysosomes in Biology and Pathology*, Vol. 5, Dingle, J. T. and Dean, R. T., Eds., North-Holland, Amsterdam, 1976, 3.
121. **Cline, M. J.,** Morphology and morphogenesis of the granulocytic series, in *The White Cell*, Cline, M. J., Ed., Harvard University Press, Cambridge, 1975, 5.
122. **Cline, M. J.,** Neutrophil metabolism and composition, in *The White Cell*, Cline, M. J., Ed., Harvard University Press, Cambridge, 1975, 39.
123. **Leffell, M. S. and Spitznagel, J. K.,** Association of lactoferrin with lysozyme in granules of human polymorphonuclear leukocytes, *Infect. Immun.*, 6, 761, 1972.
124. **Murphy, G., Reynolds, J. J., Bretz, U., and Baggiolini, M.,** Collagenase is a component of the specific granules of human neutrophil leukocytes, *Biochem. J.*, 162, 195, 1977.
125. **Bainton, D. F., Ullyot, J. L., and Farquhar, M. G.,** The development of neutrophilic polymorphonuclear leukocytes in human bone marrow, *J. Exp. Med.*, 134, 907, 1971.
126. **Beaven, M. A.,** Histamine, *N. Engl. J. Med.*, 294, 30, 1976.
127. **Beaven, M. A.,** Histamine, *N. Engl. J. Med.*, 294, 320, 1976.
128. **Ackermann, G. A.,** Cytochemical properties of the blood basophilic granulocyte, *Ann. N.Y. Acad. Sci.*, 103, 376, 1963.
129. **Cline, M. J.,** The basophil, in *The White Cell*, Cline, M. J., Ed., Harvard University Press, Cambridge, 1975, 123.
130. **Amann, R. and Martin, H.,** Blutmastzellen und heparin, *Acta Haematol.*, 25, 209, 1961.
131. **Smith, R. J. and Ignarro, L. J.,** Bioregulation of lysosomal enzyme secretion from human neutrophils: roles of guanosine 3′:5′-monophosphate and calcium in stimulus-secretion coupling, *Proc. Natl. Acad. Sci. U.S.A.*, 72, 108, 1975.
132. **Goldstein, I. M.,** Pharmacologic modulation of lysosomal enzyme release from polymorphonuclear leukocytes, *J. Invest. Dermatol.*, 67, 622, 1976.
133. **Estensen, R. D., White, J. G., and Holmes, B.,** Specific degranulation of human polymorphonuclear leukocytes, *Nature (London)*, 248, 347, 1974.
134. **Zurier, R. B., Hoffstein, S., and Weissman, G.,** Mechanisms of lysosomal enzyme release from human leukocytes. I. Effect of cyclic nucleotides and colchicine, *J. Cell Biol.*, 58, 27, 1973.
135. **Zurier, R. B., Weissman, G., Hoffstein, S., Kammerman, S., and Tai, H. H.,** Mechanisms of lysosomal enzyme release from human leukocytes. II. Effects of cAMP and cGMP, autonomic agonists, and agents which affect microtubule function, *J. Clin. Invest.*, 53, 297, 1974.
136. **Ignarro, L. J., Lint, T. F., and George, W. J.,** Hormonal control of lysosomal enzyme release from human neutrophils, *J. Exp Med.*, 139, 1395, 1974.
137. **Cline, M. J.,** Neutrophils and the inflammatory process, in *The White Cell*, Cline, M. J., Ed., Harvard University Press, Cambridge, 1975, 89.
138. **Lichtenstein, L. M.,** The mechanism of basophil histamine release induced by antigen and by the calcium ionophore A23187, *J. Immunol.*, 114, 1692, 1975.
139. **Goldstein, I. M., Horn, J. K., Kaplan, H. B., and Weissman, G.,** Calcium-induced lysozyme secretion from human polymorphonuclear leukocytes, *Biochem. Biophys. Res. Commun.*, 60, 807, 1974.
140. **Simon, J. D., Houck, W. E., and Albala, M. M.,** Release of unsaturated vitamin B_{12} binding capacity from human granulocytes by the calcium ionophore A23187, *Biochem. Biophys. Res. Commun.*, 73, 444, 1976.
141. **Estensen, R. D., Reusch, M. E., Epstein, M. L., and Hill, H. R.,** Role of Ca^{2+} and Mg^{2+} in some human neutrophil functions as indicated by ionophore A23187, *Infect. Immun.*, 13, 146, 1976.
142. **Koza, E. P., Wright, T. E., and Becker, E. L.,** Lysosomal enzyme secretion and volume contraction induced in neutrophils by cytochalasin B, chemotactic factor and A23187, *Proc. Soc. Exp. Biol. Med.*, 149, 476, 1975.
143. **Zabucchi, G. and Romeo, D.,** The dissociation of exocytosis and respiratory stimulation in leukocytes by ionophores, *Biochem. J.*, 156, 209, 1976.
144. **Zabucchi, G., Soranzo, M. R., and Rossi, F.,** Exocytosis in human polymorphonuclear leukocytes induced by A23187 and calcium, *FEBS Lett.*, 54, 44, 1975.

145. **Leffell, M. S. and Spitznagel, J. K.**, Fate of human lactoferrin and myeloperoxidase in phagocytizing human neutrophils: effects of immunoglobulin G subclasses and immune complexes coated on latex beads, *Infect. Immun.*, 12, 813, 1975.
146. **Stossel, T. P.**, Phagocytosis, *N. Engl. J. Med.*, 290, 774, 1974.
147. **Weissman, G., Zurier, R. B., Spieler, P. J., and Goldstein, I. M.**, Mechanisms of lysosomal enzyme release from leukocytes exposed to immune complexes and other particles, *J. Exp. Med.*, 134, 149, 1971.
148. **Henson, P. M.**, Secretion of lysosomal enzymes induced by immune complexes and complement, in *Lysosomes in Biology and Pathology*, Vol. 5, Dingle, J. T. and Dean, R. T., Eds., North-Holland, Amsterdam, 1976, 99.
149. **Henson, P. M.**, The immunologic release of constituents from neutrophil leukocytes. I. The role of antibody and C′ on non-phagocytosable surfaces or phagocytosable particles, *J. Immunol.*, 107, 1535, 1971.
150. **Henson, P. M.**, The immunologic release of constituents from neutrophil leukocytes. II. Mechanisms of release during phagocytosis and adherence to non-phagocytosable surfaces, *J. Immunol.*, 107, 1547, 1971.
151. **Davies, P. and Allison, A. C.**, The secretion of lysosomal enzymes, in *Lysosomes in Biology and Pathology*, Vol. 5, Dingle, J. T. and Dean, R. T., Eds., North-Holland, Amsterdam, 1976, 61.
152. **Busse, W. W. and Sosman, J.**, Histamine inhibition of neutrophil lysosomal enzyme release: an H2 histamine receptor response, *Science*, 194, 737, 1976.
153. **Ignarro, L. J.**, Glucocorticosteroid inhibition of non-phagocytic discharge of lysosomal enzymes from human neutrophils, *Arthritis Rheum.*, 20, 73, 1977.
154. **Ignarro, L. J. and Cech, S. Y.**, Lysosomal enzyme secretion from human neutrophils mediated by cyclic GMP: inhibition of cyclic GMP accumulation and neutrophil function by glucocorticosteroids, *J. Cyclic Nucl. Res.*, 1, 283, 1975.
155. **Bianco, C., Patrick R., and Nussenzweig, V.**, A population of lymphocytes bearing a membrane receptor for antigen antibody complement complexes. I. Separation and characterization, *J. Exp. Med.*, 132, 702, 1970.
156. **Haegert, D. G., Hallberg, L., and Coombs, R. R. A.**, B and T lymphocyte subpopulation in human peripheral blood, *Int. Arch. Allergy Appl. Immunol.*, 46, 525, 1974.
157. **Pernis, B., Forni, L., and Amante, L.**, Immunoglobulin spots on the surface of rabbit lymphocytes, *J. Exp. Med.*, 132, 1001, 1970.
158. **Dickler, H. B. and Kunkel, H. G.**, Interaction of aggregated γ globulin with B lymphocytes, *J. Exp. Med.*, 136, 207, 1972.
159. **Jondal, M., Holm, G., and Wigzell, H.**, Surface markers on human T and B lymphocytes, *J. Exp. Med.*, 136, 207, 1972.
160. **Brown, G., and Greaves, M. F.**, Cell surface markers for human T and B lymphocytes, *Eur. J. Immunol.*, 4, 302, 1974.
161. **Pentycross, C. R.**, Technique for lymphocyte transformation, *J. Clin. Pathol.*, 21, 175, 1968.
162. **Waithe, W. I. and Hirschhorn, K.**, An assay of lymphocyte blastogenesis based on measurement of the rate of protein synthesis, in *In Vitro Methods in Cell-Mediated Immunity*, Bloom, B. R. and Glade, P. R., Eds., Academic Press, New York, 1971, 455.
163. **Nowell, P. C.**, Phytohemagglutin: an initiator of mitosis in cultures of normal human leukocytes, *Cancer Res.*, 20, 462, 1960.
164. **Barker, B. E., Lutzner, M. A., and Farnes, P.**, Ultrastructural properties of pokeweed stimulated leukocytes, in *Proceedings of the Third Leukocyte Culture Conference*, Rieke, W. O., Ed., Appelton-Century-Crofts, New York, 1969, 587.
165. **Schellekens, P. Th. A. and Eijsvoogel, V. P.**, Lymphocyte transformation in vitro. III. Mechanisms of stimulation in the mixed lymphocyte culture, *Clin. Exp. Immunol.*, 7, 229, 1970.
166. **Bach, F. H. and Hirschhorn, K.**, Lymphocyte interaction: a potential histocompatibility test in vitro, *Science*, 143, 813, 1964.
167. **Bach, F. H. and Vognow, N. K.**, One-way stimulation in mixed leukocyte cultures, *Science*, 153, 545, 1966.
168. **Thor, D. E.**, The capillary tube migration inhibitor technique applied to human peripheral lymphocytes using the guinea pig peritoneal exudate as the indicator cell population, in *In Vitro Methods in Cell Mediated Immunity*, Bloom, B. R. and Glade, P. R., Eds., Academic Press, New York, 1971, 293.
169. **Al-Askari, S., David, J. R., Lawrence, H. S., and Thomas, L.**, In vitro studies on homograft sensitivity, *Nature (London)*, 205, 916, 1965.
170. **Soborg, M. and Bendixen, G.**, Human lymphocyte migration on a parameter of hypersensitivity, *Acta Med. Scand.*, 181, 2, 247, 1967.

171. **David, J. R. and David, R.,** Assay for inhibition of macrophage migration, in *In Vitro Methods in Cell Mediated Immunity,* Bloom, B. R. and Glade, P. R., Eds., Academic Press, New York, 1971, 249.
172. **Brunner, K. T., Eugers, H. D., and Cerottini, J. C.,** The Cr^{51} release assay used for the quantitative measurement of cell-mediated cytolysis in vitro, in *In Vitro Methods in Cell Mediated and Tumor Immunity,* Bloom, B. R. and David, J. R., Eds., Academic Press, New York, 1976, 423.
173. **Cerottini, J. C. and Brunner, K. T.,** Cell mediated cytotoxicity, allograft rejection and tumor immunity, *Adv. Immunol.,* 18, 67, 1974.
174. **Schlossman, S. F. and Chess, L.,** Immunologic functions of a subset of human null cells, in *Clinical Evaluation of Immune Function in Man,* Litwin, S. D., Christian, C. L., and Siskind, G. W., Eds., Grune & Stratton, New York, 1976, 65.
175. **Perlmann, P. and Perlmann, H.,** Contactual lysis of antibody-coated chicken erythrocytes by purified lymphocytes, *Cell. Immunol.,* 1, 300, 1970.
176. **MacLennan, I. C. M., Campbell, A. C., and Gale, D. G. L.,** Quantitation of K cells, in *In Vitro Methods in Cell Mediated and Tumor Immunity,* Bloom, B. R. and David, J. R., Eds., Academic Press, New York, 1976, 511.
177. **Waldmann, T. A., Durm, M., Broder, S., Blackman, M., Blaese, R. M., and Strober, W.,** Role of suppressor T cells in pathogenesis of common variable hypogammaglobulinemia, *Lancet,* 2, 609, 1974.
178. **Broder, S., Humphrey, R., Durm, M., Blackman, M., Meade, B., Goldman, C., Strober, W., and Waldmann, T.,** Impaired synthesis of polyclonol (non-paraprotein) immunoglobulins by circulating lymphocytes from patients with multiple myeloma, *N. Engl. J. Med.,* 293, 887, 1975.
179. **Holm, G., Mellstedt, H., Bjorkholm, M., Johnsson, B., Killander, B., Sunblad, R., and Soderberg, G.,** Lymphocyte abnormalities in untreated patients with Hodgkin's Disease, *Cancer,* 37, 751, 1976.
180. **Bobrove, A. M., Fuks, Z., Strober, S., and Kaplan, H. S.,** Quantitation of T and B lymphocytes and cellular immune function in Hodgkin's Disease, *Cancer,* 36, 169, 1975.
181. **Wybran, J. and Fudenberg, H. H.,** Thymus derived rosette-forming cells in various human disease states: cancer, lymphoma, bacterial and viral infections and other diseases, *J. Clin. Invest.,* 52, 1026, 1973.
182. **Cohen, S., Fisher, B., Yosheida, L., and Bettigole, R. E.,** Serum migration-inhibitory activity in patients with lymphoproliferative diseases, *N. Engl. J. Med.,* 290, 882, 1974.
183. **Mann, R. B., Jaffe, E. S., Braylon, R. C., Eggleston, J. C., Ransom, L., Kaiser, H., and Berard, C. W.,** Immunologic and morphologic studies of T cell lymphoma, *Am. J. Med.,* 58, 307, 1975.
184. **Bloomfield, C. D., Kersey, J. H., Brunning, R. D., and Gajl-Peczalska, K. J.,** Prognostic significance of lymphocyte surface markers in adult non-Hodgkin's malignant lymphoma, *Lancet,* 2, 1330, 1976.
185. **Piesens, W. F., Schur, P. H., and Moloney, W. C.,** Lymphocyte surface immunoglobulins. Distribution and frequency in lymphoproliferative disorders, *N. Engl. J. Med.,* 288, 176, 1973.
186. **Jaffe, E. S., Shevach, E. M., Frank, M. M., Berard, C. W., and Green, I.,** Nodular lymphoma-evidence for origin from follicular B lymphocytes, *N. Engl. J. Med.,* 290, 813, 1974.
187. **Aisenberg, A. C. and Block, K. J.,** Immunoglobulins on the surface of neoplastic lymphocytes, *N. Engl. J. Med.,* 287, 272, 1972.
188. **Shevach, E. M., Herberman, R., Frank, M. M., and Green, I.,** Receptors for complement and immunoglobulin on human leukemic cells and human lymphoblastoid cell lines, *J. Clin. Invest.,* 51, 1933, 1972.
189. **Seligmann, M.,** B cell and T cell markers in lymphoid proliferations (editorial), *N. Engl. J. Med.,* 290, 1962, 1974.
190. **Rowlands, D. T., Daniele, R. P., Nowell, P. C., and Wurzel, H. A.,** Characterization of lymphocyte subpopulations in CLL, *Cancer,* 34, 1962, 1974.
191. **Astaldi, G. and Airo, R.,** Phytohaemagglutinin in leukemia, *Lancet,* 1, 1103, 1966.
192. **Preud'homme, J. L. and Seligmann, M.,** Surface bound immunoglobulins as a cell marker in human lymphoproliferative disease, *Blood,* 40, 777, 1972.
193. **Grey, H. M., Rabellino, E., and Pirofsky, B.,** Immunoglobulins on the surface of lymphocytes. IV. Distribution in hypogammoglobulinemia and chronic lymphatic leukemia, *J. Clin. Invest.,* 50, 2368, 1972.
194. **Van Boxel, J. A., Hardin, J. A., Green, I., and Paul, W. E.,** Multiple heavy chain determinants on individual B lymphocytes in the peripheral blood of patients with Sjogren's syndrome, *N. Engl. J. Med.,* 289, 823, 1973.
195. **Leventhal, B. G., Waldorf, D. S., and Talal, N.,** Impaired lymphocyte transformation and delayed hypersensitivity in Sjorgen's syndrome, *J. Clin. Invest.,* 46, 1338, 1967.
196. **Kersey, J. H., Gajl-Peczalask, J., Hallgren, H. M., Yunis, E. J., and Nesbitt, M. E.,** Acute lymphoblastic leukemic cells with T (Thymus-derived) lymphocyte markers, *Science,* 182, 1355, 1973.

197. **Borella, L. and Sen, L.**, T and B lymphocytes in untreated acute lymphocytic leukemia, *Cancer,* 34, 646, 1974.
198. **Kaplan, J., Ravindranath, Y., and Petersen, W. D.**, T and B lymphocyte antigen positive null cell leukemias, *Blood,* 49, 371, 1977.
199. **Minowada, J., Han, T., and Ohnuma, T.**, Identification of T and B lymphocytes in human lymphatic leukemia, *Proc. Am. Assoc. Cancer Res.,* 14 (Abstr.), 81, 1973.
200. **Broder, S., Edelson, R. L., Lutzner, M. A., Nelson, D. L., MacDermott, R. P., Durm, M. E., Goldman, C. K., Meade, B. D., and Waldmann, T. A.**, The Sezary Syndrome. A malignant proliferation of helper T cells, *J. Clin. Invest.,* 58, 1297, 1976.
201. **Brouet, J. C., Flandrin, G., and Seligmann, M.**, Indications of the thymus-derived nature of the proliferating cells in six patients with Sezary syndrome, *N. Engl. J. Med.,* 289, 341, 1973.
202. **Lindstrom, F. D., Hardy, W. R., Eberle, B. J., and Williams, R. C.**, Multiple myeloma and benign monoclonal gammopathy: differentiation by immunofluorescence of lymphocytes, *Ann. Intern. Med.,* 78, 837, 1973.
203. **Solomon, A.**, Cellular regulation of humoral immunity, *N. Engl. J. Med.,* 293, 928, 1975.
204. **Gross, R. L., Lassy, A., Williams, E. A., and Newberne, P. M.**, Abnormal spontaneous rosette formation and rosette inhibition in lung carcinoma, *N. Engl. J. Med.,* 292, 439, 1975.
205. **Herberman, R. B.**, Immunologic approaches to diagnosis of cancer, *Cancer,* 37, 549, 1976.
206. **Olkowski, Z. L. and Wilkens, S. A.**, T lymphocyte levels in the peripheral blood of patients with cancer of head and neck, *Am. J. Surg.,* 30, 440, 1975.
207. **Brooks, W. H., Roseman, T. A., and Rogers, A. S.**, Impairment of rosette forming T lymphocytes in patients with primary intracranial tumors, *Cancer,* 37, 1869, 1976.
208. **Dellon, A. L., Potvin, C., and Chretien, P. V.**, Thymus dependent lymphocyte levels in bronchogenic carcinoma: correlations with histology clinical stage and clinical course after surgical treatment, *Cancer,* 35, 687, 1975.
209. **Black, M. M., Leis, H. P., Shore, B., and Zachran, R. E.**, Cellular hypersensitivity to breast cancer. Assessment by a leukocyte migration procedure, *Cancer,* 33, 952, 1974.
210. **Waldmann, T. A., Durm, M., Broder, S., Blackman, M., Blaese, R. M., and Strober, W.**, Role of suppressor T cells in pathogenesis of common variable hypogammaglobulinemia, *Lancet,* 2, 609, 1974.
211. **Geha, R. S., Schmerger, E., Merber, E., and Rosen, F. S.**, Heterosensitivity of acquired or common variable agammaglobulinemia, *N. Engl. J. Med.,* 291, 1, 1974.
212. **Dickler, H. B., Adkinson, N. F., Fisher, R. I., and Terry, W. D.**, Lymphocytes in patients with variable immunodeficiency in panhypogammaglobulinemia, *J. Clin. Invest.,* 53, 834, 1974.
213. **Willams, R. C., Deboard, J. R., Mellbye, O. J., Messner, R. P., and Lindstrom, F. D.**, Studies of T and B lymphocytes in patients with connective tissue disease, *J. Clin. Invest.,* 52, 283, 1973.
214. **Edelson, R. L.**, Membrane markers of lymphocytes in lymphomas, melanoma, and lupus erythematosus, *Int. J. Dermatol.,* 15, 577, 1976.
215. **Farid, N. R., Munro, R. E., Row, V. V., and Volpe, R.**, Peripheral thymus dependent ('T') lymphocytes in Hashimoto's and Graves' Disease, *N. Engl. J. Med.,* 288, 1313, 1973.
216. **Hedfos, E., Holm, G., and Pettersson, D.**, Lymphocyte subpopulation in sarcoidosis, *Clin. Exp. Immunol.,* 17, 219, 1974.
217. **Rocklin, R. E., Lewis, E. J., and David, J. R.**, In vitro evidence of cellular hypersensitivity to glomerular-basement-membrane antigens in human glomerulonephritis, *N. Engl. J. Med.,* 283, 407, 1970.
218. **Dixon, F. J.**, What are sensitized cells doing in glomerulonephritis? *N. Engl. J. Med.,* 283, 498, 1970.
219. **Elves, M. W., Israels, M. C. G., and Collinge, M.**, An assessment of the mixed leukocyte reaction in renal failure, *Lancet,* 1, 682, 1966.
220. **Kasakura, S. and Lowenstein, L.**, The effect of uremic blood on mixed leukocyte reactions and on cultures of leukocytes with phytohemagglutinin, *Transplantation,* 5, 283, 1967.
221. **Strickland, R. G., Korsmeyer, S., Soltis, R. D., Wilson, D., and Williams, R. C.**, Peripheral blood B and T cells in chronic inflammatory bowel disease, *Gastroenterology,* 67, 569, 1974.
222. **Knowles, M., Hughes, D., Caspary, E. A., and Field, E. J.**, Lymphocyte transformation in multiple sclerosis, *Lancet,* 2, 1207, 1968.
223. **Behan, P. O., LaMarche, J. B., Feldman, R. G., and Shermata, W. A.**, Lymphocyte transformation in the Guillian-Barre syndrome, *Lancet,* 1, 421, 1970.
224. **Gajl-Peczalska, K. J., Lim, S. D., Jacobsen, R. R., and Good, R. A.**, B lymphocytes in lepromatous leprosy, *N. Engl. J. Med.,* 288, 1033, 1973.
225. **Wybran, J., Levin, A. S., Spitler, L. E., and Fudenberg, H. H.**, Rosette forming cells, immunologic deficiency diseases and transfer factor, *N. Engl. J. Med.,* 288, 710, 1973.

226. **Buckley, R. H., Lucos, Z. J., Hassler, B. G., Smijewski, C. M., and Amos, D. B.**, Defective cellular immunity associated with chronic mucocutaneous moniliasis and recurrent staphylococcal botryomyocosis: immunological reconstitution by allogeneic bone marrow, *Clin. Exp. Immunol.*, 3, 153, 1968.
227. **Levin, G. M., Turk, J. L., Wright, D. J. M., and Grimble, A. G. S.**, Reduced lymphocyte transformation due to a plasma factor in patients with syphilis, *Lancet*, 2, 246, 1969.
228. **Pattengale, P. K., Smith, R. W., and Perlin, E.**, Atypical lymphocytes in acute infectious mononucleosis, *N. Engl. J. Med.*, 291, 1145, 1974.
229. **Mangi, R. J., Niederman, J. C., Kelleher, J. E., Dwyer, J. M., Evans, A. S., and Kantor, F. S.**, Depression of cell-mediated immunity during acute infectious mononucleosis, *N. Engl. J. Med.*, 291, 1149, 1974.
230. **Pisciotta, A. and DePrey, C.**, Inhibition of mitosis by chloramphenicol in phyhemagglutinin stimulated lymphocytes, *Blood*, 30, 457, 1967.
231. **Crout, J. E., Hepburn, B., and Ritts, R. E.**, Suppression of lymphocyte transformation after aspirin ingestion, *N. Engl. J. Med.*, 292, 221, 1975.
232. **Astaldi, G., Burgio, G. R., Krc, J., Genova, R., and Astaldi, A. A., Jr.**, L-asparaginase and blastogenesis, *Lancet*, 1, 423, 1969.
233. **Hurd, E. R. and Giuliano, V. J.**, The effect of cyclophosphamide on B and T lymphocytes in patient with connective tissue diseases, *Arthritis Rheum.*, 18, 67, 1975.
234. **Gupta, S., Grieco, M. H., and Cushman, P.**, Impairment of rosette-forming T lymphocytes in chronic marijuana smokers, *N. Engl. J. Med.*, 291, 874, 1974.
235. **Paronetto, F. and Popper, H.**, Lymphocyte stimulation induced by Halothane in patients with hepatitis following exposure to Halothane, *N. Engl. J. Med.*, 283, 1970.
236. **Riddle, P. R. and Berenbaum, M. C.**, Postoperative depression of the lymphocyte response to phytohaemagglutinin, *Lancet*, 1, 746, 1967.
237. **Horowitz, S. and Hong, R.**, *The Pathogenesis and Treatment of Immunodeficiency*, S. Karger-Basel, 1977.

WHITE CELL METABOLISM

A. J. Sbarra, R. J. Selvaraj, B. B. Paul, G. W. Mitchell, Jr., and F. Louis

Introduction

White cell metabolism has been a subject for systematic review only during the past few decades. A number of reasons for this apparent delay and intensification of interest are readily apparent. White cells are not of a single type. For example, the circulating granulocytes are of three varieties: neutrophils, basophils, and eosinophils. Only recently have techniques become available that permit the preparation of these cell types in sufficiently pure states so that meaningful studies can be carried out. Further compounding the problem is that each of these cell types can be divided into different stages of maturity and differentiation. Also to be considered is the fact that, in order to obtain cell types in sufficient quantity, the cell must, in most cases, be elicited (i.e., injection of the host with irritants such as casein, glycogen, peptones, etc.). This can result in altered metabolic activity. Finally, the isolation procedure itself can cause injury to the cell. In spite of these shortcomings, however, the biochemical activities of white cells have, in recent years, been of extreme interest to the biochemist, microbiologist, immunologist, hematologist, and cell biologist. No doubt, a major impetus for this aroused activity has been the fact that when white cells, in particular the polymorphonuclear neutrophilic leukocytes (PMN), are allowed to incubate in the presence of particulate material, an immediate and dramatic increase in metabolic activity occurs. Further, the positive correlation of these stimulated metabolic events with a physiological function, i.e., antimicrobial activity, has focused interest on the biochemical activities of these cells.

In this chapter, we will discuss the metabolic activity of the PMN at rest (in the absence of particles) and during phagocytosis (presence of particles). We will direct our attention mainly to the PMN, since most of the studies that have been carried out are with this cell-type. Some limited metabolic studies have also been carried out on lymphocytes, monocytes, and eosinophils. For comparative purposes, these cell types will also be discussed.

Metabolism of PMN in the Absence and Presence of Particulate Material

The polymorphonuclear leukocyte is characterized by its high rate of aerobic and anaerobic glycolysis with a corresponding accumulation of lactic acid. Intermediates and enzymes of the Embden-Meyerhof pathway have been isolated and identified, and for a number of the enzymes, V_{max} and K_m values have been estimated. From these data, it may be concluded that hexokinase is the rate-limiting enzyme governing these activities. Kreb's cycle activity has been found in these cells. The ratio of respiration to glycolysis, however, is low. Direct oxidation of glucose through the hexose monophosphate pathway (HMS) has also been reported. Certain enzymes of this pathway have been characterized, and it has been estimated that approximately 3% of the glucose is catabolized by this pathway. Some of the data supporting these concepts are presented in Tables 1 and 2. Included in these tables are the corresponding metabolic activities of leukocytes collected from patients with myelocytic and lymphocytic leukemia.[1,2] The metabolic pathways of two- and three-carbon compounds in PMN have been studied and may be seen in Tables 3 to 5.

A unique characteristic of PMN is the ability to phagocytize foreign particles. Molecular biochemists were attracted by this interesting phenomenon, since the addition of particulate material to PMN results in an immediate and dramatic increase in oxygen uptake. This observation was noted by Baldridge and Gerard in 1933.[4] It was

Table 1
COMPARISONS OF V_{max} and K_m VALUES OF GLYCOLYTIC ENZYMES OF NORMAL AND LEUKEMIC LEUKOCYTES

	Computed V_{max}				
Activity	Normal	Myelocytic leukmia	Lymphocytic leukemia	K_s[a]	K_c[a]
Aerobic glycolysis	75	22	8	2.5×10^{-4}	
Hexokinase	86	40	15	3.5×10^{-4}	3.0×10^{-4}
Phosphohexose isomerase	4950	4950	620	1.7×10^{-4}	
Phosphofractokinase	115	48	19	1.8×10^{-4}	2.5×10^{-4}
Aldolase	155	167	53	7.3×10^{-4}	
Triosephosphate isomerase	292	310	93	3.9×10^{-4}	
Glyceraldehyde 3 phosphate dehydrogenase	512	320	96	3.4×10^{-5}	4.1×10^{-5}
Pyruvate kinase	162	60	20	1.0×10^{-4}	
Lactic dehydrogenase	600	360	180	2.5×10^{-5}	4.9×10^{-5}
G6PDH[b]	55	21	10	1.7×10^{-5}	1.3×10^{-5}
6PGDH[c]	45	18	8	1.2×10^{-5}	2.1×10^{-5}
Phosphopentose isomerase	4800	4690	1150	1.4×10^{-3}	

Note: Velocities expressed as micromoles of triose or triose equivalents produced or converted per minute per 10^{10} cells. For purposes of comparison 1 mol of the substrates of G6PDH,[b] 6PGDH,[c] and phosphopentose isomerase is considered equivalent to 2 mol of triose.

[a] Means of normal, myelocytic leukemia, and lymphocytic leukemia values. K_s is Michaelis constant for substrate; K_c, Michaelis constant for coenzyme.
[b] Glucose-6 phosphate dehydrogenase.
[c] 6-Phosphogluconate dehydrogenase.

From Beck, W., S., *J. Biol. Chem.*, 232, 277, 1958. With permission.

essentially ignored until the 1940s when Nungester's group, at the University of Michigan, carried out extensive studies on the biochemical activities of leukocytes in the absence and presence of particulate material. They studied the metabolic activities of guinea pig exudate leukocytes in the absence and presence of *Streptococcus pneumoniae*. They extended Baldridge and Gerard's investigation to include the effect of inhibitors on both respiratory and glycolytic activity. Unfortunately, most of this work was published only in thesis form[5,6] and did not receive due attention.

A systematic study, dealing with the interaction of tubercle bacilli and phagocytes, was undertaken by Suter in the mid 1950s.[7-9] The effects of oxygen tension, pH limits, and concentration of cells were determined in resting and phagocytizing cells. The addition of heat-killed tubercle bacilli to PMN resulted in a doubling of the respiratory activity and a significant increase in HMS activity. These results are shown in Table 6. It became evident from these experiments that a comprehensive and in-depth study of host-parasite interactions at the biochemical level would be fruitful. On this premise, a number of studies were soon begun. In many of these investigations, inert particulate material, such as polystyrene latex spherules and bacteria, were used as test

Table 2
FACTORS CONTROLLING CHOICE OF ALTERNATIVE PATHWAY FOR GLUCOSE 6-PHOSPHATE (G-6-P)

Additions (*M*)	ΔF-6-P (μmol)	ΔTPNH (μmol)	Utilized G-6-P entering phosphogluconate path (%)[a]
Glucose (0.001)	0.026	<0.003[b]	<11.5
+ TPM (0.5 × 10^{-4})	0.018	0.010	35.7
+ TPN (1.5 × 10^{-4})	0.015	0.012	44.3
+ hexokinase[c]	0.097	<0.003[b]	<3.2
+ hexokinase[c] + TPN (0.5 × 10^{-4})	0.089	0.013	12.7
+ hexokinase[c] + TPN (1.5 × 10^{-4})	0.086	0.015	14.9
G 6-P (0.0005)	0.303	<0.003[b]	<1.0
+ TPN (0.5 × 10^{-4})	0.269	0.020	6.9
+ TPN (1.5 × 10^{-4})	0.265	0.022	7.7
G 6-P (0.001)	0.491	<0.003[b]	<0.6
+ TPN (0.5 × 10^{-4})	0.467	0.020	4.1
+ TPN (1.5 × 10^{-4})	0.480	0.022	4.4

Note: Each incubation contained 50 μmol of Tris buffer, pH 7.4, 4 μmol of ATP, 10 μmol of $MgCl_2$, 2 μmol of DPN, an aliquot of normal leukocyte homogenate containing the equivalent of 1.36×10^6 cells, plus the additions given above. Final volume, 3 mℓ; duration of incubation, 2 min. Δ signifies the amounts formed during total incubation.

[a] Equals (100 × ΔTPNH)/(ΔF-6-P + ΔTPNH).

[b] Limit of sensitivity of method.

[c] The amount of hexokinase added resulted in a five-fold increase in the level of hexokinase activity per incubation.

From Beck, W. S., *J. Biol. Chem.*, 232, 260, 1958. With permission.

particles. Guinea pig exudate cells, containing over 80% PMN, generally served as phagocytes.

Many of the initial studies were repeated and confirmed. Also, glucose utilization and lactic acid production were studied under aerobic and anaerobic conditions. Both increased during phagocytosis. Particle entry occurred under aerobic and anaerobic environments. At this point, it was established conclusively that a number of metabolic stimulations occurred during phagocytosis. The use of some common respiratory and glycolytic inhibitors permitted us to learn more about the significance of the stimulated metabolic activities, or "burst", accompanying phagocytosis. The glycolytic inhibitors (iodoacetic acid and sodium fluoride) inhibited the increased respiratory, HMS, and glycolytic activities. Engulfment was also inhibited. On the other hand, the generally assumed respiratory inhibitors (KCN and Antimycin A®), and an uncoupler of oxidative phosphorylation, Dinitrophenol®, did not affect particle entry or the increased

Table 3
INCORPORATION OF C^{14} INTO GLYCOGEN AND LACTATE OF RABBIT POLYMORPHONUCLEAR LEUKOCYTES AFTER INCUBATION WITH LABELED ACETATE, PYRUVATE, LACTATE, AND GLYCEROL

Expt no.	Labeled substrates	μCi	μmol	Glycogen isolated (mg)	C^{14} incorporation into glycogen (%)	Lactate produced (mg)	C^{14} incorporation into lactate (%)
1	Acetate-1-C^{14}	35.5	7.4	15.2	1×10^{-3}	14.8	0.4
	Acetate-2-C^{14}	35.5	7.4	13.5	2×10^{-3}	13.9	2.4
2	Pyruvate-1-C^{14}	12.5	4.0	7.1	3×10^{-3}	18.4	39.4
	Pyruvate-2-C^{14}	12.5	4.0	10.3	4×10^{-3}	16.3	26.0
	Pyruvate-3-C^{14}	12.5	4.0	8.5	5×10^{-3}	17.6	34.8
3	Lactate-2-C^{14}	15.7	2.4	11.0	2×10^{-3}	17.3	29.7
4	Glycerol-1(3)-C^{14}	9.1	2.4	11.2	2.8	17.8	3.5

Note: 2×10^9 cells were used in each incubation.

From Noble, E. P., Stjernholm, R. L., and Weisberger, A. S., *J. Biol. Chem.* 235, 1262, 1960. With permission.

Table 4
DISTRIBUTION OF C^{14} IN LACTATE PRODUCED BY RABBIT POLYMORPHONUCLEAR LEUKOCYTES INCUBATED WITH LABELED ACETATE, PYRUVATE, LACTATE, AND GLYCEROL

Expt no.	Labeled substrate	Radioactivity in lactate carbon atoms (%)			Recovery of C^{14} in degradation (%)
		C-1	C-2	C-3	
1	Acetate-1-C^{14}	100	0	0	104
	Acetate-2-C^{14}	15	42	43	100
2	Pyruvate-1-C^{14}	100	0	0	95
	Pyruvate-2-C^{14}	0	100	0	101
	Pyruvate-3-C^{14}	0	1	99	93
3	Lactate-2-C^{14}	0	100	0	98
4	Glycerol-1(3)-C^{14}	49	1	50	100

From Noble, E. P., Stjernholm, R. L., and Weisberger, A. S., *J. Biol. Chem.*, 235, 1262, 1960. With permission.

Table 5
DISTRIBUTION OF C^{14} IN GLUCOSE OF GLYCOGEN ISOLATED FROM RABBIT POLYMORPHONUCLEAR LEUYKOCYTES INCUBATED WITH LABELED ACETATE, PYRUVATE, LACTATE, AND GLYCEROL

Expt no.	Labeled substrate	Radioactivity in glucose of glycogen carbon atoms (%)						Recovery of C^{14} in degradation (%)
		C-1	C-2	C-3	C-4	C-5	C-6	
1	Acetate-1-C^{14}	3	3[a]		86	4	4	99
	Acetate-2-C^{14}	1	3	2	17	38	39	95
2	Pyruvate-1-C^{14}	3	2	2	87	3	3	92
	Pyruvate-2-C^{14}	2	6	3	0	87	2	94
	Pyruvate-3-C^{14}	2	5	2	3	0	88	93
3	Lactate-2-C^{14}	0	13	1	3	75	8	105
4	Glycerol-1(3)-C^{14}	3	3	0	46	0	48	99

[a] C-2 and C-3 were not individually separated for this experiment.

From Noble, E. P., Stjernholm, R. L., and Weisberger, A. S., *J. Biol. Chem.*, 235, 1263, 1960. With permission.

Table 6
OXIDATION OF GLUCOSE-1-C^{14} AND GLUCOSE-6-C^{14} BY PEC ALONE, AND DURING PHAGOCYTOSIS OF DEAD TUBERCLE BACILLI

Cells	O_2 uptake (μl)[a]	Activity in CO_2 (cpm) C_1[a]	C_6[b]	Ratio (C_1/C_6)[b]
PEC	12.7	432	14.5	29.7
	12.7	336	17.2	19.5
R1Rv	1	134	10.3	13.0
	2	123	16.5	7.5
PEC and R1Rv together	27.1	1609	23.8	67.5
	27.6	2085	29.2	71.4
Sum of means of values for PEC and R1Rv separately	14.2	512	29.3	17.5
Mean value for PEC and R1Rv together, corrected for R1Rv alone[c]	25.9	1718	13.1	131.0

[a] Oxygen uptake in experiments with PEC expressed as μl O_2/100 μg cellular P and hour.

[b] C_1 and C_6 refer to CO_2 derived from flasks containing glucose-1-C^{14} and glucose-6-C^{14} respectively. Results have been normalized to 1×10^5 cpm used.

[c] Third line minus second line.

From Stahelin, H., Karnovsky, M. L., Farnham, A. E., and Suter, E., *J. Exp. Med.*, 105, 273, 1957. With permission.

metabolic activities.[10,11] It appeared from these studies that metabolic energy, specifically glycolytic energy, is required for particle entry. These results are summarized in Table 7.

Nature of Metabolic Stimulation

In addition to the stimulated activities noted above, the incubation of PMN with particulate material also results in increased NADPH oxidase,[12,16] NADH oxidase,[17] glutathione (GSSG) reductase,[18,19] myeloperoxidase (MPO),[20] and a general activation of lysosomal enzyme activities.[21,23] Production of H_2O_2, an end product of NADPH and NADH oxidation,[24] as well as D- and L-amino acid oxidases,[25,26] is also increased in PMN stimulated by phagocytosis. The antiinflammatory drug phenylbutazone inhibits the HMS at the level of glucose-6-phosphate dehydrogenase (G6PDH) and 6-phosphogluconate dehydrogenase (6PGDH). Also, hydrogen peroxide production is inhibited, as is killing of phagocytized bacteria.[27,28] Hydrogen peroxide has long been known to be a potent antimicrobial agent. However, the amount produced by PMN neutrophils during phagocytosis does not appear to be sufficient to account for the observed bactericidal activity of these cells. If, however, one reacts sublethal concentrations of H_2O_2 and MPO with a halide, either I^-, Cl^-, or Br^-, at acid pH, significant bactericidal activity is obtained.[29,31] This antimicrobial system will be discussed in more detail later.

Since H_2O_2 appears to be an important, if not a critical, component of a functional antimicrobial system in the cell, some studies regarding its site of production have appeared. It was first postulated by Quastel and co-workers that H_2O_2 production

Table 7
EFFECT OF INHIBITORS ON PMN METABOLISM IN THE ABSENCE AND PRESENCE OF PARTICLES

	Q_{O_2} (P) (μℓ)		Activity in CO_2 (cpm): C-1[a]		Activity in CO_2 (cpm): C-6[a]		C-1:C-6		Lactate (μM)[b]		Entry
Particles	−	+	−	+	−	+	−	+	−	+	
Normal	18.7 ± 0.7	45.6 ± 2.4	211 ± 18	1406 ± 139	26 ± 4	65 ± 10	8.1	21.6	1.9	2.6	max
P→	<0.001		<0.001		<0.001				<0.02		
1 × 10⁻⁴ M Iodoacetate	19.1 ± 2	23.5 ± 3.7	180 ± 23	291 ± 166	166 ± 7	66 ± 26	2.7	4.4	—	—	min
P↓	<0.3	<0.01	<0.1	<0.01	>0.2	>0.5					
P→	>0.3		>0.5		>0.9						
2 × 10⁻² NaF	45.6 ± 2.2	56.2 ± 3.6	459 ± 37	506 ± 71	26 ± 6	36 ± 17	17.7	14.1	—	—	min
P↓	<0.001	>0.1	<0.001	<0.05		>0.3					
P→	<0.05		>0.5		<0.5						
1 × 10⁻³ M KCN	5.1 ± 1.9	22.5 ± 4.0	297 ± 53	1453 ± 95	19 ± 5	26 ± 8	15.7	55.9	—	—	max
P↓	<0.01	<0.01	0.5	0.2	>0.05	<0.001					
P→	<0.01		<0.001		>0.5						
3.3 μg Antimycin A	10.3 ± 1.4	44.8 ± 13.0	217 ± 66	1394 ± 386	19 ± 10	27 ± 7	11.4	51.6	—	—	max
P↓	0.05	>0.1	>0.1	>0.1	>0.1	>0.1					
P→			<0.01		>0.1						
1 × 10⁻⁴ M Dinitrophenol	36.1 ± 2.4	55.5 ± 8.4	241 ± 24	898 ± 103	59 ± 7	61 ± 8	3.9	14.8	—	—	max
P↓	<0.001	>0.1	<0.05	>0.5	<0.01	<0.1					
P→	<0.05		<0.01		>0.1						

Note: All results are given on the basis of 100 μg of cellular phosphorus per hour. Radioactivity data are normalized to 1 × 10^5 cpm added to the flasks as glucose. The mean and standard error of the mean is given in all cases. P refers to the probability value for difference between systems without and with particles, respectively.

[a] Glucose labeled in C-1 or C-6 used as substrate.

[b] Results expressed per 100 μg cellular phosphorous for a 30-min period in incubation.

From Stahelin, H., Karnovsky, M. L., Farnham, A. E., and Suter, E., *J. Exp. Med.*, 105, 265, 1957; Sbarra, A. J. and Karnovsky, M. L., *J. Biol. Chem.*, 234, 1359, 1959. With permission.

occurs in PMN and that it is increased in phagocytizing cells.[32] Later it was actually shown, by direct measurement, that H_2O_2 production is actually increased two- to fourfold in phagocytizing cells.[33] Somewhat later, a more sensitive assay for peroxide was developed, and it was shown that the extracellular H_2O_2 concentration in phagocytizing cells increased approximately 50-fold above base lines levels.[34] Recently, cytochemical demonstration of H_2O_2 in PMN leukocyte phagosomes has been reported by the application of a modified diaminobenzidine technique.[35] H_2O_2 synthesis in PMN leukocytes is generally thought to depend on the oxidation of reduced pyridine nucleotide(s) by oxidases. The resulting H_2O_2, according to the above, would accumulate in the phagocytic vacuole.

The precise enzymatic basis for the metabolic "burst", noted when particulate material is added to phagocytes, has been the subject of much controversy. Results from a number of laboratories indicate that the major pathway that will account for the increased oxygen uptake, HMS activation, and H_2O_2 production in phagocytizing cells is an increased oxidation of NADPH by its granule-bound oxidase.[13,14,16,36-39] This view appears valid for a number of reasons, e.g., the V_{max} of NADPH oxidase increases during phagocytosis. The oxygen consumed in the oxidation of NADPH can essentially account for the increased respiration noted in phagocytizing cells. The oxidase is insensitive to KCN (depending on the methodology used in its preparation).[16] Also, the oxidase affinity for NADPH increases; its apparent Michaelis constant decreases tenfold. This low K_m reaches a value that is close to the actual NADPH concentration in the cell. Finally, the NADP to NADPH ratio in phagocytizing cells increases three- to five fold, while the total content of nicotinamide adenine dinucleotide phosphate is not changed.[37,39]

Additional evidence that NADPH oxidase is directly involved, as a primary enzyme responsible for the burst in oxidative activity, is the observations made with phagocytic cells from patients with chronic granulomatous disease.[40] These workers measured the cyanide-insensitive NADPH oxidase activity of phagocytizing cells collected from children with this disease. They noted that phagocytic neutrophils from these patients were markedly deficient in NADPH oxidase activity. The cells were able to phagocytize normally, but they did not show the oxidative respiratory burst when challenged with particles. The finding of a deficiency of NADPH oxidase in the cells suggests that the enzyme is intimately related to the oxidative activity of the cell.

Recently, an interesting mechanism involved in the oxidation of NADPH has been postulated.[36,38,41,42] This mechanism involves a chain reaction with enzymatic and nonenzymatic steps. The enzymatic step is initiated by either an oxidase or peroxidase-oxidase. The postulated steps are given below:

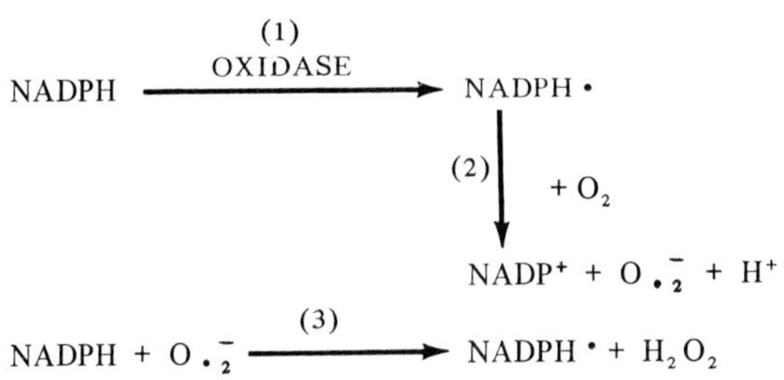

Reactions (2) and (3) are stimulated by Mn^{++} at acid pH and are nonenzymatic.

The reactions account for both oxygen consumption and H_2O_2 formation. The involvement of $O\cdot^-_2$ is demonstrated by the partial inhibition of NADPH oxidation by superoxide dismutase (SOD). This enzyme dismutates the superoxide anion ($O\cdot^-_2$) to H_2O_2:

$$O\cdot_2^- + O\cdot_2^- + 2H^+ \xrightarrow{SOD} H_2O_2 + O_2$$

Since $O\cdot^-_2$ is produced, the possibility that a one-electron oxidation of NADPH, the only hydrogen donor in the system, is postulated. The resulting free radical (NADPH) could then react with O_2 to yield $O\cdot^-_2$.

A number of different investigators have shown that Mn^{++} stimulates the oxidation of NADPH. According to Rossi and co-workers, this is probably due to the stimulatory effect of Mn^{++} on chain reactions (2) and (3) above. This finding does not indicate that NADPH oxidation is nonenzymatic. When heat-inactivated granules are used, no oxidation is noted. Whether the Mn^{++} stimulation is pertinent to the intact cell is open to question. Hohn and Lehrer[40] have shown, using atomic absorption spectrophotometric methodology, that PMN granules contain Mn^{++}, on a molar basis 7.9% as abundant as zinc, a metal in which PMN are rich. The observation that Mn^{++} is present and in relative abundance in the cell, suggests that its role in NADPH oxidation may have physiological significance.

Plasma Membrane, Lysosomal Enzymes, and Stimulated Metabolic Activity

It has been pointed out that the addition of particulate material to PMN results in an immediate and dramatic increase in several different metabolic activities. The extremely rapid metabolic stimulations suggest that they may not be directly dependent on actual particle uptake. The possibility that they may simply be the result of particle-cell interaction, by way of some signal, has been suggested. As a matter of fact, the increased oxygen uptake, oxidation of glucose by the HMP, and NADPH oxidation occur within seconds after the addition of particles to PMN.[15] The metabolic stimulation is noted only when intact PMN are used. PMN homogenates do not respond as intact cells. However, homogenates from phagocytizing cells have stimulated activity.[12]

The metabolic stimulation, or "burst", similar to that induced by phagocytizable matter, can be obtained by a number of different agents that act on the cell membrane. Antileukocyte antibodies induce, within seconds, a significant stimulation in respiration and oxidation of glucose, by way of the HMP. The metabolic changes are, as with phagocytizable particles, insensitive to rotenone, antimycin A, and cyanide. Also, in the same study, granules obtained from PMN exposed to antibodies show an increased KCN-insensitive NADPH oxidation. These results have been attributed to a modification of the PMN plasma membrane.[43]

In an interesting study,[44] the plant lectin, Concanavalin A (Con A), a substance known to excite membranes, was shown to bind to PMN, and to cause a stimulation in PMN-oxidative metabolism similar to that noted with phagocytizing cells. As with antileukocyte antibodies, cyanide, antimycin A, and rotenone did not inhibit the increased oxygen uptake, HMS, and NADPH oxidation in Con A-treated cells. By using fluorescein-labeled Con A, it was noted that the label was found predominantly at the cell surface, generally distributed in small aggregates. If sugars such as Methyl-D-glucopyranoside (which is known to compete with Con A for cell receptors) were added along with the lectin, metabolic stimulation was no longer observed. These results suggest that the binding of Con A to the surface glycoproteins of PMN leads to a change in property of the cell membrane. This change appears to stimulate the oxidative metabolism of the cell.

Cytochalasin E, a metabolite of *Rosellinia necatrix*, when added to PMN, induced metabolic stimulation similar to that noted during phagocytosis. The increased respiratory activity was again found to be insensitive to cyanide, rotenone, and antimycin A. Other cytochalasins, A and B, at similar concentrations, were not effective in stimulating oxidative metabolic activity. The metabolic changes noted with cytochalasin E are assumed to be associated with the involvement of the cell membrane in phagocytosis.[45] A number of other agents, such as surfactants, phospholipase C, fatty acids, immune complexes bound to nonphagocytizable surfaces, soluble immune complexes, and endotoxin, have also been observed to cause stimulation of intact PMN similar to that caused by bacteria and inert particulate material.[37]

Along somewhat similar lines, it has been shown[46] that guinea pig PMN undergo the phagocytosis characteristic of increased oxidative metabolism when the cell is treated with the divalent cation — specific inophore A 23187 within a specific concentration range of calcium. This appears to act as a freely mobile carrier, to equilibrate divalent cation concentrations across membranes via an electroneutral process. Contact of different substances with the cell membrane apparently results in structural changes that "trigger" the initiation of a number of biochemical events. The "trigger" or "signal" for this stimulation is unknown.

One of the most striking morphological features of the cytoplasm of PMN is the presence of an abundance of characteristically staining granules. The finding by Cohn and Hirsch,[21-23] that degranulation occurs during phagocytosis, suggested that these granules might be related to antimicrobial activity. This important observation has led to an extensive study on the origin, nature, and distribution of these granules in the PMN. Two distinct types of granules have been distinguished: azurophilic and specific. Both are produced by the Golgi complex, but at different stages of maturation and from different faces of the Golgi complex. The azurophilic granules are formed only during the progranulocyte stage. They are larger and more dense than the specific granules, which are formed during the myelocyte stage. Progranulocytes contain only azurophilic granules. Mature PMN have relatively few azurophilic granules — most of the granules present are specific. The azurophils contain approximately 90% of the cell's MPO activity. The specific granules contain essentially all of the lactoferrin and 50% of the lysozyme. In addition to MPO, the azurophilic granules also contain acid phosphatase, arylsulfatase, B-glucorinadase, esterase, and 5-nucleotidase. The finding of these lysosomal enzymes in the azurophilic granules suggests that this granule is a primary lysosome. Briefly, when microorganisms are engulfed by PMN, the granules, or lysosomes, degranulate and discharge their lysosomal enzyme into the phagocytic vacuole, where killing and digestion occur. More specific and detailed discussions of this lysosomal enzyme activity are available.[47,48]

In addition to the intracellular activities ascribed to lysosomal enzymes, it has been reported that these enzymes can be released from PMN. It is now generally well accepted that lysosomal enzyme release from phagocytic cells is a selective process. Release varies with particle size and amount ingested, and it is not associated with cell death.[49-51] Moreover, ingestion is not a necessary requirement for selective release.[50-53] Release can take place in the absence of measurable ingestion. When leukocytes are exposed to large surfaces coated with immune complexes, enzyme release occurs. Also, cells pretreated with cytochalasin B, a fungal metabolite, do not ingest particles; however, they do secrete lysosomal enzymes when appropriately stimulated. This finding has permitted researchers to separate the process of enzyme secretion from that of phagocytosis. Thus direct biochemical and morphological studies of secretory events can be evaluated without concern for possible inhibiting effects that added agents might have on phagocytosis. Such studies have shown that agents that adversely affect microtubule function reduce degranulation and lysosomal enzyme release.[54]

The biologic roles of guanosine 3′,5′-monophosphate (cyclic GMP) and adenosine 3′,5′-monophosphate (cyclic AMP) on the secretion of lysosomal enzymes during phagocytosis by human leukocytes have been examined.[55] Contact between phagocytes and particulate immunologic reactants resulted in phagocytosis and secretion of lysosomal enzymes, as expected. These events were accompanied by an accumulation of cyclic GMP and required the presence of extracellular calcium. Acetylcholine, pilocarpine, and cyclic GMP enhance epinephrine; cyclic AMP and/or dibutyryl AMP inhibit both phagocytosis and lysosomal enzyme secretion. The stimulatory action of cholinergic agents and the inhibitory action of epinephrine are accompanied by accumulation of cyclic GMP and cyclic AMP in human phagocytes. These data suggest that cyclic GMP stimulates, while cyclic AMP inhibits, some major functions of human neutrophils.

The above findings indicate not only that lysosomal enzymes are secreted from phagocytic cells, but also that their release is selective. Recently, a most interesting finding that may have some relationship with membrane function has been reported from Karnovsky's laboratory.[56,57] A suspension of intact guinea pig polymorphonuclear leukocytes was able to hydrolyze added ATP, AMP, and p-nitrophenylphosphate under physiologically appropriate conditions. The enzymatic activities noted were attributed to the presence of three ectoenzymes, with their active sites on the plasma membrane facing the external medium. A number of possible physiological roles for these ectoenzymes have been postulated. Presently, however, no definitive role can be assigned to them. Nevertheless, the finding presents interesting possibilities and certainly requires much more study.

Relationship Between PMN Metabolic Activity and Function

It has been alluded to previously that a relatively new antimicrobial system, seemingly activated as a result of the biochemical and morphological changes accompanying phagocytosis, is present in PMN.

It is known that concentrations of myeloperoxidase (MPO), H_2O_2, and halide, which are not in themselves bactericidal, form a potent bactericidal system when they are combined. The reaction has been reported to have a pH optimum in the acid range. At neutral pH, essentially no killing has been reported. The mechanism(s) by which this reaction exerts its activity is of interest. When the halide employed is iodide, it has been suggested that iodination of engulfed bacteria is the mode of action.[58] Although it is true that iodination appears to correlate in some situations with killing, iodination has also been found to occur in the absence of killing. For this reason, it is felt that iodination is not necessarily directly related to bactericidal activity.

In what appeared to be an unrelated study, Zgliczynski[59] showed that MPO prepared from leukocytes isolated from patients with chronic granulocytic leukemia, in the presence of H_2O_2 and Cl^-, could deaminate and decarboxylate amino acids, yielding aldehydes of one carbon less than the corresponding amino acid. Guinea pig leukocytes and other animal leukocytic cells were similarly found to be capable of deaminating and decarboxylating amino acids. It was suggested that the resulting aldehyde could be the actual bactericidal agent.[60,61] Later work indicated that amino acid chloramines were an intermediate product in this reaction. These chloramines can be unstable and spontaneously undergo decarboxylation and deamination. The possibility that the amino acid chloramines could themselves act as bactericidal agents was suggested.[62]

In an effort to learn more about the mechanism of this system, the susceptibility of protein-bound amino acids to enzymatic attack by MPO, in the presence of H_2O_2 and chloride ions, was investigated. 1,7-^{14}C-diaminopimelic acid (DAP) was incorporated into *Escherichia coli* W-7 proteins with little randomization of the radioactivity. Under appropriate conditions, the MPO-H_2O_2-chloride system released approximately 94% of the radioactivity from labeled bacteria. This would indicate that, in addition to decarboxylation, peptide bonds are also split during this reaction. The oxidative decarboxylation of DAP-labeled bacteria by MPO occurs under conditions similar to those observed with amino acids.[63] It appears from these data that MPO not only can decarboxylate free and bound amino acids, yielding chloramines and aldehydes, but also can actively participate in oxidative peptide cleavage. Further evidence for this has been obtained by using markers other than DAP. By using ^{14}C-amino acid mixtures, it has been shown that as much as 10% of the radioactivity incorporated into proteins are converted into TCA-soluble products by the MPO-H_2O_2-Cl^- system.

It can be postulated that a sequence of reactions occurs in the MPO-H_2O_2-Cl^- antimicrobial system and results in the formation of an MPO Cl^- H_2O_2 complex. This complex can undergo intramolecular rearrangement to form activated chlorine (Cl^+). The reactions resulting in the formation of Cl^+ were reported by Agner in 1958. The complex can participate in the chlorination of amino acids and other substrates. Chlorination of β-amino acids yields stable chloramines, while chlorination of α-amino acids results in the formation of unstable chloramines. Unstable amino acid chloramines undergo spontaneous decarboxylation and deamination, yielding aldehydes.[62]

At this point, systematic affinity studies between MPO and H_2O_2 and MPO and Cl^- at different pH were reported.[64] It was determined that for any given Cl^- concentration (50 to 400 m*M*), the affinity between MPO and Cl^- increases with a decrease in pH, and decreases with increasing H_2O_2 concentrations. These results predict that the MPO-H_2O_2-Cl^- system can function over a wide pH range, with varying H_2O_2 and Cl^- concentrations. Experimental proof that the velocity of chlorination is similar under a variety of different, but optimal, experimental conditions has been presented.[64] From this work, it may be stated that the chlorination reaction is influenced by changes in pH and H_2O_2 and Cl^- concentrations, independently and in conjunction with each other. On the basis of these data, it can be predicted that bactericidal activity will also occur at neutral pH, if sufficiently low H_2O_2 concentrations can be maintained in the reaction medium. By using sustained low concentrations of H_2O_2 (utilizing the glucose-glucose oxidase system), bactericidal activity at pH 7.4 is readily demonstrated; in fact, greater killing efficiency has been noted at pH 7.4 than at pH 5.0.[65]

The production of a free and diffusible agent with bactericidal activity by this system was only recently demonstrated. Concentrations of MPO and H_2O_2 generally used in the antimicrobial system must be increased 50- and 15-fold, respectively, for the agent to be produced. This modification results in the formation of a diffusible cidal agent (possibly Cl^+). Addition of amino acids to the modified antimicrobial system completely neutralizes Cl^+ with the formation of chloramines and leads to reduction, but not abolition, of cidal activity. Thus it appears that amino acid chloramines also act as bactericidal agents, although they are much less potent than Cl^+.[65,66]

No agent has been found that will enhance the bactericidal activity of the MPO-H_2O_2-Cl^- system. However, the findings that MPO can actually coat bacteria[67] and that chlorination of bacteria can be enhanced by preincubation with MPO, are pertinent.[64] Upon the addition of H_2O_2 and Cl^-, bacteria preincubated with MPO were killed more readily than non-MPO incubated controls. This is evidenced by the decreased requirements of MPO and H_2O_2 for equivalent bactericidal activity. From these studies, it is concluded that when MPO is adsorbed to the bacteria, a coupled reaction occurs in which the activated chlorine directly attacks the bacterial cell surface.[68]

In summary, it may be stated:

1. MPO, H_2O_2, and Cl^- form a complex that undergoes intramolecular rearrangement, yielding the chlorinium ion.
2. The chlorinium ion can interact with MPO, bacteria, and amino acids.
3. The reaction can occur over a wide pH range with various concentrations of H_2O_2 and Cl^-.
4. The chlorinium ion can attack different protein molecules to cause structural changes.

5. Preincubation of bacteria with MPO results in greater bactericidal activity.
6. Diffusible bactericidal agents are produced by the MPO-H_2O_2-Cl^- system. Their possible physiological significance is presently unknown.

Lipid Composition and Metabolism

Lipid composes approximately 5% of the net weight of the total neutrophilic mass.[69] The PMN contain about twice as much lipid as the lymphocyte, and over 40 times as much lipid as the erythrocyte. Phospholipid makes up about 33% of the total lipid content of leukocytes. Another 33% is neutral lipid and free cholesterol. Glycolipid, predominantly ceramide dihexoside, may constitute about 16% of the total lipid weight. The lipid patterns of normal human blood cells may be seen in Table 8.

Leukocytes are not able to carry out *de novo* synthesis of neutral lipids and fatty acids. They are, however, capable of chain elongation reactions.[70] Normal mature leukocytes lack acetyl CoA carboxylase, the first enzyme unique to fatty acid synthesis.[71] The distribution of fatty acids has not been extensively studied in purified leukocyte preparations. Rabbit peritoneal exudate granulocytes have a total fatty acid pattern similar to that of erythrocytes. There is a predominance of linoleic (C18:2), palmitic (C16:0), oleic (C18:1), and stearic (C18:0) acids. The phospholipid fraction contains mostly linoleic (40%) and palmitic (20%) acids. The neutral fraction contains mostly oleic and palmitic (26% each) acids.[72] If ^{32}P is administered in vivo, it labels principally leukocytic phosphatidyl ethanolamine-choline and -serine and phosphoinositol. In vitro, the ^{32}P labels mainly phosphoinositol and phosphotidic acid.[73,74]

Lymphocytes and granulocytes contain substantial amounts of glycolipids (16% of the total lipid weight). It has been reported that most of the glycolipid is in the form of dihexosylceramide, with only small amounts of mono- and trihexosides.[75] The major glycolipid has now been characterized as lactosylceramide.[76] Glycolipids appear to be predominantly localized to the cell membrane. The known capacity of these lipids to function as haptens indicates that glycolipids may play an important role in determining the immunochemical specificity of the cell surface. The relatively high content of lactosylceramide suggests that these cells have an especially important function.

From different studies on the lipid composition of human leukocytes, we may conclude that each cell type has a characteristic lipid pattern.[69] Lymphocytes and granulocytes have different lipid patterns. Leukemic cells show major differences. The true significance of these changes is not clear. Lipid metabolism in phagocytizing cells has been extensively studied.[77] From these studies, it appears that synthesis and breakdown of lipids may play an integral role in phagocytosis. The relatively large increase in cellular phospholipid, noted in phagocytizing cells, may serve to provide new membrane material for the phagocyte. Whether the cell requires replacement of membrane during phagocytosis has yet to be proven; however, the finding that phospholipids increase during phagocytosis is of extreme interest. Additional studies in this field are in order.

Nucleic Acid Metabolism

The DNA content per leukocyte is approximately the same for each cell type (0.7×10^{-12} g DNA-phosphorus per cell). The RNA content varies considerably.[78] It is generally greatest in immature leukocytes of all cell lines and decreases with cellular maturation. The RNA/DNA ratio is highest in leukocytes collected from patients with acute leukemia.

The basic features of RNA metabolism are well known for a number of different cell types. Presumably, RNA metabolism in human leukocytes has similar features. However, there is still uncertainty regarding the actual sites within these cells where RNA metabolism takes place. RNA synthesis and turnover are increased during phag-

Table 8
LIPIDS OF NORMAL HUMAN BLOOD CELLS

		Lymphocytes	Polymorphonuclear leukocytes	Erythrocytes
Wet weight	pg per cell	212	430	97
Total lipid weight	pg per cell	10.0	21.5	0.50
	Wet weight (%)	4.7	5.0	0.52
Cholesterol	Moles × 10^{-15} per cell	3.24	5.33	0.34
	Total lipid weight (%)	12.5	10	27
Phospholipids	Moles × 10^{-15} per cell	4.73	9.67	0.36
	Total lipid weight (%)	35	34	55
α,β-Unsaturated ether:lipid-P	Molar ratio	0.14	0.24	0.17
Cholesterol:lipid-P	Molar ratio	0.68	0.55	0.94

From Gottfried, E. L., *Semin. Hematol.*, 9, 241—242, 1972. By permission.

ocytosis.[79] Actinomycin D specifically blocks RNA synthesis without affecting any other metabolic parameter. The inhibition of RNA synthesis in monocytes does not affect phagocytosis. The principal features of purine, pyrimidine, and RNA metabolism in granulocytes have been summarized:[80]

1. Enzymes for *de novo* pyrimidine synthesis are found only in immature, normal, and malignant granulocytes.
2. Thymidylate synthetase and thymidine kinases are found only in immature granulocytes.

Cationic Proteins

In addition to the oxygen-dependent antimicrobial system discussed above, a number of oxygen-independent antimicrobial systems have also been described. Increased activity of lysozyme, lactoferrin, elastase, and a number of cationic proteins have all been implicated as contributors to the antimicrobial activity of the PMN. The elegant and pioneering work of Spitznagel, and somewhat later of Olsson, on the isolation and characterization of the cationic proteins of PMN is of major importance. It appears that all the cationic proteins of the PMN have antimicrobial activity. The cationic proteins are so named because they have cathodal electrophoretic mobilities greater than lysozyme at pH 4.0 in cellulose acetate. They have been noted in PMN from guinea pigs, rabbits, and humans.[81]

All the cationic proteins differ from species to species in molecular weight, amino acid composition, and enzymatic properties. The relative amounts of the human proteins are less than those found in rabbit PMN. The amount of protein required for killing is dependent upon the specific cationic protein and, to some extent, on the microorganism. The most sensitive organism can be effectively eliminated with as little as 0.3 $\mu g/m\ell$. The mechanism of action of the human cationic proteins is presently unknown. Interestingly, human cationic proteins have chymotryptic activity. Heat-inactivation does not destroy their ability to kill bacteria.[82] The role that these proteins may have in the killing of engulfed microorganisms is presently not clear. Since chicken PMN lack a peroxidase antimicrobial system, it would appear that cationic proteins would be most important in this species. However, since the PMN may be faced with literally thousands of different types of microorganisms under a variety of different environmental conditions, it is to be expected that these antimicrobial cationic proteins have a major role in controlling infections in man.

Lymphocytes, Monocytes, and Eosinophils

Lymphocytes

The metabolic and bactericidal activities of lymphocytes from AKR and CD1 mice have been studied. Spleen cell suspensions from nonleukemic AKR and CD1 mice were found to have the ability to kill *E. coli* in vitro. When these cells were incubated in the presence of particles, there was an increased flow of glucose through the HMS, increased NADPH oxidase activity, and increased formate oxidation (a measure of H_2O_2 production). These cells were also found to contain a peroxidase, spleen peroxidase (SLPO), that was bactericidal in the presence of H_2O_2 and chloride, at acidic pH.[61,83]

The predominant cell found in these spleen suspensions was identified morphologically as a lymphocyte. In addition, it has been recently demonstrated that isolated human peripheral blood lymphocytes have significant peroxidase and bactericidal activity.[84] Thus lymphocytes appear to have the major role in the observed in vitro bactericidal activity by spleen cell suspensions. Light and electron microscopic studies revealed that particles adhered to the cell membrane, or were partially embedded in the cytoplasm of spleen lymphocytes. In no instance were lymphocytes found to completely phagocytize particles. Thus, if these cells were bactericidal, the activity had to occur on the surface and/or extracellularly. A possible mechanism for such activity can be postulated from observations reported with PMN. During phagocytosis, PMN were found to selectively release lysosomal enzymes, including MPO, into the extracellular environment.[20,50,51] Further, these cells were also noted to selectively release lysosomal enzymes in the absence of actual ingestion. Because spleen cells exhibit many of the same metabolic stimulations as PMN when incubated with particles, it is possible that these cells also release their peroxidase in a similar fashion or that the enzyme could be an ectoenzyme. In any event, SLPO and metabolic H_2O_2, in the presence of extracellular chloride, could then react with bacteria that are in contact, or in close association, with the lymphocytes and could cause the death of the bacteria.

Monocytes and Macrophages

The metabolism of monocytes and macrophages is to a great extent determined by the degree of cellular maturity and the level of endocytic activity. The mononuclear phagocytes represent a diversity of cells at various levels of differentiation. The blast cells and promonocytes, the first identifiable cells of the series, are characterized by a high rate of nucleic acid synthesis. The mature macrophage (monocyte migrated into tissue) is characterized by high levels of protein synthesis and elevated levels of lysosomal enzymes. It has been reported that macrophages will enhance their function during infection, and these cells are now termed "activated" macrophages. The basis of this enhancement of activity is immunological and involves the lymphocyte.

The metabolic activities of different macrophages as compared to PMN are summarized in Table 9. It is evident that the rate of respiratory activity of resting MN phagocytes is higher than that of PMN. Glucose is oxidized through the HMP. In alveolar macrophages, the ratio of HMP to Kreb's cycle activity is lower than that obtained with the PMN. The addition of bacteria to the cell results in an increase in oxygen uptake.[85] The magnitude of stimulation is dependent on the cell type. Oxidation of 1-^{14}C-glucose is significantly increased. It would appear that the initial events involved with metabolic stimulation of both rabbit and guinea pig mononuclear phagocytes are characterized by an increased activity of the HMS. This stimulation is detectable within seconds after the addition of bacteria. Since both oxygen uptake and glucose oxidation occur almost simultaneously, a link between the two is suggested. The link appears to be mediated by a particulate NADPH oxidase that appears to be stimulated in phagocytizing macrophages. The increased oxidative metabolism in this cell is likely related to bactericidal activity. Both H_2O_2 production and peroxidase activities have been reported in these cells.[86]

In addition to the above metabolic activities noted in resting and phagocytizing cells, macrophages have been reported to contain a variety of different enzymatic activities. Lysozyme, acid phosphatase, ribonucleases, esterases, lipases, different dehydrogenases, proteases, and proteinases have all been reported to be present in macrophages.[87]

There is less available metabolic information on the mononuclear cell than on the PMN. Some distinctive features of mononuclear cell metabolism may, nevertheless, be noted. It has a high basal level of oxygen consumption. Its metabolism is primarily oxidative. It is evident that additional systematic biochemical studies are needed with this cell type.

Eosinophils

Until recently, relatively little was known about the metabolic activities of eosinophils because it was difficult to obtain sufficient numbers of pure populations of eosi-

Table 9
RATE OF RESPIRATION AND GLUCOSE OXIDATION BY RESTING AND PHAGOCYTOSING MACROPHAGES AND PMN LEUCOCYTES

		Oxygen uptake[a]			$^{14}CO_2$ from 1-^{14}C-Glc[b]		$^{14}CO_2$ from 6-^{14}C-Glc[b]	
					Bacteria[c]			
		−	+		−	+	−	+
Guinea pig								
Alveolar macrophages	(10)	32	47	(4)	12,610	25,785	3,200	3,950
		±3	±3	(4)	±3,370	±4,000	±940	±1,030
Peritoneal macrophages	(9)	23	65	(5)	28,700	75,410	375	650
		±2	±4	(5)	±4,670	±21,130	±55	±180
PMN leucocytes	(10)	7	43	(20)	21,945	92,650	135	455
		±1	±4	(20)	±3,540	±23,600	±75	±180
Rabbit								
Alveolar macrophages	(10)	26	39	(13)	5,995	22,420	1,395	2,205
		±2	±3	(13)	±600	±2,730	±215	±300
Peritoneal macrophages	(8)	29	45	(2)	9,150	45,300	195	295
		±4	±7	—	—	—	—	—
PMN leucocytes	(9)	7	26	(2)	10,865	172,615	280	615
		±1	±2	—	—	—	—	—

Note: Mean values ±SE. The number of experiments is given in parentheses.

[a] Natoms per minute per 10^7 cells.
[b] $^{14}CO_2$ cpm per μCi ^{14}C-glucose per 10 min per 10^7 cells.
[c] *B. mycoides.*

From Rossi, F., Zabucchi, G., and Romeo, D., *Mononuclear Phagocytes in Immunity, Infection and Pathology,* van Furth, R., Ed., Blackwell Scientific, Oxford, 1975, 442. With permission.

nophils for study. Some progress in this area has been made,[88,89] and studies on the metabolism of eosinophils are being reported.

It has been noted[90] that eosinophils could phagocytize bacteria; however, they were not as efficient as neutrophils. The number of particles per cell and number of cells containing particles were significantly less. Eosinophils exhibited a more pronounced oxidative response during phagocytosis. This increased activity resulted in a greater production of H_2O_2. These increased activities were attributed to an increased activity of NADPH oxidase. However, in spite of these increased oxidative activities, the cells were less bactericidal than PMN.

Oxidation of glucose-1-^{14}C, glucose-6-^{14}C, and formate-^{14}C is significantly greater in nonphagocytizing eosinophils than in neutrophils.[91] As in the previous study, the increase in glucose oxidation was greater in eosinophils than in neutrophils. Eosinophils have also been reported to contain more peroxidase than neutrophils.[92] However, the eosinophilic peroxidase has been reported to be genetically[93] and biochemically distinct from neutrophilic peroxidase.[94] In another section of this chapter, we have noted that neutrophilic myeloperoxidase is integrally involved in a major antimicrobial system within the cell. Azide has been shown to inhibit myeloperoxidase activity of the PMN and, consequently, antimicrobial activity. In the eosinophil, azide does not inhibit killing, suggesting that the eosinophilic peroxidase does not play a role in the intracellular killing mechanism of these cells.[95] It is apparent that the significance of this enzyme in this cell remains to be determined. Additional biochemical studies with this cell are needed. Preliminary studies indicate that fruitful comparative information will be forthcoming.

REFERENCES

1. **Beck, W. S.**, The control of leukocyte glycolysis, *J. Biol. Chem.*, 232, 251, 1958.
2. **Beck, W. S.**, Occurrence and control of the phosphogluconate oxidation pathway in normal and leukemic leukocytes, *J. Biol. Chem.*, 232, 271, 1958.
3. **Noble, E. P., Stjernholm, R. L., and Weisberger, A. S.**, Carbohydrate metabolism in the leukocytes. I. The pathway of two- and three-carbon compounds in the rabbit polymorphonuclear leukocyte, *J. Biol. Chem.*, 235, 1261, 1960.
4. **Baldridge, C. W. and Gerard, R. W.**, The extra respiration of phagocytosis, *Am. J. Physiol.*, 103, 325, 1933.
5. **Marinelarena, R.**, The Effect of Various Chemical Substances and Bacteria on the Glycolytic and Respiratory Activities of Leukocytes, Doctoral dissertation, University of Michigan, Ann Arbor, 1950.
6. **Alonso, D.**, Comparative Study of the Host-Resistance of Guinea Pigs and Rats, *Doctoral dissertation*, University of Michigan, Ann Arbor, 1952.
7. **Stahelin, H., Suter, E., and Karnovsky, M. L.**, Studies on the interaction between phagocytes and tubercle bacilli. I. Observations on the metabolism of guinea pig leukocytes and the influence of phagocytosis, *J. Exp. Med.*, 104, 121, 1956.
8. **Stahelin, H., Karnovsky, M. L., and Suter, E.**, Studies on the interaction between phagocytes and tubercle bacilli. II. The action of phagocytes upon ^{14}C labelled tubercle bacilli, *J. Exp. Med.*, 104, 137, 1956.
9. **Stahelin, H., Karnovsky, M. L., Farnham, A. E., and Suter, E.**, Studies on the interaction between phagocytes and tubercle bacilli. III. Some metabolic effects in guinea pigs associated with infection with tubercle bacilli, *J. Exp. Med.*, 105, 265, 1957.
10. **Sbarra, A. J. and Karnovsky, M. L.**, The biochemical basis of phagocytosis. I. Metabolic changes during the ingestion of particles by polymorphonuclear leukocytes, *J. Biol. Chem.*, 234, 1355, 1959.
11. **Sbarra, A. J. and Karnovsky, M. L.**, The biochemical basis of phagocytosis. II. Incorporation of C^{14} labelled building blocks into lipid, protein and glycogen of leukocytes during phagocytosis, *J. Biol. Chem.*, 235, 2224, 1960.
12. **Selvaraj, R. J. and Sbarra, A. J.**, Relationship of glycolytic and oxidative metabolism to particle entry and destruction in phagocytizing cells, *Nature (London)*, 211, 1271, 1966.
13. **Stjernholm, R. L. and Manak, R. C.**, Carbohydrate metabolism in leukocytes. XIV. Regulation of pentose cycle activity and glycogen metabolism during phagocytosis, *RES J. Reticuloendothel. Soc.*, 8, 550, 1970.
14. **Patriarca, P., Cramer, R., Moncalvo, S., Rossi, F., and Romeo, D.**, Enzymatic basis of metabolic stimulations in leucocytes during phagocytosis: the role of activated NADPH oxidase, *Arch. Biochem. Biophys.*, 145, 255, 1971.
15. **Rossi, F., Romeo, D., and Patriarca, P.**, Mechanism of phagocytosis associated oxidative metabolism in polymorphonuclear leukocytes and macrophages, *RES J. Reticuloendothel. Soc.*, 12, 127, 1972.
16. **Paul, B. B., Strauss, R. R., Jacobs, A. A., and Sbarra, A. J.**, The role of the phagocyte in host-parasite interactions. XXVI. KCN insensitive NADPH oxidase: its direct involvement with the stimulated respiratory and hexose monophosphate shunt activities in phagocytizing cells, *Exp. Cell Res.*, 73, 456, 1972.
17. **Gagan, R. H. and Karnovsky, M. L.**, Enzymatic basis of the respiratory stimulation during phagocytosis, *Nature (London)*, 204, 255, 1964.
18. **Reed, P. W.**, Glutathione and the hexose monophosphate shunt in phagocytizing and hydrogen peroxide-treated rat leukocytes, *J. Biol. Chem.*, 244, 2459, 1969.
19. **Strauss, R. R., Paul, B. B., Jacobs, A. A., and Sbarra, A. J.**, The role of the phagocyte in host-parasite interactions. XIX. Leukocytic glutathione reductase and its involvement in phagocytosis, *Arch. Biochem. Biophys.*, 135, 265, 1969.

20. **Paul, B. B., Strauss, R. R., Jacobs, A. A., and Sbarra, A. J.**, The role of the phagocyte in host-parasite interactions. XVIII. The function of H_2O_2, myeloperoxidase and hexose monophosphate shunt enzymes in phagocytizing cells from different species, *Infect. Immun.*, 1, 338, 1970.
21. **Cohn, Z. A. and Hirsch, J. G.**, The isolation and properties of the specific cytoplasmic granules of rabbit polymorphonuclear leucocytes, *J. Exp. Med.*, 112, 983, 1960a.
22. **Hirsch, J. G. and Cohn, Z. A.**, Degranulation of polymorphonuclear leucocytes following phagocytosis of microorganisms, *J. Exp. Med.*, 112, 1005, 1960b.
23. **Cohn, Z. A. and Hirsch, J. G.**, The influence of phagocytosis on the intracellular distribution of granule-associated components of polymorphonuclear leucocytes, *J. Exp. Med.*, 112, 1015, 1960c.
24. **Roberts, J. and Quastel, J. H.**, Particle uptake by polymorphonuclear leukocytes and Ehrlich ascites-carcinoma cells, *Nature (London)*, 202, 85, 1964.
25. **Cline, M. J. and Lehrer, R. I.**, D-amino acid oxidase in leukocytes: a possible D-amino acid linked antimicrobial system, *Proc. Natl. Acad. Sci. U.S.A.*, 62, 756, 1969.
26. **Skarnes, R. C.**, L-amino acid oxidase, a bactericidal system, *Nature (London)*, 225, 1072, 1970.
27. **Strauss, R. R., Paul, B. B., and Sbarra, A. J.**, Effect of phenylbutazone, an anti-inflammatory agent, on phagocytosis and intracellular killing by guinea pig polymorphonuclear leukocytes, *J. Bacteriol.*, 96, 1982, 1968.
28. **Kvarstein, B. and Stormorken, H.**, Influence of acetylsalicylic acid, butazolidine, colchicine, hydrocortisone, chlorpromazine and Imipramine on the phagocytosis of polystyrene latex particles by human leukocytes, *Biochem. Pharmacol.*, 20, 119, 1971.
29. **Klebanoff, S. J.**, Myeloperoxidase-halide-hydrogen peroxide antimicrobial system, *J. Bacteriol.*, 95, 2131, 1968.
30. **McRipley, R. J. and Sbarra, A. J.**, The role of the phagocyte in host-parasite interactions. XI. Relationship between stimulated oxidative metabolism and hydrogen peroxide formation and intracellular killing, *J. Bacteriol.*, 94, 1417, 1967a.
31. **McRipley, R. J. and Sbarra, A. J.**, The role of the phagocyte in host-parasite interactions. XII. Hydrogen peroxide-myeloperoxidase system in the phagocyte, *J. Bacteriol.*, 94, 1425, 1967b.
32. **Iyer, G. Y. N., Islam, M. F., and Quastel, J. H.**, Biochemical aspects of phagocytosis, *Nature (London)*, 192, 535, 1961.
33. **Paul, B. B. and Sbarra, A. J.**, The role of the phagocyte in host-parasite interactions. XIII. The direct quantitative estimation of H_2O_2 in phagocytes, *Biochim. Biophys. Acta*, 156, 168, 1968.
34. **Root, R. K., Metcalf, J., Oshino, N., and Chance, B.**, H_2O_2 release from human granulocytes during phagocytosis, *J. Clin. Invest.*, 55, 945, 1975.
35. **Briggs, R. T., Karnovsky, M. L., and Karnovsky, M. J.**, Localization of NADH oxidase on the surface of human polymorphonuclear leukocytes by a new cytochemical method, *J. Cell Biol.*, 64, 254, 1975.
36. **Rossi, F., Patriarca, P., Romeo, D., and Zabucchi, G.**, The mechanism of control of phagocytic metabolism, *Adv. Exp. Med. Biol.*, 73(Abstr.), 205, 1976.
37. **Rossi, F., Patriarca, P. L., and Romeo, D.**, Regulation of oxidative metabolism and function of phagocytes, in *Future Trends in Inflammation*, Velo, G. P., Willoughby, D. A., and Giroud, J. P., Eds., Piccin Medical Books, Padua, Italy, 1975, 103.
38. **Patriarca, P. and Dri, P.**, The NADPH oxidase activity of polymorphonuclear neutrophilic leukocytes revisited, *Adv. Exp. Med. Biol.*, 73(Abstr.), 151, 1976.
39. **Selvaraj, R. J. and Sbarra, A. J.**, The role of the phagocyte in host-parasite interactions. XII. Di- and triphosphopyridine nucleotide kinetics during phagocytosis, *Biochim. Biophys. Acta*, 141, 243, 1967.
40. **Hohn, D. C. and Lehrer, R. I.**, NADPH oxidase deficiency in X-linked chronic granulomatous disease, *J. Clin. Invest.*, 55, 707, 1975.
41. **Patriarca, P., Dri, P., Kakinuma, K., Tedesco, F., and Rossi, F.**, Studies on the mechanism of metabolic stimulation in polymorphonuclear leucocytes during phagocytosis. I. Evidence for superoxide anion involvement in the oxidation of $NADPH_2$, *Biochim. Biophys. Acta*, 385, 380, 1975.
42. **Yokota, K. and Yamazaki, I.**, Action of peroxidase with reduced nicotinamide adenine nucleotide and reduced nicotinamide adenine dinucleotide phosphate, *Biochim. Biophys. Acta*, 105, 301, 1965.
43. **Rossi, F., Zatti, M., Patriarca, P., and Cramer, R.**, Effect of specific antibodies on the metabolism of guinea pig polymorphonuclear leukocytes, *RES J. Reticuloendothel. Soc.*, 9, 67, 1971.
44. **Romeo, D., Zabucchi, G., and Rossi, F.**, Reversible metabolic stimulation of polymorphonuclear leukocytes and macrophages by concanavalin A, *Nature (London)*, 243, 111, 1973.
45. **Nakagawara, A., Takeshiga, K., and Minakami, S.**, Induction of a phagocytosis-like metabolic pattern in polymorphonuclear leucocytes by cytochalasin E, *Exp. Cell Res.*, 87, 392, 1974.
46. **Schell-Frederick, E.**, Stimulation of the oxidative metabolism of polymorphonuclear leukocytes by the calcium ionophore A 23187, *FEBS Lett.*, 48, 37, 1974.

47. **Klebanoff, S. J.**, Intraleukocytic microbicidal defects, *Annu. Rev. Med.*, 22, 39, 1971.
48. **Baggiolini, M.**, The enzymes of the granules of polymorphonuclear leukocytes and their functions, *Enzyme*, 13, 132, 1972.
49. **Zurier, R. B., Weissmann, G., Hoffstein, S., Kammerman, S., and Tai, H. H.**, Mechanisms of lysosomal enzyme release from human leukocytes. II. Effects of cAMP and cGMP, autonomic agonists and agents which affect microtubule function, *J. Clin. Invest.*, 53, 297, 1974.
50. **Henson, P.**, The immunologic release of constituents from neutrophil leukocytes. I. The role of antibody and complement on non-phagocytosable surfaces or phagocytosable particles, *J. Immunol.*, 107, 1535, 1971a.
51. **Henson, P.**, The immunological release of constituents from neutrophilic leukocytes. II. Mechanism of release during phagocytosis and adherance to non-phagocytosable surfaces, *J. Immunol.*, 107, 1547, 1971b.
52. **Hawkins, D. J.**, Neutrophilic leukocytes in immunologic reactions, evidence for the selective release of lysosomal constituents, *J. Immunol.*, 108, 310, 1973.
53. **Zurier, R. B., Hoffstein, S., and Weissmann, G.**, Mechanisms of lysosomal enzyme release from human leukocytes, *J. Cell Biol.*, 58, 27, 1973.
54. **Hoffstein, S., Zurier, R. B., and Weissmann, G.**, Mechanisms of lysosomal enzyme release from human leukocytes. III. Quantitative morphologic evidence for an effect of cyclic nucleotides and calchicine on degranulation, *Clin. Immunol. Immunopathol.*, 3, 201, 1974.
55. **Ignarro, L. and Cech, S. Y.**, Hormonal control of lysosomal enzyme release from human neutrophils. Effects of autonomic agents on enzyme release, phagocytosis and cyclic nucleotide levels, *Proc. Soc. Exp. Biol. Med.*, 151, 448, 1976.
56. **DePierre, J. W. and Karnovsky, M. L.**, Ecto-enzymes of guinea pig polymorphonuclear leukocytes. I. Evidence for ecto-adenosine monophosphatase-adenosine triphosphatase and -p-nitrophenyl phosphatase, *J. Biol. Chem.*, 249, 7111, 1974a.
57. **DePierre, J. W. and Karnovsky, M. L.**, Ecto-enzymes of the guinea pig polymorphonuclear leukocyte. II. Properties and suitability as markers for the plasma membrane, *J. Biol. Chem.*, 249, 7121, 1974b.
58. **Klebanoff, S. J.**, Iodination of bacteria: a bactericidal mechanisms, *J. Exp. Med.*, 126, 1063, 1967.
59. **Zgliczynski, J. M., Stelmaszynska, T., Ostrowski, W., Naskalski, J., and Sznajd, J.**, Myeloperoxidase of human leukaemic leukocytes. Oxidation of amino acids in the presence of hydrogen peroxide, *Eur. J. Biochem.*, 4, 540, 1968.
60. **Jacobs, A. A., Paul, B. B., Strauss, R. R., and Sbarra, A. J.**, The role of the phagocyte in host-parasite interactions. XXIII. Relation of bactericidal activity to peroxidase associated decarboxylation and deamination, *Biochem. Biophys. Res. Commun.*, 39, 384, 1970.
61. **Strauss, R. R., Paul, B. B., Jacobs, A. A., and Sbarra, A. J.**, The role of the phagocyte in host-parasite interactions. XXII. The *in vitro* bactericidal and associated metabolic activities of mouse spleen cells, *Infect. Immun.*, 5, 114, 1972.
62. **Zgliczynski, J. M., Stelmaszynska, T., and Domanski, J.**, Chloramines as intermediates of oxidation reaction of amino acids by myeloperoxidase, *Biochim. Biophys. Acta*, 235, 419, 1971.
63. **Selvaraj, R. J., Paul, B. B., Strauss, R. R., Jacobs, A. A., and Sbarra, A. J.**, Peptide cleavage and oxidative decarboxylation by the MPO-H_2O_2-halide system, *Infect. Immun.*, 9, 255, 1974.
64. **Zgliczynski, J. M. and Stelmaszynska, T.**, Chlorinating ability of human phagocytosing leucocytes, *Eur. J. Biochem.*, 56, 157, 1975.
65. **Selvaraj, R. J., Zgliczynski, J. M., Paul, B. B., Poskitt, P. K. F., Stelmaszynska, T., and Sbarra, A. J.**, Newer insights of the MPO-H_2O_2-Cl^- bactericidal system, *RES J. Reticuloendothel. Soc.*, 18, 35b, 1975.
66. **Selvaraj, R. J., Zgliczynski, J. M., Paul, B. B., Poskitt, P. K. F., and Sbarra, A. J.**, Mechanism of action of the MPO-H_2O_2-Cl^- bactericidal system, *Abstr. Annu. Meet. Am. Soc. Microbiol.*, 17, 1976.
67. **Klebanoff, S. J.**, Myeloperoxidase mediated antimicrobial systems and their role in leukocyte function, in *Biochemistry of the Phagocytic Process*, Schultz, J., Ed., Interstate Publishers, New York, 1969, 89.
68. **Selvaraj, R. J., Zgliczynski, J. M., Paul, B. B., and Sbarra, A. J.**, Enhanced bactericidal activity of myeloperoxidase coated bacteria in the MPO-H_2O_2-Cl^- System, *J. Infect. Dis.*, submitted.
69. **Gottfried, E. L.**, Lipid patterns of leukocytes in health and disease, *Semin. Hematol.*, 9, 241, 1972.
70. **Buchanan, A. A.**, Lipid synthesis by human leukocytes *in vitro*, *Biochem. J.*, 75, 315, 1960.
71. **Majerus, P. W. and Lastra, R. R.**, Fatty acid biosynthesis in human leukocytes, *J. Clin. Invest.*, 46, 1596, 1967.
72. **Elsbach, P.**, Composition and synthesis of lipids in resting and phagocytizing leukocytes, *J. Exp. Med.*, 110, 969, 1959.
73. **Forkin, B. G. and Williams, W. J.**, The incorporation of radioactive phosphorus into the phospholipids of human leukemic leukocytes and platelets, *J. Clin. Invest.*, 40, 423, 1961.

74. **Rowe, C. E.**, The biosynthesis of phospholipids by human blood cells, *Biochem. J.*, 73, 438, 1959.
75. **Miras, C. J., Mantzos, J. D., and Levis, G. M.**, The isolation and partial characterization of glycolipids of normal human leucocytes, *Biochem. J.*, 98, 782, 1966.
76. **Kampine, J. P., Martensson, E., Yankee, R. A., and Kanfer, J. N.**, Sphingolipid metabolism in leucocytes. I. Incorporation of ^{14}C-glucose and ^{14}C-galactase into glycosphinogolipids by intact human leucocytes, *Lipids*, 3, 151, 1968.
77. **Elsbach, P.**, Lipid metabolism by phagocytes, *Semin. Hematol.*, 9, 227, 1972.
78. **Davidson, J. N., Leslie, J., and White, J. C.**, Quantitative studies on the content of nucleic acids in normal and leukemic cells from bone and bone marrow, *J. Pathol. Bacteriol.*, 63, 471, 1951.
79. **Cline, M. J.**, Ribonucleic acid biosynthesis in human leukocytes. Effects of phagocytosis on RNA metabolism, *Blood*, 28, 188, 1966.
80. **Cline, M. J.**, *The White Cell*, Harvard University Press, Cambridge, Mass., 1975.
81. **Spitznagel, J. K.**, Bactericidal mechanisms of the granulocyte, in *The Granulocyte: Function and Clinical Utilization*, Alan R. Liss, New York, 1977, 103.
82. **Odeberg, H. and Olsson, E.**, Antibacterial activity of cationic proteins from human granulocytes, *J. Clin. Invest.*, 56, 1118, 1975.
83. **Paul, B. B., Poskitt, P. K. F., Selvaraj, R. J., Zgliczynski, J. M., and Sbarra, A. J.**, Mouse spleen lymphocyte bactericidal and peroxidase activities: enhancement by whole body X-irradiation, *Proc. Soc. Exp. Biol. Med.*, 152, 151, 1976.
84. **Paul, B. B., Poskitt, P. K. F., Selvaraj, R. J., and Sbarra, A. J.**, Human Peripheral Lymphocyte Peroxidase: Quantitative Assay by Both Biochemical and Antimicrobial Methods, Adlard Coles London, 1975.
85. **Rossi, F., Zabucchi, G., and Romeo, D.**, Metabolism of phagocytosing mononuclear phagocytes, in *Mononuclear Phagocytes in Immunity, Infection and Pathology*, van Furth, Ralph, Ed., Blackwell Scientific, Oxford, 1975.
86. **Romeo, D., Cramer, R., Marzi, T., Soranzo, M. R., Zabucchi, G., and Rossi, F.**, Peroxidase activity of alveolar and peritoneal macrophages, *RES J. Reticuloendothel. Soc.*, 13, 399, 1973.
87. **Cohn, Z.**, Macrophage physiology, *Fed. Proc.*, 34, 1725, 1975.
88. **Day, R. P.**, Eosinophil cell separation from human peripheral blood, *Immunology*, 18, 955, 1970.
89. **Gleich, G. J. and Loegering, D.**, Selective stimulation and purification: eosinophils and neutrophils from guinea pig peritoneal fluids, *Am. J. Lab. Clin. Med.*, 82, 522, 1973.
90. **Baehner, R. L. and Johnston, R. B., Jr.**, Metabolic and bactericidal activities of human eosinophils, *Br. J. Haematol.*, 20, 277, 1971.
91. **Mickenberg, I. D., Root, R. K., and Wolff, S. M.**, Bactericidal and metabolic properties of human eosinophils, *Blood*, 39, 67, 1972.
92. **Archer, G. T. and Hirsch, J. G.**, Isolation of granules from eosinophil leukocytes and study of their enzyme content, *J. Exp. Med.*, 118, 277, 1963.
93. **Salmon, S. E., Cline, M. J., Schultz, J., and Lehrer, R. I.**, Myeloperoxidase deficiency: immunologic study of a genetic leukocyte defect, *N. Engl. J. Med.*, 282, 250, 1970.
94. **Archer, G. T., Air, G., Jackos, M., and Morell, D. B.**, Studies on rat eosinophil peroxidase, *Biochim. Biophys. Acta*, 99, 96, 1965.
95. **Bujak, J. S. and Root, R. K.**, The role of peroxidase in the bactericidal activity of human blood eosinophils, *Blood*, 43, 727, 1974.

THE IMMUNOLOGY OF HISTOCOMPATIBILITY ANTIGENS, NON-HLA ANTIGENS AND MEMBRANE RECEPTORS ON HUMAN LEUCOCYTES

David S. Gordon

The Human Leucocyte Antigen System

The Biology and Genetics of the Human Leucocyte Antigen (HLA) System

Human leucocyte antigen (HLA) determinants are found on the surface of most, if not all, human nucleated cells. The genes coding for these determinants are located on the sixth chromosome of man. These genes are, in general, referred to as the major histocompatibility complex (MHC), and primarily by extrapolation from the functions of the MHC in the mouse, one can state that an immune response to a wide variety of stimuli in any individual probably is primarily determined by this same region. At the practical, clinical level, three major areas have benefited from investigations into this system: clinical tissue transplantation, studies of associations of disease to HLA phenotype, and blood component replacement therapy. A number of excellent reviews on the HLA system have recently been published.[1-4]

Each individual inherits one haplotype of the MHC region from each parent, and the genes in each haplotype, and their products, are codominantly expressed. The total number of determinants coded for in the MHC is unknown, but five major subregions of a haplotype are shown schematically in Figure 1. Thus, each individual would express, on nucleated cells (except perhaps spermatozoa), two gene products of each subregion, i.e., two HLA-A antigens (one from each parental halpotype), two HLA-B antigens (one from each parental haplotype), etc. The antigens HLA-A, HLA-B, HLA-C, and HLA-DR are determined serologically by using antisera, generally obtained from multiparous women, in cytotoxic or other serological tests. Because of exposure to fetal tissue of a different MHC type during pregnancy and delivery, some women respond by producing antibodies (alloantisera) specifically directed to such fetal MHC antigens. By screening sera from multiparous women against panels of cells, investigators obtain possibly useful reagents. A number of different investigators then test these reagents at workshops, and if they are found to be unique, the reagents are assigned a workshop number (i.e., BW39). If various investigators define a series of antisera to be cross reactive and they seem to be truly unique, the workshop designation is removed, a new allele at a given locus is "defined" by these antisera, and a number (i.e., A2, B27, etc.) is assigned. Over the past 10 years, a number of HLA-gene products have been described, and the list, as of October 1977, is summarized in Table 1.

The HLA-D locus has been characterized in a different fashion. Lymphocytes from one individual, when exposed to lymphocytes of another individual, will respond with protein and nucleic acid synthesis, will morphologically change (blast transformation), and will undergo mitosis. This "activity" most commonly is quantitated by the uptake of radioisotopes (i.e., tritiated thymidine) during nucleic acid synthesis. Thus differences in individuals can be shown in the "mixed lymphocyte culture" (MLC). The major area responsible for the MLC activity also resides in the MHC, and has been called the D locus. Since each haplotype of chromosome 6 has one D locus, most individuals will express two alleles of this locus. However, when members of a family intermarry, some individuals, by the laws governing genetics, will inevitably be "homozygous" for the D and other loci. Cells from these homozygous individuals have been extremely important in defining the D locus antigens in the mixed lymphocyte culture, since they carry a double dose of one antigen.

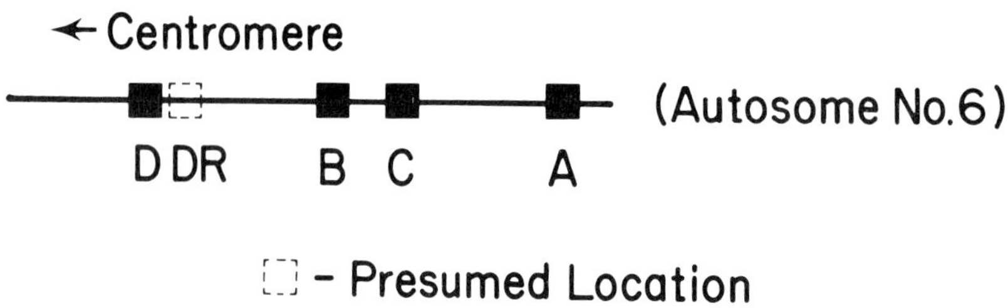

FIGURE 1. A schematic representation of the major histocompatibility complex of man.

Table 1
HUMAN LEUCOCYTE ANTIGENS[a]

Locus				
A	B	C	D	DR
A1	B5	CW1	DW1	DRW1
A2	B7	CW2	DW2	DRW2
A3	B8	CW3	DW3	DRW3
A9	B12	CW4	DW4	DRW4
A10	B14	CW5	DW5	DRW5
A11	B15	CW6	DW6	DRW6
A25	B17		DW7	DRW7
A26	B18		DW8	
A28	B27		DW9	
A29	B37		DW10	
AW19	B40		DW11	
AW23	BW16			
AW24	BW21			
AW30	BW22			
AW31	BW35			
AW32	BW38			
AW33	BW39			
AW34	BW41			
AW36	BW42			
AW43	BW44			
	BW46			
	BW47			
	BW48			
	BW49			
	BW50			
	BW51			
	BW52			
	BW53			
	BW54			

[a] As of October 1977.

Table 2
ASSOCIATIONS OF HLA-TYPE AND DISEASE SUSCEPTIBILITY[43-45]

Disease[a]	Antigens	Antigen frequencies (%) Controls	Patients	Relative risk[b]
Ankylosing spondylitis	B27	3—12	50—100	120
Reiter's syndrome	B27	3—12	65—100	36
Yersinia arthritis	B27	3—12	58—76	18
Psoriatic arthritis	B27	3—12	7—91	5
	BW38	3	7—27	12
Juvenile rheumatoid arthritis	B27	3—12	15—57	5
	DW4	13—17	45—72	10
Acute anterior uveitis	B27	3—12	37—58	9
Multiple sclerosis	DW2	15—31	35—70	5
Psoriasis	B13	2—9	2—34	5
	B17	4—11	12—36	5
	BW37	1—3	4—16	6
Dermatitis herpetiforms	B8	17—33	58—87	9
Behçet's disease	B5	9—25	18—86	7
Subacute thyroiditis	BW35	9—14	63—73	17
Coeliac disease	B8	11—29	45—89	9
	DW3[c]	96	27	73
Idiopathic haemochromatosis	A3	27—31	76—78	8.3

[a] Only those associations with $p \leq 4 \times 10^{-4}$ and where ≥75 patients have been studied are included in the table.

[b] Only diseases with a relative risk ≥5 are included. Relative risk is the risk someone with the given antigen has of developing the disease, compared to someone who is negative for the antigen.

[c] 28 patients studied.

The determinants of the DR locus (and the D locus) are unusual in that they are represented on only a portion of lymphocytes — namely, the B lymphocyte.[5,6] By analogy again to the murine systems, the determinants to which DR antisera react are probably the most closely linked to (if indeed they are not analogous to) the true immune response gene antigens (called "Ia" in the mouse). Recently, investigators have described "heteroantisera" (antisera raised by immunizing a different species, such as the monkey and rabbit, with human cellular material) directed to determinants on B lymphocytes, and thus directed, perhaps, to the antigens closely related, or analogous, to the DR loci and Ia antigens.[7] The relationship of heteroantisera and the DR alloantisera to each other is not at the moment clear, nor is the importance of defining these antigens in clinical practice apparent as yet.

HLA Antigens and Disease Association

In retrospect, perhaps it is not surprising that some of the closest associations of HLA genotype and disease are found in diseases whose pathogenesis is probably tied to abnormal immune responsiveness. The prototype example is the significantly high asociation of ankylosing spondylitis and Reiter's syndrome to HLA B-27. The incidence of HLA B-27 in the population is about 3 to 12%, whereas the incidence in patients with those diseases is uniformly greater than 50%. Table 2 demonstrates the pertinent associations in these and other diseases to HLA phenotype.

The association of HLA antigens to disease must be considered in the context of two important facts. First, the gene frequency may not be clearly defined in the general population, and the "control" population in a given study may not be the true control for the population of patients with a given disease. In this instance the analyses upon which conclusions of HLA and disease associations are drawn may be statistically sound, but biologically tenuous. Second, the associations do not necessarily prove or disprove that the disease susceptibility gene product is one and the same as the HLA antigen in question; rather, it only implies that these two determinants are closely linked.

Recent evidence developed in a murine system may be pertinent as to a possible mechanism for the observed association of HLA phenotype and disease susceptibility in some circumstances. An immune response may be directed against the immunizing antigen in combination with MHC gene products. For example, the response of lymphocytes to a virally infected cell may in fact be a response to an MHC product directly altered by the virus, perhaps implying that the MHC product is the virus receptor itself.[8] Thus one might speculate that a "pathogenic ankylosing spondylitis agent" has great affinity for the HLA B-27 gene product, and that is why the association of B-27 to that disease is so strong.

HLA in Clinical Transplantation

As the intricacies of the HLA system began to unravel, the general concepts and the actual tissue typing results were applied to clinical transplantation. It is clear that renal transplantation between monozygotic twins inevitably leads to graft acceptance if the surgical technique is sound. HLA-and-ABO compatible siblings are the next best donor-recipient pair, yet rejection episodes do occur, implicating as yet undefined genetic loci incompatibility as a factor in rejection. The least successful transplants are those between unrelated pairs (including cadaver transplants), and early series suggested HLA compatibility might not be a significant factor in the outcome of this therapeutic maneuver. However, as larger series have been conducted, a direct correlation between the number of HLA mismatches and graft failure has been observed.[3,9] In particular, the B series antigens are more important than the A, and the MLC-determined D locus antigens may be more important than either the A or B.[10] A possible explanation of this may be that the major determinant in graft survival is closest to D loci on the haplotype, next closest to B, and somewhat further from the A locus.

In bone marrow transplantation the "goodness of fit" of the MHC of the donor to recipient is absolutely crucial. In the instance where the recipient has a relatively intact immune system but bone marrow "failure" (i.e., aplastic anemia or leukemia), donor-recipient compatibility in the MHC, is necessary for the transplant to take.[9,11] In severe combined immunodeficiency, the effects of MHC incompatibility are not rejection of the graft by the host because the host is incapable of an adequate immunological response, but rather rejection of the host by the graft (graft vs. host disease), since immunocompetent tissues are being transplanted and will react to the foreign MHC products of the host. Perhaps the most crucial compatibility in bone marrow transplantation is at the D locus, an observation in keeping with the closeness of the putative immune response gene antigens to that locus.[9]

HLA in Blood Component Therapy

Early blood component therapy was limited to red cell transfusions, and the importance of ABO compatibility is well known. Many febrile transfusion reactions are probably due to recipient HLA antibodies, arising from previous transfusions and interacting with leucocytes (probably with granulocytes) contaminating the donor red cell preparation. Even packed red cells are not without white cell contamination. On the other side of the coin, individuals with high titers of HLA antibodies probably should not be used as donors of blood components, since some of these antibodies will be transfused into the recipient and could lead to transfusion reactions.[3]

The aggressive nature of today's therapy for malignant disease, particularly leukemia, dictates a constant need for platelet replacement therapy. Unlike red cells, HLA antigens are well represented on platelets.[2,9] Platelets from random donors, even if they are ABO compatible, characteristically lose their effectiveness with time. Frequently, this is because of the interaction of tranfused platelets with HLA antibodies elicited by previous platelet transfusions. In such instances HLA-compatible platelets must be taken from either random donors or siblings.[9] Adequate planning can be done if one is aware of these facts *before* transfusion therapy. Whereas HLA-identical siblings as donors are clearly advantageous for the survival of platelets, if a bone marrow transplant is anticipated from the same sibling, there is a risk of immunizing the recipient to minor histocompatibility antigens, and then an increased risk of a nontake of the bone marrow cells should the transplant be done. Therefore, in this situation, nonsibling single donor of similar HLA phenotype may be the best choice as a source of platelets.

Granulocyte transfusions are clearly efficacious in decreasing infection in neutropenic patients.[12] These cells carry HLA as well as neutrophil specific antigens.[13] Logic similar to that described above regarding platelet transfusions also applies to granulocyte tranfusions. Additionally, since the febrile nature of a transfusion reaction may, in large part, be due to the release of pyrogenic materials from neutrophils, the most severe reactions may be seen in recipients of granulocytes who in fact have high-titer antibody to HLA or other antigens on the donor cells.[3]

Membrane Receptors on White Cells

Four major membrane receptors of white cells have been intensively investigated in recent years: integral surface membrane immunoglobulin (sIg), a receptor for the Fc portion of IgG (Fc), a family of receptors for components of complement (C'R), and a receptor for sheep red blood cells (E). Table 3 demonstrates the association of these receptors with mature white blood cells normally found in human peripheral blood and bone marrow.

Integral Surface Membrane Immunoglobulin (sIg)[14-18]

The presence of sIg is the *sine qua non* of a B lymphocyte. Although assays for immunoglobulin on cells may demonstrate Ig on a wide variety of cell types, it must be recalled that the sIg definition contains the word "integral". This means that should the sIg be removed by any means (stripping the membrane, etc.), it will be resynthesized by the B lymphocyte itself and reinserted into the membrane. Therefore, for example, cytophilic Ig (derived from the milieu around the cell) bound to the Fc receptor of any of a number of cells would not be resynthesized if stripped, but might give positive results in the sIg test.

The sIg receptor is the antigen receptor on the B cell, and contact with the appropriate antigen and other factors leads to cell division and plasma cell development. The specificity of the Ig produced by the plasma cell will be the same as the specificity of the sIg on the precursor B cell. In general, the final differentiation step in the B cell series to a plasma cell is associated with a loss of membrane immunoglobulin, and at this stage virtually all of the Ig is found in the cytoplasm.

All heavy chain isotypes (IgG, IgA, IgM, IgD, and IgE) known in humans are represented on a subpopulation of B cells, and frequently are found in doublets or even triplets (e.g., IgM and IgD on the same cell). The heavy chain found first in ontogeny of B cells is IgM. As in circulating Ig, these heavy chains have associated light chains (kappa or lambda) and, except in monoclonal lymphoproliferative diseases, the ratio

Table 3
LEUCOCYTE MEMBRANE RECEPTORS

	sIg[a]	Fc[b]	C'R[c]	E	CyIg[d]
T lymphocytes	−	±[e]	±[f]	+	−
B lymphocytes	+	+	+	−	±[g]
K lymphocytes	−	+	±[h]	−[i]	−
Plasma cell	±	−	−	−	+
Granulocyte	−	+	+	−	−
Monocyte	−	+	+	−	−
Platelet	−	+	?	−	−

[a] sIg = integral surface membrane immunoglobulin.
[b] Fc = receptor for the Fc portion of IgG.
[c] C'R = receptor for complement components.
[d] CyIg = intracytoplasmic immunoglobulin.
[e] 15 to 20% of T lymphocytes may have a receptor for the Fc portion of IgG.
[f] 5% of peripheral blood T cells have a receptor for complement components.
[g] Plasmacytoid lymphocytes may have some cytoplasmic immunoglobulin.
[h] K cells probably have receptors for C_{3b}, but not for C_{3d}.
[i] Depending on the E rosette method used, K cells may or may not make E rosettes.

of kappa (κ) to lambda (λ) light chains in the total population of B cells is approximately 2:1. About 12 to 15% of all circulating lymphocytes have sIg, and true sIg is found only on B lymphocytes.

Receptors for the Fc Portion of IgG (Fc)[14-17,19-23]

An immunoglobulin molecule is represented in Figure 2. A wide variety of white cells have a receptor for the Fc portion of the IgG molecule, including granulocytes, monocytes, platelets, B lymphocytes, K lymphocytes, and a subset of T lymphocytes. As noted above, the presence of this receptor, particularly when cytophilic Ig is attached to that receptor, may, without appropriate technical precautions, confuse the laboratory determination of the cells bearing true integral membrane Ig (B cells).

The function of this receptor is clearly different for different cells. In the granulocytic and monocytic series of cells, the function of the Fc-receptor is mainly one of facilitating phagocytosis of complexes of Ig and antigen (i.e., bacteria plus specific antibacterial antibody). In the "killer" lymphocyte (K cell) the cytotoxicity of antibody-coated cells requires interaction of that antibody-coated target cell with the Fc-receptor on K cells for cytotoxicity of the target cell (antibody-dependent cellular cytotoxicity). The function of the Fc receptor on B lymphocytes, platelets, and a subset of T cells is not yet clear, but undoubtedly will be elucidated over the next few years.

Receptors for Components of Complement (C'R)[14-17,21,24-26]

Receptors for components of complement (C'R) are almost as ubiquitous on white cells as are Fc receptors The complement system is an essential partner in some, if not all, immune responses. An adequate explanation of the complement system would require at least a monograph, and is beyond the scope of this review. Concerning receptors on white cells, it is important to concentrate on some of the early steps in the complement cascade. In particular, after the very early steps (C1 → C4 → C2 →) one complement component, C3b, is generated and is of importance because of the interaction of this molecule with the membrane of white cells.

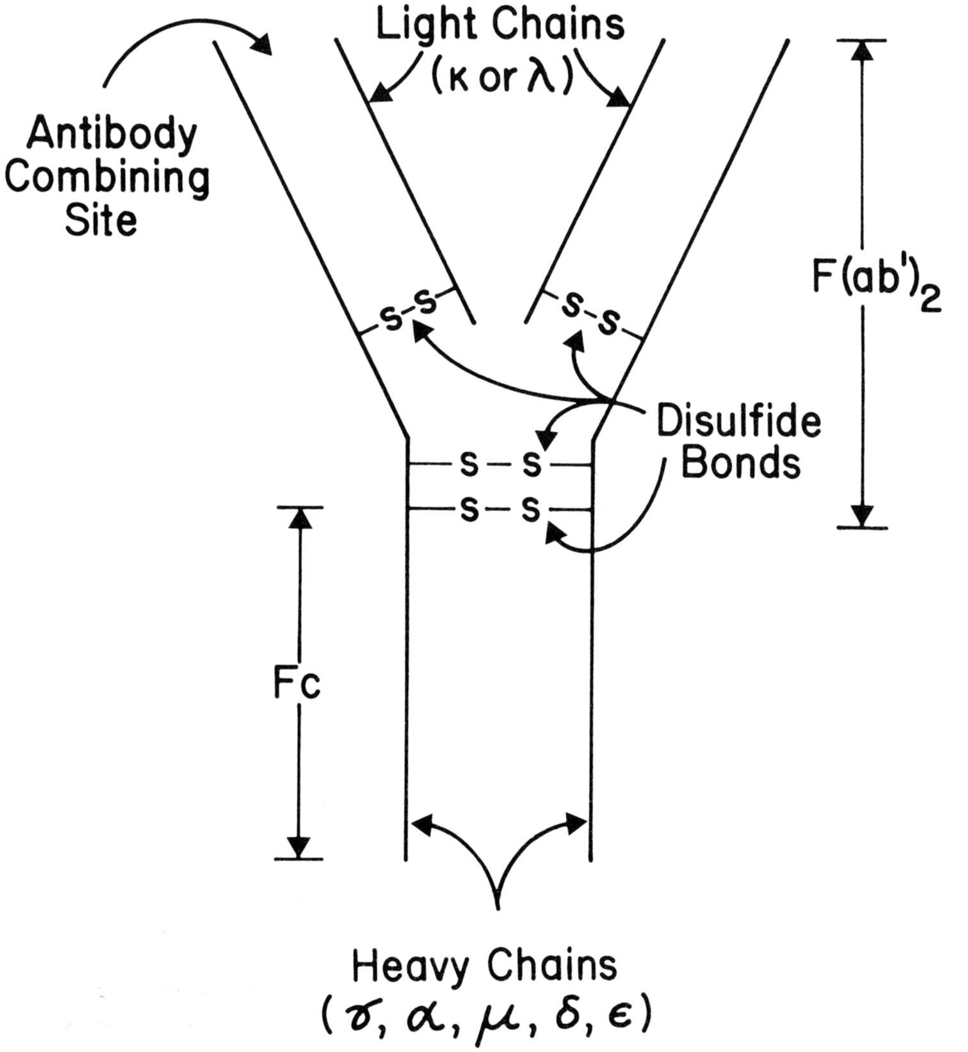

FIGURE 2. Human IgG immunoglobin.

C3b receptors (immune adherence receptors) are found on human red cells, granulocytes, monocytes, B lymphocytes, K lymphocytes, and a very small subset of T lymphocytes. In the granulocytes and monocytes, the function of C'R is probably to facilitate phagocytosis of Ig-antigen complexes in cooperation with the Fc receptors on the same cell. The function of this receptor on the other cells is currently unknown.

Receptors for the fourth component of complement (C4) are frequently found on the same cell as C3b receptors. When C3b is acted upon by a plasma inactivator, a new product is formed—C3d. C3d receptors are found on B lymphocytes and are even more frequently found on cells from B cell chronic lymphocytic leukemia than are C3b receptors, a finding contrary to the usual state of affairs on normal B lymphocytes.

The percent of cells in normal peripheral blood having C'R in most series corresponds with the number of B lymphocytes determined by the presence of sIg, and is approximately 10 to 15%. In fact, it can be directly shown that the vast majority of cells, if not all cells, bearing sIg also bear C'R. In general, however, the association of all of the known B cell receptors (sIg, Fc, and C'R), as well as newly described B cell receptors, to each other remains a subject of intense current investigation.

Receptors for Sheep Red Blood Cells (E)[14-17,27,28]

Why the human T lymphocyte has an affinity for sheep red blood cells (SRBC) remains an enigma. Nonetheless, the empirical observation that most, if not all, T lymphocytes bind SRBC, forming the so-called "E" rosette, has given clinical immunologists an important laboratory tool. Although certain nonhematopoietic cells will also bind SRBC, within the hematopoietic compartments (peripheral blood, bone marrow, spleen, and lymph nodes), this seems to be a function exclusive to T lymphocytes. Perusal of the literature to ascertain the true percent and absolute number of T lymphocytes in normal peripheral blood may be a confusing exercise in that values vary widely from series to series and laboratory to laboratory. The reason for this is probably the variety of techniques used to mark T lymphocytes. Seemingly small differences in technique, such as the amount of protein in the milieu, temperature of incubation, or ratio of sheep cells to lymphocytes can lead to significant differences in results.

The true percent in peripheral blood is probably 70 to 80%. Furthermore, it is important to consider the total absolute number of T lymphocytes in addition to the percent. For example, in B cell chronic lymphocytic leukemia, the percent of T cell lymphocytes may be quite low, but since the total number of lymphocytes in the differential is quite high, calculation of the absolute numbers of T lymphocytes leads in fact to a realization that in this disease the actual number of T cells is usually normal or elevated.

The Use of Membrane Markers in Clinical Practice

The apparent simplicity of the laboratory assays for sIg, Fc receptors, C'R, and E rosettes has led to a wide application of these methods to the study of a number of diverse diseases. Two major areas have benefited the most from these studies: immune deficiency diseases[14,17,18,25,29-32] and lymphoproliferative states.[14,17,18,25,33-37] As many as 4% of all hospitalized patients have been estimated to suffer from some form of congenital, acquired, or iatrogenic immune deficiency.[24] Though applying of the usual quantitative cellular assays alone will not necessarily shed light on the conditions of all of these patients, these assays, when used in combination with analysis of serum Ig levels, specific antibody response to immunization, assays of lymphocyte, granulocyte and monocyte function, and assays for the status of circulating complement components, will aid in diagnosis and treatment.

Unfortunately, the development of effective therapy has lapsed behind the development of diagnostic techniques. Except for gamma globulin replacement therapy in the setting of recurrent infection and depressed IgG levels, and the usefulness of an MLC- and HLA-matched bone marrow transplant in the setting of severe combined immunodeficiency, the efficacy of other therapies remains to be proven. Certainly, the evaluation of immune deficiency is a combined laboratory-clinical endeavor, beset by a number of pitfalls, many of which are technical. Therefore, it is folly to undertake the diagnosis and care of these patients unless a laboratory with standard reproducible assays and a clinician who knows how to evaluate the laboratory data work closely together.

Concerning gamma globulin replacement therapy, two matters are important. First,

Table 4
IMMUNOLOGIC MEMBRANE MARKERS IN LYMPHOPROLIFERATIVE STATES

	B Cell	T Cell	Null Cell
Acute lymphoblastic leukemia	±	+	+
Nodular lymphoma (all types)	+	−	−
Diffuse well-differentiated lymphocytic lymphoma	+	±	−
Diffuse lymphocytic lymphoma (mixed, poorly differentiated, histocytic)	+	+	+
Burkitt's lymphoma	+	−	−
Chronic lymphocytic leukemia	+	+	−
Waldenström's macroglobulinemia	+	−	−
Plasma cell myeloma	+	−	−
Cutaneous T cell lymphoma (including Sezary syndrome)	−	+	−

commercially available gamma globin contains IgG almost exclusively. Therefore, symtomatic IgA-deficient patients will very likely not benefit from replacement therapy with commercial gamma globulin.[30] Second, IgA-deficient patients have a significant incidence of serum sickness after blood component therapy, presumably because antibodies to IgA are induced by such therapy.

Hematologists responsible for diagnosing and treating patients with lymphoproliferative disease have benefited to some extent already and will probably benefit even more from membrane-marker assays. The prognosis in acute lymphoblastic leukemia is clearly worse if the immunologic type of the lymphoblast is T rather than null (negative for all markers).[38,39] Early data in non-Hodgkin's lymphoma suggest that marking the abnormal cells can supplement the standard Rappaport histopathological classification scheme in elucidating the prognosis in a given patient. Whereas all nodular lymphomas are of B-cell type, the diffuse lymphomas can be of B-cell type, T-cell type, or null. Within a given subdivision of the diffuse lymphomas (according to Rappaport), T- and null-cell types seem to do worse than B-cell types.[40] Table 4 summarizes some of the data in lymphoproliferative diseases.

One area deserving more investigation is the laboratory assessment of lymphoproliferation (peripheral blood, bone marrow, lymph node and spleen) to ascertain the malignancy or nonmalignancy in an individual case. As noted above, B-lymphoid cells may bear more than one heavy chain type in the normal state, and, furthermore, most B lymphocytes have IgM on the surface. Thus conclusions as to the monoclonality of cells derived on the basis of tests for heavy chain types may be uninformative and misleading. On the other hand, in the normal state two thirds of all B cells will bear κ light chain determinants, whereas about one third will bear λ light chains. In monoclonal proliferation, since all cells presumably are derived from a single precursor, one light chain will be represented in great excess over the other. Unfortunately, we have observed that the usual kappa and lambda light chain reagents available commercially are frequently inadequate when applied to analyses of cell populations, although they may be adequate for typing monoclonal proteins in serum and urine. The reasons for this are technical and somewhat complicated. In essence, light chain reagents made with only free light chains as the immunogen (i.e., Bence-Jones proteins) are inadequate. Suffice it to say that manufacturers are becoming aware of this problem and undoubtedly will furnish adequate reagents in the future.

Non-HLA Leucocyte Antigens

In the preceeding section, alloantisera and heteroantisera were briefly mentioned. In the former, the antisera is derived from a member of the same species immunized by previous exposure to the antigen (mother immunized by fetal tissue, immunization by blood component therapy, etc.); in the latter, human cellular material, or extracts made from cellular material, are used as the antigen, and another species is used (rabbit, monkey, etc.) as the source of the antisera.

In the not too distant future, reagents made by heteroimmunization may be extensively used in analyzing cell populations. The major difficulty has been in preparing a pure immunizing antigen, because a multitude of antigens at the immunization level leads to a multitude of specificities at the antisera level.

Nonetheless, progress, particularly in the area of reagents to quantitate T lymphocytes, is being made. Such reagents may define, for example, lymphoproliferative diseases heretofore "null" by classic membrane marker techniques, as being T cell in origin.[41] Similarly, reagents specific for B lymphocytes are now being developed and do not react directly with the usual B lymphocyte membrane markers (sIg, Fc, and C'R). These reagents are particularly interesting in that they frequently react with "null" blasts from acute myeloid and acute lymphoid leukemia, despite the fact that these cells do not mark with classic B cell membrane reagents.[7] This intrigues the basic cell biologist because it suggests that immune-response gene antigens may be present on the membrane of these cells. This observation may be important in attempts to unravel the ontogeny and cooperative efforts of hematopoietic cells. The clinical importance of these observations requires further investigation.

A series of neutrophil alloantigens, distinct from HLA antigens, has been described.[13] This polymorphic system consists of at least four different specificities and at least two independent genetic loci (NA1, NA2, NB1, and Vaz). The clinical importance of these antigens is in two areas: isoimmune neonatal neutropenia and possibly febrile transfusion reactions.[13] The importance of these antigens in clinical transplantation is not at the moment clear. A similar antigen, specific for platelets, has been described. Incompatibilities in this system have been implicated in neonatal and post-transfusion thrombocytopenia.[9,42]

REFERENCES

1. **Bach, F. H. and van Rood, J. J.,** The major histocompatibility complex-genetics and biology, *N. Engl. J. Med.*, 295, 806, 872, 927, 1976.
2. **Amos, D. B. and Ward, F. E.,** Immunogenetics of the HLA system, *Phys. Rev.*, 55, 206, 1975.
3. **Svejgaard, A., Hauge, M., Jersild, C., Platz, P., Ryder, L. P., Nielsen, L. S., and Thomsen, M.,** The HLA system. An introductory survey, in *Monographs in Human Genetics*, Vol. 7, Beckman, L. and Hauge, M., Eds., S. Karger, Basel, 1975, 1.
4. **Snell, G. B., Dausset, J., and Nathenson, S.,** The HLA complex: serology and genetics, in *Histocompatibility*, Academic Press, New York, 1976, 181.
5. **Walford, R. L., Gossett, T., Smith, G. S., Zeller, E., and Wilkinson, J.,** A new alloantigenic system on human lymphocytes, *Tissue Antigens*, 5, 196, 1975.
6. **Mann, D. L., Abelson, L., Henkart, P., Harris, S. D., and Amos, D. B.,** Specific human B lymphocyte alloantigens linked to HLA, *Proc. Natl. Acad. Sci. USA*, 72, 5103, 1975.
7. **Schlossman, S. F., Chess, L., Humphreys, R. E., and Strominger, J. L.,** Distribution of Ia-like molecules on the surface at normal and leukemic human cells, *Proc. Natl. Acad. Sci. USA*, 73, 1288, 1976.
8. **Doherty, P. C., Gotze, D., Trinchieri, G., and Zinkernagel, R. M.,** Models for recognition of virally modified cells by immune thymus-derived lymphocytes, *Immunogenetics*, 3, 517, 1976.

9. **Snell, G. B., Dausset, J., and Nathenson, S.**, The HLA complex: practical implicatons, in *Histocompatibility*, Academic Press, New York, 1976, 249.
10. **Opelz, G. and Teraski, P. I.**, Significance of mixed leucocyte culture testing in cadaver kidney transplantation, *Transplantation*, 23, 375, 1977.
11. **Storb, K., Prentice, R. L., and Thomas, E. D.**, Marrow transplantation for treatment of aplastic anemia. An analysis of factors associated with graft rejection, *N. Engl. J. Med.*, 296, 61, 1977.
12. **Lowenthal, R. M., Grossman, L., Goldman, J. M., Storring, R. A., Buskard, N. A., Park, D. S., Murphy, B. C., Spiers, A. S. D., and Galton, D. A. G.**, Granulocyte transfusions in treatment of infections in patients with acute leukemia and aplastic anemia, *Lancet*, 1, 353, 1975.
13. **Lalezari, P. and Radel, F.**, Neutrophil specific antigens: immunology and clinical significance, *Semin. Hematol.*, 11, 281, 1974.
14. **Moeller, G., Ed.**, T and B lymphocytes in humans, *Transplant. Rev.*, 16, 1, 1973.
15. International Union of Immunological Societies, (IUIS) Report, Identification, enumeration, and isolation of B and T lymphocytes from human peripheral blood, *Clin. Immunol. Immunopathol.*, 3, 584, 1974.
16. **Jondal, M.**, Surface markers on human T and B lymphocytes. IV. Distribution of surface markers on resting and blast-transformed lymphocytes, *Scand. J. Immunol.*, 3, 739, 1974.
17. **Dwyer, J. M.**, Identifying and enumerating human T and B lymphocytes. A review of techniques, problems and progress in clinical studies, *Prog. Allergy*, 21, 178, 1976.
18. **Seligmann, M., Preud'homme, J.-L., and Brouet, J.-C.**, B and T cell markers in human proliferative blood diseases and primary immunodeficiencies, with special reference to membrane bound immunoglobulin, *Transplant. Rev.*, 16, 85, 1973.
19. **Dickler, H. B.**, Lymphocyte receptors for immunoglobulin, *Adv. Immunol.*, 24, 167, 1976.
20. **Kerbel, R. S. and Davies, A. J. S.**, The possible biological significance of Fc receptors on mammalian lymphocytes and tumor cells, *Cell*, 3, 105, 1974.
21. **Lay, W. H. and Nussenzweig, V.**, Receptors for complement on leucocytes, *J. Exp. Med.*, 128, 991, 1968.
22. **Shore, S. L., Melewicz, F. M., and Gordon, D. S.**, The mononuclear cell in human blood mediating antibody dependent cellular cytotoxicity to virus-infected target cells. I. Identification of the population of effector cells, *J. Immunol.*, 118, 558, 1977.
23. **Ferrarini, M., Moretta, L., Abrile, R., and Durante, M. L.**, Receptors for IgG molecules on human lymphocytes forming spontaneous rosettes with sheep cells, *Eur. J. Immunol.*, 5, 70, 1975.
24. **Eden, A., Miller, G. W., and Nussenzweig, V.**, Human lymphocytes bear membrane receptors for C3b and C3d, *J. Clin. Invest.*, 52, 3239, 1973.
25. **Shevach, E. M., Jaffe, E. S., and Green, I.**, Receptors for complement and immunoglobulin and human and animal lymphoid cells, *Transplant. Rev.*, 16, 3, 1973.
26. **Ross, G. D., and Polley, M. J.**, Specificity of human lymphocyte complement receptors, *J. Exp. Med.*, 141, 1163, 1975.
27. **Jondal, M., Holm, G., and Wigzell., H.**, Surface markers on human T and B lymphocytes. I. A large population of lymphocytes forming nonimmune rosettes with sheep cells, *J. Exp. Med.*, 136, 207, 1972.
28. **Bentwich, Z., Douglas, S. D., Siegal, F. P., and Kunkel, H. G.**, Human lymphocyte-sheep erythrocyte rosette formation: some characteristics of the interaction, *Clin. Immunol. Immunopathol.*, 1, 511, 1973.
29. **Hobbs, J. R.**, Immunoglobulins in clinical chemistry, *Adv. Clin. Chem.*, 14, 219, 1971.
30. **Cooper, M. D., Faulk, W. P., Fudenberg, H. H., Good, R. A., Hitzig, W., Kunkel, H. G., Roitt, I. M., Rosen, F. S., Seligmann, M., Soothill, J. F., and Wedgwood, R. J.**, Meeting report of the second international workshop on primary immunodeficiency diseases in man, *Clin. Immunol. Immunopathol.*, 2, 416, 1975.
31. **Stiehm, E. R.**, Immunodeficiency disorders: general considerations, in *Immunologic Disorders in Infants and Children*, Stiehm, E. R. and Fulginitti, V. A., Eds., W. B. Saunders, Philadelphia, 1973, 145.
32. **Gordon, D. S.**, Immunoglobulin quantitation and characterization as a diagnostic tool, *South. Med. J.*, 70, 236, 1977.
33. **Jaffe, E. S., Shevach, E. M., Sussman, E. H., Frank, M., Green, I., and Berard, C. W.**, Membrane receptor sites for the identification of lymphoreticular cells in benign and malignant conditions, *Br. J. Cancer*, 31, (Suppl. 2), 107, 1975.
34. **Brouet, J. C., Labaume, S., and Seligmann, M.**, Evaluation of T and B lymphocyte membrane markers in human non-Hodgkin malignant lymphomata, *Br. J. Cancer*, 31 (Suppl. 2), 121, 1975.
35. **Aiuti, F., Lacava, V., Fiorilli, M., and Ciarla, M. V.**, Lymphocyte surface markers in lymphoproliferative disorders, *Acta Haematol.*, 50, 275, 1973.

36. **Aisenberg, A. C. and Long, J. C.**, Lymphocyte surface characteristics in malignant lymphoma, *Am. J. Med.*, 58, 300, 1975.
37. **Gordon, D. S. and Hubbard, M. R.**, Surface membrane characteristics and cytochemistry of the abnormal cells in adult leukemia, *Blood*, 51, 681, 1978.
38. **Sen, L. and Borella, L.**, Clinical importance of lymphoblasts with T markers in childhood leukemia, *N. Engl. J. Med.*, 292, 828, 1975.
39. **Brouet, J. C., Valensi, F., Daniel, M.-T., Flandrin, G., Preud'homme, J.-L., and Seligmann, M.**, Immunologic classification of acute lymphoblastic leukemias: evaluation of its clinical significance in a hundred patients, *Br. J. Haematol.*, 33, 319, 1976.
40. **Bloomfield, C. D., Kersey, J. H., Brunning, R. D., Gajl-Peczalska, K.**, Prognostic significance of lymphocyte surface markers in adult non-Hodgkins malignant lymphoma, *Lancet*, 2, 1330, 1976.
41. **Ades, E. W., Gordon, D. S., Phillips, D. J., Hubbard, M. R., Black, C. M., Martin, L. H., Lavia, M. F., and Reimer, C. B.**, Antisera for immunofluorescent enumeration of human T lymphocytes utilizing fluorescinated staphylococcal protein A, *Am. J. Pathol.*, 92, 619, 1978.
42. **Shulman, N. R., Marder, V. J., Hiller, M. C., and Collier, E. M.**, Platelet and leucocyte isoantigens and their antibodies: serologic, physiologic, and clinical studies, *Prog. Hematol.*, 4, 222, 1964.
43. **Svejgaard, A., Matz, P., Ryder, L. P., Nielsen, L. S., and Thomsen, M.**, HL-A and disease associations. A survey, *Transplant. Rev.*, 22, 1, 1975.
44. **Snell, G. B., Dausset, J., and Nathenson, S.**, Histocompatibility genes and disease, in *Histocompatibility*, Academic Press, New York, 1976, 334.
45. **Dausset, J. and Svejgaard, A., Eds.**, The data, in *HLA and Disease*, 1st ed., Williams & Wilkins, Baltimore, 1977, 54.

QUANTITATIVE DISORDERS OF LEUKOCYTES: DIFFERENTIAL DIAGNOSIS

Thomas F. Necheles

The differential diagnosis of quantitative disorders of leukocytes is presented in Table 1.

TABLE 1
QUANTITATIVE DISORDERS OF LEUKOCYTES: DIFFERENTIAL DIAGNOSIS

Leukocytosis with increased granulocytes

- Absolute increase in granulocytes
  - Physiological
    - After strenuous exercise
    - After repeated vomiting
    - In pregnancy, during labor, and in puerperium
  - Inflammatory diseases
    - Tonsillitis
    - Bronchopneumonia
    - Meningitis
    - Miliary tuberculosis
    - Early stages of viral diseases
    - Rheumatic fever
    - Abscesses
  - During convulsions
  - Hemorrhage — acute and subacute
  - Postsplenectomy
  - Postoperative periods
  - Coronary thrombosis
  - Metabolic disorders
    - Diabetic acidosis
    - Uremia
    - Gout
    - Eclampsia of pregnancy
  - Burns
  - Polyarteritis nodosa
  - Intestinal obstruction
  - Malignant disease
  - Reticuloses
  - Hodgkin's disease
  - Hematologic diseases
    - Hemolytic anemias
    - Thrombotic microangiopathy
    - Polycythemia vera
- Leuko-erythroblastic reaction
  - Some cases of severe sepsis
  - Some cases of miliary tuberculosis
  - Severe hemorrhage
  - Phosphorus and carbon tetrachloride poisoning
  - Postirradiation
  - Erythroblastosis fetalis
  - Macroglobulinemia
  - Bone marrow carcinomatosis
  - Myelomatosis
  - DiGuglielmo's syndrome
  - Leukemias

Table 1 (continued)
QUANTITATIVE DISORDERS OF LEUKOCYTES: DIFFERENTIAL DIAGNOSIS

- Gaucher's disease
- Niemann-Pick's disease
- Myelosclerosis

Leukocytosis with increased lymphocytosis

- Bacterial infections
  - Tuberculosis
  - Undulant fever
  - Whooping cough
- Viral infections
- Recovery from acute infections
- Malnutrition
- Rickets
- Carcinoma
- Macroglobulinemia

Leukocytosis with increased monocytes

- Absolute monocytosis
  - Protozoal infections
    - Malaria
    - Kala-azar
    - Trypanosomiasis
  - Bacterial infections
    - Subacute bacterial endocarditis
    - Tuberculosis
    - Typhoid
  - Rickettsial infections
    - Typhus
    - Rocky Mountain spotted fever
  - Recovery from acute infections
  - Recovery from agranulocytosis
  - Drug poisoning
  - Hodgkin's disease
  - Gaucher's disease
  - Niemann-Pick's disease
- Monocytic leukemoid reaction
  - Tuberculosis
- Atypical mononucleosis
  - Infectious mononucleosis
  - Toxoplasmosis
  - Cytomegalic virus infection
  - Postoperative open heart surgery
  - Bacterial endocarditis
  - Infectious hepatitis
  - Typhoid
  - Brucellosis

Leukopenia

- With lymphopenia
  - Congenital absence of lymphoid tissue
  - "Swiss form" of agammaglobulinemia
  - Hodgkin's disease
  - Uremia
  - Congestive heart failure
- With neutropenia

Table 1 (continued)
QUANTITATIVE DISORDERS OF LEUKOCYTES: DIFFERENTIAL DIAGNOSIS

- Bacterial infections
  - Miliary tuberculosis
  - Whooping cough
  - Typhoid
  - Syphilis
- Viral infections
- Protozoal infections
  - Kala-azar
- Endocrine disorders
  - Hyperthyroidism
  - Addison's disease
  - Pituitary insufficiency
- Hypersplenism
- Collagen diseases
  - Rheumatoid arthritis
  - Felty's syndrome
  - Disseminated SLE
  - Periarteritis nodosa
- Congestive splenomegaly
  - Cirrhosis of the liver
  - Portal vein thrombosis
  - Splenic vein thrombosis
- Reticuloses
  - Hodgkin's disease
  - Giant follicular lymphoma
  - Lymphosarcoma
  - Reticulum cell sarcoma
  - Letterer-Siwe disease
- Metastatic carcinoma
- Sarcoidosis
- Drugs and chemicals
- Gaucher's disease
- Niemann-Pick's disease
- Macroglobulinemia
- Hematologic diseases
  - Cyclic or congenital neutropenia
  - Agranulocytosis
  - Leukemia
  - Paroxysmal nocturnal hemoglobinuria
  - Sideroblastic anemia
  - Aplastic anemia
  - DiGuglielmo's syndrome
  - Myelosclerosis

With pancytopenia

- Infections
  - Miliary tuberculosis
  - Syphilis
  - Kala-azar
- Collagen diseases
  - Rheumatoid arthritis
- Sarcoidosis
- Metastatic carcinoma
- Drugs and chemicals
- Gaucher's disease
- Niemann-Pick's disease
- Lymphomas
  - Hodgkin's disease

Table 1 (continued)
QUANTITATIVE DISORDERS OF LEUKOCYTES: DIFFERENTIAL DIAGNOSIS

- Giant follicular lymphoma
- Lymphosarcoma
- Reticulum cell sarcoma
- Letterer-Siwe disease
- Congestive splenomegaly
- Hematologic diseases
  - Paroxysmal nocturnal hemoglobinuria
  - Sideroblastic anemia
  - Megaloblastic anemia
  - Aplastic anemia
  - DiGuglielmo's syndrome
  - Agranulocytosis
  - Leukemia
  - Myelosclerosis

Eosinophilia
- Familial
- Infections
  - Scarlet fever
  - Rheumatic fever
  - Erythema multiforme
- Parasitic infestation of the tissues
  - Trichinosis
  - Hydatid disease
- Skin diseases
  - Pemphigus
  - Dermatitis herpetiformis
- Allergic disorders
  - Hay fever
  - Asthma
  - Drug allergy
  - Serum sickness
- Tropical eosinophilia
- Loeffler's syndrome
- Periarteritis nodosa
- Hodgkin's disease
- Postirradiation
- Hematological diseases
  - Polycythemia vera
  - Leukemia

Basophilia
- Chicken pox
- Smallpox
- Postsplenectomy
- Hodgkin's disease
- Hematologic diseases
  - Polycythemia vera
  - Myelocytic leukemia (acute and chronic)
  - "Preleukemia" syndrome

Adapted with modifications from Harper, Trevor, A., *Peripheral Blood Film,* Butterworths, London, 1968.

QUALITATIVE DISORDERS OF THE LEUKOCYTES

Thomas F. Necheles

A number of morphological and structural anomalies have been described in circulating (and bone marrow) leukocytes. Several of these are of little significance in themselves and often reflect pathologic processes in which the leukocyte is a more or less innocent bystander. These include toxic granulation and Döhle bodies (seen frequently in severe systemic infections). There are, however, several syndromes in which changes in the leukocytes indicate a severe systemic disease and which in themselves are diagnostic. The most important are the Chediak-Higashi syndrome, Gaucher's disease, and Niemann-Pick disease. Other syndromes associated with leukocyte changes include the May-Adler anomaly and Hurler's syndrome. These, however, are of lesser importance because (1) they are usually diagnosed by changes other than those seen in the leukocytes and (2) these syndromes are quite rare.

Niemann-Pick Disease

Niemann-Pick disease is a heterogeneous group of autosomal recessive disorders of phospholipid metabolism, in which lipids accumulate in histiocytes and tissues.[1-7] The phospholipid accumulated was found to be a sphingomyelin associated with a deficient enzyme, a sphingomyelinase. The biochemical abnormality was first identified by Brady and later confirmed by others.[8-16] Two sphingomyelinase isoenzymes have been described: I and II.[17] Sphingomyelinase takes part in the hydrolytic cleavage of spingomyelin to phosphorylcholine and ceramide.

The phenotypic variation of the disease has led to attempts to classify the disorder according to clinicopathologic criteria, and five different types are now recognized[3,17] (Table 1). Sphingomyelin and other lipid measurements in various tissues of individuals are shown in Table 2. Table 3 shows sphingomyelinase values found in healthy controls and patients with Niemann-Pick disease in various tissues.

Pathophysiologic Considerations

The biochemical defect leading to accumulation of phospholipid has been identified in two out of the five types of Niemann-Pick disease. Sphingomyelinase activity is low or absent in types A and B.[15,16] The remaining three types exhibit close to normal or normal enzyme activity in nonneural tissue.[3,16] The increased tissue sphingomyelin found in these variants in spite of the normal enzyme levels leads to the speculation of increased synthesis of sphingomyelin. This hypothesis has been partially disproved.[19,20] Studies of the chemical nature of sphingomyelin synthesized in various types of Niemann-Pick disease demonstrated that it is indistinguishable from the material synthesized in normal tissue.[3,21-24]

Significantly, increased amounts of unesterified cholesterol have been found in all types of Niemann-Pick disease.[3,21] It is difficult to link the accumulation of cholesterol to the primary defect in sphingomyelin metabolism, since the catabolic pathways of these two compounds are somewhat remote. Compensatory mechanisms facilitating the storage of phospholipids have been proposed as an explanation for the increased synthesis or decreased catabolism of cholesterol.[21,26]

A generally accepted explanation of the pathophysiologic event underlying the manifestations of the disease is still lacking, although traditionally, it has been held that the accumulation of sphingomyelin in the reticuloendothelial system and other tissues is the primary event. Reticuloendothelial system and other phagocytic cells become filled with loaded secondary lysosomes.[25] Intracellular organelles undergo physical

Table 1
CLINICAL TYPES OF NIEMANN-PICK DISEASE

Age	A Early infancy	B Infancy	C 1—2 years	D 1—2 years	E Childhood
Ethnic background	High in Ashkenazi Jews	Multiracial	Multiracial	Nova Scotia	—
Viscera	Severely affected	Severely affected	Moderately affected. Late visceral changes	Moderately affected	Slight—moderate
CNS	Severe psychomotor retardation in early infancy. CSF—normal	No involvement. CSF—normal	Delayed involvement. Cerebellar involvement. Mental retardation. Spasticity. Seizures	Delayed involvement. Cerebellar mental retardation. Seizures	Normal
Enzyme activity	Severely decreased	Severe. Less than type A	Normal	Normal	Normal
Niemann-Pick cells	Numerous	Numerous	Numerous	Present	Absent
Sphingomyelin in tissues	Increased	Increased	Slightly increased	Slightly increased	Slightly increased
Course	Acute	Subacute	Subacute	Subacute	Benign
Outcome	Death in early childhood	Often death by adolescence	Often death by adolescence	Death in childhood	Benign
Other	Cherry-red spots	—	Cherry-red spots	Early jaundice	—

Table 2

TOTAL AND FRACTIONATED LIPIDS IN LIVER (mg/g wet weight), IN RED CELLS (mg/100 mℓ of packed red cells) AND IN SERUM (mg/100 mℓ of serum) IN THREE PATIENTS AFFECTED BY NIEMANN-PICK DISEASE AND IN NORMAL SUBJECTS

	Liver				Red cells				Serum			
Lipid fractions	Patient I	Patient II	Patient III	Normal[a]	Patient I	Patient II	Patient III	Normal[b]	Patient I	Patient II	Patient III	Normal[c]
Cholesterol esters	3	7	6	4	0	0	0	0	117	57	96	151
Triglycerides	10	2	10	7	32	32	30	36	272	251	106	151
FFA	1	1	0	1	0	0	0	0	47	23	0	17
Free cholesterol	14	12	20	6	124	124	127	132	163	91	105	52
Phosphatidyl ethanolamine	0	0	5	4	36	28	24	92	20	15	6	15
Phosphatidyl serine	0	0	2	2	0	0	24	0	3	2	3	2
Phosphatidyl choline	15	24	8	14	96	124	81	92	140	114	125	162
Sphingomyelin	27	21	17	3	112	92	70	48	16	17	42	23
Total phospholipids	42	45	32	23	244	244	199	232	179	148	176	202
Total lipids	70	68	68	41	400	400	356	400	800	600	500	580

[a] This value includes phosphatidylcholine and small quantities of lysophostidylcholine.
[b] Average of two subjects.
[c] Average of five subjects.

From Ciardini, O., Cardi, E., Castro, M., and Donfrancesco, A., *Clin. Chim. Acta*, 42, 18, 1972. With permission.

Table 3
SPHINGOMYELIN-CLEAVING ENZYME ACTIVITY IN HUMAN TISSUE PREPARATIONS

			Fibroblasts	
Type	Liver[a]	Spleen[b]	Bone marrow[c]	Skin[c]
A	0.0	—	—	—
A	0.54	—	0.3	0.1
A	0.61	—	—	—
A	0.26	—	0	0
A	0.46	—	—	0.1
A	0.89	—	0	0.2
A	—	1.0	—	—
A	—	1.4	—	—
A	—	—	0.0	—
A	—	—	0.0	—
B	—	3.0	—	—
B	—	7.6	—	—
B	—	3.3	—	—
B	1.3	—	2.9	2.0
B	0.9	—	3.5	1.8
B[d]	—	—	—	1.3
B	1.2	—	—	1.9
C	—	181	—	—
C	—	88	—	—
C	—	152	—	—
C	—	254	—	—
C	—	117	—	—
C	8.8	3.2[a]	30.6	—
D	—	36	—	—
D	6.7	—	30.1	—
D	5.8	—	—	—
Normal range	4.4—11.1	65—200	52 + 10	35 + 6

[a] Units per milligram of protein.
[b] Microinternational units per milligram of protein.
[c] Units per million cells.
[d] This is a patient of uncertain type who is described in the text under type B.

From Stanbury, J. B., Wyngaarden, J. B., Fredrickson, D. S., Eds., *Glucosyl-Ceramide Lipidoses in the Metabolic Basis of Inherited Disease,* 3rd ed., McGraw-Hill, New York, 1972, 730. With permission.

damage. Proliferation of lipid loaded cells leads to mechanical problems and to secondary functional disability of the affected organs. Liver, spleen, lymph nodes, bone marrow, kidneys, lungs, bones, and brain are the primary target organs. CNS involvement, the hallmark of the severe form of the disease, varies according to the type, and there seems to be no pattern either in the extent or the distribution of pathologic change within the same type. The ganglion cells are often swollen and contain cytoplasmic vacuoles that frequently do not stain with lipid dyes and stain weakly with PAS. Electron microscope studies of ganglion cells show residual bodies.[34,36] There is often loss of myelin in the white matter, and storage cells are seen around the leptomeninges, in the perivascular space, and in the endothelium of cerebral vessels. Table 5 describes the morphologic findings in plasma and formed elements of peripheral blood in Niemann-Pick disease.

Table 4
CHARACTERISTICS OF THE NIEMANN-PICK CELL

Light Microscopy[27-31]
- Reticuloendothelial, phagocytic, lymphoid cell
- 20—90 μm in diameter
- Foamy mulberry appearance
- Stains black with Sudan black stain
- Stains black with Smith-Dietrich stain
- Stains red with Oil-red-O stain
- Stains violet with Nile blue stain
- Stains violet with mercuric nitrate stain
- Stains black-blue with hematin
- Stains red with periodic acid-Schiff
- Positive for acid phosphatase

Electron Microscopy[29,32-35]
- Cytoplasmic residual bodies (lysosomes), 0.5—5 μm in diameter
- Residual bodies contain layers of osmophilic material (phosphorylcholine)
- Osmophobic layer (ceramide)

Table 5
FINDINGS IN PLASMA AND FORMED ELEMENTS OF PERIPHERAL BLOOD IN NIEMANN-PICK DISEASE

	Ref.
Increased triglyceride	3
Increased low density lipoproteins	3
Increased acid phosphatase	41
Decreased noncholine-containing phosphatids in RBC	42
Decreased sphingomyelin in RBC	43

REFERENCES

1. **Niemann, A.,** Ein unbekanntes Krankheitsbild, *Jahrb. Kinderheilk.*, 79, 1, 1914.
2. **Pick, L.,** Uber die lipoidzellige splenoheptamegalie typus Niemann-Pick als Stoffwechselerkrankung, *Med. Klin. (Munich)*, 23, 1483, 1927.
3. **Fredrickson, D. S.,** Sphingomyelin lipidosis: Niemann-Pick disease, in *The Metabolic Basis of Inherited Disease*, 2nd ed., Stanbury, J. B., Wyngaarden, J. B., and Fredrickson, D. S., Eds., McGraw-Hill, New York, 1960, 586.
4. **Bloom, W. and Kern, R.,** Spleens from Gaucher's disease and lipoid-histiocytosis; the chemical analysis, *Arch. Intern. Med. (Chicago)*, 39, 456, 1927.
5. **Brahn, B. and Pick, L.,** Zur chemischen Organalyse bei der lipoidzelligen Splenohepatomegalie typus Niemann-Pick, *Klin. Wochenschr.*, 6, 2367, 1927.
6. **McFate, R. P.,** The chemical analysis of liver and spleen from a case of lipoid histiocytosis (Niemann-Pick's disease), *Arch. Pathol. Lab. Med.*, 6, 1054, 1928.
7. **Sobotka, H., Glick, D., Reiner, M., and Tuchman, L. E.,** The lipoids of spleen and liver in various types of lipoidoses, *Biochem. J.*, 27, 2031, 1933.
8. **Klenk, E.,** Uber die Natur der Phosphatide der Milz bei der Niemann-Pickschen Krankheit, *Z. Physiol. Chem.*, 229, 151, 1934.

9. **Klenk, E.**, Uber die Natur der Phosphatide and anderer lipoide des Gehirns und der Leber bei der Niemann-Pickschen Krankheit, *Z. Physiol. Chem.*, 235, 24, 1935.
10. **Tropp, C. and Eckhardt, B.**, Sphingomyelin bei Niemann-Pickschen Krankheit, *Z. Physiol. Chem.*, 243, 38, 1936.
11. **Tropp, C. and Eckhardt, B.**, Gehirn-sphingomyelin bein Niemann Pickschen Krankheit, *Z. Physiol. Chem.*, 245, 1963, 1936.
12. **Thannhauser, S. J., Benotti, J., and Reinstein, H.**, cited by Thannhauser, S. J., in *Lipidoses: Diseases of the Intracellular Lipid Metabolism*, Grune & Stratton, New York, 1958.
13. **Teunissen, P. H. and Den Ouden, A.**, Nachtrag zu der Mitteilung: Beitrag zur Kenntnis der Chemie der Lipoidosis phosphatidica, *Z. Chem.*, 252, 271, 1938.
14. **Chargaff, E.**, A study of the spleen in a case of Niemann-Pick disease, *J. Biol. Chem.*, 130, 503, 1939.
15. **Brady, R. O., Kanfer, J. N., Mock, M. B., and Frerickson, D. S.**, The metabolism of sphingomyelin. II. Evidence of an enzymatic deficiency in Niemann-Pick disease, *Proc. Natl. Acad. Sci. U.S.A.*, 55, 366, 1966.
16. **Schneider, P. B. and Kennedy, E. P.**, Sphingomyelinase in normal human spleens and in spleens from subjects with Niemann-Pick disease, *J. Lipid Res.*, 8, 202, 1967.
17. **Callahan, J. W., Khalil, M., and Gerrie, J.**, Isoenzymes of sphingomyelin and the genetic defect in Niemann-Pick disease, type C, *Biochem. Biophys. Res. Commun.*, 58, (2), 784, 1974.
18. **Sloan, H. R., Uhlendorf, B. W., Kanfer, J. N., Brady, R. O., and Fredrickson, D. S.**, Deficiency of sphingomyelin-cleaving enzyme activity in tissue cultures derived from patients with Niemann-Pick disease, *Biochem. Biophys. Res. Commun.*, 34, 582, 1969.
19. **Crocker, A. C. and Mays, V. B.**, Sphingomyelin synthesis in Niemann-Pick disease, *Am. J. Clin. Nutr.*, 9, 63, 1961.
20. **Holtz, A. I.**, Quantitation of phospholipid analysis using P^{32} by a digital computer method in metabolic experiments on Niemann-Pick disease, *J. Am. Oil Chem. Soc.*, 44, 80, 1967.
21. **Ivemark, B. I., Svennerholm, L, Thoren, C., and Tunnell, R.**, Niemann-Pick disease in infancy: report of two siblings with clinical, histologic and chemical studies, *Acta Paediatr.*, 52, 391, 1963.
22. **Porges, E., Sojak, L., Solcaniova, E., and Cap, J.**, Beitrag zum studium des miltzsphingomyelin bei der Niemann-Pick'schen erkrankung, *J. Neurochem.*, 13, 879, 1966.
23. **Lowden, J. A., LaRamee, M. A., and Wentworth, P.**, The subacute form of Niemann-Pick disease, *Arch. Neurol. (Chicago)*, 17, 230, 1957.
24. **Svennerholm, E., Stallberg-Stenhagen, S., and Svennerholm, L.**, Fatty acid composition of sphingomyelins in blood, spleen, placenta, liver, lung and kidney, *Biochim. Biophys. Acta*, 125, 60, 1966.
25. **Hers, H. G.**, Inborn lysosomal diseases, *Gastroenterology*, 48, 625, 1965.
26. **Vandenheuvel, A.**, Study of biological structure at the molecular level with stereomodel projections. I. The lipids in the myelin sheath of nerve, *J. Am. Oil Chem. Soc.*, 40, 455, 1963.
27. **McFate, R. P.**, The chemical analysis of liver and spleen from a case of lipoid histiocytosis (Niemann-Pick's disease), *Arch. Pathol. Lab. Med.*, 6, 1054, 1928.
28. **Pearse, A. G. E.**, *Histochemistry—Theoretical and Applied*, Little, Brown, Boston, 1960.
29. **Hooghwinkel, G. J. M. and Borri, P. F.**, Pathochemie van de sphingolipidosen, *Chem., Weekbl.*, 60, 578, 1964.
30. **Bloom, W.**, The histogenesis of essential lipoid histiocytosis (Niemann-Pick's disease), *Arch. Pathol. (Chicago)*, 6, 827, 1928.
31. **Crocker, A. C. and Farber, S.**, Niemann-Pick disease: A review of 18 patients, *Medicine (Baltimore)*, 37, 1, 1958.
32. **Roos, B., Cottier, H., and Rossi, E.**, Elektronenoptische Beobachtungen bei Speicherkrankheiten, *Pathol. Microbiol. (Basel)*, 24, 278, 1961.
33. **Tanaka, Y., Brecher, G., and Fredrickson, D. S.**, Cellules de la maladie de Niemann-Pick et de quelques autres lipoidoses. (The storage cells of Niemann-Pick disease and some other lipidoses), *Nouv. Rev. Fr. Hematol.*, 3, 5, 1963.
34. **Wallace, B. J., Schneck, L., Kaplan, H., and Volk, B.W.**, Fine structure of the cerebellum of children with lipidoses, *Arch. Pathol. (Chicago)*, 80, 466, 1965.
35. **Stoekenius, W.**, Osmium Tetroxide Fixation of Lipids, in *Proceedings of the European Regional Conference on Electron Microscopy*, Nederlandsche Vereniging voor Electronen Microscope, Delft, 1960.
36. **Luse, S.**, The fine structure of the brain and other organs in Niemann-Pick disease, in *Inborn Disorders of Sphingolipid Metabolism. (Proceedings of the Third International Symposium on the Cerebral Sphingolipidoses)*, Aronson, S. M., and Volk, B. W., Eds., Pergamon Publishing, Elmsford, N.Y., 1967, 93.
37. **Rabinowicz, T., Klein, D., and Tchicaloff, M.**, Juvenile form of Niemann-Pick disease, *Pathol. Eur.*, 3, 154, 1968.

38. **Pick, L. and Bielschowsky, M.**, Uber lipoidzellige Splenomegalie (Typus Niemann-Pick) und amaurotische Idiotie, *Klin. Wochenschr.*, 6, 1631, 1927.
39. **Van Bogaert, L., Seitelberger, F., and Edgar, G. W. F.**, Etudes neuropathologiques et neurochimiques sur un cas de Niemann-Pick chez un jeune enfant, *Acta Neuropathol.*, 3, 57, 1963.
40. **Philippart, M., Martin, L., Martin, J. J., and Menkes, John H.**, Niemann-Pick disease, *Arch. Neurol. (Chicago)*, 20, 227, 1969.
41. **Hastrup, B., and Videbaek, A.**, Acid phosphatase in Niemann-Pick's disease and a therapeutic experiment with cortisone, *Acta Med. Scand.*, 149, 287, 1954.
42. **Balint, J. A., Nyhan, W. L., Lietman, P., and Turner, D. A.**, Lipid patterns in Niemann-Pick disease, *J. Lab. Clin. Med.*, 58, 548, 1961.
43. **Hooghwinkel, G. J. M., van Gelderen, H. H., and Staal, A.**, Sphingomyelin of red blood cells in lipidosis and in dementia of unknown origin in children, *Arch. Dis. Child.*, 44, 197, 1969.

CHEDIAK HIGASHI SYNDROME

Andreas Athanasiou

The Chediak-Higashi syndrome is a rare disorder inherited on an autosomal recessive basis and characterized by partial oculocutaneous albinism and giant lysosomal inclusions in leukocytes and other granule-containing cells.[1-5] A similar disease has also been described in mink, mice, and cattle.[16,17]

A central clinical feature of the Chediak-Higashi syndrome is a markedly increased susceptibility to pyogenic infections, usually caused by Gram-positive organisms, frequently (Staphylococcus aureus, and most often involving the respiratory system.

Multiple defects in the function of granulocytes have been described, including diminished bactericidal activity, abnormalities in leukocyte migration and chemotaxis, abnormal lysosomal function, impaired microtubule function, and neutropenia.[6-10]

Clinically, the disease "presents" early in childhood, with repeated infection, photophobia, nystagmus, decreased skin pigmentations, and silky hair. Most of the patients develop a lymphoma-like disease, with infiltrations of lymphoid, parenchymal, and bone marrow tissues by benign-looking mononuclear cells. Massive hepatosplenomegaly is usually present during the malignant phase of the disease, and secondary hematologic changes constitute the major cause of death in affected individuals. Other abnormalities associated with Chediak-Higashi syndrome are summarized in Table 1.

Table 1
ABNORMALITIES ASSOCIATED WITH CHEDIAK-HIGASHI SYNDROME

Abnormality	Ref.
Peripheral neuropathy	14,15
Spirocerebellar degeneration	11
Abnormal platelet function	12,13
Mental retardation	14,15
Autonomic dysfunction	14,15
Serum lipid abnormalities	20,21
Renal tubular changes	20

No unifying concept has been proposed for the syndrome. The possible relationship of Chediak-Higashi syndrome to a genetically determined alteration in lipid metabolism has been put forward, but the biochemical data available neither confirm nor deny this association.[22-26]

During the last 10 years, efforts have been made to elucidate the ultrastructural and biochemical events leading to the formation of abnormal lysosomal granules and defective bactericidal activity of the granulocyte in Chediak-Higashi syndrome. Most of the available information came from studies done in animal models with the homologous syndrome.[27-32] The number of the precursor primary (azurophile) granules is decreased, and, as maturation proceeds, they seem to undergo fusions leading to the formation of the Chediak-Higashi granule. The crystalloid present in normal primary granules appears to be missing, and the granule matrix is often arranged in a reticulated manner.[30] No abnormalities have been uncovered during the formation of the secondary granules, and a normal number of those are formed during the later stages of granulogenesis.[27] A pathogenetic correlation between the formation of the abnormal

Table 2
DISTRIBUTION OF PROTEIN AND LYSOSOMAL ENZYMES IN NORMAL AND CHEDIAK-HIGASHI SYNDROME GRANULOCYTES

Determination	No. of samples	Total activity (%)[a]	No. of samples	Total activity (%)	p[b]
Protein	9		15		
NF (nuclear fraction)		10.4 ± 1.3[d]		21.1 ± 1.9	<0.01
PGS (postgranular supernatant)		55.1 ± 1.2		52.4 ± 1.9	>0.20
GF (granular fraction)		34.4 ± 0.9		26.5 ± 1.0	<0.01
Recovery (%)[c]		90.4		91.5	
Acid phosphatase (PNP)[d]	9		15		
NF		4.7 ± 1.2		11.0 ± 2.5	<0.10
PGS		28.0 ± 1.3		26.6 ± 2.3	>0.20
GF		66.5 ± 1.3		62.4 ± 1.7	>0.10
Recovery		95.1		102.4	
Acid phosphatase (BGP)[d]	9		12		
NF		4.0 ± 0.5		8.4 ± 2.0	<0.10
PGS		17.4 ± 1.2		38.0 ± 3.2	<0.01
GF		78.5 ± 0.8		51.5 ± 3.5	<0.01
Recovery		145.1		116.4	
Alkaline phosphatase	9		11		
NF		9.0 ± 1.1		14.4 ± 2.0	<0.05
PGS		33.6 ± 3.2		36.8 ± 1.8	>0.20
GF		57.3 ± 4.0		48.8 ± 1.4	<0.05
Recovery		80.2		83.1	
B-Glucuronidase[d]	9		15		
NF		6.9 ± 1.0		15.7 ± 1.6	<0.01
PGS		12.3 ± 1.6		36.7 ± 3.7	<0.01
GF		80.6 ± 1.6		47.6 ± 3.4	<0.01
Recovery		95.1		101.5	
Myeloperoxidase[d]	9		14		
NF		7.1 ± 1.0		19.2 ± 3.1	<0.01
PGS		7.5 ± 1.0		27.1 ± 3.0	<0.01
GF		85.2 ± 1.1		53.7 ± 4.1	<0.01
Recovery		84.4		84.1	
Muramidase	9		14		
NF		8.0 ± 1.5		14.8 ± 2.5	<0.05
PGS		18.9 ± 2.9		34.7 ± 2.6	<0.01
GF		73.0 ± 3.1		47.3 ± 3.9	<0.01
Recovery		103.8		101.7	

[a] Combined activity of nuclear, granular, and postgranular supernatant fractions.
[b] Significant level of difference from normal.
[c] Total activity of nuclear, granular, and post-granular supernatant fractions compared to cell lysate fraction.
[d] Mean ± standard error.

From Kimball, H. R., Ford, G. H., and Wolff, S. M., *J. Lab. Clin. Med.*, 86, 621, 1975. With permission.

granules in Chediak-Higashi syndrome and cellular dysfunction is suggested by the failure to degranulate following ingestion of bacteria. This defect seems to be variable, and histochemical studies usually reveal the presence of decreased amounts of acid phosphatase and peroxidase within the phagolysosome.[33] Quantitative studies of lysosomal enzymes showed significant deviations from the normal pattern, as shown in Tables 2 and 3.

Table 3
LYSOSOMAL ENZYMES OF NORMAL AND CHEDIAK-HIGASHI SYNDROME GRANULOCYTES

	B-Glucuronidase[b]			Myeloperoxidase[c]			Muramidase[d]			Cathepsin[e]		
Fraction[a]	Normal	CHS	P[f]	Normal	CHS	P	Normal	CHS	P	Normal	CHS	P
No. samples	9	15		9	14		9	14		6	6	
Lysate												
Activity/10^7 cells	65.1 ± 4.5	32.2 ± 4.6	<0.01	1.04 ± 0.05	0.39 ± 0.05	<0.01	61.2 ± 4.6	52.2 ± 5.0	<0.20	237.6 ± 14.4	248.0 ± 26.5	>0.2
Activity/mg protein	75.6 ± 3.9	36.3 ± 5.3	<0.01	1.24 ± 0.10	0.42 ± 0.05	<0.01	72.5 ± 6.3	59.7 ± 6.3	<0.20	717.2 ± 74.9	641.5 ± 85.6	>0.2
Nuclear												
Activity/10^7 cells	4.4 ± 0.9	4.7 ± 0.8	>0.20	0.06 ± 0.01	0.07 ± 0.02	>0.20	5.0 ± 1.0	7.8 ± 1.9	<0.01	—	—	—
Activity/mg protein	53.6 ± 5.1	30.5 ± 6.4	<0.01	0.81 ± 0.10	0.34 ± 0.06	<0.01	60.7 ± 8.5	39.1 ± 5.8	>0.01	—	—	—
Postgranular supernatant												
Activity/10^7 cells	7.6 ± 1.3	11.6 ± 2.0	<0.01	0.07 ± 0.01	0.10 ± 0.02	<0.01	11.6 ± 1.8	19.0 ± 3.3	<0.01	—	—	—
Activity/mg protein	17.6 ± 2.5	25.6 ± 4.0	<0.01	0.16 ± 0.03	0.21 ± 0.05	<0.05	26.5 ± 3.3	43.6 ± 10.1	<0.01	—	—	—
Granular												
Activity/10^7 cells	50.4 ± 5.5	15.5 ± 2.3	<0.01	0.75 ± 0.05	0.16 ± 0.02	<0.01	45.3 ± 3.7	24.3 ± 2.3	<0.01	—	—	—
Activity/mg protein	190.2 ± 17.4	72.4 ± 13.2	<0.01	2.86 ± 0.24	0.71 ± 0.09	<0.01	175.3 + 9.4	107.4 + 9.6	<0.01	—	—	—

[a] Mean ± standard error.
[b] Activity expressed as micrograms of phenolphthalein liberated per hour.
[c] Activity expressed as microgram equivalents of horseradish peroxidase.
[d] Activity expressed as microgram equivalents of egg white lysozyme.
[e] Activity expressed as micrograms of protein equivalents released per hour.
[f] Significance level of difference from normal.

From Kimball, H. R., Ford, G. M., Wolff, S. M., *J. Lab. Clin. Med.*, 86, 621, 1975. With permission.

1. **Blume. R. S. and Wolff, S. M.,** The Chediak-Higashi syndrome studies in 4 patients and review of the literature, *Medicine (Baltimore),* 51, 247, 1972.
2. **Chediak, M.,** Nouvelle anomalie leukocytaire de caractère constitutionel familial, *Rev. Haematol.,* 7, 362, 1952.
3. **Higashi, O.,** Congenital gigantism of peroxidase granules, *Tohoku J. Exp. Med.,* 59, 315, 1954.
4. **Bequéz-César, A.,** Neutropenia cronica maligna familiar con granulociones atipicas de los leukocitos, *Bid. Soc. Cub. Ped.,* 15, 900, 1943.
5. **Steinbrinck, W.,** Über eine neue Granulocytanomalie de Leukocyten, *Dtsch. Arch. Klin. Med.,* 193, 577, 1948.
6. **Clark, R. A. and Kimball, H. R.,** Defective granulocyte chemotaxis in the Chediak-Higashi syndrome, *J. Clin. Invest.,* 50, 2645, 1971.
7. **Clark, R. A., Kimball, H. R., and Padgett, G.,** Granulocyte chemotaxis in Chediak-Higashi syndrome of mink, *Blood,* 39, 644, 1972.
8. **Root, R. K., Rosenthal, A. S., and Balestra, D. J.,** *J. Clin. Invest.,* 51, 649, 1972.
9. **Oliver, J. M.,** Impaired microtubule function correctable by cyclic AMP and cholinerg agonists in the Chediak-Higashi syndrome, *Am. J. Pathol.,* 85, (65), 395, 1976.
10. **Hinds, K. and Danes, B. S.,** Microtubular defect in Chediak-Higashi syndrome, *Lancet,* 2, 149, 1976.
11. **Sheramata, W., Kott, H. S., and Cyr, D. P.,** The Chediak-Higashi-Steinbrinck syndrome, *Arch. Neurol. (Chicago),* 25, 289, 1971.
12. **Buchanan, G. R. and Handin, R. I.,** Platelet function in the Chediak-Higashi syndrome, *Blood,* 47, 941, 1976.
13. **Bell, T. G., Meyers, K. M., Prieux, D. J., Fauci, A. S., Wolff, S. M., and Padgett, G. A.,** Decreased nucleotide and serotonin storage associated with defective function in Chediak-Higashi syndrome cattle and human platelets, *Blood,* 48, 175, 1976.
14. **Sung, J. M., Meyers, J. P., Standlan, E. M., Cowen, D., and Wolf, A.,** Neuropathological changes in Chediak-Higashi disease, *J. Neuropathol. Exp. Neurol.,* 28, 86, 1969.
15. **Lockman, L. A., Kennedy, W. R., and White, J. G.,** The Chediak-Higashi syndrome: electrophysiological and electrome microscopy observations on the peripheral neuropathy, *J. Pediatr.,* 70, 942, 1967.
16. **Leader, R. W., Padgett, G. A., and Gorham, J. R.,** Studies of abnormal leukocyte bodies in the mink, *Blood,* 22, 477, 1963.
17. **Bennett, J. M., Blume, R. S., and Wolff, S. M.,** Characterization and significance of abnormal leukocyte granules in the beige mouse: a possible homologue of Chediak-Higashi Alentian trait, *J. Lab. Clin. Med.,* 73, 235, 1969.
18. **Kritzler, R. A., Terner, J. Y., Lindenbaum, J., Magidson, J., Williams, R., Preisig, R., and Philipps, G. P.,** Chediak-Higashi syndrome, *Am. J. Med.,* 36, 583, 1964.
19. **Cat, I., Marinoni, L. P., Giralti, D. J., Almeida, B. D., Neto, A. S., Bragh, H., and Silva, A. T. D.,** Chediak-Higashi syndrome with familial idiopathic hyperlipenia, *Lancet,* 1, 1398, 1965.
20. **Saraiva, L. G., Azevedo, M., Correa, J. M., Carvalho, G., and Prospero, J. D.,** Anomalous panleukocytic granulation, *Blood,* 14, 1112, 1959.
21. **Bernard, J., Bessis, M., Seligmann, M., Chassigneaux, J., and Chomé, J.,** Un cas de maladie de Chediak-Steinbrinck-Higashi, *Presse Med.,* 68, 563, 1960.
22. **Davis, C. N. C. and Douglas, S. D.,** Defective granule formation and function in the Chediak-Higashi syndrome in man and animals, *Semin. Hematol.,* 9, 43, 1972.
23. **Davis, W. C., Spicer, S. S., Greene, W. B., and Padgett, G. A.,** Ultrastructural of BM granulocytes in normal mink and in mink with the homologue of the Chediak-Higashi trait of humans, *Lab. Invest.,* 24, 303, 1971.
24. **Davis, W. C., Spicer, S. S., Greene, W. B. and Padgett, G. A.,** Ultrastructure of cells in BM and peripheral blood of normal mink and mink with the homologue of the Chediak-Higashi trait of humans, *Am. J. Pathol.,* 63, 411, 1971.
25. **Douglas, S. D., Blume, R. S., and Wolff, S. M.,** Five ultrastructural studies of leukocytes from patients and heterozygotes with the Chediak-Higashi syndrome, *Blood,* 33, 527, 1969.
26. **White, J. G.,** The Chediak-Higashi syndrome: a possible lysosomal disease, *Blood,* 28, 143, 1966.
27. **White, J. G.,** The Chediak-Higashi syndrome: cytoplasmic sequestration in circulating leukocytes, *Blood,* 29, 435, 1967.

GAUCHER'S DISEASE

Andreas Athanasiou

Gaucher's disease is a glycolipid storage disease caused by the deficiency of a lysosomal hydrolase, β-glucocerebrosidase,[1-7] inherited as an autosomal recessive trait.

The resulting catabolic block causes glycocerebroside to accumulate in the reticuloendothelial system, producing the characteristic cells seen most often in this condition. Proliferation and deposition of these storage cells in parenchymal organs, lymph nodes, bones, bone marrow, and brain lead to the functional and anatomic abnormalities characteristic of the disease. The three recognized variants of the disorder, Type I (chronic adult nonneuropathic), Type II (acute neuropathic), and Type III (subacute neuropathic, juvenile), probably represent allelic mutations acting at the same genetic locus. Table 1 summarizes the clinicopathologic findings in the three types of Gaucher's disease. Table 2 refers to the biochemical abnormalities seen in this disorder. Serum enzymatic abnormalities in Gaucher's disease are shown in Table 3, and in Table 4 urinary amino acid concentrations in Gaucher's disease are compared to normal concentrations. The structural characteristics of the Gaucher's cell appear in Table 5, and diagnostic criteria and laboratory tests in the disease are shown in Table 6. Postulated pathophysiologic events are summarized in Table 7.

Table 1
CLINICAL TYPES OF GAUCHER'S DISEASE

	Type I	Type II	Type III
Age at onset	Older children	Early infancy	Young children
Background	Mostly Jewish	Mostly non-Jewish	Non-Jewish, Scandinavian
Hepatosplenomegaly	Pronounced	Pronounced	Pronounced
Hematologic changes	Severe thrombocytopenia. Leukopenia. Anemia	Not as severe thrombocytopenia. Leukopenia. Anemia	Severe thrombocytopenia. Leukopenia. Anemia
CNS changes	None	Psychomotor retardation. Mental retardation. Extrapyramidal cranial nerves. Gaucher's cells in brain	Seizures. Mental retardation. EEG abnormalities, cranial nerves and extrapyramidal
Acid phosphatase	Increased	Increased	Increased
Course	Mostly benign	Fulminant	Protracted
Primary cause of death	Bleeding. Pulmonary disease	Pulmonary disease. CNS	Infection. Pulmonary disease

Table 2
BIOCHEMICAL ABNORMALITIES IN GAUCHER'S DISEASE

Tissues, except brain	Ref.
Increased monohexosyl ceramides	9
Increased glucosyl ceramides	10, 11
Increased galactosyl ceramide in Type III	12
Increased C16:0 and C24:1 fatty acids	13, 14
Increased saturated lung chain fatty acids	15, 16
Increased ganglioside GM3 Type I and II	13, 14, 16
Increased sphingomyelin	17
Increased cholesteryl ester	16
Increased lactosyl ceramide in WBC	25
Brain	
Decreased galactosyl ceramide in Type II	18
Increased gal-glu cerebroside in Type III	—
Plasma	
Increased neutral plasma glycolipids Type III	19
Increased cerebrosides	—
Increased glycosyl ceramide	22
Increased transcobalamin	23
Increased alpha lipoprotein	26
Increased plasma immunoglobulins	9

Table 3
SERUM ENZYME ABNORMALITIES IN GAUCHER'S DISEASE

Enzyme	Ref.
Acid phosphatase	20
Acid phosphatase isoenzyme 5	21
β-glucosaminidase	28
β-glucuronidase	28
β-galactosidase	28
β-fucosidase	28
Lysozyme	29
Peptidase	30
Angiotensin converting enzyme	30

Table 4
URINARY AMINO ACIDS IN GAUCHER'S DISEASE

Amino acid	Gaucher's disease (n = 4)
Aspartic acid	0.063 (0.055—0.072)
Threonine	0.216 (0.149—0.280)
Serine + glutamine	—
Serine	0.937 (0.75—1.26)
Glutamic acid	0.103 (0.083—0.124)
Glycine	1.565 (1.27—1.86)
Alanine	0.363 (0.23—0.61)
Valine	0.055 (0.036—0.079)
Cystine	0.114 (0.069—0.19)
Tyrosine	0.156 (0.108—0.22)
Phenylalanine	0.107 (0.064—0.16)
Lysine	0.161 (0.11—0.213)
Histidine	1.134 (0.89—1.25)
Tryptophan	0.083 (0—0.140)

Note: Concentration expressed as μ moles amino acid excreted per milligram creatinine. All values given as mean ± SD (range) or mean (range). Student's test used for comparison of values in controls and patients.

Table 5
STRUCTURAL CHARACTERISTICS OF GAUCHER'S DISEASE

	Ref.
Reticulum cell 200—100 μm	35
Cytoplasm, "crumbled silk", "wrinkled tissue paper"	36, 37
+ PAS stain, PAS-leucofuschin stain	38, 39
+ Mallory trichrome stain	—
Secondary lysosomes and residual bodies by Gaucher's disease	40, 41
Tubules 5 μm in length, 120—200 Å diameter	9, 42
Tubules contain 10—12 fibrils arranged in helices	42

Table 6
DIAGNOSTIC CRITERIA AND TESTS IN GAUCHER'S DISEASE

	Ref.
Gaucher's cells in liver and spleen	
Increased acid phosphatase activity in plasma	31
Lipid hydrolase activity in WBC using ^{14}C-labeled glycocerebroside	32
Lipid hydrolase in cultured skin fibroblast	—
Lipid hydrolase activity in culture skin fibroblasts using monosaccharide derivatives of 4-methy *lumbelli ferone*	33
Lipid hydrolase activity in WBC using monosaccharide derivatives of 4-methy*lumbelli ferone*	34
Detection of carrier state using ^{14}C labeled glucocerebroside in leukocytes	32
Lipid hydrolase activity in cultured amniotic cells at 14-weeks gestation for detection of carrier and homozygous state	32, 34

Table 7
POSTULATED PATHOPHYSIOLOGIC EVENTS IN GAUCHER'S DISEASE

Water-insoluble glycocerebroside accumulates in Gaucher's cells
Formation of secondary lysosomes for storage of glucocerebrosides in Gaucher's cells
Increase in plasma levels of glucocerebroside
Mechanical complications in enlarged spleen, liver, nodes, bones, and kidneys
Secondary hypersplenism and hematologic sequelae
Neuronal deposition of glycolipid in Type II syndrome

REFERENCES

1. **Brady, R. O., Kanfer, J. N., and Shapiro, D.,** Metabolism of glucocerebrosides: evidence of an enzymatic deficiency in Gaucher's disease, *Biochem. Biophys. Res. Commun.*, 18(2), 221, 1965.
2. **Beutler, E. and Kuhl, W.,** The diagnosis of the adult type of Gaucher's disease and its carrier state by demonstration of deficiency of B-glucosidase activity in peripheral blood leukocytes, *J. Lab. Clin. Med.*, 76, 747, 1970.
3. **Beutler, E. and Kuhl, W.,** Detection of the defect of Gaucher's disease and its carrier state in peripheral blood leukocytes, *Lancet*, 1, 612, 1970.
4. **Kampine, J. P., Brady, R. O., Kanfer, J. N., Feld, M., and Shapiro, D.,** Diagnosis of Gaucher's disease and Niemann-Pick disease with small samples of venous blood, *Science*, 155, 86, 1967.
5. **Snyder, R. A. and Brady, R. O.,** The use of white cells as a source of diagnostic material for lipid storage disease, *Clin. Chim. Acta*, 25, 331, 1969.
6. **Beutler, E., Kuhl, W., Matsumoto, F., and Pangalis, G.,** Acid hydrolases in leukocytes and platelets of normal subjects and in patients with Gaucher's and Fabry's disease, *J. Exp. Med.*, 143, 975, 1976.
7. **Brady, R. O.,** Heritable catabolic and anabolic disorders of lipid metabolism, *Metabolism*, 26, 329, 1977.
8. **Brady, R. O., Kanfer, J. N., Bradley, R. M., and Shapiro, D.,** Demonstration of a deficiency of glucocerebroside-cleaving enzyme in Gaucher's disease, *J. Clin. Invest.*, 45, (7), 1112, 1966.

9. **Fredrickson, D. S. and Sloan, H. R.,** *Glucosyl-Ceramide Lipidoses in the Metabolic Basis of Inherited Disease,* 3rd ed., Stanbury, J. B., Wyngaarden, J. B., and Fredrickson, D. S., Eds., McGraw-Hill, New York, 1972, 730.
10. **Suomi, W. D. and Agranoff, B. W.,** Lipids in the spleen in Gaucher's disease, *J. Lipid Res.,* 6, 211, 1965.
11. **Kennaway, N. G. and Woolf, L. I.,** Splenic lipids in Gaucher's disease, *J. Lipid Res.,* 9, 755, 1968.
12. **Maloney, A. F. J. and Cumings, J. N.,** A case of juvenile Gaucher's disease with intraneuromal lipid storage, *J. Neurol. Neurosurg. Psychiatry,* 23, 207, 1960.
13. **Makita, A., Suzuki, C., Yosizana, Z., and Konno, T.,** Glycolipids isolated from the spleen in Gaucher's disease, *Tohoku J. Exp. Med.,* 88, 277, 1966.
14. **Philippart, M., Rosenstain, B. and Menkes, J. H.,** Isolation and characterization of the main splenic glycolipids in the normal organ and in Gaucher's disease: Evidence for the site of metabolic block, *J. Neuropathol. Exp. Neurol.,* 24, 290, 1965.
15. **Philippart, M. and Menkes, J.,** Isolation and characterization of the main splenic glycolipids in Gaucher's disease: evidence for the site of metabolic block, *Biochem. Biophys. Res. Commun.,* 6, 551, 1964.
16. **Kennaway, N. G. and Woolf, L. I.,** Splenic lipids in Gaucher's disease, *J. Lipid Res.,* 9, 755, 1968.
17. **Parke, D. V.,** The occurrence of lactose in the spleen cerebrosides of Gaucher's disease, *Clin. Sci.,* 22, 119, 1962.
18. **Banker, B. Q., Miller, J. Q., and Crocker, A. C.,** *The Cerebral Pathology of Infantile Gaucher's Disease in Cerebral Sphingolipidoses,* Aronson, S. M. and Volk, B. W., Eds., Academic Press, New York, 1962, 73.
19. **Hillborg, P. O. and Svennerholm, L.,** Blood level of cerebrosides in Gaucher's disease, *Acta Paediatr.,* 49, 707, 1960.
20. **Tuchman, L. R., Suna, H., and Carr, J. J.,** Elevation of serum acid phosphatase in Gaucher's disease, *J. M. Sinai Hosp., N.Y.,* 23, 227, 1956.
21. **Mercer, D. W., Peters, P. S., Glew, R. H., Lee, R. E., and Wenger, D. M.,** Acid phosphatase isoenzymes in Gaucher's disease, *Clin. Chim. Acta,* 23(4), 631, 1977.
22. **Dawson, G. and Oh, J. Y.,** Blood glucosylceramide levels in Gaucher's disease with distribution amongst lipoprotein fraction, *Clin. Chim. Acta,* 75, 149, 1977.
23. **Gilbert, H. S. and Weinreb, N.,** Increased circulating levels of Transcobalamin II in Gaucher's disease, *N. Engl. J. Med.,* 295, 1096, 1976.
24. **Lieberman, J. and Beutler, E.,** Elevation of serum angiotensin-converting enzyme in Gaucher's disease, *N. Engl. J. Med.,* 294, 1442, 1976.
25. **Klibansky, C., Ossimi, Z., Matoth, Y., Pinkhas, J., and DeVries, A.,** Accumulation of lactosyl ceramide in leukocytes of patients with adult Gaucher's disease, *Clin. Chim. Acta,* 72, 141, 1976.
26. **Frederickson, D. S.,** *Sphingomyelin lipidosis: Niemann-Pick Disease in the Metabolic Basis of Inherited Disease,* 2nd Ed., Stanbury, J. B., Wyngaarden, J. B., Frederickson, D. S., Eds., McGraw-Hill, New York, 1966, 586.
27. **Hutberg, B., Ockerman, P., and Ericksson, O.,** Urinary amino acids in storage disorders: mucopolysaccharidosis, Gaucher's disease and metachromatic lipodystrophy, *Metabolism,* 18, 713, 1969.
28. **Ockerman, P. A. and Kohlin, P.,** Acid hydrolases in plasma in Gaucher's disease, *Clin. Chem.,* 15, 61, 1969.
29. **Weinreb, J.,** Serum and splenic lysozyme in Gaucher's disease, *Clin. Res.,* 24, 295A, 1976.
30. **Silverstein, E. and Friedlan, J.,** Elevated serum and spleen angiotensin-converting enzyme (ACE) and serum lysozyme (L) in chronic Gaucher's disease, *Clin. Res.,* 24, 478A, 1976.
31. **Kampine, J. P., Brady, R. O., Kanfer, J. N., Feld, M., and Shapiro, D.,** Diagnosis of Gaucher's disease and Niemann-Pick disease with small samples of venous blood, *Science,* 155, 86, 1967.
32. **Brady, R. O., Johnson, W. C., Uhlendorf, W. B.,** Identification of heterozygous carriers of lipid storage diseases, *Am. J. Med.,* 51, 423, 1971.
33. **Ho, M. W., Seck, J., Schmidt, D., Veath, M. L., Johnson, W., Brady, R. O., and O'Brien, J. S.,** Adult Gaucher's disease: kindred studies and demonstration of a deficiency in acid β-glucosidase in cultured fibroblasts, *Am. J. Hum. Genet.,* 24, 37, 1972.
34. **Schneider, E. L., Ellis, W. C., Brady, R. O., McCullock, J. R., and Epstein, C. J.,** Infantile (type II) Gaucher's disease: in utero diagnosis and fetal pathology, *J. Pediatr.,* 81, 1134, 1972.
35. **Schlaugenhaufer, F.,** Uber meist familiar vorkommente, histologisch characteristische splenomegalien (typus Gaucher), *Arch. Pathol. Anat.,* 187, 125, 1907.
36. **Block, M. and Jacobson, L. O.,** The histogenesis and diagnosis of the osseous type of Gaucher's disease, *Acta Hemat. (Basel),* 1, 165, 1948.
37. **Pittaluga, P. G. and Goyanes, J.,** Contribution a l'etude de la cellule de Gaucher, *Arch. Mal. Coeuf.,* 26, 65, 1933.

38. **Morrison, R. W. and Hack, H. M.,** Histochemical studies in Gaucher's disease, *Am. J. Pathol.*, 25, 497, 1949.
39. **Diezel, P. B.,** Histochemische, untersuchungen an primaren lipoidosen: Amaurotische Idiotie, Gargoylismus Niemann-Pick Krankheit, mit besonderer Berucksichtignung des zentrol-nerve system, *Arch. Pathol. Anat.*, 326, 89, 1954.
40. **Adachi, M., Wallace, G. J., Schneck, L., and Volk, B. W.,** Fine structures of central nervous system in early infantile Gaucher's disease, *Arch. Pathol. (Chicago)*, 83, 513, 1967.
41. **Lorber, M. and Nemes, J. L.,** Identification of ferritin within Gaucher's cells: an electron microscopic and immunofluorescent study, *Acta Haematol. (Basel)*, 37, 189, 1967.
42. **Lee, R. E.,** The fine structure of the cerebroside occurring in Gaucher's disease, *Proc. Natl. Acad. Sci. U.S.A.*, 61, 484, 1968.

FUNCTIONS OF PHAGOCYTIC LEUKOCYTES

Paul G. Quie and Elaine L. Mills

Introduction

The primary function of polymorphonuclear neutrophil leukocytes is phagocytosis and killing of invading microbes. Defective function of phagocytes is found to be associated with multiple clinical disorders, and there is now overwhelming evidence that adequate numbers of properly functioning, mature phagocytic cells are essential for host defense against microbial disease. Therefore, this review will discuss current knowledge of the function of the phagocytic system in antimicrobial defense, with major emphasis on polymorphonuclear neutrophils.

The principal tissue-bound phagocytic cells comprise the monocyte-macrophage system, while the polymorphonuclear neutrophils are the primary phagocytes of the peripheral circulation. The morphology of polymorphonuclear leukocytes is evidence of their unique function. The multilobed nucleus allows the cells to effectively crawl through tissue spaces, and the heterogenous array of cytoplasmic granules contribute to the cells' bactericidal function. Neutrophils are released from the bone marrow as mature cells with very few mitochondria. Their total life span is measured in hours: approximately 6 hr in the circulation and 24 to 48 hr in tissue. Once neutrophils leave the bloodstream, either randomly or in response to inflammatory stimulation, they do not return.[1] Mononuclear phagocytic cells are released from the bone marrow as immature cells. They mature into macrophages with unique morphology and function after they have become located in various organ systems.

The Inflammatory Response

Acute inflammation stimulates release of neutrophil leukocytes from marginated pools and bone marrow reserves and, therefore, inflammation is accompanied by prompt leukocytosis. Humoral factors released from peripheral phagocytic cells sustain increased production of neutrophils by the bone marrow, so that inflammation and infection are usually accompanied by persistent increase in the numbers of circulating neutrophils until the inflammatory stimulus is gone.[2] Monocytes are also found in areas of inflammation, but arrive after neutrophils. Monocytes are the primary cells involved in granuloma formation.[3] Methods for evaluating the quantity of circulating neutrophils and the capacity of phagocytic cells to respond during inflammation are listed in Table 1.

The physiologic mechanisms utilized by circulating phagocytic cells in response to inflammation and in host defense against infection are shown in Table 2. These leukocyte functions can be measured individually in vitro by acceptable laboratory methods, but they are, of course, highly interdependent in vivo as they accomplish the ultimate function of the phagocytic system, i.e., defense against microbial disease.

Adhesiveness

Polymorphonuclear leukocytes normally circulate with erythrocytes at the periphery of the bloodstream, and are in a steady state of margination and circulation. The cells leave the circulation in random fashion, and the majority of their life span is spent in tissue spaces. Circulating neutrophils are exquisitely sensitive to inflammatory stimuli, and respond by adherence to the walls of capillaries and small venules and diapedes through spaces between endothelial cells. The capacity for adhesiveness appears to be contolled by prostaglandins, since small concentrations of aspirin and corticosteroids (prostaglandin synthetase inhibitors) decrease neutrophil adhesiveness. An assay of

Table 1
QUANTITATIVE ASSAYS OF NEUTROPHILS

Location	Method of Evaluation	Ref.
Circulating neutrophils	WBC and differential every other day for several weeks	2
Bone marrow reserve	Steroid test	4
Marginated pool	Epinephrine test	5

Table 2
MEASURABLE LEUKOCYTE FUNCTION ESSENTIAL FOR HOST DEFENSE AGAINST INVADING MICROBES

Function	Ref.
Adhesiveness	6
Locomotion	7
Chemotaxis	7
Phagocytosis	8
Oxidative metabolism	9
Microbial killing	10

Table 3
PHARMACOLOGIC AGENTS AND CLINICAL CONDITIONS THAT INFLUENCE NEUTROPHIL ADHESIVENESS

Increased adhesiveness	Decreased adhesiveness
Rheumatoid arthritis	Dysgammaglobulinemia
Lupus erythematosis	Corticosteroids
Acute inflammation	Indomethacin
Acute infection	Aspirin
Myocardial infarction	Ethanol
	Epinephrine

granulocyte adhesiveness has been developed by MacGregor et al., which allows quantitation of the cells with capacity for adherence to nylon wool.[6] This assay has been utilized in clinical studies, and abnormalities of neutrophil adhesiveness have been found in numerous clinical conditions. In addition, several pharmacologic agents have been shown to influence adhesiveness.[6] Table 3 lists these conditions.

Chemotaxis

Small molecular weight factors released during the inflammatory reaction attract polymorphonuclear neutrophils toward the highest concentration of these factors. The chemotactic attractants termed "cytotaxins" are derived from a variety of sources and are listed in Table 4. Excellent reviews of chemotactic attractants are found in a recent monograph and a review.[7,11]

Table 4
CYTOTAXINS FOR HUMAN POLYMORPHONUCLEAR LEUKOCYTES

Activated complement components C_3 fragment, C_5 fragment, and $C_{\overline{567}}$
Bacterial peptides
Tissue factors
Neutrophil products
Synthetic peptides
Lymphocyte products
Bradykinin

Table 5
CHEMOTAXIS ASSAY METHODS

Response to chemoattractants in Boyden chambers[12]
Distance of migration "leading front"[13]
Ratio of migrating versus nonmigrating cells[12]
Migration of radiolabeled cells[14]
Distance of migration under agarose[15]

The standard method for measuring neutrophil and monocyte chemotaxis is an assay which measures the capacity of neutrophils or monocytes to migrate into micropore filters in response to chemotactically active factors. After incubation for periods ranging from 30 min to 3 hr, either the distance migrated by a "leading front" of phagocytic cells is measured, or the cells that have migrated to the bottom of the filter are counted. The capacity of cells for random or spontaneous migration can also be observed by incubating leukocytes in chemotactic chambers with buffer instead of chemotactically active factors. Precise evaluation of chemotaxis can be obtained by radiolabeling neutrophils, and measuring the amount of radioactive activity that reaches a second filter in the chemotaxis chambers.

Random migration, chemokinesis, and chemotaxis may also be measured by observing distance of migration under agarose. This method measures the capacity of neutrophils (or monocytes) to migrate spontaneously or, in response to chemotactic factors, through the interphase between agarose and a plastic surface. Methods currently employed for measuring chemotaxis are listed in Table 5.

It is the gradient of attractant factors that brings about directed locomotion of phagocytic cells toward the center of an inflammatory process. The interaction of cytotaxins with the leukocyte membrane stimulates a cellular response which results in cytoplasmic contraction and relaxation in sequential regions of neutrophils or monocytes. There is also a shift in calcium concentration and in surface charge in sequential segments of the cell, as it migrates in response to a concentration gradient of cytotaxin. A recent symposium report in the *American Journal of Pathology* provides an excellent review of chemotaxis in health and disease.[16-19]

Recognition and Engulfment

Phagocytosis occurs when microbes or other particles are recognized as "non-self", and there is attachment of the particle to the phagocytic membrane. This usually requires alteration of the microbial surace so that it is appetizing for the phagocyte. This process is termed opsonization. Opsonization influences the surface of microbes by neutralizing antiphagocytic factors. In addition, the opsonin serves as a ligand so that

Table 6
PHAGOCYTOSIS ASSAY METHODS

Phagocytic index[2]
Uptake of radiolabeled bacteria[24]
Uptake of oil red O[8]
Bacterial killing[10]
Chemiluminescence[25]

attachment and stimulation of the phagocytic membrane occurs. Opsonins include heat-stable serum factors (primarily antibacterial antibodies), and heat-labile factors (primarily components of the complement system). Antibodies neutralize specific antiphagocytic factors on the surface of microbes such as streptococcal M protein, or polysaccharides of encapsulated organisms. Specific antibacterial antibodies are effective opsonins if they are present in sufficiently high concentrations. Under physiological conditions, however, activated complement C_3 is a primary opsonin. The opsonically active fragment of C_3 may be produced by classical pathway activation of C_3, or by alternative pathway activation of C_3. The activated C_3 fragment promotes efficient phagocytosis of many microbial species even in the absence of specific antibacterial antibodies.

Once the phagocytic cell membrane has been perturbated by recognition and attachment of a particle, there is stimulation of cytoplasmic contractile proteins. An actin-binding protein reacts with actin, and this protein is polymerized into microfilaments.[8] Contraction of the cytoplasmic microfilaments results in pseudopodia, which surround the particles, and there is engulfment of the attached particles. Once particles are interiorized within the phagocytic vacuoles, there is rapid degranulation, and cytoplasmic granular contents are contributed to the phagocytic vacuole.[20,21] Two excellent reviews of phagocytosis in health and disease have recently been published.[22,23] Methods for measuring capacity for phagocytosis are listed in Table 6.

The energy required for particle engulfment is provided primarily by glycolysis, although under certain experimental conditions in which glucose utilization is blocked, bacteria can be ingested normally.[26] These auxiliary energy sources mobilized during phagocytosis are not well understood. It is clear, however, that the process of engulfment is quite independent from stimulation of oxidative metabolism, since neutrophils of patients with defective oxidative metabolism engulf particles normally.[27]

Respiratory Metabolism

Perturbation of the neutrophil plasma membrane by particle attachment, or by a soluble activating agent, initiates a sudden surge in cellular oxidative metabolism.

The rapid sequence of metabolic events that follows stimulation and involves the uptake of large amounts of oxygen, is known as the "respiratory burst". The sequence begins with a 10- to 15-fold increase in oxygen consumption over resting levels.[28] Oxygen uptake is rapid and is not inhibited by cyanide, an agent which inhibits mitochondrial respiration.[29] During the respiratory burst there is also a tenfold rise in glucose metabolism via the hexose monophosphate shunt.[30] Since most of the glucose oxidized by this pathway can be reutilized, there is little change in the rate of glycolysis and only a slight increase in total glucose consumption. As stimulated neutrophils take up exogenous oxygen, large amounts of H_2O_2 are being released into the surrounding medium.[31,32] The amount of H_2O_2 which accumulates accounts for 30 to 70% of the oxygen consumed.

Concomitant with H_2O_2 generation, another product of oxygen reduction, the superoxide anion, is also released into the medium of respiring neutrophils.[33,34] Super-

Table 7
BACTERIAL PRODUCTS OF OXYGEN REDUCTION

Product	Symbol	Generation
Superoxide	OH	$OH + e^- \rightarrow O_2^-$
Hydrogen peroxide	$H_2O_2^-$	$O_2 + O_2^- \xrightarrow{2H+} {}^1O_2^-* + H_2O_2^-$
Hydroxyl radical	·OH	$O_2^- + H_2O_2 \xrightarrow{H+} \cdot OH + OH^- + O_2$
Singlet oxygen	$^1O_2*$	$O_2 + O_2^- \xrightarrow{2H+} {}^1O_2* + H_2O_2$
		$20Cl^- + H_2O_2^- \xrightarrow{MPO} {}^1O_2* + 2Cl^- + H_2O_2$

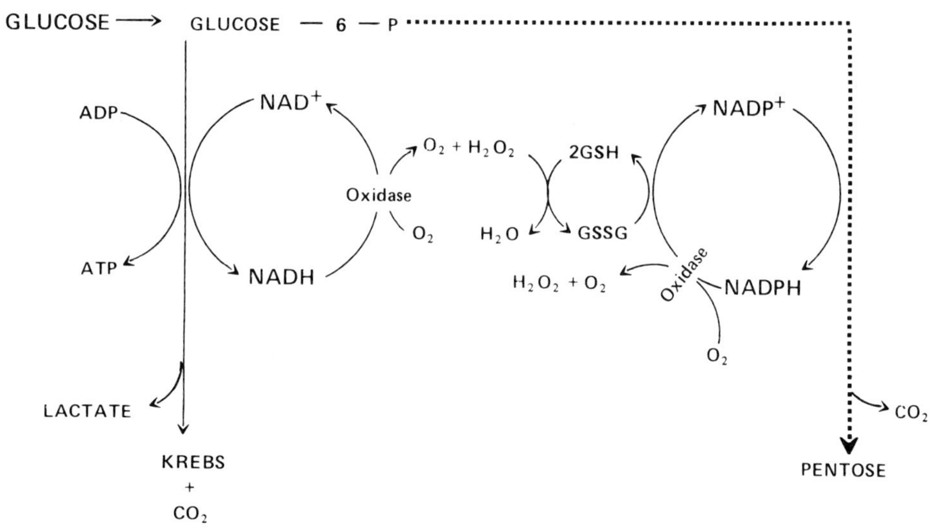

FIGURE 1. A simplified scheme of the oxidative metabolism associated with onset of phagocytosis. The respiratory burst is associated with increased glucose consumption, a tenfold augmentation in hexose monophosphate shunt activity (----) and production of large amounts of superoxide (O_2^-) and H_2O_2.

oxide, a highly reactive product of the one electron reduction of oxygen, has been reported to account for as much as 70% of the oxygen consumed during the respiratory burst.[35] The recent observation that 40 to 60% of the H_2O_2 produced in stimulated neutrophils is derived from superoxide, would account for the conversion of oxygen to large amounts of both H_2O_2 and superoxide.[36] There is recent evidence that stimulated neutrophils generate yet another radical of oxygen reduction, the hydroxyl radical.[37] While the hydroxyl radical has not been directly quantitated, indirect measurements indicate that it is present in these cells and could be accounted for by a reaction between superoxide and hydrogen peroxide (Table 7).

Perturbation of the neutrophil plasma membrane by an appropriate stimulus is thought to activate an enzyme that, in turn, initiates the respiratory burst. The initiating enzyme responsible for oxygen consumption is a cyanide-insensitive oxidase which has yet to be identified. The two most likely candidates are the pyridine nucleotide oxidases, nicotinamide adenine dinucleotide (NADH) oxidase, and nicotinamide adenine dinucleotide phosphate (NADPH) oxidase, which are known to exist in neutrophils (Figure 1). The NADH oxidase, an enzyme associated with the neutrophil plasma membrane,[38] and NADPH oxidase, an enzyme associated with the azurophil gran-

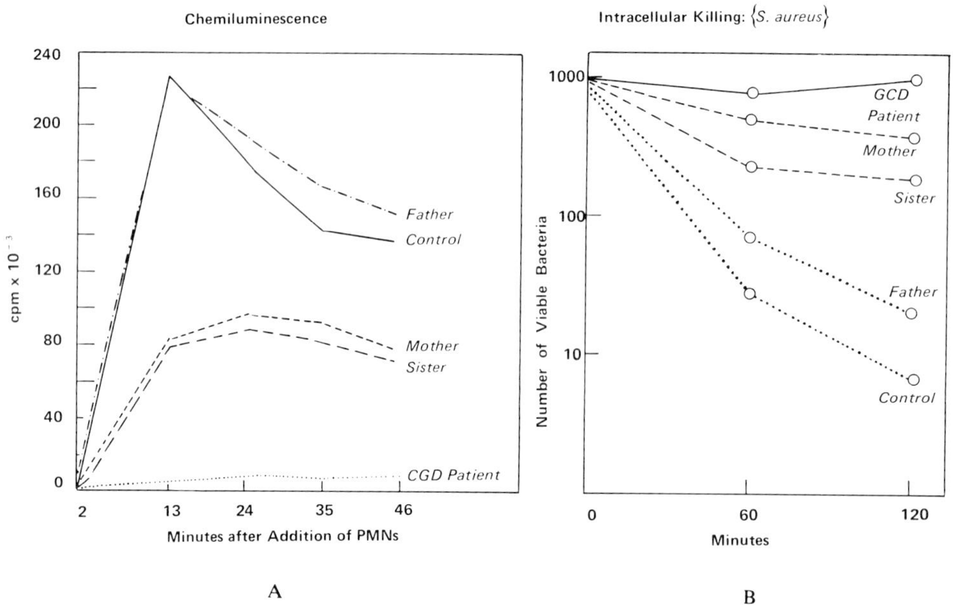

FIGURE 2. Chronic granulomatous disease. (A) The chemiluminescence response of neutrophils from a patient with chronic granulomatous disease and members of his family. GGD = chronic granulomatous disease proband. Mother and sister = chronic granulomatous disease carriers, (B) Intracellular killing of *S. aureus* comparing neutrophils of a patient with chronic granulomatous disease and members of his family. CGD = chronic granulomatous disease proband. Mother and sister = chronic granulomatous disease carriers.

ules,[39] are both cyanide insensitive. To explain the concomitant increase in oxygen uptake and activation of the hexose monophosphate (HMP) shunt during membrane stimulation, two metabolic sequences have been proposed.

In the sequence initiated by NADH oxidase, the enzyme consumes oxygen, using NADH as the preferred reducing agent. The enzyme transfers electrons to oxygen to form superoxide.[34] However, since activation of the HMP shunt is NADPH specific, a proposal that NADH is the initiating oxidase would not be valid unless a pathway to transfer electrons between the two pyridine nucleotides could be devised. The most likely pathway is a pair of reactions in which glutathione is the substrate. One of these reactions involves generation of H_2O_2 by NADH oxidase, and rapid removal of H_2O_2 by reduced glutathione to form oxidized glutathione. This is followed by conversion of oxidized glutathione back to reduced glutathione by glutathione reductase, an NADPH-requiring enzyme. The reactions are

$$2GSH + H_2O_2 \rightarrow GSSG + 2H_2O$$

$$GSSG + 2NADPH \rightarrow 2GSH + 2NADP$$

The overall reaction is the removal of a molecule of H_2O_2 by two molecules of NADPH. Activation of the hexose monophosphate shunt serves to regenerate NADPH consumed in the reduction of H_2O_2. There is experimental evidence indicating that the glutathione cycle could account, at least in part, for the stimulation of the hexose monophosphate shunt in respiring neutrophils.

The second proposed mechanism is that stimulation of respiration begins with activation of NADPH oxidase.[40] This activation is said to be caused by the conversion of

Table 8
NONPARTICULATE ACTIVATION OF NEUTROPHIL RESPIRATION

Phospholipase C
Antineutrophil antibodies
Concanavalin A
Detergents (deoxycholate, fatty acids)
Kallikrein
C_{5a} fragment
Phorbol myristate acetate
Ionophore (A23187)
Cytochalasin E
Fluoride

NADPH oxidase from a form with a relatively low affinity for NADPH, to a form with a much higher affinity for the nucleotide. At concentrations of NADPH known to be present in neutrophils, this conversion would result in increased oxidase activity and stimulation of the respiratory burst. Despite intensive research in this area, it is impossible from our present knowledge to decide which of these two enzyme systems accounts for stimulation of granulocyte oxidative metabolism.

The respiratory burst associated with phagocytosis can be initiated by a variety of particles. Microorganisms such as bacteria, fungi, and mycoplasma, or microbial products such as zymosan, must all be opsonized by incubation with plasma or serum before respiratory stimulation occurs. Polystyrene latex particles, on the other hand, do not require prior opsonization to stimulate neutrophil respiration. While it appears that all particulate stimuli will invariably induce phagocytosis, phagocytosis may occur without stimulating respiration. This is evident from the finding that neutrophils ingest certain organisms in the absence of any measurable increase of oxidative metabolism.[41]

Studies with a number of soluble compounds that do not form particulate substances would indicate that phagocytosis and activation of oxidative metabolism are independent processes. Such diverse agents as phospholipase C,[42] antinuclear antibodies,[43] concanavalin A,[44] and certain detergents, including deoxycholate[45] and fatty acids,[46] all initiate oxygen uptake and HMP shunt activity. A number of other soluble activating agents have been demonstrated as effective respiratory stimulants: kallikrein, C_{5a} (a complement fragment), phorbol myristate acetate (an ester of a polycyclic alcohol derived from croton oil), cytochalasin E, calcium ionophores, and fluoride ions all stimulate respiration in the absence of phagocytosis[47] (Table 8).

Microbicidal Mechanisms

Studies of inherited leukocyte abnormalities have shown that oxidative processes play a major role in the armamentarium of neutrophils against both bacteria and fungi:[48,49] (Table 9). Patients with chronic granulomatous disease (CGD) have severe infections produced by these microbes, their leukocytes fail to show phagocytosis-stimulated oxidative metabolism, and they are markedly defective in microbicidal activity for both bacteria and fungi. Their leukocytes also fail to generate products of oxygen reduction such as H_2O_2 and superoxide.[50] Patients with leukocytes deficient in the enzyme myeloperoxidase (MPO) also have more frequent infections, their neutrophils are defective in generation of certain products of oxygen reduction, and they have delayed bactericidal and fungicidal activity.[51]

Patients with Chediak-Higashi syndrome (CHS) have frequent and severe pyogenic infections, which appear to result from the combined effects of neutropenia, defective chemotaxis, and bactericidal activity. Their peripheral blood leukocytes contain characteristic large cytoplasmic inclusions that have been shown to be abnormal azurophilic

Table 9
CONGENITAL CONDITIONS ASSOCIATED WITH NEUTROPHIL BACTERICIDAL DEFECTS

Chronic granulomatous disease
Myeloperoxidase deficiency
Chediak-Higashi syndrome
Glucose-6-phosphate dehydrogenase deficiency
Leukocyte alkaline phosphatase deficiency
Down's syndrome (subgroup)

granules containing MPO and acid phosphatase.[52] Degranulation is defective in these cells because of delayed and incomplete fusion of the giant granules with phagocytic vesicles.[53] After 60-min incubation of these cells with *Staphylococcus aureus*, many phagocytic vesicles still contain no peroxidase. Therefore, it is not surprising that CHS leukocytes kill *S. aureus*, streptococci, and pneumococci poorly after 2 hr of incubation and require another 2 hr of incubation for normal killing to occur. There are several lines of evidence to suggest that delayed microbial killing in CHS neutrophils may result from defective granulation. The delay observed in degranulation parallels the delay in bacterial killing. In phagocytic vacuoles in which delayed release of granule enzymes can be demonstrated, there is concomitant morphological evidence of bacterial destruction, where as vesicles that have not fused with cytoplasmic granules contain intact bacteria. Since the large granules contain virtually all of the myeloperoxidase in the neutrophil, the phagocyte is essentially myeloperoxidase deficient during the first hour of phagocytosis. Thus, a major bactericidal system, MPO-halide-H_2O_2, which will be discussed later, is all but nonfunctional.

Complete absence of glucose-6-phosphate dehydrogenase (G-6-PD) activity has also been associated with severe infections.[54] While neutrophil microbial ingestion appears to be normal, there is little stimulation of HMP shunt activity and less than 25% normal H_2O_2 production during phagocytosis. There is evidence that patients with absent G-6-PD have normal NADH and NADPH oxidase activity, but decreased supply of the cellular substrates NADH and NADPH. This would explain the markedly decreased HMP shunt activity and H_2O_2 production, and the observed decreased microbicidal activity for *Staphylococcus aureus*, *Escherichia coli*, and Serratia.

A clinical syndrome that includes recurrent bacterial infections and a minimal bactericidal defect has been associated with a deficiency in neutrophil alkaline phosphatase.[55,56] The function of leukocyte alkaline phosphatase is unknown, and this evidence suggests that it may participate in microbicidal processes.

The bactericidal defect of CGD is found only with catalase-positive bacteria and fungi:[57] H_2O_2 generating organisms such as streptococci and *S. pneumoniae* are killed by these neutrophils at rates comparable to that of normal controls. Leukocytes that cannot take up oxygen normally to generate H_2O_2 may utilize the H_2O_2 supplied by the engulfed catalase-negative bacteria to activate the HMP shunt. The generated H_2O_2 could be utilized in the MPO-H_2O_2-halide microbicidal system to accomplish intracellular killing.

From the foregoing considerations of clinical syndromes, it is apparent that oxidative processes play a major role in intracellular microbicidal activity. Recent investigations of leukocyte oxidative metabolism has made it apparent that phagocytizing cells generate several products of oxygen reduction. Hydrogen peroxide and superoxide have been measured directly, while the hydroxyl radical has been quantitated by an indirect assay.[46] There is indirect but compelling evidence for the presence of singlet oxygen in the phagocytic vacuole.[58,59]

The superoxide anion, a free radical formed by the univalent reduction of molecular oxygen, is a powerful oxidation-reduction agent. In the presence of an acid pH, it is exceedingly unstable and disproportionates spontaneously to generate the electronically excited species, singlet oxygen.[60] The highly reactive properties of superoxide, its abundant supply in stimulated phagocytes, and the striking temporal relationship between its production and oxygen consumption, as well as the fact that patients with intracellular killing defects (CGD) generate virtually no superoxide, are all suggestive evidence that this radical, or one of its derivatives, is involved in microbial killing.[61,62] The contribution of superoxide to bacterial killing has been studied in a number of different in vitro and in vivo systems.[63] While these studies support the participation of superoxide in the bactericidal event, the evidence suggests that superoxide itself has little bactericidal activity. Similarly, hydrogen peroxide alone has limited bactericidal activity, but hydrogen peroxide acting in concert with MPO and a halide, form a potent antimicrobial system.[48] The hydroxyl radical, a potentially bactericidal agent, has been demonstrated in phagocytizing neutrophils, and could be generated in the phagocytic vacuole by a reaction between superoxide and hydrogen peroxide.[37] In addition to the hydroxyl radical, this reaction is known to generate still another product of oxygen reduction, singlet oxygen.

Evidence for the generation of singlet oxygen in phagocytizing neutrophils first came with the observation that these cells produce chemiluminescence.[38] Allen postulated that singlet oxygen ($^1O_2^*$) is generated in these cells by two potential methods: the nonenzymatic disproportionation of superoxide, and the reaction of MPO-H_2O_2-halide system of the phagocyte (Table 7). The generated $^1O_2^*$, a potent electrophilic reactant, could attack electron-dense regions of the target microorganisms such as unsaturated lipids, nucleic acids, and amino acid residues. Oxidation of these substances by singlet oxygen could generate electronically excited carbonyl groups, which relax by means of photon emission. The dissipation of excess energy from a biochemical reaction in the form of light emission, rather than heat, is termed chemiluminescence. This light, measurable with a beta-spectrophotometer, forms the basis of the chemiluminescence assay.

Studies of the spectral analysis of phagocytizing granulocytes have shown light emission over a broad region of the visible light spectrum.[59,64] These findings are consistent with oxidation of a variety of particle constituents producing a heterogenous group of electronically excited species. These species could relax to ground state with light emission in multiple regions of the visible spectrum.

Both in vivo and in vitro evidence suggests that chemiluminescence and microbial killing are related. The granulocytes of CGD patients have a severe intracellular killing defect and produce virtually no chemiluminescence.[65] Leukocytes from MPO-deficient patients have a characteristic lag phase in killing bacteria and a parallel lag in chemiluminescence.[66] Agents which specifically quench singlet oxygen, such as 2,5-dimethyl furan and bilirubin, have been reported to significantly inhibit normal killing of *Staphylococcus aureus.*[67]

There is some evidence that bacteria possess virulence factors which inhibit neutrophil oxidative metabolism. Certain pigmented strains of *Sarcina lutea* are much more resistant to intracellular killing that are nonpigmented mutant strains.[68] The pigmented strains contain carotenoids that are thought to be singlet oxygen quenchers. Similarly, catalase may provide protection for *S. aureus* against neutrophil bactericidal activity.[69] A high-catalase producing staphylococcal strain was found to be ingested normally, but it killed relatively poorly, and iodinated less well than a low-catalase strain. Addition of exogenous catalase decreased the ability of neutrophils to kill and to iodinate

Table 10
NONOXYGEN BACTERICIDAL FACTORS OF GRANULOCYTES

Lysozyme
Lactoferrin
Acid pH
Cationic proteins
Myeloperoxidase

Table 11
ACQUIRED NEUTROPHIL BACTERICIDAL DEFECTS

Severe bacterial infections
Severe thermal injuries
Malignancy
Certain viral infections
Protein-calorie malnutrition
Radiation (in acute leukemia)

the low-catalase strain. Catalase may be protective by destroying hydrogen peroxide, but the mechanism of the inhibition is unknown.

Human neutrophils also possess important nonoxygen-dependent microbicidal systems (Table 10). These systems appear to be responsible for the intracellular killing of *Pseudomonas aeruginosa* and certain Candida species, and are independent of both oxygen and MPO. Even though these organisms are catalase positive, they are killed at a normal rate within leukocytes of CGD patients, or within leukocytes incubated under anaerobic conditions.[70] Several granule-derived proteins, which are released into phagocytic vacuoles during phagocytosis, are responsible for this nonoxygen-dependent cidal activity. Lysozyme[71] is such a protein with limited microbicidal activity, and lactoferrin, a protein that is bacteristatic rather than bactericidal,[72] may function by binding iron, an essential substrate for certain microorganisms. A group of highly cationic (basic) proteins exhibit antibacterial activity with specificity for such organisms as *Streptococcus faecalis*, *S. aureus*, and *Escherichia coli*.[73,74]

Clinical conditions associated with transient defects in intracellular killing are outlined in Table 11.

Patients with severe, overwhelming infections have a high percentage of circulating cells that have morphologic changes, i.e., Döhle bodies, cytoplasmic vacuoles, and toxic granules. There is a direct relationship between the percentage of cells with these changes and depressed microbial killing.[75,76] Patients with severe burns have similar evidence of neutrophil dysfunction. In patients with malignancy there may be transient abnormality of function, but there does not appear to be a correlation between dysfunction and clinical manifestations. Radiation may have a subtle adverse effect on development of neutrophil function, since there is diminished microbicidal capacity of neutrophils from patients receiving spinal column irradiation during therapy of acute leukemia.[77] Patients with protein-calorie malnutrition have primarily cell-mediated immune deficiency, but depressed intracellular bacterial killing by neutrophils has also been described in patients with severe protein-calorie malnutrition.[78]

Summary

The phagocytic system is essential for host defense against invasion by microorganisms and recovery from microbial disease. Since phagocytosis does not occur in the absence of inflammation, phagocytic function is considered in the context of the inflammatory process. Invading microbes, or any material the body recognizes as "non-self", can initiate the complex interreactions between phagocytic cells and various humoral mediators to produce the inflammatory response. Invading microbes, or tissue responding to foreign material, release freely diffusible active factors of small molecular weight into the center of an inflammatory process. Circulating neutrophils and monocytes are attracted to these sites by these leukoattractants (chemotactic factors) and rapidly accumulate in areas of inflammation in massive numbers.

Phagocytosis is a complex process that involves attachment of particles to the phagocytic plasma membrane, engulfment of the particle by armlike cellular projections, which surround the particle to form a phagocytic vacuole, and killing and digestion of the engulfed material. Attachment and ingestion are greatly facilitated by a highly complex system of humoral factors termed opsonins. The opsonic factors, derived principally from complement and immunoglobulin, assist phagocytosis by neutralizing antiphagocytic factors on the microbial surface and increasing the affinity of microbes for phagocytic cells to permit binding of the organisms to phagocytic plasma membranes. A normal opsonization system is necessary for efficient phagocytosis of most microorganisms. Oxidative processes comprise the major intracellular killing mechanisms of the neutrophil. Several highly reactive products of oxidative metabolism are known to be generated in phagocytizing leukocytes, and they may act singly or in concert to produce their cidal effect. The final event of the phagocytic process, digestion of the foreign material, is accomplished by activated hydrolytic enzymes derived from the cytoplasmic granules.

Patients with disorders of the phagocytic system not only have greatly increased susceptibility to infection, but also have clinically more severe microbial disease. Fortunately, most patients do not have a complete absence of normal phagocytic microbicidal activity. While they frequently respond poorly to antimicrobial therapy and usually require surgical drainage of infected lesions, complete recovery is the rule with optimal medical management. On the other hand, patients who have virtually no circulating phagocytic cells usually do not recover from sepsis.

Recent appreciation of the central role the phagocytic system exerts on host defense has lead to the utilization of clinical modalities that attempt to improve or restore phagocytic function. Such attempts are the expanded use of leukocyte transfusions in granulocytopenic patients and the aggressive use of nutritional supplementation in malnourished patients.

REFERENCES

1. **Williams, W. J., Beutler, E., and Erslev, A. J.,** *Hematology*, 1st ed., McGraw-Hill, New York, 1972.
2. **Wintrobe, M. M.,** *Clinical Hematology*, 5th ed., Lea & Febiger, Philadelphia, 1974.
3. **van Furth, R.,** Origin and kinetics of monocytes and macrophages, *Semin. Hematol.*, 7, 125, 1970.
4. **Dale, D. C., Fauci, A. S., Guerry, D., and Wolff, S. M.,** Comparison of agents producing a neutrophilic leukocytosis in man, *J. Clin. Invest.*, 56, 808, 1975.
5. **Storti, E., Lusvarghi, E., Grignaffini, G. F., and Sgandurra, A.,** Biological and clinical significance of the Adrenaline® test in haematology, *Hematologia*, 1, 27, 1967.
6. **MacGregor, R. R., Spagmolo, P. J., and Lentneh, A. Z.,** Inhibition of granulocyte adherence by ethanol, prednisone, and aspirin measured with an assay system, *N. Engl. J. Med.*, 291, 642, 1974.
7. **Wilkinson, P. C.,** *Chemotaxis and Inflammation*, 1st ed., Churchill Livingstone, Edingburgh, 1974.
8. **Stossel, T. P., Mason, R. J., Hartwig, J., and Vangham, M.,** Quantitative studies of phagocytosis by polymorphonuclear leukocytes: use of emulsions to measure the initial rate of phagocytosis, *J. Clin. Invest.*, 51, 615, 1972.

9. **Klebanoff, S. J.,** Antimicrobial mechanisms in neutrophilic polymorphonuclear leukocytes, *Semin. Hematol.*, 12, 117, 1975.
10. **Quie, P. G., White, J. G., Holmes, B., and Good, R. A.,** In vitro bactericidal capacity of human polymorphonuclear leukocytes: diminished activity in chronic granulomatous disease of childhood, *J. Clin. Invest.*, 46, 668, 1967.
11. **Ward, P. A.,** Complement-derived inflammatory mediators, the C_5-cleaving enzymes in biological reactions, in *The Phagocytic Cell in Host Resistance,* Bellanti, J. A. and Dayton, D. H., Eds., Raven Press, New York, 1975, 117.
12. **Hill, H. R., Gerrard, J. M., Hogan, N. A., and Quie, P. G.,** Hyperactivity of neutrophil leukocyte response during active bacterial infection, *J. Clin. Invest.*, 53, 996, 1974.
13. **Zigmond, S. J. and Hirsch, J. G.,** Effects of cytochalasin B on polymorphonuclear leukocyte locomotion, phagocytosis, and glycolysis, *Exp. Cell Res.*, 73, 383, 1972.
14. **Gallin, J. I., Clark, R. A., and Kimball, H. R.,** Granulocyte chemotaxis: an improved in vitro assay employing ^{51}Cr-labeled granulocytes, *J. Immunol.*, 111, 233, 1973.
15. **Nelson, R. D., Quie, P. G., and Simmons, R. D.,** Chemotaxis under agarose: a new and simple method for measuring chemotaxis and spontaneous migration of human polymorphonuclear leukocytes and monocytes, *J. Immunol.*, 115, 1650, 1975.
16. **Ward, P. A., Johnson, K. J., and Kreutzer, D. L.,** Regulatory dysfunction in leukotaxis, *Am. J. Pathol.*, 88, 701, 1977.
17. **Quie, P. G. and Cates, K. L.,** Clinical conditions associated with defective polymorphonuclear leukocyte chemotaxis, *Am. J. Pathol.*, 88, 711, 1977.
18. **Stossel, T. P.,** Phagocytosis: clinical disorders of recognition and ingestion, *Am. J. Pathol.*, 88, 741, 1977.
19. **Snyderman, R. and Pike, M. C.,** Macrophage migratory dysfunction in cancer: a mechanism for subversion of surveillance, *Am. J. Pathol.*, 88, 727, 1977.
20. **Cohn, Z. A. and Hirsch, J. G.,** The influence of phagocytosis on the intracellular distribution of granule-associated components of polymorphonuclear leukocytes, *J. Exp. Med.*, 112, 1015, 1960.
21. **Elsbach, P.,** Lipid metabolism by phagocytes, *Semin. Hematol.*, 9, 227, 1972.
22. **Bellanti, J. A. and Dayton, D. H., Eds.,** *The Phagocytic Cell in Host Resistance,* 1st ed., Raven Press, New York, 1975.
23. **Humbert, J. R., Miescher, P. A., and Jaffe, E. R., Eds.,** *Neutrophil Physiology and Pathology,* 1st ed., Grune & Stratton, New York, 1975.
24. **Verhoef, J., Peterson, P. K., Kim, Y., Sabath, L. D., and Quie, P. G.,** Opsonic requirements for staphylococcal phagocytosis. Heterogeneity among strains, *Immunology,* 33, 191, 1977.
25. **Grebner, J. V., Mills, E. L., Gray, B. H., and Quie, P. G.,** Comparison of phagocytic and chemiluminescence response of human polymorphonuclear leukocytes, *J. Lab. Clin. Med.*, 89, 153, 1977.
26. **Stossel, T. P.,** Phagocytosis (second of three parts), *N. Engl. J. Med.*, 290, 774, 1974.
27. **Holmes, B., Page, A. R., and Good, R. A.,** Studies of the metabolic activity of leukocytes from patients with a genetic abnormality of phagocyte function, *J. Clin. Invest.*, 46, 1422, 1967.
28. **Weening, R. S., Roos, D., and Loos, J. A.,** Oxygen consumption of phagocytizing cells in human leukocyte and granulocyte preparations: a comparative study, *J. Lab. Clin. Med.*, 83, 570, 1974.
29. **Sbarra, A. J. and Karnovsky, M. L.,** The biological basis of phagocytosis. I. Metabolic changes during the ingestion of particles by polymorphonuclear leukocytes, *J. Biol. Chem.*, 234, 1355, 1959.
30. **Evans, W. H. and Karnovsky, M. L.,** The biochemical basis of phagocytosis. IV. Some aspects of carbohydrate metabolism during phagocytosis., *Biochemistry,* 1, 159, 1962.
31. **Homan-Müller, J. W. T., Weening, R. S., and Roos, D.,** Production of hydrogen peroxide by phagocytizing human granulocytes, *J. Lab. Clin. Med.*, 85, 198, 1975.
32. **Root, R. K., Metcalf, J., Oshino, N., and Chance, B.,** H_2O_2 release from human granulocytes during phagocytosis. I. Documentation, quantitation, and some regulating factors, *J. Clin. Invest.*, 55, 945, 1975.
33. **Curnutte, J. T. and Babior, B. M.,** Biological defense mechanisms. The effects of bacteria and serum on superoxide production by granulocytes, *J. Clin. Invest.*, 53, 1662, 1974.
34. **Johnston, R. B., Keele, B. B., Misra, H. P., Lehmeyer, J. E., Webb, L. S., Baehner, R. L., and Rajagopalan, K. V.,** The role of superoxide anion generation in phagocytic bactericidal activity. Studies with normal and chronic granulomatous disease leukocytes, *J. Clin. Invest.*, 55, 1357, 1975.
35. **Goldstein, I. M., Roos, D., Kaplan, H. B., and Weissmann, G.,** Complement and immunoglobulins stimulate superoxide production by human leukocytes independently of phagocytosis, *J. Clin. Invest.*, 56, 1155, 1975.
36. **Root, R. K. and Metcalf, J.,** Relationship between O_2^- and H_2O_2 production and utilization by human granulocytes, *Clin. Res.*, 23, 311A, 1975.
37. **Tauber, A. I. and Babior, B. M.,** Evidence for hydroxyl radical production by human neutrophils, *J. Clin. Invest.*, 60, 374, 1977.

38. **Briggs, R. T., Drath, D. B., Karnovsky, M. L., and Karnovsky, M. J.,** Localization of NADH oxidase on the surface of human polymorphonuclear leukocytes by a new cytochemical method, *J. Cell Biol.*, 67, 566, 1975.
39. **Rossi, F. and Zatti, M.,** Biochemical aspects of phagocytosis in polymorphonuclear leucocytes. NADH and NADPH oxidase by the granules of resting and phagocytizing cells, *Experientia*, 20, 21, 1964.
40. **Paul, B. B., Strauss, R. R., Jacobs, A. A., and Sbarra, A. J.,** Direct involvement of NADPH oxidase with the stimulated respiratory and hexose monophosphate shunt activities in phagocytizing leukocytes, *Exp. Cell Res.*, 73, 456, 1972.
41. **Miller, R. M., Garbus, J., and Hornick, R.,** Lack of enhanced oxygen consumption by polymorphonuclear leukocytes on phagocytosis of virulent *Salmonella typhi*, *Science*, 175, 1010, 1974.
42. **Patriarca, P., Cramer, R., Marussi, M., Moncalvo, S., and Rossi, F.,** Phospholipid splitting and metabolic stimulation in polymorphonuclear leukocytes, *J. Reticuloendothelial Soc.*, 10, 251, 1971.
43. **Rossi, F., Zatti, M., Patriarca, P., and Cramer, R.,** Effect of specific antibodies on the metabolism of guinea-pig polymorphonuclear leukocytes, *J. Reticuloendothelial Soc.*, 9, 67, 1971.
44. **Romeo, D., Zabucchi, G., and Rossi, F.,** Reversible metabolic stimulation of polymorphonuclear leukocytes and macrophages, *Nature London New Biol.*, 243, 111, 1973.
45. **Graham, R. C., Jr., Karnovsky, M. J., Shafer, A. W., Glass, E. A., and Karnovsky, M. L.,** Metabolic and morphological observations on the effect of surface-active agents on leukocytes, *J. Cell Biol.*, 32, 629, 1967.
46. **Kakinuma, K.,** Effects of fatty acids on the oxidative metabolism of leukocytes, *Biochim. Biophys. Acta*, 348, 76, 1974.
47. **Cheson, B. D., Curnutte, J. T., and Babior, B. M.,** The oxidative killing mechanisms of the neutrophil, in *Progress in Clinical Immunology*, Vol. 3, Schwartz, R. S., Ed., Grune & Stratton, New York, 1977, 8.
48. **Klebanoff, S. J.,** Antimicrobial mechanisms of neutrophil polymorphonuclear leukocytes, *Semin. Hematol.*, 12, 117, 1975.
49. **Karnovsky, M. L.,** Chronic granulomatous disease — pieces of a cellular and molecular puzzle, *Fed. Proc.*, 32, 1527, 1973.
50. **Babior, B. M., Kipnes, R. S., and Curnutte, J. T.,** Biological defense mechanisms. The production by leukocytes of superoxide, a potential bactericidal agent, *J. Clin. Invest.*, 52, 741, 1973.
51. **Klebanoff, S. J. and Hamon, C. B.,** Role of myeloperoxidase-mediated antimicrobial systems in intact leukocytes, *J. Reticuloendothelial Soc.*, 12, 170, 1972.
52. **Wolff, S. M., Dale, D. C., Clark, R. A., Root, R. K., and Kimball, H. R.,** The Chediak-Higashi syndrome: studies of host defense, *Ann. Intern. Med.*, 76, 293, 1972.
53. **Root, R. K., Rosenthal, A. S., and Balestra, D. J.,** Abnormal bactericidal, metabolic, and lysosomal functions of Chediak-Higashi syndrome leukocytes, *J. Clin. Invest.*, 51, 649, 1972.
54. **Baehner, R. L., Johnston, R. B., Jr., and Nathan, D. G.,** Comparative study of the metabolic and bactericidal characteristics of severely glucose-6-phosphate dehydrogenase-deficient polymorphonuclear leukocytes and leukocytes from children with chronic granulomatous disease, *J. Reticuloendothelial Soc.*, 12, 150, 1972.
55. **Strauss, R. G., Bove, K. E., Jones, J. F., Mauer, A. M., and Fulginiti, V. A.,** An anomaly of neutrophil morphology with impaired function, *N. Engl. J. Med.*, 290, 478, 1974.
56. **Repine, J. E., Clawson, C. C., and Brunning, R. D.,** Primary leucocyte alkaline phosphatase deficiency in an adult with repeated infections, *Br. J. Haematol.*, 34, 87, 1976.
57. **Kaplan, E. L., Laxdal, T., and Quie, P. G.,** Studies of polymorphonuclear leukocytes from patients with chronic granulomatous disease of childhood, *Pediatrics*, 41, 591, 1968.
58. **Allen, R. C., Stjernholm, R. L., and Steele, R. H.,** Evidence for the generation of an electronic excitation state(s) in human polymorphonuculear leukocytes and its participation in bactericidal activity, *Biochem. Biophys. Res. Commun.*, 47, 679, 1972.
59. **Cheson, B. D., Christensen, R. L., Sperling, R., Kohler, B. E., and Babior, B. M.,** The origin of the chemiluminescence of phagocytizing granulocytes, *J. Clin. Invest.*, 58, 789, 1976.
60. **Stauff, J.,** Chemiluminescence of some reactions with molecular oxygen, *Photochem. Photobiol.*, 4, 1199, 1965.
61. **Weening, R. S., Wever, R., and Roos, D.,** Quantitative aspects of the production of superoxide radicals by phagocytizing human granulocytes, *J. Lab. Clin. Med.*, 85, 245, 1975.
62. **Curnutte, J. T. and Babior, B. M.,** Biological defense mechanisms: the effect of bacteria and serum on superoxide production by granulocytes, *J. Clin. Invest.*, 53, 1662, 1974.
63. **Johnston, R. B., Jr., Keele, B. B., Misra, H. P., Lehmeyer, J. E., Webb, L. S., Baehner, R. L., and Rajagopalan, K. V.,** The role of superoxide anion generaton in phagocytic bacterial activity. Studies with normal and chronic granulomatous disease leukocytes, *J. Clin. Invest.*, 55, 1357, 1975.

64. **Lint, T. F., Brendzel, A. M., and Anderson, B. R.,** Studies of the spectral characteristics of the chemiluminescent emissions from human polymorphonuclear leukocytes and isoated myeloperoxidase, *Fed. Proc. Abstr.*, 36, 1071, 1977.
65. **Stjernholm, R. L., Allen, R. C., Steele, R. H., Waring, W. W., and Harris, J. N.,** Impaired chemiluminescence during phagocytosis of opsonized bacteria, *Infect. Immun.*, 7, 313, 1973.
66. **Rosen, H. and Klebanoff, J. S.,** Chemiluminescence and superoxide production by myeloperoxidase deficient leukocytes, *J. Clin. Invest.*, 58, 60, 1976.
67. **Weiss, S. J., Bain, G., and LoBuglio, A. F.,** The role of singlet oxygen in the antibacterial mechanism of the human neutrophil., *Clin. Res. Abstr.*, 24, 579, 1976.
68. **Krinsky, N. I.,** Singlet excited oxygen as a mediator of the antibacterial action of leukocytes, *Science*, 180, 363, 1974.
69. **Mandell, G. L.,** Catalase, superoxide dismutase and virulence of *Staphylococcus aureus*, *J. Clin. Invest.*, 55, 561, 1975.
70. **Lehrer, R. I.,** Functional aspects of a second mechanism of candidacidal activity by human neutrophils, *J. Clin. Invest.*, 51, 2566, 1972.
71. **Salton, M. R. J.,** The properties of lysozyme and its action on microorganisms, *Bacteriol. Rev.*, 21, 82, 1957.
72. **Masson, P. L., Heremans, J. F., and Schonne, E.,** Lactoferrin, an iron-binding protein of neutrophilic leukocytes, *J. Exp. Med.*, 130, 643, 1969.
73. **Welsh, I. R. H. and Spitznagel, J. K.,** Distribution of lysosomal enzymes, cationic proteins, and bactericidal substances in subcellular fractions of polymorphonuclear leukocytes, *Infect. Immun.*, 4, 97, 1971.
74. **Odeberg, H. and Olsson, I.,** Antibacterial activity of cationic proteins from human granulocytes, *J. Clin. Invest.*, 56, 1118, 1975.
75. **McCall, C. E., Katayama, I., Cotran, R. S., and Finland, M.,** Lysosomal and ultrastructural changes in human "toxic" neutrophils during bacterial infection, *J. Exp. Med.*, 129, 267, 1969.
76. **Solberg, C. O. and Hellum, K. B.,** Neutrophil granulocyte function in bacterial infections, *Lancet*, 2, 727, 1972.
77. **Baehner, R. L., Neiburger, R. G., and Johnson, D. E.,** Bactericidal defect in blood of children with acute lymphoblastic leukemia, *N. Engl. J. Med.*, 289, 1209, 1973.
78. **Douglas, S. D. and Schopfer, K.,** Phagocyte function in protein-calorie malnutrition, *Clin. Exp. Immunol.*, 17, 121, 1974.

THE LEUKEMIAS

Thomas F. Necheles

The leukemias are a group of neoplastic diseases of the bone marrow, involving any one or more cell lines and characterized by morphologically recognizable disorders of proliferation and/or maturation. The leukemias are usually classified into "acute" and "chronic" forms; traditionally, this division has been based both on cell morphology and cell survival after onset of the disease. More recently, classifications based on survival have become meaningless, since the average survival of children with acute lymphoblastic leukemia (ALL) is longer than that of patients with chronic myelocytic leukemia (CML). Currently, classification of the leukemias is based almost exclusively on morphological criteria (Table 1), with occasional assistance from special histochemical stains (Table 2). In the past several years, ALL has been subdivided into a number of subgroups on the basis of immunological surface markers (Table 3). These subgroups are, in general, not recognizable on morphological grounds. Recognition of the various subgroups of ALL assumes importance in terms of prognosis and, eventually, in developing modified forms of therapy. CML has also been subdivided on the basis of the presence or absence of the Ph′ chromosome.

The etiology of the leukemias is still uncertain, although a number of factors such as radiation exposure, congenital chromosomal abnormalities, treatment with immunosuppressive agents, and immunological abnormalities have all been linked with an increased incidence of leukemia. There is considerable experimental evidence that at least some types of leukemia may be caused by viruses, but the evidence here is still controversial. In fact, we may be indulging in a considerable oversimplification in looking for *one* single etiological agent for the various types of leukemia.

The clinical manifestations of the leukemias (Table 4) are, in general, related to the replacement of the normal bone marrow by leukemic elements (with resultant cytopenias), to infiltration of various organs, and, in some patients, to immunologic abnormalities resulting from replacement of normal lymphoid cell populations. The laboratory manifestations (Table 5) also vary as to the cell type affected. Thus anemia in CML is much less frequent than in AML, reflecting to some extent the loss of differentiation in the leukemic "stem" cell in AML vs. that in CML. Ancillary laboratory tests (Table 6) are occasionally useful in establishing the diagnosis of leukemia, especially in patients with CML, where confusion with "leukemoid" reactions may occasionally be a problem.

There is no description of current treatment programs or of survival because these are rapidly evolving, and any discussion would soon be outdated.

Table 1
MORPHOLOGICAL CLASSIFICATION OF THE LEUKEMIAS

I. "Acute" leukemia
  A. Acute "stem" cell leukemia
  B. Acute lymphoblastic leukemia
    1. Prolymphoblastic (? = "stem" cell leukemia)
    2. Prolymphocytic leukemia
    3. Burkitt's cell leukemia
    4. Lymphosarcoma cell leukemia
    5. Plasma cell leukemia
  C. Acute myelogenous leukemia
    1. "Pure" myelogenous
    2. Myelomonocytic
    3. Promyelocytic
    4. Erythroleukemia
    5. Eosinophilic leukemia
    6. Basophilic leukemia
  D. Acute monocytic leukemia
  E. Leukemic reticuloendotheliosis ("hairy cell" leukemia)

II. "Chronic" leukemia
  A. Chronic myelogenous leukemia
    1. Granulocytic
    2. Eosinophilic
    3. Basophilic
  B. Chronic monocytic leukemia
  C. Chronic lymphocytic leukemia

Table 2
HISTOCHEMICAL FEATURES OF THE ACUTE LEUKEMIAS

Staining reaction	ALL	AML	Acute myelomonocytic leukemia	Erythroleukemia
PAS	Present as coarse granules or blocks in a variable number of cells	Negative or diffusely positive	Negative or fine granulation	Strongly positive — granular
Naphthol AS-D chloroacetate esterase	Negative	Positive	Negative	Negative
Naphthol AS-D acetate esterase	Negative or weakly positive	Positive (not inhibited by fluoride)	Strongly positive (inhibited by fluoride)	Weakly positive
Alpha naphthyl acetate esterases	Negative	Negative	Strongly positive	Strongly positive
Sudan black	Negative	Positive	Positive	Positive
Peroxidase	Negative	Positive	Usually negative	Positive

Reproduced from Necheles, T. F., *The Acute Leukemias*, Stratton Intercontinental Medical Book Corp., N.Y., N.Y., 1979. With permission.

Table 3
IMMUNOLOGIC CLASSIFICATION OF ACUTE LYMPHOBLASTIC LEUKEMIA

	"Common"	Null-cell	T-cell	B cell		
				Burkitt's	Non-Burkitt's	
Frequency (%)	58	20	20	2		<1
E-C rosettes	—	—	+	—	—	+
Mitotic rate	Low	?	High	High	?	?
Surface Ig	—	—	—	+	+	+
Thy antigen	—	—	+	—	—	+ (?)
ALL antigen(s)	+	—	—	?	+	?
WBC	Low	High	High	High	High or low	High
Sex	M = F	?	M > F	M = F	?	?
Origin	Marrow	?	Thymus	Nasopharynx	?	?
Remissions	Long	Long	Short	Shortest	?	?

Note: Adapted from data presented by Pinkel at the Karnofsky Lecture, Am. Soc. Clin. Oncology, April 1978 and Chessells et al. Additional unpublished data included from our own experience. Further subcategories such as "Suppressor-T-Cell leukemia" and "Pre-B-cell" leukemia may also become important clinical entities.

Reproduced from Necheles, T. F., *The Acute Leukemias,* Stratton Intercontinental Medical Book Corp., N.Y., N.Y., 1979. With permission.

Table 4
CLINICAL MANIFESTATIONS OF THE LEUKEMIAS (% OF PATIENTS)

	AML	ALL	CML	CLL
Symptoms				
Fatigue	88	92	83	50
Fever without infection	41	71	—	—
Purpura	30	51	35	—
Bone pain	20	79	—	—
Weight loss	47	66	61	—
Infection	26	17	—	25
Asymptomatic	—	—	15	25
Physical findings				
Splenomegaly	60	86	95	74
Hepatomegaly	54	74	48	45
Lymphadenopathy	47	76	64	83
Bone tenderness	65	69	78	27
Skin bleeding	46	50	27	—

Adapted from Wintrobe, M. M. et al., *Clinical Hematology,* 7th ed., Lea & Febiger, Philadelphia, 1974. With permission.

Table 5
LABORATORY MANIFESTATIONS OF THE LEUKEMIAS (% OF PATIENTS)

	AML	ALL	CML	CLL
Total leukocyte count				
<10,000/cmm	44	40	—	—
>100,000/cmm	15	11	62—90	32
Platelet count				
<50,000/cmm	39	62	—	—
>150,000/cmm	17	8	—	—
Thrombocytopenia	83	92	13	39
Thrombocytosis	—	—	57	—
Anemia	97	98	55	84

Adapted from Wintrobe, M. M. et al., *Clinical Hematology*, 7th ed., Lea & Febiger, Philadelphia, 1974. With permission.

Table 6
ANCILLARY LABORATORY TESTS USEFUL IN THE DIAGNOSIS OF THE LEUKEMIAS

Cytogenetics (especially useful in the diagnosis of "typical" chronic myelocytic leukemia)
Leukocyte alkaline phosphatase stain (especially useful in the diagnosis of CML)
Serum vitamin B_{12} levels
Serum muramidase (elevated in monocytic and myelomonocytic leukemias, normal in myelocytic and lymphocytic variants)
Serum protein electrophoresis on polyacrylamide gel (may be useful in distinguishing CLL from lymphosarcoma cell leukemia)
Electron microscopy (may be helpful in classifying some especially undifferentiated cases of acute leukemia)

PLASMALYMPHOCYTIC PROLIFERATIVE DISORDERS

W. Pruzanski

Introduction

The immune system may be divided into two functionally related compartments of lymphoid tissue differentiation — T and B. T lymphocytes (thymus-derived) are primarily responsible for cellular immunity, whereas B lymphocytes (bursa-derived) are the precursors of immunoglobulin-producing cells. Other populations such as "null" lymphocytes and "double-marker" lymphocytes have also been recognized.

Abnormal proliferation of any of these lymphocyte types may lead to the development of malignant disease. In this chapter, only B lymphocyte-related disorders will be discussed. The great majority of abnormally proliferating clones of B lymphocytes synthesize and secrete homogeneous immunoglobulins and/or their fragments — so-called M components (Table 1). However, in pathologic conditions, so-called nonproducers and producers-nonsecretors have also occasionally been observed. Since M components are composed of physicochemically and antigenically identical molecules, they present as narrow bands on the electropherogram and as rather short, strongly curved precipitation lines on immunoelectrophoresis (IEP).

B lymphocytes related proliferative disorders are listed in Table 2. Whereas some of them, after reaching a certain point of proliferation, run a prolonged, stationary course, the majority are progressive and often fatal. In each of these disorders, the abnormal clone has its own degree of differentiation and characteristic membrane markers.[1]

M Components

The appearance of an M component in a serum electropherogram suggests that an abnormal clone that synthesizes this homogeneous immunoglobulin has reached at least 5×10^9 cells. It is not yet known what triggers such clonal proliferation and the synthesis of M components. Prolonged antigenic stimulation has been suggested, similar to that used in the rabbit's model; however, only in a very small proportion of M components (maybe 2%) was antibody activity detected. These included cold agglutinins and M components with antibody activity against DNP, TNP, heparin, cardiolipin, bacterial antigens, antistreptolysin, IgG (rheumatoid factor) lipoproteins, and others.[2-5] Presence of familial M components has been well documented,[6,7] raising an important question about genetic predisposition and/or common environmental factors in the production of M components.

The prevalence of M components, in a general population over 25 years of age, was found to be 0.9%.[8] Surveys of two large series of hospital patients (7200 and 5327 patients, respectively) showed the same prevalence — 0.8%.[9-11] In the survey of 6995 persons, all 64 individuals with M components were examined, and only 7 were found to have a malignant disease.[8] Further clinical information was obtained, in 55 of 64 individuals, 5½ years later.[12] Of the 16 who died, only 5 had had malignant diseases. No change in the serum concentration of M components was detected in the survivors, and malignant disease had not developed in any. Thus, in the great majority of individuals with M components, the condition was still benign after 5½ years. Among 13,400 healthy young adults in another study, the prevalence of M components was 0.15%. Of 20 individuals with M components, only 4 had malignant diseases.[13]

It seems, therefore, that when an M component is detected incidentally, especially in a young individual, the chance that the condition is benign is very high. The fact that, in some series of M components, 38 to 73% of the patients had multiple myeloma and

Table 1
M COMPONENTS

IgG
IgG HL's[a]
IgG with deleted parts of heavy and/or light chains
γ-HCD[b] protein
IgA monomers and polymers
IgA HL's
α-HCD[c] protein
IgM
IgM — low molecular weight (7S, 11S, etc.)
μ-HCD[d] protein
BJP's,[e] monomers, and polymers
BJP - related low molecular weight polypeptides
Homogeneous Ig's complexing with heterogeneous Ig's and/or other components
IgD
IgE

[a] Half-molecules.
[b] γ-Heavy chain disease.
[c] α-Heavy chain disease.
[d] μ-Heavy chain disease.
[e] Bence Jones proteins.

Table 2
CLASSIFICATION OF CONDITIONS ASSOCIATED WITH M COMPONENTS

A. Uncontrolled (neoplastic) proliferation of an M-component producing clone
   1. Multiple myeloma, solitary plasmacytoma, PCL[a]
   2. MW,[b] 7S IgM syndrome
   3. Heavy chain diseases (γ, α, μ)
   4. Immunoglobulin-related amyloidosis
   5. CLL[c]
   6. Some nonHodgkin's lymphomas
B. Proliferation of an M-component producing clone with a long stationary phase ("controlled")
   1. BMI[d]
   2. Chronic cold agglutinin disease
   3. Some patients with α-HCD
   4. Some patients with "essential" cryoglobulinemia
C. Unknown relationship
   1. Associated with neoplasms of cell types not known to produce immunoglobulins
   2. Autoimmune-collagen diseases
   3. Infections (viral, bacterial, and parasitic)
   4. Chronic liver diseases
   5. Lichen myxedematosus
   6. PG[e]
   7. SCLS[f]
   8. Miscellaneous diseases associated with M components
D. Transient (self-limited) proliferation of an M-component producing clone
   1. Transient M components (see Table 23)

[a] Plasma cell leukemia.
[b] Waldenström's macroglobulinemia.
[c] Chronic lymphocytic leukemia.
[d] Benign monoclonal immunoglobulinopathy.
[e] Pyoderma gangrenosum.
[f] Systemic capillary leak syndrome.

Table 3
CLASSIFICATION OF 1255 SERUM M COMPONENTS ACCORDING TO CLASS AND TYPE

Class and type of M component	No. (%)
IgG	
κ	459 (36.6)
λ	273 (21.8)
IgA	
κ	102 (8.1)
λ	83 (6.6)
IgM	
κ	83 (6.6)
λ	42 (3.3)
Unidentified	39 (3.1)
BJP	
κ	66 (5.3)
λ	57 (4.5)
IgD	
κ	1 (0.08)
λ	11 (0.9)
Biclonal[a]	16[a] (2.5)
Unidentified[b]	7 (0.6)

[a] Sixteen pairs or 32 M components (excluding cases with Bence Jones proteinemia in addition to whole-molecular M component).
[b] Very small but definite spikes of γ mobility — probably IgG.

From Ameis, A., Ko, H. S., and Pruzanski, W., Originally published in *CMA Journal* 114:889, May 22, 1976. With permission.

18% had other malignant disease,[14] does not contradict this statement. Those series were composed mainly of patients referred for special studies.

The majority of M components belong to the IgG class (Table 3). Approximately two thirds of M components have κ light chains, but the ratio of κ to λ light chains varies in different classes of M components and among various diseases. For example, κ light chains were found in 63% of patients with IgG myeloma, 53% of IgA myeloma, but in only 8% of IgD myeloma. M components with κ light chains predominated in Waldenström's macroglobulinemia (MW) cancer, lymphoma, leukemia, and connective tissue diseases. In contrast, M components with λ light chains predominated in immunoglobulin-related (primary) amyloidosis.[14]

The distribution of various classes of M components in nonmyelomatous malignant diseases differs from that in multiple myeloma (Table 4). In lymphoma and leukemia, almost half of the M components belong to the IgM class. The proportion of IgM M components in patients with cancer and with connective tissue diseases is also high. A much higher prevalence of Bence Jones proteinemia was observed in immunoglobulin-related (primary) amyloidosis (48%) than in multiple myeloma (16%). The incidence of Bence Jones proteinemia in nonmyelomatous diseases was very low. In patients who could not be classified into any of the groups of diseases in which M components are

Table 4
CLASSES OF M COMPONENTS ASSOCIATED WITH VARIOUS DISEASES (1244 PATIENTS)

Diagnosis	No. patients with M protein	(%)	Patients (%)						
			IgG	IgA	IgD	IgM	LCD[a]	Biclonal	Unidentified[b]
Plasma cell neoplasia (myeloma and macroglobulinemia)	677	(54.4)	56.9	18	1.8	6.9	15.7	0.7	0
Malignant lymphomas, Hodgkin's disease, and CLL	98	(7.9)	35.7	9.2	0	42.9	1.0	3.1	8.2
Other leukemias	12	(1.0)	50.0	0	0	16.7	25	0	8.3
Cancer	72	(5.8)	62.5	12.5	0	13.9	0	0	9.7
Collagen-vascular diseases	53	(4.3)	69.8	7.5	0	17.0	0	0	5.7
Immunoglobulin-related (primary) amyloidosis	31	(2.5)	35.5	12.9	0	3.2	48.4	0	0
Other benign conditions, including BMI	301	(24.2)	72.8	12.3	0	11.3	0	1.3	2.3

[a] LCD = Light chain disease.
[b] Very small but definite spikes of γ mobility — probably IgG.

From Ameis, A., Ko, H. S., and Pruzanski, W., Originally published in *CMA Journal* 114:889, May 22, 1976. With permission.

Table 5
MINIMAL INCIDENCE OF M COMPONENTS IN CANCER[a]

	No. of cases	(%)	Incidence[b] in Ontario, 1966 (%)[84]	Incidence[c] in Toronto, 1975 (%)[85]
Colon and rectum	53	16.3	14.0	5.7
Prostate	48	14.8	6.3	2.6
Breast	46	14.2	13.1	16.8
Lung	40	12.3	8.5	13.2
Adenocarcinoma (site unknown)	17	5.2	2.2[d]	2.9[d]
Stomach	13	4.0	4.7	0.9
Bladder	11	3.4	4.4	2.4
Cervix	8	2.5	4.4	4.1
Pancreas	8	2.5	2.5	Not recorded
Kidney	7	2.2	1.5	1.2
Uterus	7	2.2	2.7	3.4
Tongue	6	1.8	0.5	0.7
Esophagus	5	1.5	1.1	1.4
Skin	5	1.5	20.5	14.5
Thyroid[e]	5	1.5	0.8	0.6
Larynx and epiglottis	5	1.5	1.1	2.5
Melanoma	5	1.5	1.3	1.3
Sarcoma	4	1.2	0.8	0.8
Biliary tract	4	1.2	Not recorded	Not recorded
Others	28	8.4	Incomplete data	Incomplete data
Total	325	100	—	—

[a] Compiled from several sources; references available upon request.
[b] Based on 23,099 cases.
[c] Based on 6,304 cases.
[d] Includes other cancers site unknown.
[e] In one, gliobastoma was found as well.

usually detected and were labeled as "others" or as having "unclassified benign" conditions, the proportion of IgM M components was not high, and no Bence Jones proteinemia was detected.[14] In approximately half of these patients, the serum concentration of M components exceeded 1.0 g/dℓ at the time of detection, and in many the concentration exceeded 2.0 g/dℓ.

Among the patients with cancer and M components, those with carcinoma of the colon, prostate, breast, and lung composed 58% of the whole group (Table 5). It should be stressed, however, that the real incidence of M components in cancer cannot be estimated with certainty. Firstly, no routine search for the presence of M components has been conducted in patients with various cancers. Secondly, the proportion of patients with cancer and M components was almost never calculated as a percentage of the total number of patients with a given neoplasm. When such calculation was done (Table 6), the incidence of M components seemed to be similar to that found at random in a general population.[15]

Bence Jones proteinuria was found in more than 70% of the patients with multiple myeloma (Table 7). In other diseases, the prevalence varied from 37 to 78% with an overall prevalence of 48%. The amount of Bence Jones protein (BJP) in the urine

Table 6
FREQUENCY OF M COMPONENTS IN PATIENTS WITH NEOPLASTIC DISEASES AND IN ASYMPTOMATIC ADULTS

	M proteins per sera tested	(%)
Multiple myeloma	253/255	(99.2)
Diffuse lymphomas and CLL	45/641	(7.0)
Nodular lymphomas	4/292	(1.4)
Hodgkin's disease	1/218	(0.5)
Cancer	32/5043	(0.6)
Asymptomatic adults ≥ 25 years	64/6995	(0.9)

Reprinted from Bergsagel, D. E. and Pruzanski, W., *Immunodiagnosis of Cancer,* McIntire, K. R. and Herberman, R. B., Eds., Marcel Dekker, New York, 1977. By courtesy of Marcel Dekker, Inc.

depends on several factors, such as the rate of synthesis and of degradation, size of the molecules, glomerular permeability, tubular reabsorption, renal catabolism, and the urinary volume. Therefore, the finding of serum M component and/or Bence Jones proteinuria does not make it possible to distinguish a neoplastic process from a benign condition, nor is the serum concentration of M component very helpful, although in multiple myeloma and MW, the concentration is usually higher than in other diseases. The concentration of immunoglobulins, other than M components, is usually low in multiple myeloma and MW. Low levels of immunoglobulins were only rarely observed in patients with cancer, connective tissue disorders, and unclassified benign disorders. It is not clear whether the suppression of immunoglobulin production can be taken as definite evidence of malignant process. However, the patients with M components and low concentrations of normal immunoglobulins should be checked repeatedly for malignant disease, and the finding of an M component always warrants extensive investigation (Table 8). A diagnosis of "benign" M component should be made by exclusion only.[16,17] Malignant disease may develop in patients with these seemingly benign conditions; therefore, all patients with M components should be followed up for long periods of time. Transient M components have been described and will be discussed later on.

Laboratory Investigation of M Components (Table 9)

Electrophoresis

Electrophoresis is a screening procedure for the analysis of immunoglobulin abnormalities. Its sensitivity depends on the medium in which the proteins are separated, the buffer, the electrical current, and the dye used for staining. When cellulose acetate membrane is used, the electropherogram will detect most M components, the great majority of which will show as narrow bands of γ, β, or, rarely, of fast anodal mobility. In an early stage of the disease, or in remission, M components may produce faint bands, or no bands at all. Because of a low concentration, IgD M component and homogeneous light chains may not be visible, even in the advanced stage of disease (Figure 1). In this case plate isoelectric focusing, or use of nigrosin for staining, may increase the rate of detection of discrete bands.

Calculation of the concentration of M component, from the electropherogram, as a percentage of the total serum protein, has routinely been used in most laboratories. The procedure is simple; however, there are several disadvantages limiting its accuracy. Since the calculation involves two factors, i.e., estimation of the total serum protein

Table 7
INCIDENCE OF BENCE JONES PROTEINURIA AS TESTED BY ELECTRO- AND IMMUNOELECTROPHORESIS OF CONCENTRATED URINE

Disease		No. of urines tested	No. of positive urines	(%)
Multiple myeloma	IgG(κ)	151	106	70
	IgG(λ)	100	59	59
	IgA(κ)	40	21	53
	IgA(λ)	38	26	68
	LCD(κ)	59	59	100
	LCD(λ)	47	47	100
	IgD(κ)	1		
	IgD(λ)	6	6	86
	IgM	2	1	—
TOTAL		444	325	73
MW		24	14	58
Lymphoma with M components		16	7	44
Immunoglobulin-related (primary) amyloidosis		31	24	78
Cancer with M components		27	11	41
CLL with M components		11	8	73
Acute myelogeneous leukemia with M components		3	2	—
Acute myelomonocytic leukemia with M components		3	1	—
Connective tissue diseases with M components		32	13	41
Others including benign monoclonal gammopathy		76	28	37
TOTAL		223	108	48

Table 8
SUGGESTED INVESTIGATION OF M COMPONENTS

Presumptive diagnosis	Tests
A. Multiple myeloma, MW, heavy chain diseases	A. Bone marrow, skeletal survey, electro- and immunoelectrophoresis of serum and urine, immunoquantitation, general hematological tests
B. Cancer, lymphoma, leukemia	B. All group A tests and radiological study of various organs, lymphangiography, liver and spleen scan, lymph node or other organ biopsy
C. Amyloidosis	C. All group A tests and biopsy of the rectum and/or of other involved organs
D. Chronic liver diseases	D. All group A tests and liver function tests, LE cells test, latex fixation tests for rheumatoid factor
E. Collagen-autoimmune diseases	E. All group A tests and LE cells tests, ANF, DNA binding, latex fixation for rheumatoid factor, total hemolytic complement, C3, C4, etc.
F. Skin diseases	F. All group A tests and skin biopsy
G. Others — including benign and transient M components	G. By exclusion of groups A F; use clinical judgment; follow up and repeat estimation of the concentration of M components is necessary.

Table 9
IMMUNOLOGICAL AND IMMUNOCHEMICAL TESTS FOR STUDY OF M COMPONENTS

Serum	Urine and other fluids	Cells
Total protein	Total protein	Membrane markers on peripheral blood lymphocytes[a]
Electrophoresis	Electrophoresis	E and EAC rosettes and Fc receptor[a]
IEP	IEP	Mitogen stimulation, etc.[a]
Immunoquantitation	Immunoquantitation (optional)	
Cryoglobulin		
Pyroglobulin		
Sia test		
Cold agglutinins		
Viscosity (serum and whole blood)		
Antibody activity[a]		
Cytotoxic activity[a]		
Purification and characterization of M components[a]		
Analytical ultracentrifugation[a]		

[a] These tests are presently performed for research purposes only. Many other specialized, but less common, tests have not been included in the list.

and reading the electropherogram, the possibility of technical error is greater. Also, it is not always possible to accurately distinguish the M protein and the neighboring, normal proteins. This is especially true in the case of broad-based, IgA M components and in the case of small spikes. Even when the spike is well defined, there is always

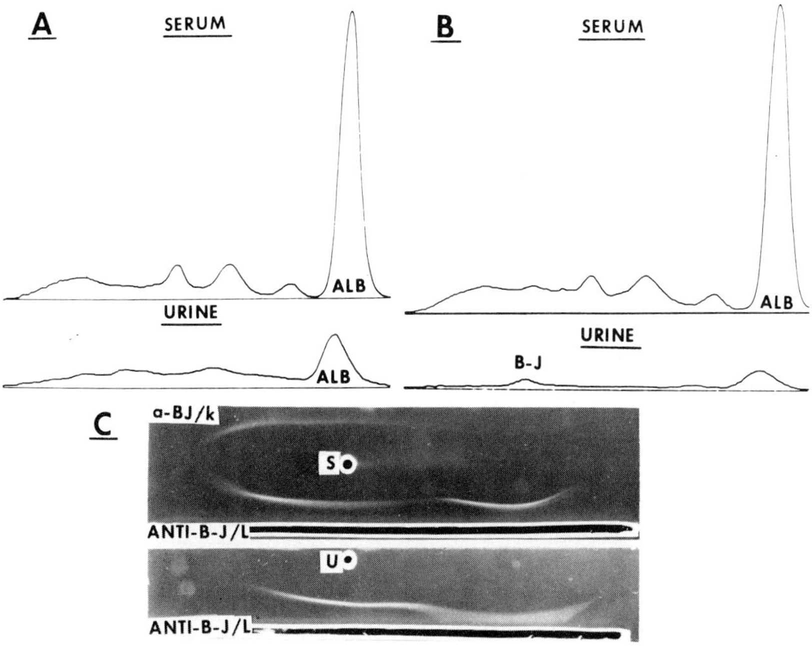

FIGURE 1. Electropherograms in LCD. (A) ''Normal'' serum and urine electropherograms. Lambda type BJP was detected in these samples by IEP. (B) Another example of ''normal'' serum pattern with a faint abnormality in the urine. (C) IEP.

some proportion of normal immunoglobulins, of identical electrophoretic mobility, located in the area occupied by the spike. Nevertheless, the fact that the electrophoretic technique is readily available, easy to use, and reproducible, makes it one of the most popular tools in clinical immunology.

Immunoelectrophoresis (IEP)

IEP is used for identifying the class and type of M component(s), as well as for the analysis of the subclasses, subtypes, detection of various parts of immunoglobulin molecules, etc. IEP may reveal the presence of M component even when it is not visible in the electropherogram (Figure 1).

The accuracy of IEP depends on the availability of high quality antisera. The concentration of antibody and the ''purity'' of antisera, i.e., the detection of specific antigens only, are crucial for correct interpretation of IEP. Immunoelectrophoretic analysis depends also on the number of antisera that are used in each case. For example, the use of antifree κ and antifree λ antisera significantly increased the incidence of detection of free light chains in the serum, in addition to complete M components.[14] Use of anti-Fc and anti-Fab antisera may be helpful in the detection of heavy chain disease protein. Since the precipitating properties of antigen-antibody complexes depend, among other things, upon the concentration of the components, appropriate dilution of sera with M components, or of antisera used, may facilitate identification of the heavy and/or light chains. In a high percentage of IgM M components, the light chains are not easily identifiable in IEP. In such cases, either concentration of IgM by the euglobulin precipitation technique, or reduction of the protein, will allow easy assessment of the light-chain type. Light chains of IgA M proteins that are otherwise unidentifiable can sometimes be identified by reduction and alkylation of the serum.

Immunoquantitation

Measurement of immunoglobulins is usually done with immunoquantitation plates, which consist of a medium, usually agar or agarose, evenly mixed with appropriate antiserum. The fluid sample, in which Ig is to be measured, diffuses through the medium, and a ring of precipitation is formed. The diameter of the precipitation ring is proportionate to the logarithm of the antigen concentration in the sample, or, alternatively, the area of precipitation is proportionate to the antigen concentration. The accuracy of these techniques is far from being perfected. The quality of the medium, per se, seems to influence the rate of diffusion. The antibody concentration in the antiserum, incorporated to the medium, influences precipitation and thus affects the visibility of rings. Time and temperature of incubation play a role in development of the precipitation ring in some immunoplates. Other factors important to the accuracy of immunoquantitation are the concentration and some characteristics of the immunoglobulin to be measured. Immunoquantitation plates are limited in accuracy, for both the lowest and the highest concentration of immunoglobulins. Since the lowest concentration is usually about 3 to 5 mg/dℓ (using ultralow level plates), this limitation is of no clinical significance. More important is the upper limit of accuracy of immunoplates, which is different for each immunoglobulin. Above the upper limit (usually stated by each company), accurate measurement cannot be obtained with immunoplates. In such cases, many laboratories use diluted sera; however, the dilution, per se, introduces an additional error. Purified immunoglobulin in a buffer, quantitated on immunoplates, gives a different reading from that obtained when an identical quantity of the same immunoglobulin is dissolved in the whole serum.

Immunoplates may give false high and low readings. The former is observed when immunoglobulin is present in the serum in two or more forms of different, lower than normal, molecular weights, for example, when low molecular weight IgM such as 11S, 7S, or μ-HCD protein is present, in addition to 19S IgM. Likewise, the presence of 7S IgG, together with lower molecular weight, γ-related globulins, such as incomplete molecules, half molecules, Fc fragment, or γ-HCD protein, produce disproportionately large precipitation rings and falsely high readings. The reason for this is that these low molecular weight molecules diffuse faster through the medium than normal molecules. When low molecular weight globulins are present in the serum, along with "normal" molecular weight immunoglobulins, two precipitation rings, a dense ring located centrally and a faint precipitation ring located peripherally, are often observed on immunoplates (Figure 2). Such double precipitation rings should always raise the possibility that there are low molecular weight immunoglobulin-related fragments in the serum. Occasionally, low molecular weight proteins produce a weak precipitation reaction, and the ring is almost invisible. In such cases, immersion of immunoplates into 7% acetic acid for 1 min will render the precipitation ring clearly visible.

False low readings may be observed when the serum is hyperviscous, or when high molecular weight polymeric forms of immunoglobulins are present in the serum. There is some evidence that large amounts of immune complexes (IgM/IgG, IgG/IgG) may slow down the diffusion of the involved immunoglobulins as well.

Another technique, used in some laboratories, is the one-dimensional single electroimmunodiffusion, or rocket electrophoresis.[18] In this method, appropriate antiserum is incorporated into the medium, an antigen is added to small wells, and then electrophoresis is performed. This technique detects small amounts of antigen.

Proteinuria

Examination of the urinary proteins may give important information as to the presence of BJP, their fragments, and whole M components in the urine. Neither the heat precipitation test, nor dipsticks, should be used for detection of Bence Jones protein-

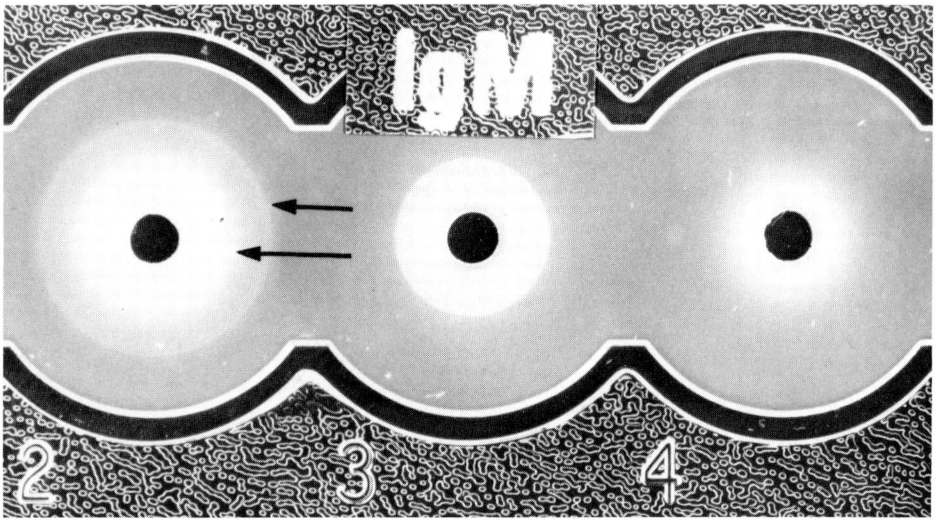

FIGURE 2. Immunoquantitation plate against IgM. Pattern 2 shows two rings: the inner one corresponds to 19S IgM and the outer one to the low molecular weight IgM-related globulin. Pattern 3 — one ring in 19S IgM MW. Pattern 4 — IgM in healthy individual.

uria. The former may give both false negative and false positive results,[19] while the latter does not detect BJP.[20] Urine investigation should include estimation of the total urinary protein excreted in 24 hr, appropriate concentration of urine, and then electrophoresis and immunoelectrophoresis of the concentrate. The degree of concentration depends on the total protein value. When the total protein is below 200 mg per 24 hr, concentration of 500 times, or more, is often necessary to detect small amounts of BJP. The urinary electropherogram easily shows abnormal bands corresponding to BJP or to other M proteins (Figure 3). Final identification is made by IEP, applying antisera against BJP of kappa or lambda types. The type of BJP in the urine usually corresponds to the type of light chain of the serum M protein. Rarely have two BJP's of different types been found in the urine, whereas serum has contained either a single M component or two M components with the same type of light chain. Exceedingly rare are cases in which light chains of serum M proteins and urinary BJP were of different antigenic type.

Not rarely, whole M components are found in the urine (Figures 3 and 4) as well as in the serum. This finding signifies increased glomerular permeability of the kidneys. In addition, two or three bands (spikes) of proteins related to BJP may be observed on urine EP. In such a case, there are either monomers and various polymers of BJP and/or variable and constant parts of BJP that have different EP mobilities.

Electrophoresis of concentrated urine may show several bands of cathodal post-gamma mobility that have diagnostic importance, especially for leukemias. Although these bands represent nonimmunoglobulin, low molecular weight proteins, they are mentioned here, since they present as spikes that resemble BJP's. The most important in this group is lysozyme (LZM), an enzyme produced mainly by monocytes and found in neutrophils as well. This enzyme is present in normal urines in minute quantities, not exceeding 2 $\mu g/m\ell$. In monocytic and myelomonocytic leukemia, and occasionally in chronic myelogeneous leukemia, the level of lysozyme in the plasma increases markedly and, when the tubular mechanism of reabsorption becomes saturated, spillover to the urine occurs. The excretion of LZM in the urine may reach values higher than 1300 $\mu g/min$.[21] When such urine is concentrated, LZM is visible as a band of post-

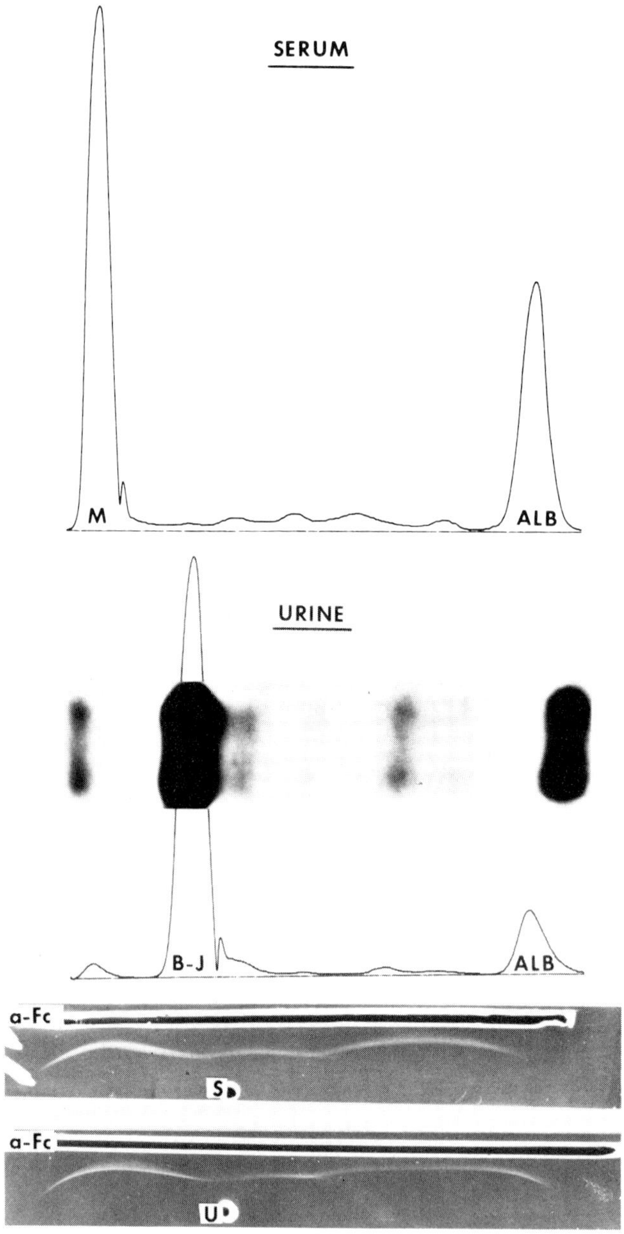

FIGURE 3. Electropherogram in IgG multiple myeloma; with one spike in the serum and two spikes in the urine. IEP detected monoclonal IgG with Fc and F′c fragments in the serum and similar fragments along with BJP in the urine.

gamma mobility (Figure 5). Bands of LZM may also be pronounced in abnormalities of the tubular reabsorptive mechanism, such as in adult Fanconi syndrome, myeloma, cadmium poisoning, and others.

Another postgamma protein was recently described in chronic myelocytic leukemia.[22] This so-called cationic leukemia antigen (CLA) is excreted by cells of the neutrophil series and appears in the urine as a postgamma protein of slightly less cathodic mobility than LZM.

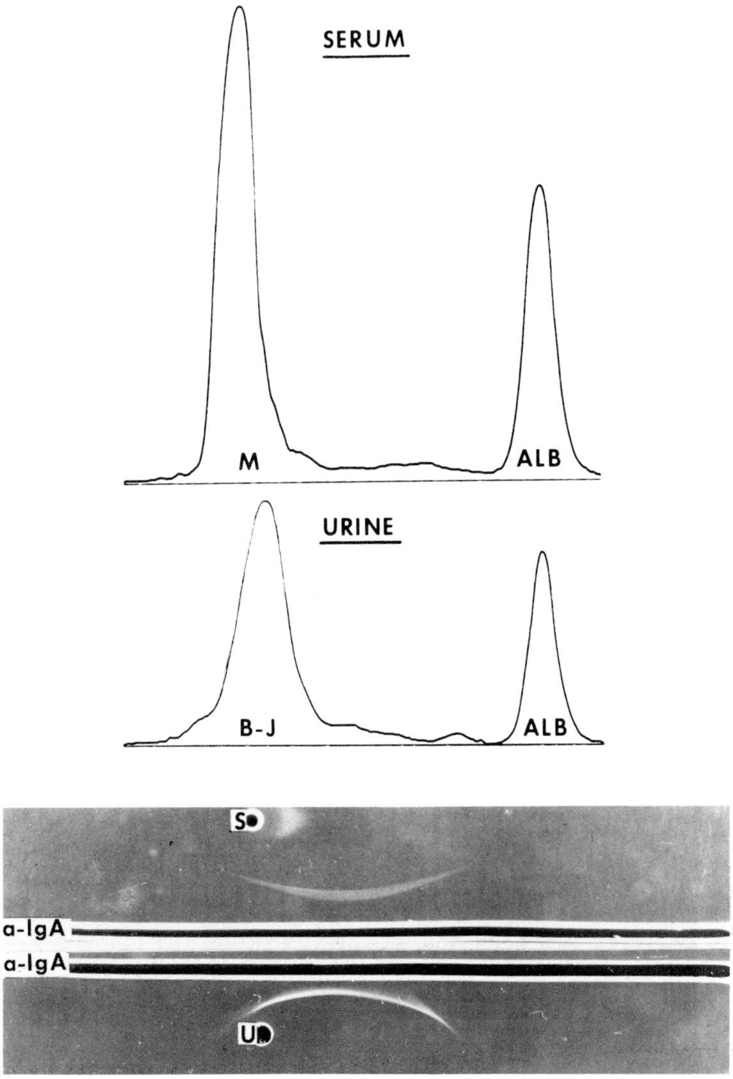

FIGURE 4. Electropherogram in IgA multiple myeloma. IEP detected BJP and monoclonal IgA in the urine.

Multiple Myeloma

Multiple myeloma is the most common malignant plasma cell neoplasm. No cause of neoplastic transformation of plasma cells has yet been discovered. The abnormality affects not only plasma cells, but also lymphocytes. A significantly low percentage of B lymphocytes having normal surface immunoglobulins and a high percentage of lymphocytes having idiotypic (with the corresponding M component) immunoglobulin on the surface have been noted in the peripheral blood of myeloma patients.[23-25] In 99% of the cases, morphologically more-or-less immature plasma cells synthesize and secrete either homogeneous immunoglobulins (IgG, IgA, IgD, and, very rarely, IgE or IgM) and/or the light chain κ or λ proteins (Table 10). In less than 1% of patients, the neoplastic plasma cells either synthesize, but do not secrete, or do not synthesize immunoglobulins at all.[26]

The annual incidence of multiple myeloma in various countries is between 2.0 and

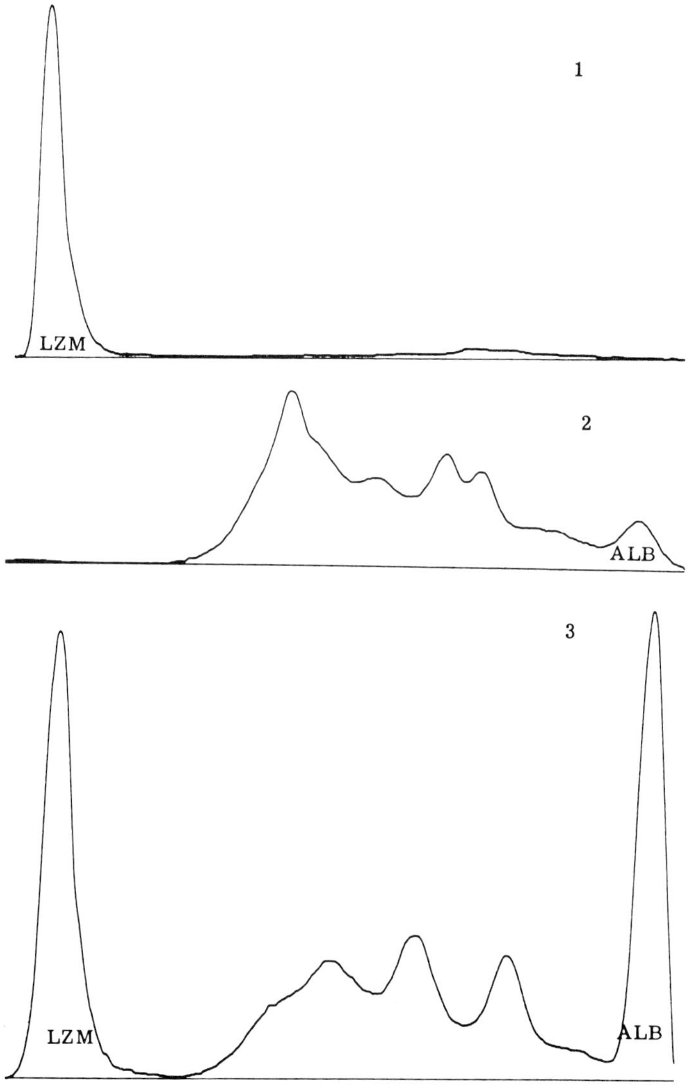

FIGURE 5. Electropherogram of urinary proteins in three cases of myelomonocytic leukemia. Pattern 1 shows a spike of postgamma mobility identified as LZM (muramidase). Patterns 2 and 3 show spikes of LZM, along with other proteins, especially of α-β mobility (tubular pattern).

3.1 per 100,000.[27-29] The disease probably affects males and females equally and seems to occur more frequently in black patients than in whites.[29,30] The disease is infrequent before the fifth decade of age. Familial multiple myeloma in one or more generations,[6] as well as multiple myeloma developing in spouses,[7] have been described.

Although the clinical picture of the advanced disease is well known, diagnosis in the early stages, or when the classical picture is overshadowed by one of the complications, may be difficult (Table 11).[31] It seems that the course and the prognosis of multiple myeloma relate, to some extent, to the class of heavy chains and the type of light chains of M components synthesized by the neoplastic cells (Table 12).[31]

As seen in Table 11, in the early stage, multiple myeloma may be asymptomatic or may present with rather vague manifestations. Appearance of M components may precede other manifestations by many years. When the disease progresses, most patients

Table 10
PREVALENCE OF M COMPONENTS IN MULTIPLE MYELOMA

Class		No.	(%)
IgG	κ — 242	385	61
	λ — 143		
IgA	κ — 65	122	19
	λ — 57		
LCD	κ — 59	106	17
	λ — 47		
IgD	κ — 1	12	1.9
	λ — 11		
Biclonal		5	0.8
IgM		2	0.3
IgE		0	0

From Pruzanski, W. Originally published in *CMA Journal* 114:896, May 22, 1976. With permission.

complain of bone pain, especially in the back, tiredness and weakness, frequent infections, etc. Various complications may develop, producing a multitude of clinical manifestations. The majority of, if not all, patients with advanced multiple myeloma have microscopic, and occasionally macroscopic, plasma cell infiltrates in various organs, particularly in the spleen, liver, nodes, and kidneys.[32,33] However, some patients present with especially extensive macroscopic extraskeletal involvement of various organs.[32,33] More than half of the patients with IgD myeloma have lymphadenopathy, hepatomegaly, and/or splenomegaly.[34]

Durrie and Salmon analyzed various features of multiple myeloma, in relation to the total tumor mass, and correlated them with therapeutic response and survival.[35] They found (Table 13) that the serum concentration of M components, anemia, hypercalcemia, and the extent of osteolytic lesions correlated well with the neoplastic cell mass. According to their classification of multiple myeloma into three stages, the therapeutic response and survival are best in stage one and worst in stage three. This emphasizes the importance of early diagnosis of multiple myeloma.

Anemia, usually mild to moderate, is observed in the majority of patients. It is usually of the normocytic, normochromic type, but microcytosis, hypochromia, poikilocytosis, and, rarely, macrocytic megaloblastic anemia have been described in multiple myeloma. Marked anemia, associated with a high myeloma cell mass, is a poor prognostic sign. Leukopenia and thrombocytopenia are quite common in multiple myeloma and are caused by the disease, per se, and/or by chemotherapy-induced bone marrow suppression. Occasionally leukocytosis and/or thrombocytemia are observed. Increased numbers of plasma cells in the peripheral blood have been noted in almost all patients when the buffy coat technique is used, but in some cases, large numbers of immature plasma cells denote development of plasma cell leukemia.[36] In the advanced stage of multiple myeloma, occurrence of acute blast cell leukemia or myelomonocytic leukemia, with high serum and urinary LZM, has been observed.[37]

M components may interact with various coagulation factors, leading to bleeding and thrombotic phenomena. Various abnormalities, such as low level of several coagulation factors, interference with fibrinogen polymerization and abnormal fibrinogen-

Table 11
CLINICAL MANIFESTATIONS AND LABORATORY FEATURES OF MULTIPLE MYELOMA

Stage	Clinical manifestations	Laboratory findings
Early	Asymptomatic, or fatigue, recurrent infection, solitary plasmacytoma	One or more of the following: elevated ESR, rouleaux formation, anemia, proteinuria, anticomplement activity, low concentration of some immunoglobulins, M components, intra- or extramedullary tumor, bone marrow plasmacytic infiltration
Developed	Skeletal pain (back, ribs, other), pathologic fractures, recurrent infection, bleeding, bruising, anorexia, nausea, vomiting	M components in serum in 99%, Bence Jones proteinuria in 70%, osteolytic lesions and/or osteoporosis, bone marrow plasmacytic infiltration, anemia, bleeding/clotting abnormalities, azotemia and other renal manifestations, hypercalcemia, cryoglobulinemia, intra- or extramedullary tumors, hyperviscosity
Advanced	Same as in the previous stage and PCL, blast cell leukemia or mono- or myelomonocytic leukemia	Same as in the previous stage, and high peripheral WBC count with leukemic cells, thrombocytopenia, pancytopenia, cellular bone marrow
	Acute terminal phase with fever and general deterioration	

Complications that May Present as Main Clinical Manifestations

Hyperviscosity syndrome	Renal syndrome
Cryoglobulinemia	Chronic progressive renal failure
Amyloidosis	Acute renal failure
Hypercalcemia	Adult Fanconi's syndrome
Bleeding/clotting abnormalities	Salt-losing nephritis
Polyneuropathy	Renal tubular acidosis
Extramedullarly forms (organomegaly, lymphadenopathy, etc.)	Nephrotic syndrome Chronic pyelonephritis
Plasma cell (or another) leukemia	Terminal acute phase

From Pruzanski, W., Originally published in *CMA Journal* 114:889, May 22, 1976. With permission.

fibrin conversion, coating of collagen by the protein, etc., were noted in multiple myeloma, especially of IgA class.[38]

The majority of patients with multiple myeloma have bone marrow infiltrated with plasma cells of various maturity. The percentage of abnormal marrows increases when repeat aspirations are performed in the same patient, or when a bone biopsy is done. Occasionally, an admixture of plasma cells with plasmacytoid lymphocytes, immunob-

Table 12
COMPARISON OF SEVERAL MANIFESTATIONS OF MULTIPLE MYELOMA IN RELATION OF CLASS OF M COMPONENT

Variable	IgG	IgA	LCD κ	LCD λ	IgD
Mean age at diagnosis (years)[a]	62, 62	64, 65	61	61	56
Sex, male to female	1:1	1:1	1:1	1:1	3:1
Blood urea nitrogen value ⩾ 30 mg/dℓ (%)	14	33	61	53	67
Serum calcium value ⩾ 11 mg/dℓ (%)	8—33	47—59	39	29	30
Osteolytic lesions (%)	57	65	78	83	79
Mean concentration of serum M component (g/dℓ)	4.3	2.8	±[b]	±[b]	1.7
Light chains ratio; κ to λ	2:1	2:1	1.2:1	1.2:1	1:9
Bence Jones proteinuria (%)	60—70	70	100	100	92
Median survival time (months)	κ, 35	κ, 22	24	7	9
	λ, 25	λ, 19	—	—	—

[a] Means of two series.
[b] ± = Almost none detectable.

From Pruzanski, W., Originally published in *CMA Journal* 114:889, May 22, 1976. With permission.

Table 13
MYELOMA STAGING OF DURIE AND SALMON

Stage[a]	Hemoglobin (g/dℓ)	Calcium (mg/dℓ)	Skeletal survey	M component (g/dℓ)	Myeloma cell mass (X 10^{12})
I, with all criteria met	>10.0	⩽12.0	Normal or one lytic lesion	IgG <5.0, or IgA <3.0, or urine BJP <4 g/day	<0.6
II	Fitting neither stage I nor stage III				0.6—1.2
III, with one or more criteria met	<8.5	>12.0	Many lytic lesions	IgG >7.0, or IgA >5.0, or urine BJP >12 g/day	>1.2

[a] Each stage may be subclassified as follows: (A) serum creatinine value, <2.0 mg/dℓ or blood urea nitrogen value, <30 mg/dℓ and (B) serum creatinine value, ⩾2.0 mg/dℓ or blood urea nitrogen value, ⩾30 mg/dℓ.

From Durie, B. G. M. and Salmon, S. E., *Cancer,* 36, 842, 1975. With permission.

lasts, and, rarely, eosinophils is observed. Intra- and extracellular crystal-like material, representing excessive production of M component, or small droplets of cryoglobulin can be found in the marrow aspirates.

Biochemical variables of importance in multiple myeloma are

1. Blood urea nitrogen and creatinine — up to 70% of patients with multiple mye-

Table 14
RENAL ABNORMALITIES IN MULTIPLE MYELOMA AND OTHER PLASMA-LYMPHOCYTIC DISEASES

Slow progressive renal failure
Acute renal failure (dehydration, iatrogenic, other)
Nephrotic syndrome (especially in amyloidosis)
Renal tubular acidosis
Fanconi syndrome
Salt-losing nephritis

Pathomechanisms of Renal Disease in Multiple Myeloma

Glomerular damage
Myeloma kidney
Plasmalymphocytic interstitial infiltrate
Hypercalcemia and hypercalciuria
Hyperuricemia and uricosuria
Amyloidosis
Pyelonephritis
Bleeding and coagulation defects
Ig/Lp complexes and foam cell formation
Hyperviscosity
Acute tubular damage due to complexes of pyelography dye and BJP, dehydration, etc.

loma eventually develop azotemia, a poor prognostic sign; impairment of renal function is a serious and often life-threatening situation in multiple myeloma. Precipitation of BJP's, along with other plasma proteins in the tubules, leads to the production of casts, degeneration of the tubule endothelial layer, and appearance of giant multinucleated cells (myeloma kidney). This tubular blockage may lead to the deterioration of renal functions, acidification defects, and occasionally to the development of adult Fanconi syndrome. Several other mechanisms contribute to the development of various renal abnormalities (Table 14).
2. Calcium — hypercalcemia occurs in up to 60% of multiple myeloma patients.
3. Uric acid — hyperuricemia is quite frequently observed, but gouty attacks are rare.
4. Hypoalbuminemia, unrelated to the extent of albuminuria, has been noted in many patients with advanced multiple myeloma and seems to be a poor prognostic sign.
5. Other rarer abnormalities include elevation of alkaline phosphatase or of acid phosphatase.[39] Impairment of the liver function has been noted in some cases of multiple myeloma with liver involvement.

Increased plasma volume, related to the elevation in the total serum protein, has been recorded in many patients with multiple myeloma. It may lead to congestive heart failure and to the dilution and fall of the hemoglobin concentration. Reduced anion gap [(Na + K) − (Cl + CO_2cp)] has been reported in patients with multiple myeloma, but its biological significance is unknown.

The immunological study of multiple myeloma uses several tests, which are listed in Table 9. Their aim is to assess the class and type of the M component, its concentration, and its certain characteristics such as cryoprecipitation, cold agglutinin activity, and viscosity. It is notable that the frequency with which each class of immunoglobulins is produced by multiple myeloma parallels quite well the rate of physiological synthesis of these immunoglobulins (Table 15). Thus it seems that plasma cell clones,

Table 15
FREQUENCY OF M-COMPONENT CLASSES PRODUCED BY PLASMA CELL NEOPLASMS

A.	M components containing both heavy and light chains	(%)
	1. IgG	52
	2. IgA	31
	3. IgM	12
	4. IgD	2
	5. IgE	<0.01
B.	M components containing only light chains (κ or λ)	11
C.	M components containing only heavy chain-related fragments (γ, α, or μ)	<1
D.	Two or more M components (biclonal, triclonal gammopathy)	0.5
E.	No M components in serum or urine	1

From Pruzanski, W. and Ogryzlo, M. A., *Adv. Clin. Chem.*, 13, 335, 1970. With permission.

producing each class of immunoglobulins, are equally susceptible to neoplastic transformation. Characterization of the M components and estimation of their concentration are important for the assessment of therapeutic response and prognosis (vide supra). Approximately 5% of M components in myeloma are cryoprecipitable. Various aspects of cryoglobulinemia will be discussed later. Occasionally pyroglobulinemia — clotting of the serum at 56°C — has been observed in multiple myeloma.[40]

Radiological study of multiple myeloma should include complete skeletal survey. About 60 to 79% of the patients present with osteolytic lesions,[41] with or without diffuse osteoporosis; 20 to 25% of the patients have osteoporosis only; and about 3% have osteosclerotic lesions; whereas the rest may have radiologically normal bones. Production of osteolytic lesions has been related to the expansive growth of the malignant plasma cells, but recently an osteoclast-stimulating factor has been detected in supernatants, from the short-term cultures of myeloma marrow cells. This factor may contribute to the lytic activity.[42] Osteoblastic (sclerotic) lesions have been noted in various classes of myeloma.[43] Notably, there is an association of these lesions with the involvement of the neurological system, especially with peripheral neuropathy. Interestingly, two of five reported patients with IgE myeloma had osteosclerotic bone lesions.[44]

Other tests, such as liver and spleen scan, lymphangiography, or rectal biopsy, are indicated when one searches for amyloidosis, internal organ involvement, etc.

The treatment of multiple myeloma includes continuous or intermittent use of chemotherapeutic agents (Melphalan, Cyclophosphamide, Chlorambucil, BCNU, procarbazine, etc.), with or without steroids. Irradiation of the severely involved areas and specific therapy for various complications should always complement chemotherapy. The interested reader is referred to the pertinent publications.[45,46]

A few unusual clinical manifestations or laboratory features of multiple myeloma require separate mention:

1. IgM multiple myeloma is an entity in which characteristic features of myeloma are

present, but the M component has μ heavy chains. More than 50 cases of this disease have been suspected, but only about 20 have been documented, with 11 reported in detail. The age of the patients varied from 32 to 69 years, and there was no predominance of either sex. Bone marrow showed plasmacytosis, usually over 15%. Osteolytic lesions, with or without osteoporosis, were found in all patients. Hyperviscosity was noted in 5 of 11 patients, and bleeding phenomena were frequent. Lymphadenopathy and/or organomegaly were noted in one third of the patients. Plasma cell leukemia was noted in two patients. Of 11 patients, 10 died within 24 months after diagnosis. The duration of the disease, from first symptom to death, ranged from 6 months to 9 years.

2. Five patients with unusual half molecule (HL) IgG M components were reported.[47] There were three patients with extramedullary plasmacytoma, one with multiple myeloma, and one with plasma cell leukemia. Deletion of the third constant domain was detected by biochemical study of the M components. Recently a patient with plasma cell leukemia was found to have IgA_1/λ_1 half-molecular M component.[48] Various "broken" molecules, with deletions in heavy and/or light chains, have also been detected in patients with M components.
3. Two patients with renal failure, one due to multiple myeloma and another due to glomerulonephritis, developed multiple-organ-system disease with deposition of kappa light chains in the tissues.[49]
4. Several cases of multiple myeloma, xanthomatosis, and lipid abnormalities have been described.[50,51] Recently, in one such patient with multiple myeloma and nodular xanthomatosis, lipemia and heparin-M component interaction were detected, along with heparin resistance and delayed triglyceride and apolipoprotein removal. Another patient with myeloma and diffuse plane xanthomata had normal lipids and cryoglobulinemia. The cryoprecipitate had orange color and contained IgG/K M component, β- and pre-β-lipoproteins, carotenoids, and cholesterol.[51]

Plasma Cell Leukemia (PCL)

The acute leukemic form of immunocytic dyscrasia is rare and almost without exception is a fatal disease.[36] In only one instance has a prolonged remission been observed. This form, behaving as do other acute leukemias, has given rise to controversial opinions regarding its relationship to multiple myeloma, the degree of maturity of proliferating plasmacytes, and the production of M components.

The incidence of PCL among myeloma patients is close to 2%. No difference among the sexes has been found. The mean age for the total group of 57 patients was 59.5 years.[36] The youngest patient was 42 years old and the oldest was 82.

The majority of patients complained of general weakness, weight loss, and fatigue. The most frequent symptom was pain in the lower back, usually related to vertebral collapse, as in myeloma patients. Pain in the sternum or ribs was common. Hemorrhagic phenomena such as petechiae, epistaxis, and bleeding from the gums and gastrointestinal tract were as common in PCL as in other acute leukemias; these symptoms may be attributed to thrombocytopenia and coagulation disorders. Hepatomegaly and splenomegaly were recorded in half of the patients. Enlarged lymph nodes were noted in 26% of patients. Skin infiltrates, lingual nodules, jaundice, lethargy, congestive heart failure, renal failure, and enlargement of testicles were also observed.

Normocytic, normochromic, or hypochromic anemia was noted in almost all patients, with a mean hemoglobin of 7.4 g%. The anemia was much more prominent than is usually observed in myeloma and resembled that occurring in acute leukemia. The average white blood cell count was 51,000/mm^3 (range 4,000 to 262,000/mm^3). The number of plasma cells in the peripheral blood varied from 6 to 99% (760 to 224,000/mm^3), with an average of 56%. Sometimes plasma cells of different maturity

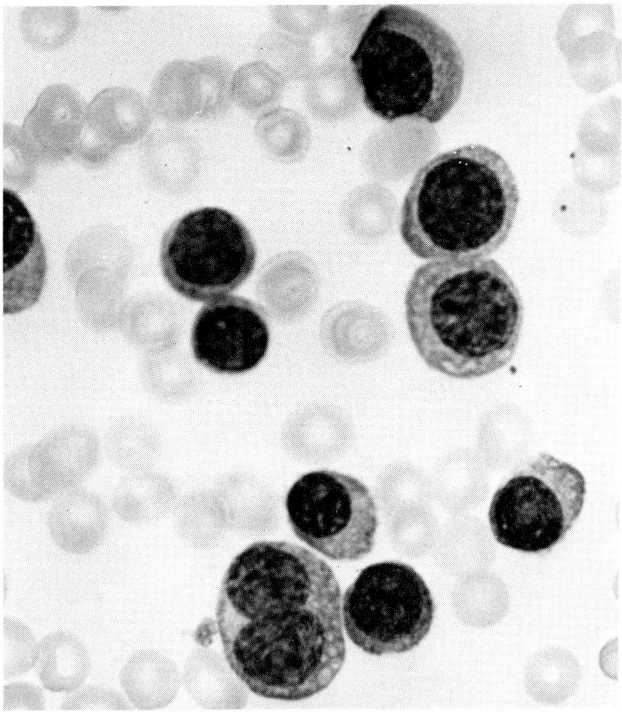

FIGURE 6. Peripheral blood smear in PCL. Immature plasma cells are seen.

were observed (Figure 6). Increased numbers of normoblasts, lymphocytes, and eosinophils were also noted. The platelet count was frequently reduced with a mean of 86,000/mm^3. The erythrocyte sedimentation rate was usually greatly increased, but occasionally was normal. The blood urea nitrogen level was elevated in 19 patients. Uric acid levels were high in eight patients. Serum calcium was normal in eight patients and high in seven others.

Proteins were studied in serum and/or urine in 54 of the 57 patients with PCL.[36] The total serum protein was more than 8.0 g% in 30 patients, normal in 13, slightly low in 8 and not stated in 6. Serum electrophoresis, performed in 43 patients, revealed a normal pattern in only 4. In 37 cases, spikes of M components of various mobility were observed. Hypogammaglobulinemia as the only abnormality was noted in two patients. All these findings are comparable to the frequency and distribution of M components in multiple myeloma. IEP was performed in a limited number of cases. A normal pattern was found in one, BJP in four, "paraproteinemia" in one, and IgG M component in two patients. In two cases IgE M component, and in another IgD/L, were reported. Cryoglobulin was demonstrated in 3 of 20 serum specimens examined. Rapid gelling of the serum was observed in two cases.

Proteinuria was found in two thirds of the patients, the Bence Jones heat test being positive in almost all of them. Altogether, 95% of the patients examined showed some serum and/or urine protein abnormality. This proportion is comparable to that reported in multiple myeloma.

Bone marrow was completely replaced by proliferating plasmacytes in 24 of the 57 patients. In the others a mean of 69% was observed with variations from 10 to 92%. Plasma cells were described as very immature, proplasmacytes, plasmablasts, etc. Some contained azurophilic granules in the cytoplasm, others were multinucleated,

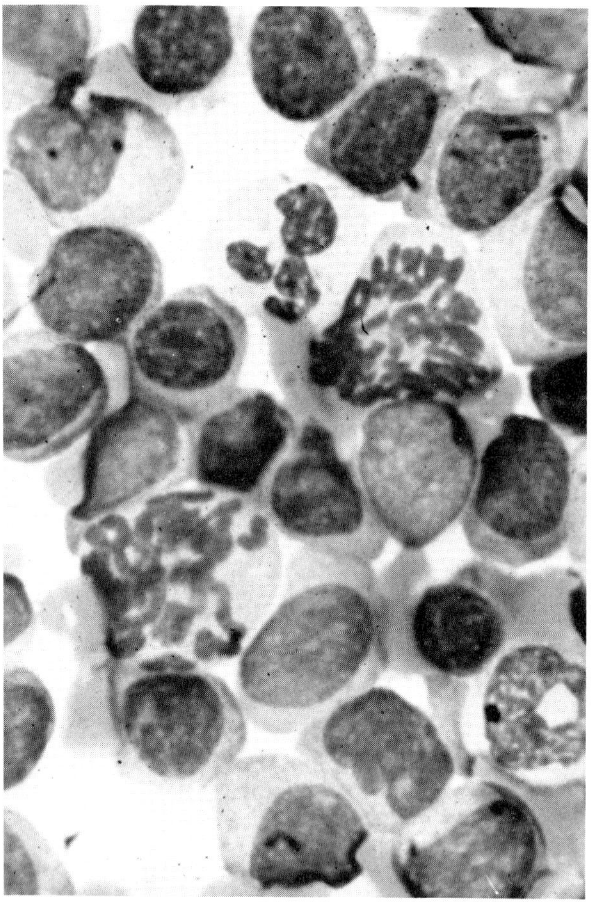

FIGURE 7. Bone marrow smear in PCL with many immature plasma cells and mitotic figures.

and many exhibited multiple mitoses or vacuoles (Figure 7). Rarely, the cells were lymphoid-like, or small and round, with basophilic cytoplasm. Usually the same cells were observed in both the peripheral blood and the bone marrow, but occasionally more mature forms were found in the latter. X-ray surveys of the skeleton were negative in 24 cases. Among 33 others with osteolytic lesions and/or osteoporosis, the skull, vertebrae, and ribs were the most frequently involved sites. The pelvis and bones of the extremities were less frequently involved.

Various chemotherapeutic agents were used in PCL. Remissions of 1 to 3 months were common and, in one patient, a remission of 18 months was noted. The average duration of the disease, from the onset of subjective complaints to death, was 4.8 months. The total duration of recognized disease ranged from 2 weeks to 2 years. The course of plasma cell leukemia, therefore, is usually rapid regardless of the therapy given, and the survival time does not seem to be related to the degree of anemia, number of peripheral white cells, percentage of plasmacytes, or the appearance of the bone marrow. Neither was there any correlation between the maturity of proliferating plasma cells or the type of M components produced and the course of the disease. However, the relatively small series does not permit one to draw firm conclusions.

Macroglobulinemia-Myeloma Double Gammopathy

More than 30 cases have been reported in which one of the M components was an IgM and the other belonged to either the IgG or IgA class.[52] The frequency of such double gammopathy, among patients with M components, is about 0.5%. IgM was present in the serum together with IgG in 17 patients and with IgA in 7 patients. The light chains of both M components were of the same type in 18 of these 24 cases: kappa in 14 and lambda in 4. In 6 other patients, either a combination of three M components or a whole immunoglobulin and a heavy chain disease protein were observed. Among 20 patients for whom the sex and age were stated, 12 were male and 8 were female. The age varied from 42 to 88 years, with a mean of 66.2

The clinical picture was described well in 21 patients. In only one patient was it that of multiple myeloma. Three patients had a solitary plasmacytoma, and one had plasma cell leukemia. In five patients, the clinical picture was compatible with MW. Two patients had lymphosarcoma. None of the others had definite clinical manifestations of a systemic malignant disease. Skin lesions, polyarthralgia, anemia, and chronic thyroiditis were observed. In some patients, osteolytic lesions were rather incidentally detected. One patient with low concentration of serum M component was clinically well.

Therefore, it would appear that the clinical picture in these patients is not directly related to the type or the concentration of the serum M components. In some patients, the clinical picture resembled a collagen or an autoimmune disease. It is possible that M components in these patients developed as a result of chronic antigenic stimulation and that they do not represent a malignant condition, per se.

Waldenström's Macroglobulinemia (MW)

MW is a malignant disease of B lymphocytes that produce IgM and retain a certain capacity to differentiate and mature into plasmacytes. Lymphocytes in MW can carry both IgM and IgD on the membrane.[1] It seems that MW occupies an intermediate position between multiple myeloma and chronic lymphocytic leukemia.

MW affects both sexes. In some series males have predominated, composing up to two thirds of the patients. Usually the patients are older than 50 years at the time of diagnosis; the average age in some series is 60 years. However, the disease may affect young people as well. It seems that some familial predisposition to this disease exists, since families with several cases of MW, and others with MW and IgM M components in several individuals, have been observed.[53]

The initial clinical manifestations are usually vague; weakness, fatigue, and weight loss are the most frequent (Table 16).[54,55] Bleeding and visual disturbances are common. Central or peripheral neurologic manifestations and, occasionally, psychiatric disorders may develop. Lymphadenopathy and hepatomegaly and/or splenomegaly have been found in more than 50% of patients. Ocular changes often seen are engorged, sausage-like veins and hemorrhages. Hyperviscosity syndrome and coma may occur. Rarer clinical manifestations, such as hemolysis, amyloidosis, malabsorption, and nephrotic syndrome, have also been described.

More than 70% of the patients have moderate to severe anemia. A very high erythrocyte sedimentation rate is common. The peripheral leukocyte count is usually normal; however, lymphocytosis has often been observed. In 20% of MW patients, thrombocytopenia has been found. Cryoglobulinemia or cryogelglobulinemia has been noted in 15% or more of patients and, in some, IgM pyroglobulins have been observed. Cold agglutinins, IgM/IgG cryocomplexes with rheumatoid factor activity, and false-positive VDRL reaction have also been described in MW.

Electrophoretic analysis of serum from these patients shows abnormal spikes of γ or β mobility, identified by IEP as IgM monoclonal proteins. The concentration of IgM in the serum usually exceeds 1000 mg/dℓ, and decreased concentrations of IgG

Table 16
MAIN CLINICAL MANIFESTATIONS AND LABORATORY DATA OF PATIENTS WITH MW[54,55]

Symptoms and signs	Patients (%)	Laboratory tests	Patients (%)
Fatigue, weakness, and/or weight loss	89	Anemia (<12.0 g/dℓ)	73
Musculoskeletal pain	16	Leukopenia (<3000) or (<5000)[a]	13;22.5[a]
Bleeding phenomena	44	Thrombocytopenia (<120,000)	20
Neurological manifestations	18	ESR ≥80	56
Psychiatric manifestations	4	ESR ≤5	7
Ocular changes	45	Azotemia (BUN > 25 mg/dℓ)	18
Hyperviscosity syndrome	21	Hypoalbuminemia (<3.5 g/dℓ)	47
Lymphadenopathy	36	Cryoglobulinemia	16
Hepatomegaly	66	Cold agglutinins (high titer)	18
Splenomegaly	46	Bence Jones proteinuria	71
		Hyperviscous serum (η rel ≥ 3.0)	70

[a] Taken from two series.

and IgA are often recorded. Usually the IgM is a pentameric 19S molecule. When IgM of low molecular weight is present in the serum, immunoquantitation plates show a higher concentration of IgM than that calculated from electrophoresis. In some cases, free light chains, IgM subunits and heavy-chain fragments of IgM have also been detected in MW. In one series, a disproportionately high concentration of IgM, calculated by immunoquantitation plates and indicating the presence of low molecular weight IgM, was observed in 49% of patients.[55] In a few instances, the concentration of an IgM M component calculated from electrophoresis exceeded greatly that calculated by immunoquantitation. In one such instance, an IgM/IgG complex was detected, and in another the serum was hyperviscous.

Bence Jones proteinuria is usually reported in one third of MW patients, but some investigators have detected it in almost all cases. In our series, more than 70% of the urine samples tested contained BJP (Figure 8).[55] Hyperviscous sera were observed in 11 of 19 patients (58%) in one series.[55] In another series, serum viscosity was elevated in 26 of 34 patients, but hyperviscosity syndrome was observed in 13 patients only.[54] In some patients with MW, abnormal chromosomes may be detected in the bone marrow and peripheral leukocytes. Poor response of peripheral blood lymphocytes to mitogenic stimulation by phytohemagglutinin has also been reported.

Bone marrow is usually infiltrated by plasma cells, lymphocytes, intermediate forms, and, occasionally, mast cells. Lymph nodes and other organs are often infiltrated as well, and the pattern may then resemble that of lymphoma. Kidney tissue studied by biopsy and immunofluorescence showed deposits of IgM on the endothelial aspect of the basement membrane. Nephrotic syndrome, with deposits of an IgM/IgG/C3 complex in the kidneys, has also been reported.

Differentiation of MW from malignant lymphoma may be difficult. Development of lymphosarcoma, reticulum cell sarcoma, or chronic lymphocytic leukemia, in the course of MW, has been well documented. In one study, 50 of 360 patients with MW (14%) had lymphomatous tumors in various organs such as bones, lungs, skin, and brain.[56] Nonlymphoplasmacytic malignant tumors have been noted in 8 to 12% of patients with MW. In some, multiple tumors have been observed. In one series of 40 patients with MW, 22 had another neoplasm during life; in more than 50%, the second tumor originated in lymphoid tissue.[54] Chronic cold-agglutinin syndrome may be associated with MW. Several patients with IgM M components were found to have plasmacytic, rather than lymphocytic, infiltration in the bone marrow, and osteolytic le-

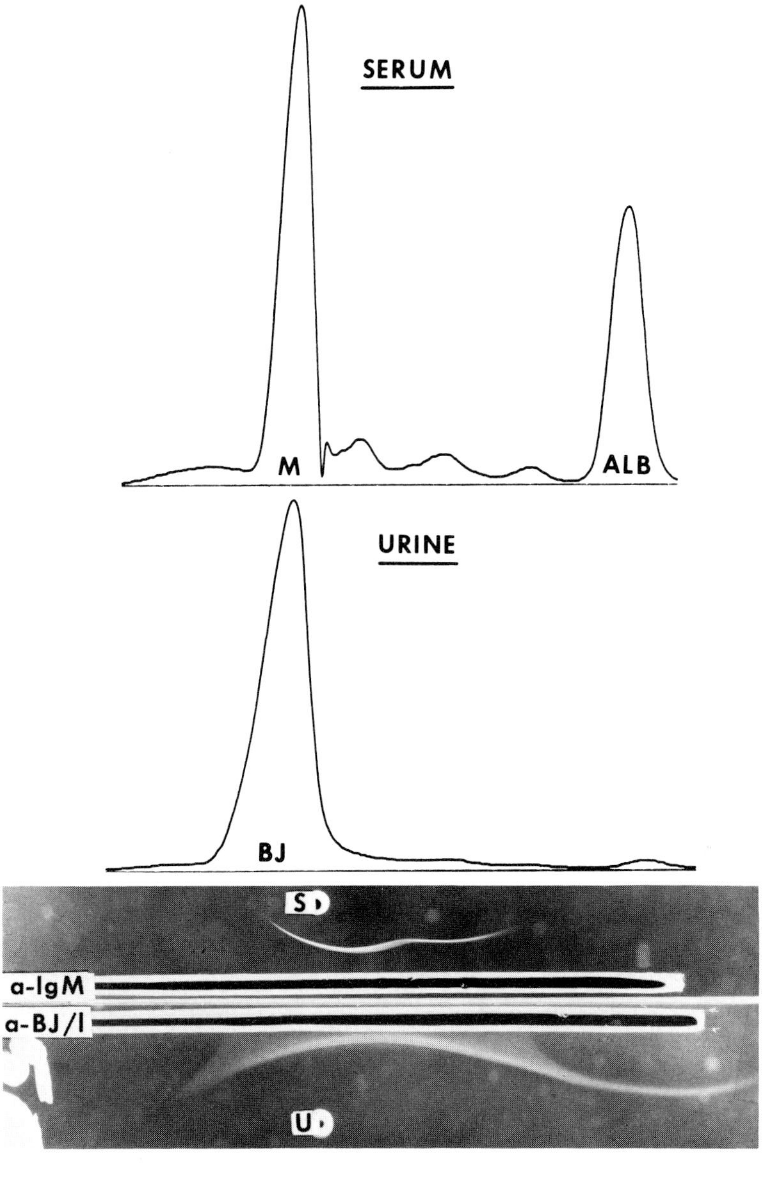

FIGURE 8. Electropherogram of serum and urine proteins in MW. Bimodal pattern of precipitation line in the serum immunoelectropherogram corresponds to IgM of at least two molecular weights — normal (19S) and low.

sions. They were considered to have IgM myeloma.[57] In some instances, however, biopsy of the lytic lesions revealed lymphosarcoma cells and not plasmacytoma.[54]

Patients with MW are usually treated with steroids, chlorambucil, cyclophosphamide, melphalan, and other chemotherapeutic agents in various combinations. Hyperviscosity syndrome and cryoglobulinemia, or cryogelglobulinemia, respond favorably to plasmapheresis. The rate of infection in MW is much lower than that in multiple myeloma.

The clinical course is variable. Asymptomatic, delayed-progressive, and progressive forms of macroglobulinemia, or, alternatively, benign and malignant forms have been described. The classification into one of these forms may depend on the time the patient is examined during the course of the disease. Most patients survive for a long time. Survival times of a group of 68 patients ranged from 2 to 10 years. In another series of ten treated patients, the mean survival time was 55 months from appearance of the first symptom and 34 months from time of diagnosis. Favorable response to chlorambucil was stressed by the authors. In one series, no relapses were observed in patients treated with chlorambucil, but all the patients whose treatment was discontinued had relapses, and the authors suggested that chlorambucil be continued indefinitely.

When treated with chemotherapeutic agents, patients may be divided into responders and nonresponders. In one series the criteria of response were (1) 50% decrease in IgM serum concentrations; (2) reduction in serum viscosity to an asymptomatic value; and (3) 50% reduction in the size of lymph nodes, liver, and spleen. According to these criteria, remission was achieved in only 40% of their patients. The mean survival time in the responders group was 49.2 months and in the nonresponders 24.1 months.[54]

In our series, the mean survival time from the time of diagnosis was 49.5 months for the patients who died, and 43 months for those who are still being followed up.[55] Shorter survival time seemed to be related to the appearance of azotemia, hypoalbuminemia, and abnormal liver function, but not to the presence of anemia, serum concentration of IgM, or Bence Jones proteinuria. Death is usually due to severe anemia, bleeding, cryopathy, coma, or infection. Terminal leukemia has been observed in several patients.

Viscosity, Hyperviscosity and Hyperviscosity Syndrome

Blood viscosity is related to the synergistic interaction of plasma and cellular elements. Viscosity, as a property of fluid to resist flow, is influenced by several factors such as the concentration and intrinsic viscosity of individual proteins in solution, number of cellular elements, and their resistance to the deformation (sickle cells, spherocytosis), and others.[58,59]

In relation to the immunoglobulin system, the measurement of viscosity is especially important because of the so-called hyperviscosity syndrome (Table 17) that may complicate various plasmalymphocytic diseases. Hyperviscosity syndrome usually occurs when the relative viscosity of plasma (or serum) (η rel) exceeds four units; however, there is no direct correlation between the viscosity units and the severity of the clinical manifestations. One of the reasons may be that whole blood viscosity is different from the fluid phase viscosity and depends on the cellular elements as well. Another factor may be the individual resistance of the vascular wall to the flow of the hyperviscous fluid.

Hyperviscosity syndrome has been observed mainly in MW.[54,55] In some series, over 30% of the patients presented with clinical manifestations of hyperviscosity.[54] It also occurs in IgG[60] and IgA myeloma,[61] lymphomas with M components, mainly of IgM class, and in collagen-vascular diseases with high concentration of immune complexes, especially of the intermediate type.[62]

In MW the concentration of IgM need not be very high to cause hyperviscosity. Levels of 3 to 4 g/dℓ of IgM were found to be associated with the syndrome.[54,55] In multiple myeloma, hyperviscosity usually develops when the concentration of IgG M component exceeds 5.0 g/dℓ.[60] The majority of hyperviscous IgG and IgM M components were found to be euglobulins giving a positive Sia precipitation test,[63] and some were cryoprecipitable. In IgA myeloma and in other diseases with hyperviscosity, an interaction of the M components with coagulation factors and with the platelets has been recorded and was found to lead to various bleeding and clotting abnormalities.

Measurement of viscosity is a simple procedure, if properly performed. The Ostwald viscosimeter, based on the falling-ball principle, is one of the most popular tools be-

Table 17
CLINICAL PICTURE OF THE HYPERVISCOSITY SYNDROME[a]

Subjective
- Weakness, fatigue, anorexia

Hematologic
- Bleeding, especially from nose, gums, and surgical or traumatic cuts, gastrointestinal, urinary, or genital tract

Ocular
- Sausage-like engorged veins, retinal hemorrhages, occasionally papilledema, retinal vein thrombosis, visual disturbances, blindness

Neurologic
- Dizziness, headaches, seizures, somnolence, stupor, coma; nystagmus, cerebrovascular accidents; EEG changes of a diffuse and occasionally focal type; Hearing loss

Psychiatric
- Confusion, personality changes, "neurotic" or occasionally "psychotic manifestations"

Cardiovascular
- Congestive heart failure, usually digitalis-resistant
- Increased plasma volume
- Raynaud's-like vasospastic phenomena
- Arterial occlusions

Renal
- Glomerular deposits of immunoglobulins?
- Impaired acidification?
- Proximal tubular dysfunction?

[a] The patients may present with only one or a few clinical manifestations.

Modified from Fahey, J. L., Barth, W. F., and Solomon, A., *JAMA*, 192, 120, 1965. With permission. Copyright 1965, American Medical Association.

cause of its low price, simplicity, short time required for measurement, and reproducibility. Its disadvantages are that no shear-rate-dependent viscosity can be measured, and when whole blood is used, the technique becomes cumbersome. For more accurate shear-related measurements, the so-called rotating disc viscosimeter should be used. For example, the Wells-Brookfield synchrolectric microviscometer (Brookfield Engineering Lab, Inc., Stoughton, Mass.) is well equipped to test shear-related, temperature-controlled viscosity of biological fluids.

Hyperviscosity syndrome is often life-threatening and requires prompt therapy. Plasmapheresis, performed with either individual plastic bags or with a cell separator, is the procedure of choice. It should be carefully monitored by repeat measurements of plasma (or whole blood) viscosity. Red blood cells should be returned to the patient and often supplemented by red blood cell transfusions, appropriately diluted with physiological fluids and/or normal plasma. In the case of concomitant cryoglobulinemia, one should be careful to separate red blood cells of the patient at 37°C before returning them to the circulation.

Cryoglobulinemia

The term cryoglobulinemia denotes a group of conditions in which one or more of serum proteins precipitate, gel, or crystallize (Figure 9), in vitro, at temperatures below

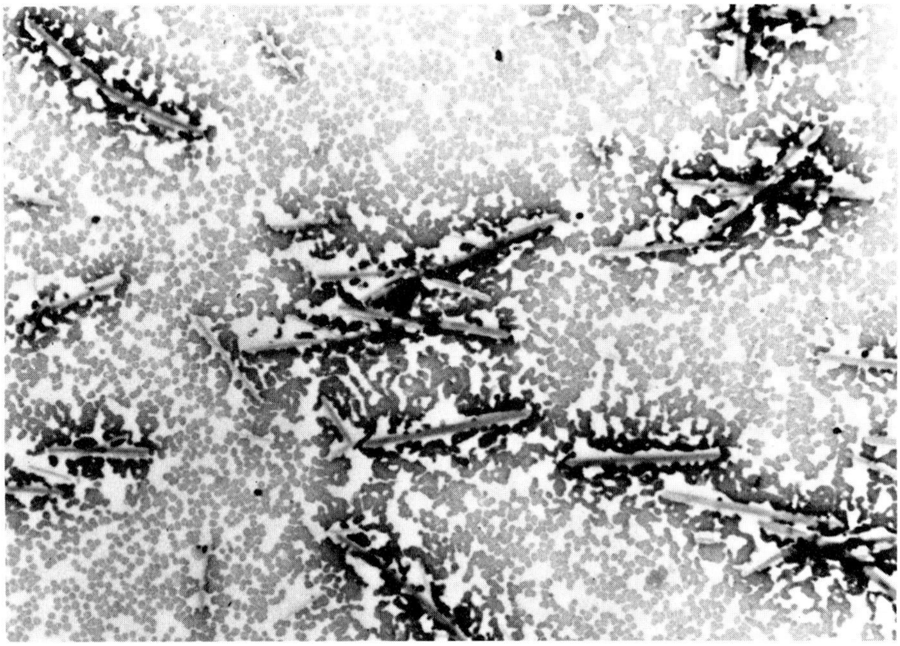

FIGURE 9. Needle-shape crystals of IgG cryocrystalglobulin detected in the peripheral blood smear.

that of the human body. Thus the terms of cryoprecipitation, cryogelation, and cryocrystallization are used, respectively, to describe these phenomena.[64,65] Cases of cryoglobulinemia differ in regard to the temperature at which the process starts, concentration of the precipitate (gel, crystals), optimum pH, and ionic strength at which the maximal amount of the material precipitates (gels, crystallizes). From the viewpoint of the immunochemical structure, cryoglobulins may be divided into monoclonal and mixed. The former are composed of a homogeneous immunoglobulin, whereas the latter usually represent immune complexes with or without additional plasma proteins. In the homogeneous group IgM/K cryoglobulins are the most common; however, cryoprecipitable (or gelling, crystallizing) IgM/λ, IgG's (especially γ3), IgA's, and BJP's have also been described. In the group of immune cryocomplexes, the most common are IgM/IgG and IgG/IgG complexes. However, many others such as IgA/IgG, IgM/IgA/IgG, or IgG/Lp have been described.[66] Cryocomplexes occasionally exhibit biological activity such as cold agglutination of the red blood cells, rheumatoid factor activity, positive VDRL, and others. Occasionally, fibrinogen, α_2-macroglobulin, DNA, various components of complement, or lipids coprecipitate with cryoproteins. The significance of such coprecipitation is unknown.

From the clinical standpoint, monoclonal cryoglobulinemia occurs most often in plasmalymphocytic neoplastic disorders (MW, multiple myeloma, chronic cold agglutinin disease), or presents as an "essential" disorder. The latter may eventually develop into a more obvious plasmalymphocytic neoplasia. Mixed cryocomplexes occur in collagen-vascular diseases, autoimmune disorders, Peetoom-Meltzer syndrome (arthralgia purpura-weakness syndrome), infections, membranous glomerulonephritis, occasionally in malignant diseases, and others.[66] Clinical manifestations of cryoglobulinemia include cold intolerance, Raynaud's phenomena, purpura, vasculopathy with skin ulcerations and gangrene, retinal hemorrhages, bleeding tendency, thrombotic phenomena such as cerebral vessels thrombosis, and temperature-related hyperviscosity (Figure 10). In the so-called Peetoom-Meltzer syndrome (purpura-weakness-polyar-

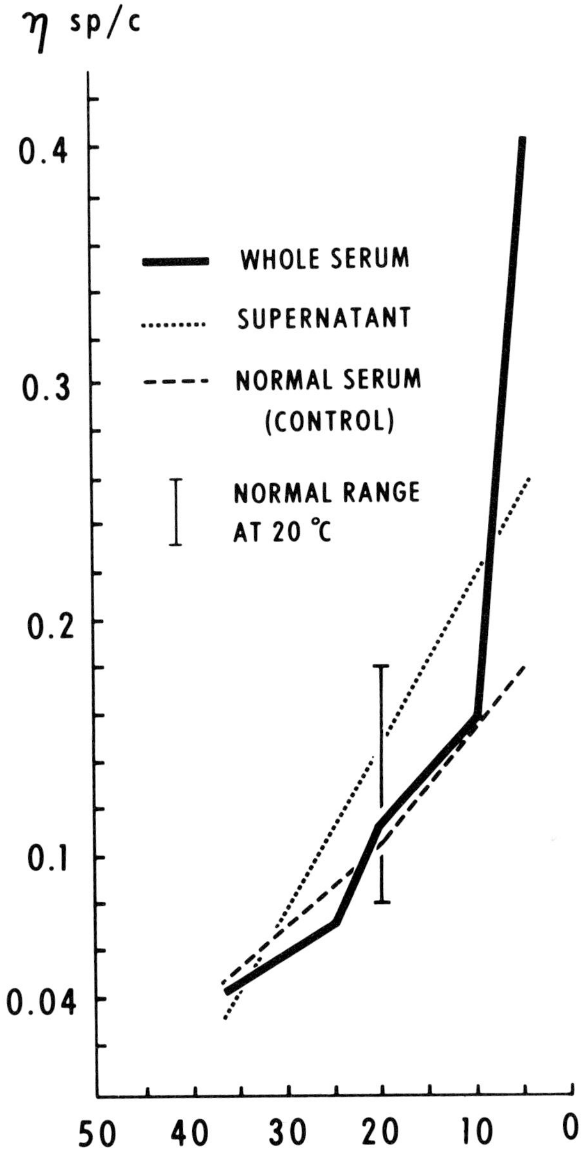

FIGURE 10. Temperature-related serum hyperviscosity in a case of cryoglobulinemia.

thralgia syndrome), pain, stiffness, and swelling of the joints, hepatic involvement with abnormal liver functions, glomerulitis with impaired renal functions, neurological manifestations, and involvement of other organs have been described. In this syndrome cryoprecipitable immune complexes of IgM/IgG or IgG/IgG type have usually been found.[66] Cold urticaria may develop during the course of cryoglobulinemia and may be passively transferred to a healthy donor by the patient's serum or by purified cryoglobulin. Mast cell degranulation occurs and is mediated by activation of C_4 and C_3 on rewarming. Often, anemia, elevated sedimentation rate, rouleaux formation, and so-called cryoglobulin-inclusion cells (Figure 11) are observed in cryoglobulinemia.

The detection of cryoglobulin is simple, if the procedure is properly performed. The blood should be withdrawn into a warm syringe and the tubes should be immersed

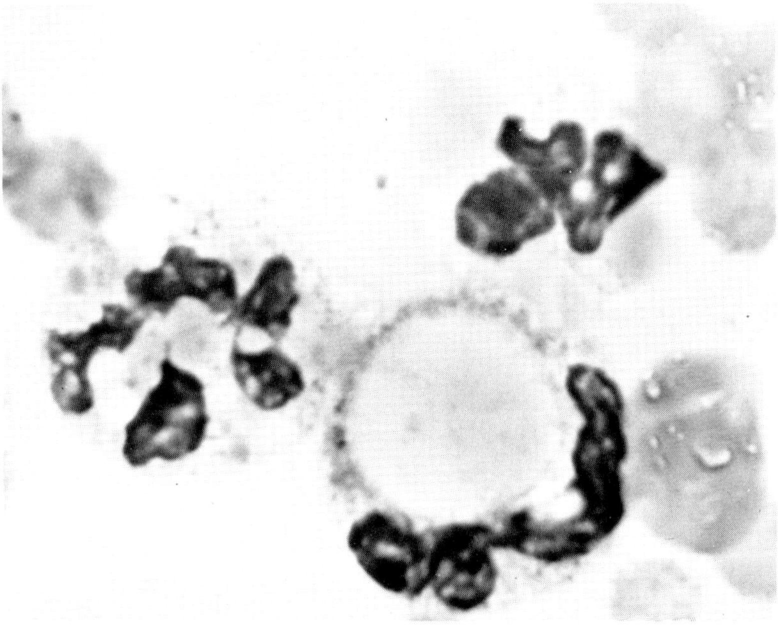

FIGURE 11. Cryoglobulin inclusion cells in the peripheral blood smear in a patient with cryoglobulinemia.

immediately in a 37°C water bath, or put in an incubator. After clotting, the serum is quickly separated and held at 4°C for at least 1 week. Occasionally, a very slow cryoprecipitation (gelling, crystallization) may be observed, starting after 3 to 5 days of cooling. Cryoprecipitation may be enhanced by mild acidification of the serum. Cryocrit (percent of cryoglobulin) may be estimated by using calibrated tubes.

Treatment of cryoglobulinemia should primarily be directed against the underlying condition. However, if severe, cryoglobulin-related, clinical manifestations develop, plasmapheresis is the therapy of choice. In isolated cases, penicillamine, antihistaminics, colchicine, steroids, immunosuppressants, and other agents have been used with variable results.

Cold-Reacting Autoantibodies

Cold Agglutinins

Cold agglutinins[67] are antibodies that agglutinate red cells most strongly (or only) at temperatures below that of the human body. Cold autoagglutinins are assigned I specificity when they react more strongly with the red cells of adults than with those of infants (umbilical cord cells). Conversely, i specificity is assigned when the agglutinin reacts more strongly with cord cells than with adult cells. Specificities, such as Pr and several others, have been described as well. The serum of healthy adults and infants contains low titer IgM auto-anti-I. This antibody reacts only at low temperatures and probably does not interact with red cells in vivo even at the moderately low temperatures of the blood in small skin vessels. Thus this cold agglutinin, present in almost all normal subjects, is active as an autoantibody, in vitro only.

Cold agglutinins, active at dilutions up to several million at 4°C, are found in some patients with chronic cold hemagglutinin disease or lymphoreticular neoplasms. Antibodies, developing in association with mycoplasma pneumonia (anti-I) or infectious mononucleosis (anti-i), are usually present in much lower titer. That some of the latter

Table 18
DISEASES ASSOCIATED WITH COLD AGGLUTININS

Polyclonal cold agglutinins	Monoclonal cold agglutinins
Mycoplasma pneumonia	Chronic cold hemagglutinin disease
Infectious mononucleosis	MW
Cytomegalovirus infection	Hodgkin's and non-Hodgkin's lymphoma
Subacute bacterial endocarditis	CLL
Listeriosis	Plasmacytoma and multiple myeloma
Mumps orchitis	Chronic myelogeneous leukemia
Syphilis	Kaposi's sarcoma
Tropical diseases (trypanosomiasis, malaria, tropical eosinophilia)	Severe combined immunodeficiency[a]
	Mycoplasma pneumonia (rare)
Collagen-vascular and immune complex diseases	
Angioimmunoblastic lymphadenopathy	

[a] In association with a leukemia-like B lymphocyte proliferation.
Modified from Pruzanski, W. and Shumak, K. H.

Reprinted, by permission from *The New England Journal of Medicine,* 297, 538, 1977.

patients can have hemolytic anemia illustrates the critical importance of thermal amplitude.

Cold agglutinins that occur in some infections, e.g., mycoplasma pneumonia, are usually immunochemically heterogeneous (Table 18). Most often, diffuse hypergammaglobulinemia is detected, and immunoelectrophoretic analysis of eluates from red cells, which have been incubated with cold agglutinin, reveals heterogeneous IgM with both kappa and lambda light chains. However, in a few patients with mycoplasma pneumonia, the antibody manifested restricted electrophoretic heterogeneity. In contrast, in chronic cold hemagglutinin disease, serum electrophoresis usually reveals a narrow γ or β band, and IEP detects monoclonal IgM. Cold agglutinins with anti-I specificity almost invariably have kappa light chains, whereas cold agglutinins with anti-i specificity usually have lambda light chains.[68]

Although most cold agglutinins are IgM's, IgA and IgG cold agglutinins have also been found in patients with chronic cold hemagglutinin disease. The cold agglutinins in patients with infectious mononucleosis have been reported to be IgG or mixed IgG-IgM. Complexes eluted from the red cells were composed of incomplete anti-i (or anti-I) IgG antibody, which could react with the red cells only by complexing with anti-IgG IgM. Similar IgM/IgG cold agglutinins were observed in angioimmunoblastic lymphadenopathy.

Most, if not all, monoclonal cold agglutinins are found in patients with lymphoreticular neoplasms. The underlying cellular proliferation may be very slowly progressive, as in classical, chronic cold hemagglutinin disease (CHAD), or rapid, as in reticulum cell sarcoma.

CHAD is probably a variant of MW, in which the IgM M component has cold agglutinin activity. No histological features distinguish CHAD from MW. In CHAD, cold agglutinins usually have I specificity, whereas in other lymphoproliferative neoplasms in which cold agglutinins are observed, either anti-I or anti-i can occur. In either case, the cold agglutinins cause variable degrees of chronic hemolytic anemia, with acute exacerbations related to cold exposure.

Except for the occasional occurrence of hyperviscosity syndrome resulting from a high M-protein concentration, all other clinical manifestations related to cold agglutinins are dependent on exposure to cold. As blood flows through the capillaries of the skin and subcutaneous tissue, its temperature falls to as low as 28°C, if the ambient temperature is low. If the cold antibody is active at these temperatures, it agglutinates the cells and fixes complement. The agglutinates obstruct the circulation and result in acrocyanosis. The toes, ear lobes, and tip of the nose, as well as the fingers, may be affected. Gangrene of these areas occurs infrequently, only because the agglutination is rapidly reversible on warming.

In patients with cold agglutinins, anemia is often mild because of C3B inactivator, which is present in the blood. The number of cells that hemolyse is related to the rate of fixation of C3. With cold stress, the capacity of C3B inactivator is exceeded, and red cells with C3B on their surface are either rosetted and phagocytosed, or, after fixation of the remaining complement components, are lysed, resulting in hemoglobinemia and hemoglobinuria.

The important principle of management of a patient with cold agglutinin disease is the maintenance of an ambient temperature, above the maximum temperature at which his antibody reacts. In this way, one can almost always prevent the attachment of antibody to the patient's red cells.

If the antibody has a high thermal amplitude, warming of the patient is insufficient to prevent hemolysis. Such patients pose difficult therapeutic problems. Administration of steroids and/or splenectomy are less useful than in patients with warm antibody autoimmune hemolytic anemia. Immunosuppressive agents such as chlorambucil are sometimes beneficial, but they are of no value in an acute condition.

Blood transfusions should be used only when severe anemia develops, since transfused cells not protected by C3d are more susceptible to lysis than the patient's own cells. Washed, packed red cells only should be transfused. Crossmatching, in the presence of high thermal amplitude cold agglutinins, should be done strictly at 37°C to avoid reactions due to the autoantibody, and thus allow the detection of red cell alloantibodies. During blood transfusion, it is safer to warm the patient than the blood.

Another procedure, which may be used in life-threatening hemolysis, is plasmapheresis to quickly remove significant quantities of antibody. The problem, peculiar to plasmapheresing patients with cold agglutinins, is that once the blood is removed from the patient, massive agglutination may make the procedure technically impossible. However, plasmapheresis can be successfully carried out by using a blood warmer to keep the blood at 37°C as it is being withdrawn from the patient. It is then possible to centrifuge the blood at room temperature, remove the plasma (containing most of the antibody), rewarm the cells to 37°C with the blood warmer, and return the cells to the patient.

It has recently been discovered that cold agglutinins react with Ii antigens on the membrane of many types of normal and neoplastic cells, in addition to red cells. In vitro, in the presence of complement, the interaction of cold agglutinins with these cells leads to their death and sometimes to lysis. Cold agglutinins were found to be cytotoxic to normal human T and B lymphocytes, polymorphonuclears, macrophages, and monocytes. Cold agglutinins also agglutinate platelets in the cold. Cytotoxic activity of cold agglutinins has also been detected against lymphoblasts, chronic lymphocytic leukemia cells, myeloblasts, and some neoplastic cells.

Cold Cytotoxins Reacting with Antigens not Detectable on Red Cells

Antibodies, different from cold agglutinins cytotoxic to human lymphocytes in vitro, have been detected in collagen vascular diseases and malignancy, in renal transplant recipients, and even in healthy individuals after immunization. Some of these cytotoxins are warm antibodies, but the majority react optimally, or only, in the cold.[67]

Cold lymphocytotoxins (CLC) are found in up to 90% of patients with systemic lupus erythematosus (SLE). Some authors reported preferential reactivity of CLC with thymic lymphocytes and poor reactivity with lymphocytes from patients with B lymphocyte CLL. Others observed that CLC in SLE sera killed B and T lymphocytes equally as well, but separate B- and T-cell specificities were found in some of these sera. The cytotoxicity of CLC from patients with SLE appears to be unrelated to HLA antigens.

Most CLC in SLE are IgM antibodies, but some are IgG. IgM CLC, detected in cryoprecipitates from SLE sera, were found to be different from IgM anti-IgG antibody.

CLC have also been detected in other collagen diseases including rheumatoid arthritis, scleroderma, and polymyositis. Similar antibodies have been found in the serum of some patients with pernicious anemia. CLC are not rare in dysproteinemia. In some cases, the CLC were of the same immunoglobulin class as the M component.

Cold-reacting cytotoxins, to polymorphonuclear leukocytes and monocytes, have been found in the serum of some patients with rheumatoid arthritis, Felty's syndrome, and SLE. The majority of these sera were also cytotoxic to lymphocytes.

γ-Heavy Chain Disease (HCD)

γ-HCD is a neoplastic disease of B-lineage lymphocytes that synthesize IgG Fc fragment-related γ-HCD protein.[69,70] Clinically, it presents as a lymphoma-like condition, with frequent infections and a high incidence of autoimmune phenomena. About 40 patients have been reported to date. Available clinical material indicates that males predominate 1.7:1, and that the mean age at the onset is about 57 years, ranging from 9 years to 76 years. Only five patients younger than 30 years have been reported. The onset has been insidious in about 60%, and abrupt in 40%, of the patients. Fever is very common (75%) and is often associated with malaise, tiredness, weakness, dyspnea, and bleeding. Frequent infections have been recorded in two thirds of the patients. Physical examination shows peripheral and internal lymphadenopathy in almost all patients, whereas hepatomegaly and splenomegaly were recorded in over 70%. Swollen, soft palate and/or uvula were observed in 40%.

Rheumatoid arthritis, systemic lupus erythematosus, thyroiditis, Sjögren's syndrome, myasthenia gravis, hemolytic anemia, and pulmonary fibrosis were observed in some patients with γ-HCD. Amyloidosis was recorded in only two patients. In a few patients, active tuberculosis preceeded the onset of the disease. Only one patient had osteolytic lesions with hypercalcemia, and another had high serum calcium and normal bones.

Anemia (usually normochromic, normocytic) was noted in all patients and in more than 60% was accompanied by high erythrocyte sedimentation rate, leukopenia, and lymphocytosis. Atypical lymphocytes and/or immature plasma cells were observed in peripheral blood smears from more than 70% of the patients. Eosinophilia was recorded in 30% and thrombocytopenia in 45%. Two patients presented with terminal plasma cell leukemia. Hyperuricemia developed in 57% of the patients. Renal function tests were usually normal. Bone marrow showed, in 70% of patients, increased concentration of often abnormal-looking lymphocytes and/or plasma cells. However, normal marrow, erythroid, or myeloid hyperplasia have also been observed.

The total serum protein was almost always normal, but albumin was often low.

Serum electropherograms showed hypogammaglobulinemia in 80% of patients. In addition, an M component, usually of β mobility, was observed in 67% of patients. IEP, using anti-IgG or anti-Fc antisera (but not anti-Fab or others) invariably showed an abnormal IgG-related precipitation line, usually of faster (anodal) than normal IgG mobility. Special immunochemical studies have shown that γ-HCD protein has a large deletion in the heavy chain, starting near the amino-terminal end, and a complete deletion of light chains. Analytical ultracentrifugation showed that the sedimentation-coefficient varies in individual cases from $S_{20,w}$ – 2.8 to 4.1, and molecular weight ranges from 45,000 to 69,000 daltons. γ_1 Subclass was the most common among γ-HCD proteins, but γ_3 subclass was more often observed than γ_2.

Proteinuria was detected in half of the patients, and with the notable exception of one patient, Bence Jones proteinuria has not been encountered. γ-HCD protein is very commonly detected in the urine, in concentrations reaching 20 g per day.

Most patients with γ-HCD have lower than normal concentrations of IgG, IgA, and IgM. Poor antibody response to bacterial antigens, lymphocytotoxic antibodies, abnormal responsiveness to mitogen stimulation and in mixed-leukocyte culture, and impaired cell-mediated immunity with negative skin-testing responses were recorded in the patients with γ-HCD.

Lymph nodes and other organs and tissues were infiltrated by a mixture of lymphocytes, plasmacytoid lymphocytes, plasma cells, eosinophils, and reticulum cells. Occasionally, the histological picture resembled that of malignant lymphoma. Biosynthetic studies have shown that γ HCD is synthesized by lymphocytic cells and is not a product of postsynthetic degradation. Normal karyotype was observed in a few investigated patients.

Therapy for γ-HCD is neither uniform nor standardized. Various chemotherapeutic agents such as cyclophosphamide, melphalan, vincristine, nitrogen mustard, procarbazine, and steroids were used, in various combinations, with or without spleen or lymph node irradiation. Remissions, with decrease in the size of the involved organs, have been observed in some patients, but a tendency towards spontaneous waxing and waning of the enlarged lymph nodes has also been observed.

In the fatal cases, the duration of life from diagnosis ranges from 3 weeks to several years; infections are the most common cause of death. The mean survival time from the first symptom was 28.5 months (for 24 patients) and a little over 21 months from the diagnosis (for 20 patients).

α-Heavy Chain Disease (HCD)

α-HCD is a plasmalymphocytic, proliferative disorder in which neoplastic B-lineage lymphocytes synthesize α-heavy chain related protein.[71] Two clinical forms have been described. The common, digestive form, has been reported in about 100 patients, and the rare respiratory form was observed in three patients only. The disease usually starts in the second or third decade of life and has mainly been observed in geographical areas where hygiene is poor and there is a high degree of intestinal infestation. Most of the patients originated from North Africa, the Middle East, South America, southern Europe, and occasionally the Far East.

The main, clinical manifestations were chronic diarrhea with severe malabsorption and steatorrhea, abdominal pain, vomiting, and weight loss. Ascites, swollen mesenteric nodes, clubbing, signs of hypopotassemia, and hypocalcemic tetany have also been described, as well as signs of protein-loosing enteropathy, hypoalbuminemia, and anemia. Occasionally, a prodromal period lasting for years and simulating the irritable colon, preceeded the full-blown clinical picture.

More than half of the patients presented with anemia, two thirds had low potassium, and about 40% had hypoalbuminemia. Alkaline phosphatase was often elevated. Jejunal bacterial overgrowth was very common and giardia lamblia was detected in about one fourth of the patients. Serum electropherograms often showed low albumin and low γ-globulin. When the α-HCD protein was present in sufficient concentration, a broad α_2- or β-mobility band was observed. IEP detected an abnormal precipitation line of α_2-β mobility when anti-IgA antiserum was used. The diagnosis was made by a specific antiserum to Fab α portion, which recognizes IgA-related protein only when the light chains are present. α-HCD protein was invariably of α_1 subclass and appeared as a diamer of 3-4S, often in conjunction with heavier polymers. The urine may contain some α-HCD protein, and characteristically there was no Bence Jones proteinuria. High concentration of α-HCD protein, bound to a secretory chain (it also contains J chain), has been detected in the jejunal fluid. Deletion of the variable and first constant region of α_1 chain, and absence of the light chains, are the main structural defects of α-HCD protein.

Radiologically, α-HCD presented with hypertrophy of the small intestinal folds and strictures, and filling defects. The pathologic picture showed nodular formation and thickening of mucosa in the small intestine, predominantly in the duodenum and jejunum. Histologically, massive infiltration of the intestinal wall by lymphocytes, immunoblasts, plasma cells, and macrophages was observed.

The course of the disease is either continuous-progressive or with exacerbation and partial remissions. In most cases, steroids, chemotherapeutic agents, and cobalt irradiation were used in various combinations and led to transient and incomplete remissions. Complete remissions were documented in a few patients treated by chemotherapy or solely with tetracycline. Autopsy occasionally shows truly malignant lymphoma in the intestinal wall and/or the mesenteric lymph nodes.

μ-Heavy Chain Disease (HCD)

μ-HCD was first described in a patient with chronic lymphocytic leukemia,[72] and 12 additional cases have since been reported.[73] The true incidence of μ-HCD is unknown.

μ-HCD was reported in eight men and five women, ranging in age from 37 to 80 years. More than half of them suffered from a malignant lymphoproliferative disorder, six having CLL and one having reticulum cell sarcoma. One patient presented with rheumatoid-like amyloid arthropathy and other manifestations of widespread amyloidosis, and another had carpal tunnel syndrome caused by amyloidosis.

The course of the disease was variable. Survival has varied from 3 months to 19 years after the onset of symptoms. One patient presented with persistent proteinuria and had vacuolated plasma cells in the bone marrow, 10 years prior to the development of chronic lymphocytic leukemia and 12 years before dying of malignant histiocytoma. Five patients were treated with steroids, with or without chlorambucil, and two had splenic irradiation. One patient has received intermittent courses of prednisone with melphalan and cyclophosphamide, with no evidence of clinical response.

Immunochemical diagnosis of μ-HCD is difficult. Serum electrophoresis in patients with μ-HCD shows either a normal pattern, or some elevation of α_1-α_2 area. In three patients, small M components were observed and attributed to the presence of BJP. IgG and IgA concentrations were low in six of eight patients. Immunoquantitation plates failed to quantitate μ-HCD protein, since a diffuse, hazy area of precipitation was usually observed. Thus the picture may be interpreted as hypogammaglobulinemia and/or light chains disease, the correct diagnosis is made by IEP, using specific anti-μ and anti-light chains antisera.

BJP's, all of kappa type, were detected by serum IEP in six patients with μ-HCD. Invariably BJP was of slower mobility than μ-HCD protein, except in one case in which a bimodal pattern was noted. In one patient, an IgA M component was also found. Bence Jones proteinuria was detected in eight patients, seven of kappa and one of lambda type. Small quantities of μ-HCD protein were found in the urine of one patient.

Bone marrow usually showed lymphocytosis, with a peculiar vacuolization of the neoplastic lymphocytes. Lymphoplasmacytic infiltration of the lymph nodes and the spleen, and periportal lymphocytic infiltration of the liver, have also been noted. In two patients, an immunofluorescence study of the bone marrow showed that the cytoplasm of plasma cells contained both μ- and κ-chain antigenic determinants. In another case, double labeling of bone marrow cells showed membrane-bound μ antigenic determinants, but not light chain determinants, and the cytoplasm contained μ chains only. In one case, bone marrow cells cultured in vitro were found to synthesize a μ-HCD fragment of 55,000 daltons. The fragment was detected intracellularly and secreted as disulfide-linked polymers. No light chains bound to the μ-HCD fragment were detected.

The mechanism of production of μ-HCD protein is not clear. The presence of light chains in the cells, producing μ-HCD protein, suggests that light chains are available for assembly, but are not used. The failure to assemble may be caused by a deficiency of structured features in the μ chains themselves, which are required for assembly. Such a deficiency in the μ chains would be consistent with the evidence that the chains of μ-HCD protein are smaller than normal μ chains.

Partial structural studies of μ-HCD fragments were performed in two cases. In one, a polymer with S_{20w} value up to 11.5S and a molecular weight of 365,000 daltons was detected. Sequence studies of the amino terminal end of the μ-HCD protein implied complete deletion of the F $(ab')_2$ μ fragment.[36] Another μ-HCD fragment of 55,000 daltons had a deletion of only 130 amino acid residues from the amino-terminal end. It seems, therefore, that the structure of various μ-HCD proteins may be different, with deletions occurring in different positions of the heavy chain.

Immunoglobulin-Related Amyloidosis

Until a few years ago, amyloidosis[74,75] was defined as a chronic, usually irreversible condition in which amorphous, congo red-positive, green birefringent material was deposited in various organs and tissues. Electron microscope studies have shown that amyloid is composed of more or less characteristic fibrils, mixed with ring-shaped elements called P component.

Amyloidosis was labeled "secondary" if it developed following chronic infections, rheumatoid arthritis, chronic liver diseases, etc. When no underlying condition could be found, it was labeled as a "primary generalized amyloidosis" (PGA). Differences in the organ distribution between the primary and the secondary varieties have been noted, with more common involvement of the heart, nerves, tongue, skin, and joints in the latter, and of the kidneys, liver, and spleen in the former variety. However, marked overlapping in the organ distribution prompted some investigators to introduce the term "mixed pattern". These and other clinical varieties of amyloidosis are tabulated in Table 19.

In the last few years, substantial knowledge of the immunochemical and biochemical characteristics of the amyloid fibrils has accumulated. On the basis of the nature of the fibrils, amyloidosis can be classified as (1) immunoglobulin-related, corresponding mainly to the PGA, (2) AA protein-related, corresponding mainly to the secondary amyloidosis, and (3) neuroendocrine system-related varieties. In each variety circulating in the blood, precursors of fibrils have been reported: immunoglobulin light chains, SAA, and polypeptides of neuroendocrine origin, respectively. Recently, a new fibrilary material was detected in senile cardiac amyloidosis. This substance, called Asca, was found to be different from all other known amyloid fibrils. In all varieties of

Table 19
CLINICOPATHOLOGIC CLASSIFICATION OF AMYLOIDOSIS

Nonfamilial
- Primary generalized, or with limited clinical expression
- With plasma-cell dyscrasia (multiple myeloma, MW, γ- and μ-HCD
- Secondary (infections, arthropathies, collagen diseases, lymphoma, cancer)
- Senile (heart, pancreas, others)
- Localized nodular
- Corneal
- Medullary carcinoma of thyroid (sporadic)

Familial
- With polyneuropathy
  - Leg
  - Arm
  - Mixed
- With corneal lattice dystrophy and cranial neuropathy
- Familial Mediterranean fever
- With nephropathy
- Urticaria, deafness, nephropathy
- Cutaneous
- Medullary carcinoma of thyroid and pheochromocytoma
- With hereditary cerebral hemorrhage

From Pruzanski, W. and Katz, A. Originally published in *CMA Journal* 114:889, May 22, 1976. With permission.

amyloidosis described above, amyloid fibrils are mixed with the so-called P component, a 9.5 S α_1 glycoprotein, present in normal sera. Similarity of the P component to the CRP has been noted, raising the question of whether these substances, so-called pentraxins, are not an additional precursor system. The issue is complicated by the fact that protein AA was also detected, in some amyloid fibrils in PGA and myeloma-related amyloidosis, and that light chain fragments were found, together with the AA protein, in amyloid fibrils from patients with secondary amyloidosis.

A brief historical review is warranted to put these new discoveries into proper perspective. It was not until 1961 that the relationship between M components, Bence Jones proteinuria, and PGA was recognized. Further studies have shown that the aminoacid sequence of amyloid fibrils in PGA is similar, if not identical, to that of the light chains and/or of their variable regions, and that some BJP's may be converted into amyloid-like substance in vitro by proteolytic digestion in an acid milieux. Also, polypeptide related to λ light chains was detected in amyloid fibrils of a patient with PGA. The patient's serum, and 5% of sera with M components tested, contained protein antigenically related to the amyloid-fibril material. Consequently, the concept of immunoglobulin-related amyloidosis has evolved.

It became obvious, however, that in secondary amyloidosis, and in some cases of PGA, the structure of amyloid fibrils did not resemble that of the light chains. Furthermore, conversion of substances other than light chains, such as γ-HCD, calcitonin, parathormone, insulin, and glucagon, into amyloid-like material in vitro was achieved by proteolytic digestion, or by acidification and heating.

In 1971, another substance, presently called AA, was found in the amyloid fibrils. AA, a low molecular weight protein of 7000 to 9000 daltons, is the major component of amyloid fibrils in secondary amyloidosis and in Familial Mediterranean Fever-related amyloidosis. The site of synthesis of AA is unknown. Its presence in plasmacy-

Table 20
CLINICAL MANIFESTATIONS OF IMMUNOGLOBULIN-RELATED AMYLOIDOSIS

	PGA (%)[a]	MRA (%)[b]
Fatigue	67	65
Weight loss	55	62
Edema	46	41
Dyspnea	30	33
Paresthesiae	26	26
Light-headedness or syncope	30	7
"Hoarseness"	12	16
Purpura	17	15
Pain	5	34

[a] Of 132 patients.
[b] Of 61 patients.

toid cells in the human lymphoid tissues, Kupffer cells of the liver and normal mononuclear cells of the peripheral blood, suggested its relationship to the immunoglobulin system.

A few years after the discovery of AA, a substance antigenically related to it, called SAA, was detected in human serum. This protein of α-β electrophoretic mobility has a molecular weight of 160,000 to 180,000 daltons. SAA has been found in normal sera, in sera from patients with various types of amyloidosis, in hypogammaglobulinemia, and in many other disorders. SAA levels increase with old age, pregnancy, and acute infections. No elevation of SAA was noted in inherited systemic amyloidosis, with lattice corneal dystrophy, or in patients with medullary carcinoma of the thyroid.

SAA is an acute-phase reactant, which increases rapidly after the beginning of an infection or a fever and promptly decreases to normal levels after recovery. Its rise and fall paralled that of the CRP and of the white cell count. In view of these observations, some pessimism was expressed regarding the diagnostic and prognostic value of SAA.

In this chapter, only immunoglobulin-related amyloidosis (primary and myeloma-related) will be discussed. Amyloidosis complicates about 15% of the cases of multiple myeloma, and has been described in plasma cell leukemia, MW, γ-HCD, μ-HCD, and various lymphomas. So-called primary amyloidosis may present in a generalized form, involving various tissues and organs, or in a more limited form, with clinical expression in one or a few organs only.[74]

The mean age of the patients with immunoglobulin-related (primary) amyloidosis (PGA), at the time of diagnosis, was 55 years in one series and 62 years in another. PGA may present with a variety of manifestations (Tables 20—22). Occasionally, one of these predominates and the involvement of other organs is asymptomatic. For example, nephrotic syndrome, heart disease, hepatomegaly, peripheral neuropathy, hemorrhagic diathesis, diarrhea and malabsorption, skin involvement, or lymphadenopathy may be the main presenting features of the disease.

The diagnosis of amyloidosis is made on histologic grounds. Involvement of rectum and gingiva is common; thus these sites, as well as kidney, liver, spleen, and bone marrow, are common sites of biopsy.

Most, if not all, patients with PGA and myeloma-related amyloidosis (MRA) present with M components in the serum and/or BJP in the urine.[77] In one series, 94% of the

Table 21
PHYSICAL FINDINGS IN IMMUNOGLOBULIN-RELATED AMYLOIDOSIS[74,75]

	PGA (%)[a]	MRA (%)[b]
Hepatomegaly	44	41
Splenomegaly	30	27
Lymphadenopathy	14	15
Nephrotic syndrome	36	11
Congestive heart failure	27	25
Salivary gland enlargement	18[c]	0[c]
Carpal tunnel syndrome	17	29
Peripheral neuropathy	17	5
Orthostatic hypotension	16[c]	8[c]
Rheumatoid-like syndrome	15[c]	29[c]
Macroglossia	14	24
Skin involvement	7	8
Diarrhea and malabsorption	6	4
Acute renal failure	0	21[c]
Hypothyroidism	0	7[c]
Plasmacytomas	0	29[c]

[a] Of 166 patients.
[b] Of 75 patients.
[c] Recorded in one series only.

Table 22
INITIAL LABORATORY FINDINGS IN IMMUNOGLOBULIN-RELATED AMYLOIDOSIS

	PGA (%)	MRA (%)
Hemoglobin (<12.0 g/dℓ)	29	52
White blood count (<4000/mm³)	3	7
ESR (>50 mm in first hr)	54	48
Platelet count (<100,000/mm³)	4	16
Platelet count (>500,000)	5	5
Proteinuria (>150 mg/day)	90	98
Creatinine (≥2.0 mg/dℓ)	51	44
Hyperuricemia	22	31
Albumin (<3.0 g/dℓ)	76	69
Elevated SGOT	38	46
High alkaline phosphatase	49	41
BSP(>5%/hr)	38	46

patients with PGA, and 93% with MRA, had M components in the serum and/or the urine. In another series, the authors divided amyloidosis into four patterns: pattern "one" and "mixed", corresponding primarily to immunoglobulin-related amyloidosis, pattern "two", corresponding to "secondary" or "AA"-related amyloidosis, and "localized" pattern.[77] M components were noted in 100% of the patients with pattern "one", 87% of pattern "mixed", 53% of pattern "two", and all three patients with "localized" amyloidosis. Forty-six percent of all patients had Bence Jones proteinemia as the only serum abnormality. There was a higher proportion of lambda type proteins, as compared to multiple myeloma. However, some patients with secondary or localized amyloidosis have been reported to have M components also,[77] although other investigators have not found M components in secondary, hereditary, or localized types of amyloidosis.

In one series, Bence Jones proteinemia was found in 56% of the patients with PGA and in 77% of those with MRA. Sixty-eight percent of the BJP's in PGA, but only 25% of the BJP's in MRA, were of the λ type.[74] The concentrations of immunoglobulins other than M components are often abnormally low in patients with PGA, but on rare occasions are elevated. In one series, the concentration of IgG in 80%, IgA in 67%, and IgM in 84% of patients was more than 1 SD below the normal mean value. Plasmacytic infiltration of the bone marrow has frequently been observed in PGA and was present in 90% of our patients.

The findings of plasmacytic infiltration of the bone marrow, M components in the serum, Bence Jones proteinuria, and a decrease in concentration of serum immunoglobulins, other than M components, make PGA very similar to multiple myeloma, the main distinction being the absence of osteolytic lesions in the former.

There is no successful treatment for amyloidosis. However, in amyloidosis secondary to various chronic diseases, regression of amyloid deposits in various organs has been observed after vigorous treatment of the underlying condition. Improvement of the nephrotic syndrome, in some patients with PGA, was achieved by administration of melphalan alone or with prednisone, penicillamine, and fluoxymesterone. However, no improvement was found in other, similarly treated, patients with PGA and the nephrotic syndrome. Several patients with secondary amyloidosis or familial Mediterranean fever have received renal transplants; in one patient, no recurrence of amyloidosis was noted 12 months after the transplant, and in a second patient who died 5 months after transplantation, no amyloid was found in the kidney at autopsy. It has been reported that the production of casein-induced amyloidosis in mice may be prevented by simultaneous administration of colchicine. This drug has also been reported to reduce the frequency of attacks of familial Mediterranean fever, an entity known to be associated with amyloidosis.

The mean survival time from diagnosis of PGA has been reported to be 13 months, with death usually being caused by cardiac, renal, or hepatic failure. In our own series, the mean survival time was 28 months.

Papular Mucinosis with M Components

Papular mucinosis (scleromyxedema or lichen myxedematosus) is an uncommon disease with characteristic disfiguring cutaneous lesions, which usually has a benign course. The clinical manifestations vary, and several types have been described:

1. A generalized lichenoid eruption with discrete papules over the entire body, especially the hands, forearms, upper trunk, face, and neck
2. A discrete papular eruption on the trunk and extremities
3. Localized or generalized lichenoid plaques over the whole body
4. Urticarial plaques and nodular eruptions

Almost invariably, patients with papular mucinosis have plasma-cell dyscrasia and an M component in the serum. About 30 such cases have been reported.[78] The M components usually have slow γ mobility on electrophoresis, and most belong to the IgG class. In all but four cases in which the light chains were typed, the type was λ. Male patients predominated 2:1, and the mean age at diagnosis was 48 years (range, 28 to 68 years).

The total serum protein values reported in 17 patients ranged from 6.0 to 8.0 g/dℓ. The albumin value was usually normal, being less than 3.0 g/dℓ in four patients only.

In 22 patients, the M component was of the IgG class. Light chains of ten IgG M components were of the λ type, four were of the κ type, and light chain types were not reported for the other patients. No evidence for common, idiotypic determinants was found in the investigation of four IgG M components. Two M components were of the IgA class and two of the IgM class. In other cases, M components were not identified. The electrophoretic mobility of the M components was slow γ in 21 instances, mid-γ in one, and β in two. The concentration of M components was usually low, with a mean of 0.85 g/dℓ (range, 0.4 to 1.1 g/dℓ). The mean concentration of IgG calculated in eight patients was 1140 mg/dℓ (range, 610 to 2000 mg/dℓ). IgA and IgM concentrations were usually normal.

Urinalysis was normal in 20 patients, and proteinuria was detected in two. Hematologic investigation generally yielded normal results. Anemia was reported in four patients, high erythrocyte sedimentation rate was noted in three, and eosinophilia of 6 to 18% was observed in three. Mild plasmacytic infiltration of the bone marrow was detected in eight patients, and moderate plasmacytic infiltration (above 10%) was noted in two. Normal bone marrow was reported in 13 patients; however, in two of them, bone marrow cells synthesized M component in vitro. Radiologic survey of the skeleton yielded normal findings in 18 patients; two other patients, 65 and 68 years old, had osteoporosis.

Immunofluorescent study of the skin demonstrated IgG in a few instances, but not in others. In one patient, IgG was synthesized in skin tissue culture despite a negative immunofluorescence pattern.

A few patients presented with additional manifestations. In one patient, amyloidosis was found along with papular mucinosis; peculiar crystalline-like material was noted in various tissues. Pachydermoperiostosis was observed in one case. The mother of one of the patients was found to have an M component. One 58-year-old patient had attacks of confusion; angiography revealed atheromatous changes in the brain vessels. Another patient had had myocardial infarction, cerebrovascular accident, polyneuritis, and hepatomegaly. Thus some patients with papular mucinosis and M components, as well as some in whom M components have not been described, have coronary artery disease or cerebrovascular accidents.

Several patients were treated with chemotherapeutic agents such as nitrogen mustard, methotrexate, cyclophosphamide, melphalan and chlorambucil. Prednisone or ACTH were given to a few patients. In two patients treated with melphalan, subjective and objective improvement was observed, but another patient died in a coma 20 days after initiation of melphalan therapy. A patient with MW and papular mucinosis improved while treated with chlorambucil.

In 14 of 18 patients who were reported to be alive at the time this chapter was written, the mean duration of the disease was 4.4 years (range: 5 months to 13 years). In three of the four patients who had died, the duration of the disease was 1, 3, and more than 7 years. The cause of death was myocardial infarction in one, meningeal bleeding in one, pulmonary embolism and coma in one, and encephalopathy and coma in one.

Autopsies were performed in only a few instances. In a 35-year-old man who had died following progressive mental deterioration, deposits of Mayer's mucicarmine-positive material were found around eccrine sweat glands, in the wall of cutaneous blood vessels, and within cutaneous nerve bundles, but not in muscle or subcutaneous fat. Similar deposits were detected in the heart vessels, in the perivascular connective tissue of the kidney and Bowman's capsule, in adrenal glands, and in the pancreas. The mucinous material in the perivascular spaces and in the connective tissue was often accompanied by fibroblastic proliferation.

In another patient, a 36-year-old man, numbness of all extremities and incoordination progressed to paralysis and coma and terminated in death. At autopsy, mucicarmine-positive material was detected in the renal papillae, bronchial epithelium, and ductal epithelium of the pancreas. The brain showed multiple infarctions.

If deposits of mucicarmine-positive material, similar to those found in the skin, are also present in the internal organs of some or maybe all patients with papular mucinosis, the conclusion would be that this condition is a systemic, rather than solely cutaneous, disease. The relation of this disease to plasmacytic dyscrasias has not yet been elucidated. However, the presence of M components in many patients with this disease implies profound abnormality of the immune system, leading to abnormal proliferation of the plasmalymphocytic cells of B lineage. As in other B-lymphocyte dyscrasias, steroids and immunosuppressive agents seem to be the drugs of choice. Indeed, in some patients treated with these drugs, subjective and objective improvement was achieved. In others, however, no obvious improvement was observed, and some deteriorated rapidly and died. Although there are insufficient data to draw statistically meaningful conclusions, some investigators have suggested that chemotherapy may have an adverse effect on the patient with papular mucinosis. The disease seems to have a prolonged, "benign" course, different from that of multiple myeloma. There is no study available of the functional characteristics of T- and B-lymphocytes in this disease; thus the significance of immunoglobulin abnormalities in papular mucinosis remains to be elucidated.

Pyoderma Gangrenosum (PG)

PG is another dermatological condition in which M components have been detected.[79] IgG components were found in some patients, and IgA or IgM M components were found in others. However, there was a clear predominance of IgA. An interaction of an M component with red blood cells, with agglomeration of the latter, has been observed.

Systemic Capillary Leak Syndrome (SCLS)

A few patients who suffered from recurrent episodes of generalized angioedema, resulting from increased systemic capillary permeability, have recently been reported.[80] A remarkable shift of plasma from the intravascular to the extravascular space occurs, leading to shock and even death. Five of six reported patients were males. In five of six patients, M components of the IgG class were detected in the serum. The relationship of these M components to the pathogenesis or the clinical manifestations of SCLS has not yet been elucidated.

Benign Monoclonal Immunoglobulinopathy (BMI)

BMI is a condition in which a homogeneous immunoglobulin — an M component — is synthesized for many years, at the same rate, by an abnormal clone of B-lineage cells.[1] Thus the main characteristic of neoplastic proliferation, namely progression of the disease, is missing. The concentration of an M component does not change over the years, there are no osteolytic lesions, no organomegaly, and no other manifestations of plasmalymphocytic disease. The finding of an M component is often incidental. Bone marrow shows either no plasmalymphocytosis, or only a mild (3 to 6%) increase in the number of plasma cells, which are usually dispersed and do not appear in the form of sheets, or groups, characteristic for multiple myeloma. However, similarly to the classical myeloma cells, these plasma cells, "dispersed" throughout the bone marrow (usually less than 5×10^{11} cells), were found to synthesize homogeneous M component. Usually there is no suppression in the synthesis of other immunoglobulins other than M components.

The great majority of patients with BMI do not suffer from any disease, or may

Table 23
CONDITIONS IN WHICH TRANSIENT M COMPONENTS WERE DETECTED IN HUMANS

Immunization	Injections of transfer factors
Pneumococcal pneumonia	Wiskott-Aldrich syndrome
Infectious mononucleosis	Acute leukemias
Acute hepatitis	Multiple sclerosis
Gantrisin hypersensitivity	Parathyroid adenoma
Immunodeficiency syndromes	Cancer of breast
Bone marrow and thymus transplants	"Healthy" individuals

present with an unrelated condition such as diabetes, osteoarthritis, A-S C-V disease, etc. BMI is the most common abnormality in the synthesis of immunoglobulins, being detected in about 0.9% of a random population over 25 years of age,[8] and in a much higher frequency at an older age. It is probably 100 times more common than multiple myeloma. Only in a very few instances did BMI convert into a neoplastic plasmalymphocytic disease such as multiple myeloma, lymphoma, or macroglobulinemia. However, such conversion was reported as many as 15 years or more after the detection of an M component.

Thus BMI may represent a prolonged, latent "premalignant" phase of plasmalymphocytic neoplasia. Theoretically, one may speculate that such neoplasia develops in BMI only when another event, "the second signal", occurs. The prevalence of classes of M components in BMI resembles that of plasmalymphocytic neoplastic disorders, with IgG/K being the most common followed by IgG/λ, IgA, and IgM. However, in contradistinction to the neoplastic disorders, light chain disease has almost never been described in BMI. Usually, the concentration of M components in BMI is less than 2.0 g/dℓ, but occasionally higher concentrations have been observed. BJP can be found in the urine in less than one third of BMI patients and usually is present in low quantities.

Patients with BMI should not be treated, but should be monitored carefully. Serum and urine electrophoresis should be repeated, twice or three times a year. Appearance of elevated sedimentation rate, mild anemia, proteinuria, skeletal pain, increase in the concentration of M components, decrease in the concentration of other immunoglobulins, or appearance of Bence Jones globulin in the urine require repeat bone marrow aspiration, radiological examination of the bones, and reassessment of the condition.

Transient M Components

It has been shown that rabbits, hyperimmunized with streptococcal polysaccharides, or bacterial vaccines from pneumococci, meningococci, or other microorganisms, exhibit narrow M component-like bands on serum electrophoresis. These proteins were identified as homogeneous (monoclonal) immunoglobulins.[81,82] After the immunization was discontinued, the concentration of these M components decreased slowly, and eventually there was complete disappearance of abnormal bands. Furthermore, some of the rabbits that produced large amount of homogeneous immunoglobulins also exhibited features of a myeloma-like disease. Counterparts to this experimental model have also been described in human beings. As a consequence of these observations, a concept of "transient" M components has emerged, suggesting that the production of M components is not always progressive and uncontrolled in a malignant sense.[83] Table 23 lists several conditions in which transient M components were documented in human beings.

REFERENCES

1. Multiple myeloma and related immunoglobulin-producing neoplasma, in *UICC Tech. Rep. Ser.*, Vol. 13, Warner, N. L., Potter, M., and Metcalf, D., Ed., International Union against Cancer, Geneva, 1974.
2. **Freedman, M., Merrett, R., and Pruzanski, W.**, Human monoclonal immunoglobulins with antibody-like activity, *Immunochemistry*, 13, 193, 1976.
3. **Potter, M.**, Myeloma proteins (M-components) with antibody-like activity, *N. Engl. J. Med.*, 284, 831, 1971.
4. **Seligmann, M. and Brouet, J. C.**, Antibody activity of human myeloma globulins, *Semin. Hematol.*, 10, 163, 1973.
5. **Farhangi, M. and Osserman, E. F.**, Myeloma with xanthoderma due to an IgG/λ monoclonal anti-Flavin antibody, *N. Engl. J. Med.*, 294, 177, 1976.
6. **Maldonado, J. E. and Kyle, R. A.**, Familial myeloma. Report of eight families and a study of serum proteins in their relatives, *Am. J. Med.*, 57, 875, 1974.
7. **Kyle, R. A., Heath, C. W., Jr., and Carbone, P.**, Multiple myeloma in spouses, *Arch. Intern. Med.*, 127, 944, 1971.
8. **Axelsson, U., Bachmann, R., and Hällen, J.**, Frequency of pathological proteins (M-components) in 6,995 sera from an adult population, *Acta Med. Scand.*, 179, 235, 1966.
9. **Hobbs, J. R.**, Disturbances of the immunoglobulins, *Sci. Basis Med. Annu. Rev.*, 106, 1966.
10. **Hobbs, J. R.**, Paraproteins, benign or malignant? *Br. Med. J.*, 3, 699, 1967.
11. **Takatsuki, K.**, personal communication, 1971.
12. **Axelsson, U. and Hällen, J.**, A population study on monoclonal gammopathy. Follow-up after 5 and one-half years on 64 subjects detected by electrophoresis of 6995 sera, *Acta Med. Scand.*, 191, 111, 1972.
13. **Fine, J. M., Lambin, P., and Leroux, P.**, Frequency of monoclonal gammopathy in 13,400 sera from blood donors, *Vox Sang.*, 23, 336, 1972.
14. **Ameis, A., Ko, H. S., and Pruzanski, W.**, M components — a review of 1242 cases, *Can. Med. Assoc. J.*, 114, 889, 1976.
15. **Migliore, P. J. and Alexanian, R.**, Monoclonal gammopathy in human neoplasia, *Cancer*, 21, 1127, 1968.
16. **Williams, R. C., Jr., Bailly, R. C., and Howe, R. B.**, Studies of "benign" serum M-components, *Am. J. Med. Sci.*, 257, 275, 1969.
17. **Zawadzki, Z. A. and Edwards, G. A.**, Nonmyelomatous monoclonal immunoglobulinemia, *Prog. Clin. Immunol.*, 1, 105, 1972.
18. **Laurell, C. B.**, Antigen-antibody crossed electrophoresis, *Anal. Biochem.*, 10L, 358, 1965.
19. **Bernier, G. M., and Putnam, F. W.**, Polymerism, polymorphism and impurities in Bence Jones proteins, *Biochim. Biophys. Acta*, 86, 295, 1964.
20. **Smith, J. K.**, The significance of the "protein error" of indicators in the diagnosis of Bence Jones proteinuria, *Acta Haematol.*, 30, 144, 1963.
21. **Pruzanski, W. and Wilson, D. R.**, Renal handling of endogeneous lysozyme in man, *J. Lab. Clin. Med.*, 90, 61, 1977.
22. **Tischendorf, F. W., Ledderose, G., Wilmanns, W., Tischendorf, M. M., and Tischendorf, G. W.**, Cationic leukocyte antigen in urine of patients with chronic myelocytic leukemia, *Nature (London)*, 245, 379, 1973.
23. **Lindström, F. D., Hardy, W. R., Eberle, B. J., and Williams, R. C., Jr.**, Multiple myeloma and benign monoclonal gammopathy. Differentiation by immunofluorescence of lymphocytes, *Ann. Intern. Med.*, 78, 837, 1973.
24. **Abdou, N. I. and Abdou, N. L.**, The monoclonal nature of lymphocytes in multiple myeloma. Effect of therapy, *Ann. Intern. Med.*, 83, 42, 1975.
25. **Mellstedt, H., Petterson, D., and Holm, G.**, Monoclonal B-lymphocytes in peripheral blood of patients with plasma cell myeloma. Relation to activity of the disease, *Scand. J. Haematol.*, 16, 112, 1976.
26. **Preud'homme, J. L., Hurez, D., Danon, F., Brouet, J. C., and Seligmann, M.**, Intracytoplasmic and surface bound immunoglobulins in nonsecretory and Bence Jones myeloma, *Clin. Exp. Immunol.*, 25, 428, 1976.
27. **Martin, N. H.**, The incidence of myelomatosis, *Lancet*, 1, 237, 1961.
28. **Kyle, R. A., Nobrega, F. T., and Kurland, L. T.**, Multiple myeloma in Olmsted County, Minnesota, 1945—1964, *Blood*, 33, 739, 1969.
29. **McPhedran, P., Heath, C. W., Jr., and Garcia, J.**, Multiple myeloma incidence in metropolitan Atlanta, Georgia: racial and seasonal variations, *Blood*, 39, 866, 1972.
30. **MacMahon, B. and Clark, D. W.**, Incidence of multiple myeloma, *J. Chronic Dis.*, 4, 508, 1956.

31. **Pruzanski, W.**, Clinical manifestations of multiple myeloma: relation to class and type of M component, *Can. Med. Assoc. J.*, 114, 896, 1976.
32. **Edwards, G. A. and Zawadzki, Z. A.**, Extraosseous lesions in plasma cell myeloma. A report of six cases, *Am. J. Med.*, 43, 194, 1967.
33. **Pasmantier, M. W. and Azar, H. A.**, Extraskeletal spread in multiple plasma cell myeloma. A review of 57 autopsied cases, *Cancer*, 23, 167, 1969.
34. **Jancelewicz, Z., Takatsuki, K., Sugai, S., and Pruzanski, W.**, IgD multiple myeloma. Review of 133 cases, *Arch. Intern. Med.*, 135, 87, 1975.
35. **Durie, B. G. M. and Salmon, S. E.**, A clinical staging system for multiple myeloma, *Cancer*, 36, 842, 1975.
36. **Pruzanski, W., Platts, M. E., and Ogryzlo, M. A.**, Leukemic form of immunocytic dyscrasia (plasma cell leukemia). A study of ten cases and a review of the literature, *Am. J. Med.*, 47, 60, 1969.
37. **Rosner, F. and Grünwald, H.**, Multiple myeloma terminating in acute leukemia. Report of 12 cases and review of the literature, *Am. J. Med.*, 57, 927, 1974.
38. **Vigliano, E. M. and Horowitz, H. I.**, Bleeding syndrome in a patient with IgA myeloma: interaction of protein and connective tissue, *Blood*, 29, 823, 1967.
39. **Frenkel, E. P. and Tourtellotte, C. D.**, Elevated serum acid phosphatase associated with multiple myeloma. Case report with tissue enzyme assay, *Arch. Intern. Med.*, 110, 117, 1962.
40. **Patterson, R., Weiszer, I., Rambach, W., Roberts, M., and Suszko, I. M.**, Comparative cellular and immunochemical studies of two cases of pyroglobulinemia, *Am. J. Med.*, 44, 147, 1968.
41. **Kyle, R. A.**, Multiple myeloma, Review of 869 cases, *Mayo Clin. Proc.*, 50, 29, 1975.
42. **Mundy, G. R., Raisz, L. G., Cooper, R. A., Schechter, G. P., and Salmon, S. E.**, Evidence for the secretion of an osteoclast stimulating factor in myeloma, *N. Engl. J. Med.*, 291, 1042, 1974.
43. **Talerman, A. and Bateson, E. M.**, Multiple myeloma associated with bone sclerosis an peripheral neuropathy, *Br. J. Radiol.*, 43, 698, 1970.
44. **Rogers, J. S., Jr., Spahr, J., Judge, D. M., Varano, L. A., and Eyster, M. E.**, IgE myeloma with osteoblastic lesions, *Blood*, 49, 295, 1977.
45. **Farhangi, M. and Osserman, E. F.**, The treatment of multiple myeloma, *Semin. Hematol.*, 10, 149, 1973.
46. **Bergsagel, D. E.**, The treatment of plasma cell myeloma, *Br. J. Haematol.*, 33, 443, 1976.
47. **Spiegelberg, H. L., Heath, V. C., and Lang, J. E.**, IgG half-molecules: clinical and immunologic features in a patient with plasma cell leukemia, *Blood*, 45, 305, 1975.
48. **Bernier, G. M., Berman, J. H., and Fanger, M. W.**, Plasma cell leukemia with excretion of half-molecules of immunoglobulin A (α_1 λ_1), *Ann. Intern. Med.*, 86, 572, 1977.
49. **Randall, R. E., Williamson, W. C., Jr., Mullinax, F., Tung, M. Y., and Still, W. J. S.**, Manifestations of systemic light chains deposition, *Am. J. Med.*, 60, 293, 1976.
50. **Cohen, L., Blaisdell, R. K., Djordjevich, J., Ormiste, V., and Dobrilovic, L.**, Familial xanthomatosis and hyperlipidemia and myelomatosis, *Am. J. Med.*, 40, 299, 1966.
51. **Wilson, D. E., Flowers, C. M., Hershgold, E. J., and Eaton, R. P.**, Multiple myeloma, cryoglobulinemia and xanthomatosis. Distinct clinical and biochemical syndromes in two patients, *Am. J. Med.*, 59, 721, 1975.
52. **Pruzanski, W., Underdown, B., Silver, E. H., and Katz, A.**, Macroglobulinemia-myeloma double gammopathy. A study of four cases and a review of the literature, *Am. J. Med.*, 57, 259, 1974.
53. **Seligmann, M., Danon, F., Mihaesco, C., and Fudenberg, H. H.**, Immunoglobulin abnormalities in families of patients with Waldenström's macroglobulinemia, *Am. J. Med.*, 43, 66, 1967.
54. **MacKenzie, M. R. and Fudenberg, H. H.**, Macroglobulinemia: an analysis for forty patients, *Blood*, 39, 874, 1972.
55. **Krajny, M. and Pruzanski, W.**, Waldenstrom's macroglobulinemia: review of 45 cases, *Can. Med. Assoc., J.*, 114, 899, 1976.
56. **Wood, T. A. and Frenkel, E. P.**, An unusual case of macroglobulinemia, *Arch. Intern. Med.*, 119, 631, 1967.
57. **Solomon, A. and Fahey, J. L.**, Plasmapheresis therapy in macroglobulinemia, *Ann. Intern. Med.*, 58, 789, 1963.
58. **Fahey, J. L., Barth, W. F., and Solomon, A.**, Serum hyperviscosity syndrome, *JAMA*, 192, 120, 1965.
59. **Bloch, K. J. and Maki, D. G.**, Hyperviscosity syndromes associated with immunoglobulin abnormalities, *Semin. Hematol.*, 10, 113, 1973.
60. **Pruzanski, W. and Watt, J. G.**, Serum viscosity and hyperviscosity syndrome in IgG multiple myeloma. Report on 10 patients and a review of the literature, *Ann. Intern. Med.*, 77, 853, 1972.
61. **Tuddenham, E. G. D., Whittaker, J. A., Bradley, J., Lilleyman, J. S., and James, D. R.**, Hyperviscosity syndrome in IgA multiple myeloma, *Br. J. Haematol.*, 27, 65, 1974.
62. **Pruzanski, W.**, Hyperviscosity and immunoglobulin complexes, *Ann. Intern. Med.*, 80, 107, 1974.

63. **Pruzanski, W. and Russell, M. L.**, Serum viscosity and hyperviscosity syndrome in IgG multiple myeloma — the relationship to Sia test and to concentration of M component, *Am. J. Med. Sci.*, 271, 145, 1976.
64. **Grey, H. M. and Kohler, P. F.**, Cryoimmunoglobulins, *Semin. Hematol.*, 10, 87, 1973.
65. **Dotten, D. A., Pruzanski, W., Olin, J., and Brown, T. C.**, Cryocrystalglobulinemia, *Can. Med. Assoc. J.*, 114, 909, 1976.
66. **MacKechnie, H. L., Ogryzlo, M. A., and Pruzanski, W.**, Heterogeneity of IgM/IgG cryocomplexes: immunological-clinical correlation, *J. Rheumatol.*, 2, 225, 1975.
67. **Pruzanski, W. and Shumak, K. H.**, Biological activity of cold-reacting autoantibodies. I and II, *N. Engl. J. Med.*, 297, 538, 1977.
68. **Pruzanski, W., Cowan, D. H., and Parr, D. M.**, Clinical and immunochemical studies of IgM cold agglutinins with lambda type light chains, *Clin. Immunol. Immunopathol.*, 2, 234, 1974.
69. **Frangione, B. and Franklin, E. C.**, Heavy chain diseases: clinical features and molecular significance of the disordered immunoglobulin structure, *Semin. Hematol.*, 10, 53, 1973.
70. **Bloch, K. J., Lee, L., Mills, J. A., and Haber, E.**, Gamma heavy chain disease — an expanding clinical and laboratory spectrum, *Am. J. Med.*, 55, 61, 1973.
71. **Rambaud, J. C. and Seligmann, M.**, Alpha-chain disease, *Clin. Gastroenterol.*, 5, 341, 1976.
72. **Forte, F. A., Prelli, F., Yount, W. J., Jerry, L. M., Kochwa, S., Franklin, E. C., and Kunkel, H. G.**, Heavy chain disease of the (γM) type. Report of the first case, *Blood*, 36, 137, 1970.
73. **Pruzanski, W., Katz, A., Hasselback, R., and Parr, D. M.**, Multiple myleoma (light chain disease) with rheumatoid-like amyloid arthropathy and μ heavy chain fragment in the serum, *Am. J. Med.*, 65, 334, 1978.
74. **Pruzanski, W. and Katz, A.**, Clinical and laboratory findings in primary generalized and multiple-myeloma-related amyloidosis, *Can. Med. Assoc. J.*, 114, 906, 1976.
75. **Kyle, R. A. and Bayrd, E. D.**, Amyloidosis: review of 236 cases, *Medicine (Baltimore)*, 54, 271, 1975.
76. **Pruzanski, W.**, Amyloidogenesis — theories and facts (editorial), *J. Rheumatol.*, 4, 219, 1977.
77. **Isobe, T. and Osserman, E. F.**, Amyloidosis, plasma-cell dyscrasia, monoclonal immunoglobulins and Bence-Jones proteins, *N. Engl. J. Med.*, 290, 473, 1974.
78. **Danby, F. W., Danby, C. W. E., and Pruzanski, W.**, Papular mucinosis with IgG(K) M component, *Can. Med. Assoc. J.*, 114, 920, 1976.
79. **Cream, J. J.**, Pyoderma gangrenosum with a monoclonal IgM red cell agglomerating factor, *Br. J. Dermatol.*, 84, 223, 1971.
80. **Atkinson, J. P., Waldmann, T. A., Stein, S. F., Gelfand, J. A., MacDonald, W. J., Heck, L. W., Cohen, E. L., Kaplan, A. P., and Frank, M. M.**, Systemic capillary leak syndrome and monoclonal IgG gammopathy: studies in a sixth patient and a review of the literature, *Medicine (Baltimore)*, 56, 225, 1977.
81. **Haber, E.**, Antibodies of restricted heterogeneity for structural study, *Fed. Proc.*, 29, 66, 1970.
82. **Krause, R. M.**, Factors controlling the occurrence of antibodies with uniform properties, *Fed. Proc.*, 29, 59, 1970.
83. **Pruzanski, W. and Ogryzlo, M. A.**, The changing pattern of diseases associated with M components, *Med. Clin. North Am.*, 56, 371, 1972.
84. **MacKay, E. N. and Sellers, A. H.**, The Ontario cancer incidence survey, 1964—66: a new approach to cancer data acquisition, *Can. Med. Assoc. J.*, 109, 489, 1973.
85. Cases of Malignant Disease Distribution by Site of Malignancy and Sex, Ont. Cancer Inst. Annu. Rep., 1975.
86. **Bergsagel, D. E. and Pruzanski, W.**, Immunoglobulins in diagnosis and monitoring of neoplasia, in *Immunodiagnosis of Cancer*, McIntire, K. R., and Herberman, R. B., Eds., Marcel Dekker, New York, 1977.
87. **Pruzanski, W. and Ogryzlo, M. A.**, Abnormal proteinuria in malignant diseases, *Adv. Clin. Chem.*, 13, 335, 1970.

Quality Control in Hematology

THE SYSTÈME INTERNATIONAL d'UNITÉS: SI

O. W. van Assendelft

The Système International d'Unités (International System of Units; SI) has been adopted by the Conférence Generale des Poids et Mesures (Général Conference of Weights and Measures; CGPM) to arrive at "a practical system of units of measurement, suitable for adoption by all signatories to the Metre Convention." SI is no more or less than an expanded version of the CGS (centimeter, gram, second) system proposed in 1873, the MKS (meter, kilogram, second; Giorgi) system proposed in 1901, and the MKSA (meter, kilogram, second, ampere) system proposed in 1950.

The SI[1,2] consists of three classes of units. Seven well-defined dimensionally independent units form the base of the SI: these are the SI base units,* given in Table 1. From these base units, units can be formed according to algebraic relations linking corresponding quantities: these are SI derived units, examples of which are shown in Table 2. The 11th CGPM admitted, in 1960, a third class of units for which it declined to state whether they were base or derived units: these are SI supplementary units, shown in Table 3. Additionally, special names and symbols have been accepted for certain derived units. Examples are given in Table 4. In Tables 1 to 4 the accepted symbols are also given. Finally, prefixes have been designated to form multiples and submultiples of SI units. These prefixes are shown in Table 5. Compound prefixes, formed by the juxtaposition of two or more SI prefixes, are not to be used; for example, 1 nm but not 1 mμm.

Among the base units of the International System, the unit of mass is the only one whose name, for historical reasons, contains a prefix. Names of decimal multiples and submultiples of the unit of mass are formed by attaching prefixes to the word "gram" (CIPM [1967], Recommendation 2).

Any measurement result in science, medicine, or technology can be adequately and unambiguously expressed with the SI. However, the CIPM (1969) recognized that users of SI will wish to employ with it certain units that are not part of it but are important and are widely used. These units are given in Table 6. The combination of units of this table with SI units to form compound units should, however, be authorized only in limited cases; in particular, the kilowatt-hour should eventually be abandoned.

In view of existing practice, the CIPM (1969) considered it was preferable to keep for the time being, for use with those of the SI, the units listed in Table 7.

On the other hand, the use of CGS units with special names (Table 8) is definitely discouraged.

Implementation of the SI in expressing results of clinical laboratory measurements has been a major concern of the Commission on Quantities and Units in Clinical Chemistry, a Committee of the Section on Clinical Chemistry of the International Union of Pure and Applied Chemistry (IUPAC), as well as of the Expert Panel on Quantities and Units, part of the Committee on Standards of the International Federation of Clinical Chemistry (IFCC). Recommendations were first published in 1966[3] and approved by IUPAC and IFCC in 1974.[4] The Recommendations have also been endorsed, in part, by the International Committee for Standardization in Haematology (ICSH) and the World Association of Societies of Pathology (Anatomic and Clinical)

* The base units are sometimes referred to in the literature as "basic units." This is incorrect. Base units are not fundamental units but have been selected as the units on which the SI is based.

Table 1
NAMES AND SYMBOLS OF SI BASE UNITS

Physical quantity	Unit name[a]	Unit symbol
Length[b]	Meter[a]	m
Mass[c]	Kilogram[a]	kg
Time[d]	Second	s
Electric current[e]	Ampere	A
Thermodynamic temperature[f]	Kelvin	K
Luminous intensity[g]	Candela	cd
Amount of substance[h]	Mole	mol

[a] Although the spelling in official ISO Recommendations is always metre and kilogramme, the simpler US spelling has been chosen.

[b] "Unit of length. The meter is the length equal to 1 650 763.73 wavelengths in vacuum of the radiation corresponding to the transition between the levels $2p_{10}$ and $5d_5$ of the krypton-86 atom." (11th CGPM [1960], Resolution 6.)

[c] "Unit of mass. The kilogram is the unit of mass" [and not of weight or of force]; "it is equal to the mass of the international prototype of the kilogram" (3rd CGPM [1901]).

[d] "Unit of time. The second is the duration of 9 192 631 770 periods of the radiation corresponding to the transition between the two hyperfine levels of the ground state of the cesium-133 atom." (13th CGPM [1967], Resolution 1).

[e] "Unit of electric current. The ampere is that constant current which, if maintained in two straight parallel conductors of infinite length, of negligible circular cross section, and placed 1 meter apart in vacuum, would produce between these conductors a force equal to 2×10^{-7} newton per meter of length." (CIPM [1946], Resolution 2 approved by the 9th CGPM, 1948).

[f] "Unit of thermodynamic temperature." The definition of the unit of thermodynamic temperature was given in substance by the 10th CGPM (1954, Resolution 3) which selected the triple point of water as fundamental fixed point and assigned to it the temperature 273.16 °K by definition. The 13th CGPM (1967, Resolution 3) adopted the name "kelvin" (symbol K) instead of "degree Kelvin" (symbol °K) and in its Resolution 4 defined the unit of thermodynamic temperature as follows:

"The kelvin, unit of thermodynamic temperature, is the fraction 1/273.16 of the thermodynamic temperature of the triple point of water." (13th CGPM [1967], Resolution 4).

The 13th CGPM (1967, Resolution 3) also decided that the unit kelvin and its symbol K should be used to express an interval or a difference of temperature. In addition to the thermodynamic temperature (symbol T), expressed in kelvins, use is also made of Celsius temperature (symbol *t*) defined by the equation:

$$t = T - T_0$$

where T_0 = 273.15 K by definition. The Celsius temperature is expressed in degrees Celsius (symbol °C). The unit "degree Celsius" is thus equal to the unit "kelvin" and an interval or a difference of Celsius temperature may also be expressed in degrees Celsius.

[g] "The candela is the luminous intensity, in the perpendicular direction, of a surface of 1/600 000 square meter of a blackbody at the temperature of freezing platinum under a pressure of 101 325 newtons per square meter." (13th CGPM [1967] Resolution 5).

[h] "Unit of amount of substance." Following proposals of IUPAP, IUPAC, and ISO, the CIPM gave in 1967, and confirmed in 1969, the following definition of the mole, adopted by the 14th CGPM (1971, Resolution 3):

"The mole is the amount of substance of a system which contains as many elementary entities as there are atoms in 0.012 kilogram of carbon 12."

"When the mole is used, the elementary entities must be specified and may be atoms, molecules, ions, electrons, other particles, or specified groups of such particles."

Note that this definition specifies at the same time the nature of the quantity whose unit is the mole. The name of this quantity, adopted by IUPAP, IUPAC, and ISO is in French "quantité de matière," in English "amount of substance," and in German "Stoffmenge." The French name recalls "quantitas materiae" by which in the past the quantity now called mass used to be known; we must forget this old meaning, for mass and amount of substance are entirely different quantities.

Table 2
NAMES AND SYMBOLS OF SOME SI DERIVED UNITS

Physical quantity	Unit name	Unit symbol
Area	square meter	m^2
Volume	cubic meter	m^3
Mass concentration	kilogram per cubic meter	$kg \cdot m^{-3}$
Substance concentration	mole per cubic meter	$mol \cdot m^{-3}$
Mass fraction	kilogram per kilogram[a]	kg/kg
Substance fraction	mole per mole[a]	mol/mol
Volume fraction	cubic meter per cubic meter[a]	m^3/m^3

[a] These kinds of quantities are dimensionless, and the coherent unit is unity. The units kg/kg, mol/mol, and m^3/m^3 are permissible alternatives.

Table 3
NAMES AND SYMBOLS OF SI SUPPLEMENTARY UNITS

Physical quantity	Unit name	Unit symbol
Plane angle	radian[a]	rad
Solid angle	steradian[b]	sr

[a] "The radian is the plane angle between two radii of a circle which cut off on the circumference an arc equal in length to the radius."

[b] "The steradian is the solid angle which, having its vertex in the center of a sphere, cuts off an area of the surface of the sphere equal to that of a square with sides of length equal to the radius of the sphere."

Table 4
SI DERIVED UNITS WITH SPECIAL NAMES AND THEIR SYMBOLS

Physical quantity	Unit name	Unit symbol	Expression in terms of other units	Expression in terms of SI base units
Frequency	hertz	Hz		s^{-1}
Force	newton	N		$m \cdot kg \cdot s^{-2}$
Pressure, stress	pascal	Pa	N/m^2	$m^{-1} \cdot kg \cdot s^{-2}$
Energy, work, quantity of heat	joule	J	$N \cdot m$	$m^2 \cdot kg \cdot s^{-2}$
Power, radiant flux	watt	W	J/s	$m^2 \cdot kg \cdot s^{-3}$
Quantity of electricity, electric charge	coulomb	C	$A \cdot s$	$s \cdot A$
Electric potential, potential difference, electromotive force	volt	V	W/A	$m^2 \cdot kg \cdot s^{-3} \cdot A^{-1}$
Capacitance	farad	F	C/V	$m^{-2} \cdot kg^{-1} \cdot s^4 \cdot A^2$
Electric resistance	ohm	Ω	V/A	$m^2 \cdot kg \cdot s^{-3} \cdot A^{-2}$
Conductance	siemens	S	A/V	$m^{-2} \cdot kg^{-1} \cdot s^3 \cdot A^2$
Magnetic flux	weber	Wb	$V \cdot s$	$m^2 \cdot kg \cdot s^{-2} \cdot A^{-1}$
Magnetic flux density	tesla	T	Wb/m^2	$kg \cdot s^{-2} \cdot A^{-1}$
Inductance	henry	H	Wb/A^2	$m^2 \cdot kg \cdot s^{-2} \cdot A^{-2}$
Luminous flux	lumen	lm		$cd \cdot sr$ [a]
Illuminance	lux	lx		$m^{-2} \cdot cd \cdot sr$ [a]

[a] In this expression the steradian (sr) is treated as a base unit.

Table 5
SI PREFIXES

Factor	Prefix	Symbol	Factor	Prefix	Symbol
10^{-1}	deci	d	10	Deca	da
10^{-2}	centi	c	10^2	Hecto	h
10^{-3}	milli	m	10^3	Kilo	k
10^{-6}	micro	μ	10^6	Mega	M
10^{-9}	nano	n	10^9	Giga	G
10^{-12}	pico	p	10^{12}	Tera	T
10^{-15}	femto	f	10^{15}	Peta	P
10^{-18}	atto	a	10^{18}	Exa	E

Table 6
UNITS IN USE WITH THE SI

Name	Symbol	Value in SI unit
minute	min	1 min = 60 s
hour[a]	h	1 h = 60 min = 3 600 s
day	d	1 d = 24 hr = 86 400 s
degree	°	1° = (π/180) rad
minute	′	1′ = (1/60)° = (π/10 800) rad
second	″	1″ = (1/60)′ = (π/648 000) rad
liter[a]	ℓ[a]	1 ℓ = 1 dm^3 = $10^{-3}m^3$
tonne[a]	t	1 t = 10^3 kg

[a] The symbol of this unit is included in Resolution 7 of the 9th CGPM (1948). The litre is defined in Resolution 6 of the 12th CGPM (1964). The U.S. has accepted the symbol l for liter.

Table 7
UNITS TO BE USED WITH THE SI FOR A LIMITED TIME

Name	Symbol	Value in SI units
nautical miles[a]		1 nautical mile = 1 852 m
knot		1 nautical mile per hour = (1852/3600) m/s
angstrom	Å	1 Å = 0.1 nm = 10^{-10}m
are[b]	a	1 a = 1 dam^2 = 10^2m^2
hectare[b]	ha	1 ha = 1 hm^2 = 10^4m^2
barn[c]	b	1 b = 100 fm^2 = $10^{-28}m^2$
bar[d]	bar	1 bar = 0.1 MPa = 10^5Pa
standard atmosphere[e]	atm	1 atm = 101 325 Pa
gal[f]	Gal	1 Gal = 1 cm/s^2 = $10^{-2}m/s^2$
curie[g]	Ci	1 Ci = $3.7 \times 10^{10}s^{-1}$
rontgen[h]	R	1 R = 2.58×10^{-4}C/kg
rad[i]	rad	1 rad = 10^{-2}J/kg

[a] The nautical mile is a special unit employed for marine and aerial navigation to express distances. The conventional value given above was adopted by the First International Extraordinary Hydrographic Conference, Monaco, 1929, under the name "International nautical mile."

[b] This unit and its symbol were adopted by the CIPM in 1879 (Proces-Verbaux CIPM, 1879, p. 41).

[c] The barn is a special unit employed in nuclear physics to express effective cross sections.

[d] This unit and its symbol are included in Resolution 7 of the 9th CGPM (1948).

[e] Resolution 4 of 10th CGPM (1954).

[f] The gal is a special unit employed in geodesy and geophysics to express the acceleration due to gravity.

[g] The curie is a special unit employed in nuclear physics to express activity of radionuclides (12th CGPM [1964], Resolution 7).

[h] The rontgen is a special unit employed to express exposure of X or γ radiations.

[i] The rad is a special unit employed to express absorbed dose of ionizing radiations. When there is risk of confusion with the symbol for radian, rd may be used as symbol for rad.

Table 8
CGS UNITS WITH SPECIAL NAMES

Name	Symbol	Value in SI units
erg[a]	erg	1 erg = 10^{-7} J
dyne[a]	dyn	1 dyn = 10^{-5} N
poise[a]	P	1 P = dyn·s/cm² = 0.1 Pa·s
stokes	St	1 St = 1 cm²/s = 10^{-4}m²/s
gauss	Gs, G	1 Gs corresponds to 10^{-4}r
oersted[b]	Oe	1 Oe corresponds to $\frac{1000}{4\pi}$ A/m
maxwell[b]	Mx	1 Mx corresponds to 10^{-8}Wb
stilb[a]	sb	1 sb = 1 cd/cm² = 10^{4}m²
phot	ph	1 ph = 10^{4}lx

[a] This unit and its symbol were included in Resolution 7 of the 9th CGPM (1948).
[b] This unit is part of the so-called "electromagnetic: 3-dimensional CGS system" and cannot strictly speaking be compared to the corresponding unit of the International System, which has four dimensions when only electric quantities are considered.

1. The liter is preferred as the unit of volume.
2. The systematic use of factors that are powers of 10, with exponents that are whole multiples of 3, is preferred. In other words, the use of hecto, deca, deci, and centi is discouraged.
3. In constructing multiples or fractions of base or derived units, only one prefix should be used. The prefix should be used in the numerator only, an exception being made in the case of the kilogram.
4. In all cases where an elementary entity may be given for a component, the physical quantity amount of substance (mole) should be preferred over mass (kilogram), especially the quantity substance concentration (mol·l^{-1}) should be preferred over mass concentration (kg·l^{-1}).

Of these rules, the third and, especially, fourth have not been generally accepted. Table 9 shows some examples of hematological laboratory results expressed in accepted or recommended SI units.

The IUPAC and IFCC recommendations[4] have also addressed uniformity of chemical and biochemical nomenclature in the clinical laboratory. In principle, a report of a determined quantity should include information on (1) the system, (2) the component, (3) the kind of quantity, (4) the numerical value, and (5) the unit.[4,5] Thus it is recommended that, for example, serum iron be reported as Serum-Iron (II + III), substance concentration = .. μmol/ℓ; abbreviated: S-Iron (II + III), substc. = ... μmol/ℓ. Proposals for abbreviations for description of the system are given in Table 10 and for quantity names in Table 11.[6]

Table 9
SOME HEMATOLOGICAL LABORATORY RESULTS EXPRESSED IN "CONVENTIONAL" AND IN SI UNITS

Component	Units: Conventional	Units: SI	Conversion factor conventional to SI unit
Carboxyhemoglobin	%	fraction	0.01
Erythrocytes (RBC)	$10^6/\mu\ell$	$10^9/\ell$	10^6
Erythrocyte diameter	..μ	μm	1
Hematocrit (PCV)	%	fraction	0.01
Hemoglobin (blood)	g/dℓ	g/ℓ[a]	10
	g/dℓ	mmol/ℓ (Fe)[b]	0.621
Iron (serum)	μg/dℓ	μmol/ℓ	0.179
Iron binding capacity	g/dℓ	mol/ℓ	0.179
Iron saturation	%	fraction	0.01
Leucocytes (WBC)	$10^3/\mu\ell$	$10^9/\ell$	10^6
Leucocytes, differential count	%	fraction	0.01
MCH	μμg	pg	1
	pg	fmol (Fe)[b]	0.621
MCHC	g/dℓ	g/ℓ	10
	g/dℓ	mmol/ℓ (Fe)[b]	0.621
MCV	μ3	fℓ	1
Methemoglobin	%	fraction	0.01
Prothrombin time	s	s	1
Reticulocytes			
Relative	0/00	fraction	0.001
Absolute	$10^3/\mu\ell$	$10^9/\ell$	10^6
Thrombocytes	$10^3/\mu\ell$	$10^9/\ell$	10^6
Vitamin B_{12}	μμg/mℓ	pmol/ℓ	0.738
	ng/dℓ	pmol/ℓ	7.378

[a] ICSH recommendation 1976.

[b] Although ICSH recommends g/ℓ, mmol/ℓ is acceptable as long as the elementary entity (monomer, tetramer) is clearly specified: e.g., Hb or Fe, 4Hb or 4Fe.[5]

Table 10
ABBREVIATIONS FOR DESCRIPTION OF THE SYSTEM

System	Abbreviation	System	Abbreviation
Arterial	a	Leucocyte	Lkc
Blood	B	Leucocytes	Lkcs
Capillary	c	Plasma	P
Day, daily, 24 hr	d	Protein	Prot
Erythrocyte	Ery	Patient	Pt
Erythrocytes	Erys	Serum	S
Fasting	f	Cerebrospinal fluid	Sp
Feces	F	Urine	U
		Venous	v

Table 11
ABBREVIATIONS FOR QUANTITY NAMES

Quantity	Abbreviation	Quantity	Abbreviation
Amount of substance	ams.	Mole fraction	molfr.
Clearance	clear.	Specific	spf.
Content	cont.	Substance concentration	substc.
Mass concentration	masc.		
Mass fraction	masfr.	Volume	vol
Molality	molal.	Volume fraction	volfr.

REFERENCES

1. National Bureau of Standards, The International System of Units (SI), NBS Spec. Publ. 330, U. S. Department of Commerce, National Bureau of Standards, 1974.
2. National Bureau of Standards, NBS Guidelines for Use of the Metric System, NBS Publ. LC 1056, U. S. Department of Commerce, National Bureau of Standards, 1975.
3. **Dybkaer, R. and Jorgensen, K.**, *Quantities and Units in Clinical Chemistry,* Williams & Wilkins, Baltimore, 1967.
4. IUPAC and IFCC, Quantities and Units in Clinical Chemistry. Recommendation 1973, *Pure Appl. Chem.*, 37, 519, 1974, IUPAC and IFCC, List of Quantities in Clinical Chemistry. Recommendation 1973, *Pure Appl. Chem.*, 37, 549, 1974.
5. ICSH, IFCC, and WAPS, Recommendations for use of SI in clinical laboratory measurements, *Z. Klin. Chem. Klin. Biochem.*, 11, 93, 1973.
6. World Health Organization, *The SI for the Health Professions,* World Health Organization, Geneva, 1977.

PRINCIPLES OF TOTAL QUALITY CONTROL

Russell J. Eilers

A total quality control system should be effective in developing, maintaining, and improving clinical laboratory services in order to assure that satisfactory services are provided to the physician as economically as possible. The system is based on general principles that have evolved from the application of quality control engineering within other diverse industries.[1]

In the phrase "quality control," the word "quality" means the degree of excellence necessary for the performance of each test in terms of the functional use of that laboratory test result by the physician to solve the individual patient-care problem for which it was ordered. The cost of the procedure to the patient must also be considered. The word "control" represents the management activities of (1) setting standards for the quality needed, (2) appraising conformance to these standards, (3) acting when the standards are not met, and (4) planning for improvements in the standards.

For the clinical laboratory, the technological and human elements of quality control can be divided into six phases (see Table 1).

Cost of Quality Control

A total quality control system provides a means of measuring and optimizing the costs of quality control activities. For analysis, the cost items can be distributed within the following four categories:

1. Prevention cost items
   A. Quality planning by management staff for each assay from specimen drawing and receipt of materials through laboratory processing to output of result in a reliable format for physician interpretation
   B. Process control audit report review by management to assure control is established, to improve processing, and to provide technical support when necessary for planning and maintaining quality control
   C. Research and development costs for the quality control plan and reliability checkout for each new or revised assay before putting into operation
   D. Design and development costs for special materials or equipment for quality control
   E. Quality training of staff
   F. Miscellaneous expenses: clerks, secretaries, aides, rent, and telephone for quality control section
2. Appraisal cost items
   A. Test and inspection of purchased materials and equipment
   B. Instrument maintenance and calibration services
   C. Supervisor review of process
   D. Laboratory result review before release
   E. Material and labor costs for process control testing
   F. Material and labor costs for personnel proficiency testing
   G. Cost of developing quality control audit reports for management
   H. Cost of staff time and subscription fees in quality control study (inspection and accreditation and proficiency testing) of external agencies (mandatory and voluntary)
3. Internal failure costs

Table 1
TOTAL QUALITY CONTROL

Phase	Human elements	Technical elements
Design control	Combination of health care problems to be served Staff organizational chart	Selection of assay methods and instruments for health care problems Functional facility design based on units with which laboratory interacts (emergency room, operating room, intensive care, outpatient clinics, etc.)[2] Breakdown of assay methods into stat, inpatient, outpatient, and reference; latter to be sent out for efficiency
Input control	Education and training specifications required for each worker category Task and function analysis to determine category of worker required for each position in organizational chart[6] Staff education program on new methods and instruments	Material and instrument specification[3-5] American Chemical Society chemicals Standard reference materials, clinical reference methods, physical standards from National Bureau of Standards American Association of Clinical Chemists recommended method Cost effectiveness of assay systems Specimen collection specifications (type, anticoagulants, amount, time relation to meals, patient position, stability, drug interference)[7]
Process control	New employee orientation program and assignment of quality control tasks Linking quality control and proficiency testing to personnel records Staff review quality control and proficiency testing results In-house education for deficiencies	Internal quality control program (procedure manual defining number of controls and calibrators for each assay method and control limits range and action to be followed) Instrument maintenance program[8] Quality control study programs Proficiency testing program of interlaboratory peer comparisons Regional quality control program to refine precision of assays and check accuracy with peers
Output control	Proficiency testing of clerical functions Physician contact for verification of unusual or diagnostic test results	Consistent report format (patient identification, physician, specimen source, date collected, terminology, abbreviations, symbols, SI units, reference value)[9] Results grouped for physiological significance, specific organ function, or disease evaluation Flagging abnormal results for physician Logical and accessible location in medical chart for laboratory reports with administrative and record-keeping value
Reliability control	Nursing unit rounds to discuss specimen collection and report receipt problems	Laboratory manual for physicians and nursing unit providing specifications for specimen collection; laboratory

Table 1 (continued)
TOTAL QUALITY CONTROL

Phase	Human elements	Technical elements
	Physician contact on rounds, in conference, and by telephone to discuss vagaries of laboratory assays, unusual results, and significance for patient care Written interpretations of result patterns, e.g., peripheral smear, urine sediment, immuno- and electrophoretic patterns, panels of tests	assay methods used; and reference values for defined patient populations, including confidence limits, related accuracy, precision, specificity, and sensitivity of method Laboratory rounds to discuss specimen and method problems Laboratory bulletins to announce assay method revisions or new methods and their pathophysiologic significance
Verification control	On-site review by peers Personnel recertification by continuing education credits and proficiency examinations	Inspection and accreditation program based on general standards and detailed check limits[10,11] Documented workload studies based on time-engineered studies (College of American Pathologists workload recording method)[12] Cost analysis mechanism based on detailed charter of accounts[13]

A. Scrap and rework costs for loss of a specimen or complete batch of samples due to quality control criteria not met and necessity to rerun with new materials and/or specimens
B. Down-time costs for overtime due to equipment or supply failure
C. Material reprocurement costs of additional procurement personnel required to handle rejected materials or supplies when quality control criteria are not met
D. Procedure change cost for personnel to change an instrument, reagent component, or material in order for the assay to meet process control criteria.

4. External failure costs
   A. Costs to investigate a physician complaint of a questionable result
   B. Costs to correct a report or modify report format
   C. Costs to expedite pickup of specimen or delivery of report which is late due to staff communication failure

Medical laboratories tend to invest most of their funds in prevention and appraisal costs in order to minimize the expense of repeating tests on batches or individual specimens or investigating the complaints of physicians about supposed laboratory error. Even minimal failures in the latter two categories above are devastating to the relationships and reputation of the laboratory with physicians and hospitals. The motto of a clinical laboratory must be "to prevent poor quality rather than to correct poor quality."

Overall total quality control costs must be kept within reasonable bounds based on cost benefit to the consumer patient. Does an increased cost of an element for quality control in the first or second categories above have a significant effect on failure costs in the third and fourth? If not, is it scientifically valid and/or possible to replace this element or reduce another element of quality control cost in the same category? This can be evaluated by analyzing sections of the laboratory performing similar procedures or the individual analyte assays in order to optimize the costs of categories and relating these analyses to defined bases over periods of time. Reference bases such as total processing cost, net value of output (laboratory charges), or cost per unit of test or workload unit may be used. The goal would be to obtain maximum benefit at the lowest cost in categories 3 and 4 with minimal cost in categories 1 and 2.

A general guideline in quality control engineering is that quality control costs for a particular product should not exceed 10% of the direct costs of production of that product. However, for many analytes in the medical laboratory this guideline cannot be met. A goal of quality control cost of 10 to 20% total direct cost for an analytic result processed in an optimum batch size may be more realistic. The consumer patient wants maximum quality of test result for least cost.

REFERENCES

1. **Feigenbaum, A. V.,** *Total Quality Control, Engineering and Management,* McGraw-Hill, New York, 1961.
2. **Thomas, R. G., Ed.,** *Manual for Laboratory Planning and Design,* College of American Pathologists, Chicago, 1974.
3. **Meinke, W. W.,** Standard reference materials for clinical measurements, *Anal. Chem.,* 43, 28A, 1971.
4. **Zeif, M. and Michelotti, F. W.,** Clinical chemistry: a challenge for high purity standards and reagents, *Clin. Chem.,* 17, 833, 1971.
5. **Eilers, R. J., Schaffer, R., Beeler, M. F., Hanson, D. J., Earenson, E., Gilbert, R. K., and Barnett, R. N.,** Clinical Analytical Chemistry Panel, in Standard Reference Materials and Meaningful Measurements, National Bureau of Standards Spec. Publ. 408, U.S. Government Printing Office, Washington, D.C., 1975, 465.
6. **Hedrick, W.** *Job Restructuring For The Clinical Laboratory,* Kettering Medical Center, Kettering, Ohio, 1976.
7. **Sacker, L. S.,** Specimen collection, in *Quality Control in Haematology,* Lewis, S. M. and Coster, J. F., Eds., Academic Press, London, 1975, 211.
8. **Hamlin, W. G., Duckworth, J. K., Gilmer, P. R., Jr., and Stevins, M. V.,** *Laboratory Instrument Maintenance and Function Verification,* College of American Pathologists, Skokie, Ill., 1974.
9. **Burns, E. L., Hanson, D. J., Schoen, J., Barnett, R. N., Minckler, T., Winter, S.,** Communication of laboratory data to the clinician, *Am. J. Clin. Pathol.,* 61, 900, 1974.
10. Commission on Laboratory Inspection and Accreditation, *Standards For Accreditation of Medical Laboratories,* College of American Pathologists, Skokie, Ill., 1974.
11. Commission on Laboratory Inspection and Accreditation, *Checklist for Inspection,* Sect. 1—9, College of American Pathologists, Skokie, Ill., 1976.
12. Laboratory Management and Planning Committee, *Laboratory Workload Recording Method,* 4th ed., College of American Pathologists, Skokie, Ill., 1977.
13. Laboratory Management and Planning Committee, *Introduction to Cost-finding in the Department of Pathology,* College of American Pathologists, Skokie, Ill., 1974.

QUALITY CONTROL BASED ON STATISTICAL ANALYSIS OF COMPLETE BLOOD COUNT DATA

Brian S. Bull

Quality control information useful for both the calibration and the control of automated and manual whole blood analyzers can be recovered as a by-product of routine complete blood counts. Reliance on a statistical analysis of patient data for quality control is a highly attractive proposition. In most laboratories, large amounts of raw data are readily available, the cost of analysis is trivial, and the alternative — the use of partially stabilized whole blood preparations — poses significant drawbacks.

Population Statistics vs. Whole Blood Preparations

Primary reliance on partially stabilized whole blood preparations for quality control of the component tests of the complete blood count means large, continuing, day-to-day costs not only for the preparations themselves, but also for a technologist's time. The use of population statistics involves no expense for supplies and negligible technologist time, especially if the computations are automated. Whole blood preparations are unstable and, consequently, must frequently be replaced. While they can serve effectively for drift control, they cannot be used for calibration because of their instability. Certain population statistics (such as the mean red cell indices) show sufficient stability to enable their use not only for drift control, but also for calibration.

As a corollary of the above, a laboratory utilizing partially stabilized whole blood preparations as its primary means of quality control must have frequent recourse to reference methods in order to validate each new batch of standard.[1] Laboratories utilizing population statistics must resort to the use of reference methods only if major shifts in the composition of the patient population occur.

Population Statistics Applied To Quality Control

Quality control based on population statistics can be summarized very simply. The true mean (or mode or median, etc.) value of a measurable population parameter (mean corpuscular volume [MCV], hemoglobin, mean corpuscular hemoglobin concentration [MCHC], etc.) is determined by using a reference method to measure that parameter in a large sample of the population. This population mean forms a standard against which the means of smaller batches selected randomly from the same population can be compared. If the apparent mean of a smaller batch differs from the known true mean of the population, drift in the analytical instrument has occurred and recalibration is necessary. The precise calibration adjustment required is indicated by the numerical difference between the batch mean and the known true mean of the population. Obviously, the population data must meet certain criteria if it is to be used satisfactorily in a quality control approach such as that outlined above. A consideration of these criteria will clarify why this is a superb approach for controlling the six red cell-related determinations (MCV, mean corpuscular hemoglobin [MCH], MCHC, hemoglobin, hematocrit, and red cell counts), but is not yet satisfactory for the white cell counting procedure.

Obligatory Population Characteristics for Statistical Quality Control

The following population characteristics are necessary for statistical quality control:

1. The distribution of the data items in question must be approximately Gaussian or

must be susceptible to Gaussian transformation. Fortunately, for practical purposes, the distribution of all of the red cell related parameters is Gaussian.[2]
2. The number of samples required for each batch (N) must be small in relation to the total number of data items available daily if quality control information is to be produced at satisfactorily frequent intervals throughout the day. For maximum utility, N should be substantially less than 50. An N of 20 is adequate for the analysis of all of the red cell indices.
3. The standard deviation (SD) of the population must be small for the particular determinant under study. Ideally, it should not be greater than three to five times the sensitivity desired for the quality control procedure. For the red cell indices, the standard deviation is 6 to 7%, permitting satisfactory quality control in the 1 to 2% range.
4. Age, sex, etc. should have no known effects on the parameter being measured. If such effects exist, the population must be segregated according to the factors known to influence the population means, thereby at least doubling the N required. In the case of the complete blood count (CBC), the primary red cell-related parameters (i.e., hemoglobin (Hgb), hematocrit (Hct), and red blood cell (RBC) count) are affected by sex. However, the red cell indices are not affected by this factor and are therefore ideal for the purpose. Statistical control using only the indices can also be extended to the Hgb, Hct, and RBC count by the simple method of calibrating the Hgb determination against a cyanmethemoglobin standard. If the Hgb determination is known to be correct and the mean indices of a batch match the known mean indices of the population, then all six red cell related parameters must be in control. This will always be true because of the invariant mathematical relationship among the red cell indices and the primary determinations on which they are based.

Examination of the white cell count demonstrates why it cannot presently be controlled effectively by the application of population statistics. Although the distribution of white cell counts is non-Gaussian, it is not sufficiently assymetrical to preclude statistical treatment. There are no known effects of sex on the population mean, and an abundant amount of data is available in most laboratories. However, the standard deviation of white cell counts in the population is too large (approximately 20%) for the apparent population mean deduced from small ($N < 50$) random population subsets to be considered reliable. Thus, statistical controls on this parameter remain ineffective.

Statistical Techniques Applied To CBC Data

The population statistics which have been used most frequently for statistical quality control are the various measures of central tendency, such as the mean, median, mode, etc. A variety of techniques are available for the determination of these measures on small population subsets. It is extremely likely that some of the techniques described for the various clinical chemistry determinations, such as the "number plus" technique[3] or the "average of normals" procedure,[4] can also be applied to hematologic data. However, the techniques detailed in Table 1 have arbitrarily been limited to those for which there is published documentation of effectiveness when applied to data from the CBC.

Table 1
STATISTICAL APPROACH TO HEMATOLOGIC QUALITY CONTROL

Statistic	Equivalent or related statistical technique	Portions of CBC monitored[a]	Refs.
Mean, $\overline{X}$[b]	Average value	MCV, MCH, MCHC, Hgb	5—7
Median, $\overline{X}_{MED}$[c]	Central value in a distribution	MCV, MCH, MCHC	6
Mode, $\overline{X}_{MOD}$[d]	Value of most frequent occurrence	MCV, MCH, MCHC, WBC	5
Windowed mean, $\overline{X}_{WND}$[e]	Average of "normal values"	Hgb, Hct, RBC count and indices	8, 9, 14
Trimmed mean, $\overline{X}_{TR}$[f]	Average of all values in a data batch after "highest" and "lowest" have been discarded	MCV, MCH, MCHC	6
Moving average mean, $\overline{X}_{MA}$[g]	The mean of each batch of N samples as modified by combination with weighted information from the previous batch mean	MCV, MCH, MCHC	6
$\overline{X}_{J}$[h]	A sophisticated variation of a trimmed mean in which the trimming function can be precisely tailored to the data distribution	MCV, MCH, MCHC	6, 11
$\overline{X}_{B}$[i]	A measure that both trims outliers and behaves like a moving average	MCV, MCH, MCHC	1, 6, 12

[a]MCV, mean corpuscular volume; MCH, mean corpuscular hemoglobin; MCHC, mean corpuscular hemoglobin concentration, Hgb, hemoglobin; WBC, white blood cell count; Hct, hematocrit; RBC, red blood cell count.

[b]$\overline{X}$, the arithmetic mean is severely affected by the random presence of blood samples from sick patients. As a result, the number of samples (N) required is too large (>50) for optimal usefulness on complete blood count (CBC) results. Other approaches are much more effective and require minimal additional computation.

[c]$\overline{X}_{MED}$, unlike the mean, the median is not heavily influenced by the presence of outliers. However, to obtain an adequate approximation of the population the median value requires an N that is too large to be useful in practice.

[d]$\overline{X}_{MOD}$, the mode is virtually unaffected by the presence of outliers. Therefore, it has a significant advantage over the mean. Unfortunately, it is difficult to determine precisely in any straightforward fashion. The imprecision which results from various approximation techniques negates much of its value.

[e]$\overline{X}_{WND}$, the influence of outliers is decreased by eliminating all values outside of "normal." Because the data window is fixed, detection of analyzer drift is delayed significantly. The magnitude of the apparent drift as measured by the statistic will always be less than the true drift (see Reference 10). Furthermore, the N required is relatively large, as many of the values fall outside the data window and are discarded.

[f]$\overline{X}_{TR}$, this statistic is similar to $\overline{X}_{WND}$. It has the advantage that the trimming function moves with the data as the analyzer drifts, thereby enabling early and rapid detection of the drift. The primary drawback of this statistic lies in its inflexibility, as a set number of values must be discarded from the ends of the distribution.

[g]$\overline{X}_{MA}$, incorporation of information from previous batches decreases the range of this statistic and thus allows for smaller batch sizes. It does not diminish the effect of outliers or lessen the effect of normal values. As a result, this statistic is relatively insensitive at drift detection.

[h]$\overline{X}_{J}$, if used in an unmodified state, this statistic is very similar to $\overline{X}_{TR}$. However, if a moving average form of this statistic is employed, the reduction in N typical of a moving average is combined with the decreased outlier contribution provided by trimming. The combination is only slightly less effective than $\overline{X}_{B}$; however, it is more complex to calculate.

[i]$\overline{X}_{B}$. this statistic is used for the same purpose as a moving average $\overline{X}_{J}$, although it achieves both the trimming and the moving average functions in a novel fashion that renders it more sensitive to drift. In addition, it is easier to calculate. For detailed programming instructions suitable for programmable calculators or computers, see Reference 13. Despite the fact that this computation monitors only the red cell indices, the quality control that results can be extended to the hemoglobin, hematocrit, and red cell count simply by calibrating one of these primary determinations against a known standard. The most convenient approach is to calibrate the hemoglobin determination against a standard solution of cyanmethemoglobin.

REFERENCES

1. **Gilmer, P. R., Williams, L. J., Koepke, J. A., and Bull, B.,** Calibration methods for automated hematology instruments, *Am. J. Clin. Pathol.*, 68, 1, 1977.
2. **Bull, B. S. and Elashoff, R. M.,** The use of patient-derived hematology data in quality control, in *Proc. San Diego Biomedical Symposium,* Vol. 13, San Diego Biomedical Symposium, San Diego, 1974.
3. **Hoffman, R. G. and Waid, M. E.,** The number plus method of quality control of laboratory accuracy, *Am. J. Clin. Pathol.*, 40, 236, 1963.
4. **Hoffman, R. G. and Waid, M. E.,** The "average of normals" method of quality control, *Am. J. Clin. Pathol.*, 43, 134, 1965.
5. **Prangnell, D. R. and Johnson, P. H.,** A new method of quality control for the Coulter Model S Counter, *J. Clin. Pathol.*, 30, 487, 1977.
6. **Bull, B. S., Elashoff, R. M., Heilbron, D. C., and Couperus, J.,** A study of various estimators for the derivation of quality control procedures from patient erythrocyte indices, *Am. J. Clin. Pathol.*, 40, 457, 1963.
7. **Cavill, I.,** Quality control in routine haemaglobinometry, *Am. J. Clin. Pathol.*, 24, 701, 1971.
8. **Dorsey, D. B.,** Quality control in hematology, *Am. J. Clin. Pathol.*, 40, 457, 1973.
9. **Kuse, R. and Hausmann, K.,** Aufdeckung von Reagenzienfehlern durch interne Qualitatscontrolle fur den Coulter Counter S, *Blut*, 32, 297, 1976.
10. **Dixon, K. and Northam, B. E.,** Quality control using the daily mean, *Clin. Chim. Acta*, 30, 453, 1970.
11. **Andrews, D. S., Bickel P., and Hampel, S.,** *Survey and Advances,* Princeton University Press, Princeton, N.J., 1972.
12. **Bull, B. S.,** A statistical approach to quality control, in *Quality Control in Hematology,* Lewis, S. M. and Coster, Eds., Academic Press, New York, 1976.
13. **Korpman, R. A. and Bull, B. S.,** The implementation of a robust estimator of the mean for quality control on a programmable calculator or a laboratory computer, *Am. J. Clin. Pathol.*, 65(2), 252, 1976.
14. **Duckmanton, J.,** A quality control programme for haematology based on the averaging of mean cell constants, *Aust. J. Med. Technol.*, 14, 13, 1973.

Computer Aids to Diagnosis

COMPUTER AIDS TO DIAGNOSIS

Ralph L. Engle, Jr. and Betty J. Flehinger

Introduction

Computers may perform a variety of functions as aids in the diagnostic process, and experimental systems have been used for over 20 years. The most striking example of new computer-based diagnostic technique is in the field of radiology, where computerized tomography has developed to the point at which it has changed the practice of medicine by providing information to the physician that was not previously available. The computer has not yet found general use in hematologic diagnosis, although several research programs are under way. This review of how computers might be used in hematologic diagnosis borrows heavily from work done in other fields of medicine and discusses briefly the systems under development for computer-aided hematologic diagnosis.

Following a set of definitions for use in the rest of the article, this chapter contains a functional classification of computer aids to diagnosis. Three dimensions of categorization are considered. The first, based on *type of information,* refers to the purposes of the programs. The second, *style of interaction,* separates those programs that operate sequentially from the single function programs, and further discriminates on the basis of degree of user control compared to computer control of program functions. Finally, *internal mechanisms* classify programs in terms of how heavily they use statistics and decision theory in contrast to direct simulation of the behavior of physicians.

Selected programs illustrating these classifications are listed in Table 1. This list is by no means exhaustive and, although it is not limited to the field of hematology, it is slanted toward programs that might be applicable to hematologic problems. Although their names do not appear in the table, mention should be made of the important theoretical contribution of Ledley and Lusted, who provided the groundwork for many of the programs listed.[1]

The last section of this chapter is a brief description of three distinct computer programs, each of which is intended to span all of hematologic diagnosis.

Definitions

Diagnosis — Diagnosis is the sequence of procedures and decisions, based upon the whole body of medical knowledge, which assigns a patient's condition to a category in the classification of diseases and draws conclusions about significant auxiliary information, such as location, stage, complications, and response to treatment.

Descriptors — Descriptors are all the characteristics of the individual that are observed or measured by specified methods and are utilized in the diagnostic process, e.g., sex and leukocyte count.

Findings — Findings are the possible observations for each descriptor, chosen to have clinical significance in the diagnostic process, e.g., for sex, male and female, for leukocyte count, six findings, i.e., less than 3000, 3000 to 4999, 5000 to 9999, 10,000 to 49,999, 50,000 to 99,999, and greater than 100,000.

Disease — Diseases are abnormal conditions that exhibit some common findings when observed in different individuals and are thought to have a common pathogenesis and similarity in prognosis and response to treatment.

Computer aid to diagnosis — A computer aid to diagnosis is a program or procedure, utilizing computer technology, which relates the findings of an individual patient

Table 1
COMPUTER AIDS TO DIAGNOSIS BY FUNCTIONAL CLASSIFICATION

Topic	Type of information[a]	Style of interaction[b]	Internal mechanisms[c]	Ref.
Blood chemistry analysis (SMAC®)	A	A	A1	
Arrhythmia detection	A	A	A1	2
Multiphasic screening	B	B	A2,D2	3
Leukocyte differential count (Hemalog D)	C	A	B1	4
Leukocyte differential count (CYDAC®)	C	A	B1	5
Erythrocyte classification	C	A	B1	6
Computed tomography	C	A	B2	7
Brain scans	C	A	B2	8
Electrocardiogram	C	A	D3	9
Echocardiogram	C	C	B2	10
Leukocyte differential count (HEMATRAK®, LARC®)	C	C	D2	11, 12
Pediatrics	D	A	C1	13
100 Common diseases	D	A	C3	14
Blood chemistry (SMA® 12)	D	A	D1	15
Hyperthyroidism	D	A	D2	16
Polycythemia vera	D	A	D3	17
Congenital heart disease	D	A	D3	18
Liver disease	D	A	D3	19
Psychiatry	D	B	A3	20
Psychiatry	D	B	C1	21
Hematology	E	A	C2	22, 23
Acute abdomen	E	A	C4,D3	24
Edema	E	B	A3	25
Hematology	E	B	A3	26
Electrolyte and acid/base	E	B	A3,A5	27
Carbohydrate intolerance (CDSS)	E	B	A3,C3	28, 29
Jaundice	E	B	D4	30
Acute renal failure	E	B	D4	31
Megoloblastic anemia	E	B	D4	32
Antimicrobial therapy (MYCIN)	E	C	A3	33
Internal medicine (DIALOG®)	E	C	A3,C3	34
Glaucoma (CASNET)	E	C	A3,C3	35
Hematology (HEME)	E	C	C4,D3	36, 37
Congenital heart disease and bone tumors	E	C	D4	38
Ischemic heart disease	E	C	E1	39
Shock	E	C	E2	40

to the body of medical knowledge and thus helps to assign the patient's condition to a position in the classification of diseases.

Functional Classification of Computer Aids to Diagnosis

Type of Information

A. **Simple flagging of abnormal findings** — Examples range from indications on blood chemistry or hematology report forms to arrhythmia detection during patient monitoring.

B. **Organized summaries of findings in individual patients** — Information obtained from diverse sources, including history, physical examination, and laboratory tests, is presented in a uniform, useful, and time-saving format.

C. **Display and interpretation of the output of a physical measuring device** — Examples include computed tomography, automated blood cell and leukocyte differential counters, and electrocardiogram interpreters.

D. **Simple diagnostic decision making** — These include computer programs that accept as input the findings of individual patients, and provide as output a list of suggested diagnoses or other characterizations of the patient's illness.

E. **Complex consultation** — These computer programs accept as input the findings of individual patients and provide as output several kinds of information, including suggested diagnoses, confirming tests, prognosis, and recommended treatment.

Style of Interaction

A. **No user options and no sequential interaction** — This style arises in systems that perform a fixed single or multiple function. From the user's standpoint, there is no variability or freedom of choice.

B. **Sequential interaction controlled by computer program** — The program determines which questions are asked and what information is provided at every decision point. The order of operations, whether fixed or variable, is under program control.

C. **User options within program-controlled sequences** — Within the limits of system capability, the user is permitted to select the findings he enters and the output he receives. The sequence in which these selections are made is partly determined by the user and partly by the program.

Internal Mechanisms

A. **Direct simulation of physician** — These mechanisms represent the designer's conception of the thoughts and actions of a physician.

1. Logical switch activated when predetermined boundaries are exceeded. The physician sets the boundaries.
2. Information storage and retrieval system designed to compile and print out data specified by a physician.
3. Sequence or network of decision modules. Each module represents the physician's opinion about one or more simple actions to result from a specified set of findings. Interconnections between modules determine the order in which these actions take place. The entire network, assembled in a discipline often called artificial intelligence, is intended to represent the physician's behavior in response to any possible set of circumstances.

B. **Direct computation and use of computer graphics** — This category contains the devices that depend upon the ability of a computer to carry out extensive arithmetic operations rapidly and accurately.

1. Feature extraction and classification according to predetermined criteria. This refers to interpretation of the output of physical measuring devices like microscopes and scanners
2. Computational manipulation of physical measurements resulting in graphical displays, such as computed tomography

C. **Algorithms for combining weights to simulate physician's thought** — In systems of this type, the physician's opinion about the impact of individual findings on decisions about diagnosis, treatment, or other actions is quantified in a system of weights. The algorithms determine how the computer responds to any input it may receive.

1. Diagnostic score equal to count of a patient's findings that match the findings thought to characterize a disease
2. Diagnostic score equal to weighted average of values representing the significance of a patient's findings in relation to the diagnosis of a disease
3. Threshold logic in which a decision is triggered whenever the sum of a specified set of weights exceeds a predetermined value
4. Bayes' Theorem with parameters which represent the physician's opinion about the frequencies of findings in diseases and of diseases in the population (Bayes' Theorem is a formula that expresses the probability that a patient has a specified disease as a function of the frequency of that disease in the population and the frequency of the patient's findings in the disease)

D. **Algorithms based on statistics** — These programs contain the following ingredients: a predetermined organization of diseases, a set of findings considered relevant to the diagnosis of those diseases, and a data base about the findings present in a large number of patients known to have each of the diseases. Using this information and statistical theory, the programs classify new patients in the disease structure.

1. Simple matching of a patient's findings with those of the subpopulation known to have each disease
2. Classical methods of discriminant analysis, including maximum likelihood. (Discriminant analysis proceeds in two stages; in the first stage, statistical computations determine those combinations of findings, discriminant functions, which best separate the patients in the data base according to their diseases; in the second or identification stage, patients with unknown disease are classified through the use of the discriminant functions)
3. Bayes' Theorem with frequency values estimated from data or combining physician's opinions with estimates from data (see C. 4. above)
4. Decision-theoretic and information-theoretic methods that include cost benefit analysis and lead to optimization of the sequence of observations

E. **Clustering algorithms** — These programs utilize only the detailed data on the findings of a large number of previous patients. Statistical methods are implemented to infer a disease structure and decision criteria from that historical data.

1. Selection of subpopulations that closely match a patient under consideration, with analysis of the response of these subpopulations to various treatments; this is used to prognosticate for the patient in question
2. Numerical taxonomy or the use of statistical methods to develop a meaningful classification of diseases, based only on the findings of a large number of patients

Computer-Aided Diagnostic Systems in the Field of Hematology

Three computer-aided diagnostic systems intended to span the subspecialty of hematology have been developed. Hematology has long been appealing as a field for computers because of the large amount of objective data that is available. All these systems were designed primarily to assist medical personnel in the diagnosis of hematologic disorders. They may also be useful as teaching aids and as models for studying the diagnostic process.

Lipkin and Hardy, who were among the earliest workers in the field of computer-aided diagnosis, developed a system in 1952 for the diagnosis of hematologic diseases using McBee marginal punch cards to match the findings about a patient with a predetermined set of findings thought to characterize each of the 27 hematologic diseases in the system.[41] A hand-operated mechanical sorting process selected those diseases with findings which best matched those of a patient, and a score was calculated for the patient's findings in relation to each of the selected diseases. Using these same principles, a group of investigators organized by Zworykin and Lipkin developed a computer program to sort the data and print out information about the matching of a patient's findings with findings characteristic of diseases. The first demonstration in 1957 of this system on a computer applied to 20 hematologic diseases. Later, the group developed a larger system.[22-23] The judgment of a panel of physicians was used to estimate weights for each of 540 findings in each of 75 hematologic diseases, and algorithms were developed to utilize these weights to calculate scores for a patient's findings in relation to each disease. The user of this system enters a list of numerical codes corresponding to the patient's findings. He receives as computer output, first, lists of those diseases that were ruled out or definitively diagnosed because of single findings or small clusters of findings; second, a list, in order of score, of those diseases for which relatively high scores were calculated; and third, for all relevant diseases, lists of patient findings that favor the diagnosis, unrelated findings, and findings to be tested.

Reich, Geer, and Bleich have developed a system that attempts to simulate directly the sequence of diagnostic thoughts and actions of a hematologist.[26] They wrote specific decision rules for diagnosing each of 174 hematologic diseases and combined them into a network of branching logic modules that leads to a diagnosis. The physician, using a teletype or a cathode-ray tube terminal, responds to a sequence of computer questions about the patient's findings. The computer prints out an evaluation note that indicates the diagnosis and the findings that led to the diagnosis. Once the diagnosis is made, the computer also prints out a brief descriptive summary of the disease and its subcategories, a statement on the pathophysiology of the disease, additional laboratory tests that might be useful, commonly prescribed treatment, complications, and references to the medical literature.

Flehinger and Engle[36] and Engle et al.[37] have written several versions of HEME, a program that uses Bayes' Theorem for diagnosis-oriented analysis of hematologic diseases. The data base contains a list of diseases with their frequencies, a list of findings, and, for each finding relevant to the diagnosis of a disease, two probabilities. The first is the probability that a patient with the disease also has the findings, and the second is the probability that a patient who does not have the disease does have the finding. In using the program, a physician enters a list of patient findings. The computer uses Bayes' Theorem to calculate the probability of each disease in the system, prints out the most likely diagnoses in order of probability, and, at the user's option, discusses the relationship of tested and untested findings to any selected disease. The latest, unpublished version of HEME deals with two levels of diagnosis and relates 140 specific diseases in 19 broad categories to 656 findings.

REFERENCES

1. **Ledley, R. S. and Lusted, L. B.**, Reasoning foundations of medical diagnosis. Symbolic logic, probability, and value theory aid our understanding of how physicians reason, *Science*, 130, 9, 1959.
2. **Vetter, N. J. and Julian, D. G.**, Comparison of arrhythmia computer and conventional monitoring in coronary-care units, *Lancet*, 1, 1151, 1975.
3. **Collen, M. F., Rubin, L., and Davis, L.**, Computers in multiphasic screening, in *Computers in Bromedical Research*, Stacy, R. W. and Waxman, B. D., Eds., Academic Press, New York, 1965, 339.
4. **Mansberg, H. P., Saunders, A. M., and Groner, W.**, The Hemalog D white cell differential system, *J. Histochem. Cytochem.*, 22, 711, 1974.
5. **Prewitt, J. M. S. and Mendelsohn, M. L.**, The analysis of cell images, *Ann. N.Y. Acad. Sci.*, 128, 1035, 1966.
6. **Bentley, S. A. and Lewis, S. M.**, The morphological classification of red cells using an image analysis computer, *Br. J. Haematol.*, 32, 205, 1976.
7. **Evens, R. G.**, New frontier for radiology: computed tomography (Hickey Memorial Lecture), *Am. J. Roentgenol.*, 126, 1117, 1976.
8. **Barber, D. C.**, Digital computer processing of brain scans using principal components, *Phys. Med. Biol.*, 21, 792, 1976.
9. **Pipberger, H. V., McCaughan, D., Littmann, D., Pipberger, H. A., Cornfield, J., Dunn, R. A., Batchlor, C. D., and Berson, A. S.**, Clinical application of a second generation electrocardiographic computer program, *Am. J. Cardiol.*, 35, 597, 1975.
10. **Saffer, S. I., Nixon, J. V., and Mishelevich, D. J.**, Sample method for computer-aided analysis of echocardiograms, *Am. J. Cardiol.*, 38, 34, 1976.
11. **Dutcher, T. F., Benzel, J. E., Egan, J. J., Hart, D. J., and Christopher, E. A.**, Evaluation of an automated differential leukocyte counting system, *Am. J. Clin. Pathol.*, 62, 525, 1974.
12. **Arkin, C. F., Sherry, M. A., Gough, A. G., and Copeland, B. E.**, An automatic leukocyte analyzer, *Am. J. Clin. Pathol.*, 67, 159, 1977.
13. **Barness, L. A., Tunnessen, W. W., Jr., Worley, W. E., Simmons, T. L., and Ringe, T. B. K., Jr.**, Computer-assisted diagnosis in pediatrics, *Am. J. Dis. Child.*, 127, 852, 1974.
14. **Brodman, K. and van Woerkom, A. J.**, Computer-aided diagnostic screening for 100 common diseases, *JAMA*, 197, 901, 1966.
15. **Ramirez, G, Dinio, R. C., and Pribor, H. C.**, Pattern recognition of multiple tests values as a diagnostic tool, *Comput. Biol. Med.*, 2, 39, 1972.
16. **Kulikowski, C. A.**, Pattern recognition approach to medical diagnosis, *I.E.E.E. Trans. Systems Sci. Cybernetics* Vol. ssc-6, 173, 1970.
17. **Bishop, C. R. and Warner, H. R.**, A mathematical approach to medical diagnosis: application to polycythemic states utilizing clinical findings with values continuously distributed, *Comput. Biomed. Res.*, 2, 486, 1969.
18. **Warner, H. R., Toronto, A. F., Veasy, G., and Stephenson, R.**, A mathematical approach to medical diagnosis. Application to congenital heart disease, *JAMA*, 177, 177, 1961.
19. **Lincoln, T. L. and Parker, R. D.**, Medical diagnosis using Bayes' Theorem, *Health Services Res.*, 2, 34, 1967.
20. **Spitzer, R. L. and Endicott, J.**, DIAGNO II: further developments in a computer program for psychiatric diagnosis, *Am. J. Psychiatry*, 125, 12, 1969.
21. **Greist, J. H., Klein, M. H., and Erdman, H. P.**, Routine on-line psychiatric diagnosis by computer, *Am. J. Psychiatry*, 133, 1405, 1976.
22. **Lipkin, M., Engle, R. L., Jr., Davis, B. J., Zworykin, V. K., Ebald, R., and Sendrow, B. S.**, Digital computer as aid to differential diagnosis, *Arch. Int. Med.*, 108, 56, 1961.
23. **Lipkin, M., Engle, R. L., Jr., Flehinger, B. J., Gerstman, L. J., and Atamer, M. A.**, Computer-aided differential diagnosis of hematologic diseases, *Proc. N. Y. Acad. Sci.*, 161, 670, 1969.
24. **Horrocks, J. C., McCann, A. P., Staniland, J. R., Leaper, D. J., and de Dombal, F. T.**, Computer-aided diagnosis: description of an adaptable system and operational experience with 2,034 cases, *Br. Med. J.*, 2, 5, 1972.
25. **Pauker, S. G., Gorry, G. A., Kassirer, J. P., and Schwartz, W. B.**, Towards the simulation of clinical cognition. Taking a present illness by computer, *Am. J. Med.*, 60, 981, 1976.
26. **Reich, P. R., Geer, D. E., and Bleich, H. L.**, A computer program for the diagnosis of hematologic disorders, *Am. J. Hematol.*, 3, 127, 1977.
27. **Bleich, H. L.**, The computer as a consultant, *N. Engl. J. Med.*, 284, 141, 1972.
28. **Shane, L. L., Marler, E., and Bauman, W. A.**, Computer simulation of medical logic in clinical decision support system, *N.Y. State J. Med.*, 72, 1636, 1972.

29. **Moore, F. J. and Goertzel, G.,** An experimental clinical decision support system, *Proc. 8th IBM Med. Symp.*, 85, 1967.
30. **Knill-Jones, R. P., Stern, R. B., Girmes, D. H., Maxwell, J. D., Thompson, R. P. H., and Williams, R.,** Use of sequential Bayesian model in diagnosis of jaundice by computer, *Br. Med. J.*, 1, 530, 1973.
31. **Gorry, G. A., Kassirer, J. P., Essig, A., and Schwartz, W. B.,** Decision analysis as the basis for computer-aided management of acute renal failure, *Am. J. Med.*, 55, 473, 1973.
32. **Peters, R. J.,** Zero order and non-zero order decision rules in medical diagnosis, *IBM J. Res. Dev.*, 21, 449, 1977.
33. **Shortliffe, E. H., Davis, R., Axline, S. G., Buchanan, B. G., Green, C. C., and Cohen, S. N.,** Computer-based consultations in clinical therapeutics: explanation and rule acquisition capabilities of the MYCIN system, *Comput. Biomed. Res.*, 8, 303, 1975.
34. **Pople, H. E., Jr., Myers, J. D., and Miller, R. A.,** DIALOG: a model of diagnostic logic for internal medicine, *Proc. 4th Int. Joint Conf. Artificial Intelligence*, 2, 848, 1975.
35. **Weiss, S., Kulikowski, C. A. and Safir, A.,** *Comput. Biol. Med.*, 8, 25, 1978.
36. **Flehinger, B. J. and Engle, R. L., Jr.,** HEME: a self-improving computer program for diagnosis-oriented analysis of hematologic diseases, *IBM J. Res. Dev.*, 19, 557, 1975.
37. **Engle, R. L., Jr., Flehinger, B. J., Allen, S., Friedman, R., Lipkin, M., Davis, B. J., and Leveridge, L. L.,** HEME: a computer aid to diagnosis of hematologic disease, *Bull. N.Y. Acad. Med.*, 52, 584, 1976.
38. **Gorry, G. A. and Barnett, G. O.,** Experience with a model of sequential diagnosis, *Comput. Biomed. Res.*, 1, 490, 1968.
39. **Rosati, R. A., McNeer, J. F., Starmer, C. F., Mittler, B. S., Morris, J. J., Jr., and Wallace, A. G.,** A new information system for medical practice, *Arch. Intern. Med.*, 135, 1017, 1975.
40. **Friedman, H. P., Goldwyn, R. M., and Siegel, J. H.,** The use and interpretation of multivariate methods in the classification of stages in serious infectious disease processes in the critically ill, in *Perspectives in Biometrics*, Vol. 1, Elashoff, R., Ed., Academic Press, New York, 1975.
41. **Lipkin, M. and Hardy, J. D.,** Differential diagnosis of hematologic diseases aided by mechanical correlation of data, *Science*, 125, 551, 1957.

Index

INDEX

A

B

C

D

E

F

G

H

I

J

K

L

M

N

O

P

Q

R

S

T

U

V

W

X